METAL IONS IN BIOLOGY AND MEDICINE

LES IONS MÉTALLIQUES EN BIOLOGIE ET EN MÉDECINE

Volume 2

Sponsored by/*Sous le haut patronage de :*

- American College of Nutrition
- Anticancer Research
- Food and Drug Administration
- International Society of Trace Elements Research in Human
- Société Francophone d'Étude et de Recherche sur les Éléments Trace Essentiels
- Société Internationale pour le Développement des Recherches sur le Magnésium

The Organizing Committee wishes to thank LABCATAL and MERAM for their support in the realization of this book

METAL IONS IN BIOLOGY AND MEDICINE

LES IONS MÉTALLIQUES EN BIOLOGIE ET EN MÉDECINE

Volume 2

Proceedings of the Second International Symposium on Metal Ions in Biology and Medicine held in Club Poseidon, Loutraki (Greece) on May 18-22, 1992

Deuxième Symposium International sur les Ions Métalliques en Biologie et en Médecine, Club Poséidon, Loutraki (Grèce), 18-22 mai 1992

Edited by
Jane Anastassopoulou
Philippe Collery
Jean-Claude Étienne
Theophile Theophanides

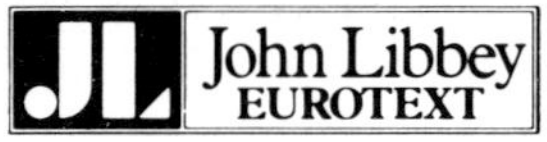

British Library Cataloguing in Publication Data
A catalogue record
for this book is
available from the
British Library

ISBN 0-86196-340-7

The first volume of this series was published in May 1990
Eds. Ph. Collery, L.A. Poirier, M. Manfait, J.C. Étienne.

Editions John Libbey Eurotext
6, rue Blanche, 92120 Montrouge, France.
Tél. : (1) 47.35.85.52 - Fax : (1) 46.57.10.09

John Libbey and Company Ltd
13, Smith Yard Summerley Street, London SW 18 4HR, England
Tél. : (01) 947.27.77

John Libbey CIC
Via L. Spallanzani, 11
00161 Rome, Italy
Tel. : (06) 862.289

Foreword

All of us have heard about drugs and vitamins since our young age, but not about metal ions. However, in many cases, minerals are more important than vitamins. It is known that, calcium builds strong bones, iron is vital to red blood to form heme, and potassium, sodium, magnesium and calcium are necessary to cells. Plants are green, because of magnesium. The magnesium intake will interact with ATP adenosine triphosphate to liberate energy. Not many people know that zinc helps many enzymatic reactions and skin problems.

Metal ions control many diseases too. Until the end of last century several diseases were cured with metal ions, such as, the mercurials, for example as antiseptics, the arsenicals, the antimony salts, the zinc salts, etc. It is also known that, stress and exposure to environmental pollution raises our requirements for zinc, calcium, magnesium and iron. There's also the opposit case of harmful minerals, such as lead, cadmium and mercury. The discovery of sulfamides and antibiotics reduced the importance of metal ions in infectious diseases until the platinum coordination compounds were found to have antitumor activity (cis-platinum). The antitumor activity of cis-platinum generated enough research and interest in metal ions so that we have today several important gatherings on studies of metal ions in biological systems and in biomedical applications. There is a growing volume of literature too, on the importance of metal ions in biochemical and physiological or life processes. The chemistry of metal ions is providing new insights into DNA, protein and membrane chemistry, as well as, the physiopathology of diseases.

Jane Anastassopoulou
Theophile Theophanides
May 18, 1992

Avant-propos

Nous avons tous entendu parler des médicaments et des vitamines depuis notre enfance, mais jamais des ions métalliques. Cependant, dans bien des cas, les ions minéraux jouent un rôle plus important que les vitamines. Nous savons tous que le calcium est nécessaire à l'ossification, le fer indispensable à la formation de l'hémoglobine, et les ions potassium, sodium, magnésium et calcium indispensables aux cellules. Les plantes sont vertes grâce à la chlorophyle. Le magnésium ingéré interagit ensuite avec l'ATP (adénosine triphosphate) et libère de l'énergie. Peu de gens savent que le zinc participe à de multiples réactions enzymatiques et joue un rôle important en dermatologie.
Les ions métalliques possèdent de multiples indications thérapeutiques. Jusqu'à la fin du siècle dernier, le traitement de nombreuses maladies reposait sur les ions métalliques, tels les sels de mercure, par exemple comme antiseptiques, les sels d'arsenic, les sels d'antimoine, les sels de zinc, etc. Nous savons également que les agressions dues à la pollution atmosphérique augmentent nos besoins en zinc, calcium, magnésium, fer... Les ions métalliques ont aussi des effets nocifs (le plomb, le cadmium et le mercure). La découverte des sulfamides et des antibiotiques a réduit l'importance des ions métalliques en pathologie infectieuse jusqu'à la découverte des composés de coordination du platine, tel le cisplatine, avec ses propriétés antitumorales. Cette activité antitumorale du cisplatine a suscité un intérêt croissant ainsi que des recherches nouvelles sur les ions métalliques. Ainsi, à l'heure actuelle se tiennent de très nombreuses réunions sur les ions métalliques dans les systèmes biologiques et leurs applications biomédicales. De plus en plus de travaux sont réalisés sur l'importance des ions métalliques dans les processus biochimiques, physiologiques ou vitaux. La chimie des ions métalliques nous permet de mieux cerner aujourd'hui celle de l'ADN, des protéines et des membranes et d'aller plus loin dans la compréhension des mécanismes physiopathologiques des maladies.

Jeanne Anastassopoulou
Théophile Théophanides
18 mai 1992

List and addresses of editors

Jane Anastassopoulou, National Technical University of Athens, Chemical Engineering Laboratory of Physical Chemistry (Radiation Chemistry-Biospectroscopy), Zografou 15773, Zografou campus, Athens, Greece.

Philippe Collery, CHRU, médecine interne/cancérologie, Département des maladies respiratoires, hôpital Maison Blanche, 45, rue Cognacq-Jay, 51092 Reims Cedex, France.

Jean-Claude Étienne, CHRU, médecine interne, hôpital Robert-Debré, rue Alexis-Carrel, 51092 Reims Cedex, France.

Théophile Théophanides, National Technical University of Athens, Chemical Engineering Laboratory of Physical Chemistry (Radiation Chemistry-Biospectroscopy), Zografou 15773, Zografou Campus, Athens, Greece.

CONTENTS/SOMMAIRE

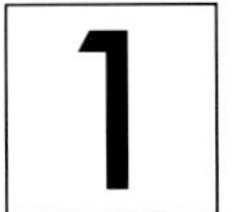

BASIC RESEARCH METAL-BIOLOGICAL MOLECULE INTERACTIONS

LECTURES

POSTERS

2 *ANALYSIS*

LECTURES

POSTERS

3 *CANCER*

LECTURES

POSTERS

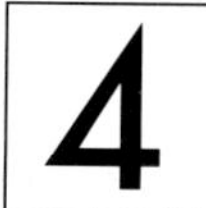

NEPHROLOGY, CARDIOLOGY, HYPERTENSION

LECTURES

POSTERS

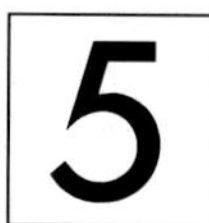

PHARMACOLOGY, TOXICOLOGY

LECTURES

POSTERS

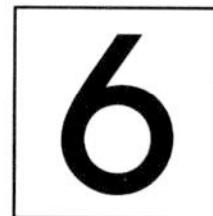

NUTRITION

LECTURES

POSTERS

7 *EPIDEMIOLOGY*

LECTURES

POSTERS

1 BASIC RESEARCH METAL-BIOLOGICAL MOLECULE INTERACTIONS

Metal Ions in Biology and Medicine, vol. 2. Eds. J. Anastassopoulou, Ph. Collery, J.C. Etienne, Th. Theophanides. John Libbey Eurotext, Paris © 1992, p. 3

Perspectives in supramolecular chemistry : from molecular recognition towards molecular devices and self-organisation

Jean-Marie Lehn

Université Louis Pasteur, Strasbourg and Collège de France, Paris, France

Molecular recognition rests on the *molecular information* stored in the interacting species. Together with *catalysis* and *transport*, and in combination with polymolecular organisation, it opens ways towards *molecular* and *supramolecular* devices, defined as structurally organised and functionally integrated chemical systems built on supramolecular architectures. The development of such devices requires the design of molecular components performing a given function (*e.g.* photoactive, electroactive, ionoactive, thermoactive or chemoactive) and suitable for assembly into an organised array. Of special interest is the possibility to design devices that may form by *molecular organisation.*

Supramolecular chemistry has relied on more or less preorganised molecular receptors for effecting molecular recognition, catalysis and transport processes. A step beyond consists in the design of systems undergoing *molecular self-organisation*, i.e. systems capable of spontaneously generating a well-defined supramolecular architecture by *self-assembling* from their components in a given set of conditions.

The *molecular information* necessary for the process to take place must be stored in the components and acts through selective molecular interactions. Thus, these *programmed molecular systems* operate via molecular recognition.

Several approaches to self-assembling systems have been pursued:

1) the formation of helical metal complexes, the *double-stranded helicates*, that result from the spontaneous organisation of two linear polybipyridine ligands into a double helix by binding of specific metal ions;
2) the generation of *mesophases* and *liquid crystalline polymers* of supramolecular nature from complementary components, amounting to macroscopic expression of molecular recognition;
3) the molecular recognition directed formation of *ordered solid state structures.*

Endowing photo-, electro- and iono-active components with recognition elements opens perspectives towards the design of *programmed molecular and supramolecular systems* capable of molecular recognition directed self-assembly into organized and functional supramolecular devices. Such systems may be able to perform highly selective operations of recognition, reaction, transfer and structure generation for signal and information processing at the molecular and supramolecular levels.

Metal Ions in Biology and Medicine, vol. 2. Eds. J. Anastassopoulou, Ph. Collery, J.C. Etienne, Th. Theophanides. John Libbey Eurotext, Paris © 1992, pp. 4-9

How metal ions may influence the structure and the biological activities of natural oligopeptides

Henryk Kozlowski

Institute of Chemistry, University of Wroclaw, F. Joliot-Curie 14, 50-383 Wroclaw, Poland

Many essential metal ions are potential factors which can critically influence the structure of the natural oligopeptides stabilizing the specific ligand conformations and affecting their biological activities. Peptides contain a variety of potential donor centers and their complexes can exist in a virtually infinitive variety of conformations with varying steric and energetic constrains to co-ordination.

The most important donor center is generally the N-terminal nitrogen, which is usually a primary $-NH_2$ group although it may be a secondary nitrogen as in proline unit. Many biologically active peptides are actually derivatives starting with the pyroglutamyl residue which contains an amido-N, **e.g.** gonadoliberin (LHRH) or thyrotropin releasing hormone (TRH). This is generally a much less effective donor than the $-NH_2$ group.

The peptide side chains can contain a variety of donor centers. The most important among them are pyridine-like imidazole nitrogen of His, the sulphur atom of Cys and Met, the carboxylate oxygens of Asp, the amino nitrogen of Lys and phenolic oxygen of Tyr. All these donors are present in many natural oligopeptides playing the critical role in their biological activities.

Some metal ions, in particular Pt(II), Pd(II), Cu(II) or Ni(II), can promote ionization of the amide hydrogen of the peptide bond, -CONH-, to form very stable metal-N^- bond. This kind of co-ordination increases dramatically the variety of complexes formed. Pt(II) and Pd(II) are able to co-ordinate in this fashion already by pH<3, Cu(II) by pH 5 and Ni(II) around pH 8-9.

The details of the metal-peptide interactions were discussed very recently in two extensive chapters, by Pettit **et al.** (1991a) and Sovago (1990).

In this work the main concern will be devoted to metal ions like Cu(II), Ni(II) and Zn(II), which play essential role in biological systems.

NATURAL OLIGOPEPTIDES WITH NON-COORDINATING SIDE CHAINS

Copper(II) complexes of short peptides with apparently non-coordinating side chains behave, in general, like tetraglycine :

$NH_2-CH_2-CONH-CH_2-CONH-CH_2-CONH-CH_2-COO^-$,

which binds metal ion *via* consecutive nitrogen donors starting at N-terminal amino group. However, various effects deriving from the different peptide sequences have been reported. A particularly dramatic effect on the peptide stability for the complexes having tetraglycine-like coordination is found for the natural vasopressin-like nonapeptides, (vasopressin, vasotocin and oxitocin (Kozlowski **et al.** 1989, Bal **et al.** 1992).

Arg[8]-Vasopressin:

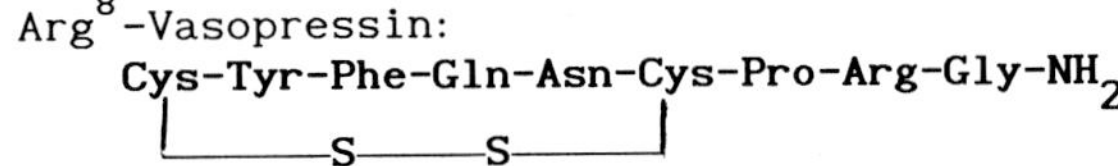

is a peptide neurohormone possessing a 20-membered ring linked by a disulfide bridge with a tripeptide side chain. This ring appears to be ideally suited to accommodate a Cu(II) ion with glycine-like 4N coordination $\{NH_2, 3xN^-\}$. This complex is 4 orders of magnitude more stable when compared to that of tetraglycine (Table 1). The ideal fitting of the peptide ring to Cu(II) ion leads to very distinct stereoselectivity when non-bonding side chain in vasopressin is replaced by one of opposite chirality. When D-Val residue is incorporated into the peptide backbone in place of L-Gln, the 3N complex, $(CuH_{-2}L)$, becomes the most stable species at intermediate pH while 4N complex, $(CuH_{-3}L)$, is about 100 times weaker than the respective species of the natural peptide (Table 1). This unusual behavior of vasopressin-like peptides towards cupric ions suggests the biological implications of the metal ion coordination in natural systems.

Even more astonishing behavior was found very recently for Cu(II) complexes with the C-terminal pentapeptide fragment of atrial natriuretic factor (ANF): **Asn-Ser-Phe-Arg-Tyr-NH$_2$** (C-ANF-NH$_2$). This fragment is necessary for most of the biological actions of the peptide. Some relations between the activity of the ANF and the physiological manifestation of copper deficiency were detected (Bathena **et al.**, 1988). This peptide, which does not exhibit any favored conformation in the aqueous solutions forms extremely stable complexes with Cu(II) ions in which the binding sites are the same as in tetraglycine or tetraalanine (Bal **et al.**, 1992a, Table 1).

Table 1. Logarithms of stability constants of cupric complexes at 25°C and I=0.1 M (KNO_3) with chosen peptides.

peptide	log *K[a]			
	1N	2N	3N	4N
C-ANF-OH[b]	-1.82	-6.89	-14.06	-20.47
C-ANF-NH$_2$[b]	-1.93	-6.91	-13.35	-20.08
AVP[c]	-2.48	-8.26	-14.36	-20.51
D-VAVP[c]	-2.63	-8.06	-13.75	-22.17
Gly$_4$	-2.89	-8.39	-15.28	-24.57
Ala$_4$	-3.36	-8.58	-16.22	-25.43
Ala-AVP[d]	-2.87	-8.04	-15.42	-24.58

[a] log *K= log β_{xN} - log β_{H_2L} (β_{HL} for Gly$_4$ and Ala$_4$), where xN corresponds to the species with x nitrogen atom coordinated. The constant describes the reaction of removal of protons from the ligand molecule by metal ion.

[b] from Bal **et al.**, 1992a, [c] from Kozlowski **et al.**, 1989, [d] from Bal **et al.**, 1992b

It is clear from the results collected in Table 1 that some intraligand interactions within C-ANF peptide stabilize the 4N complex. These interactions, however, are not observed in the metal-free ligand systems. The unusually high stabilization of the 4N complex causes that it is the major species already at physiological pH while in the systems with Ala$_4$ or Gly$_4$ its concentration is dominant at pH well above 9. Again the high stability of the Cu(II) complexes with ANF fragment may potentially be an important factor for the biological functions of this peptide.

Many biologically active peptides (**e.g.** neurohormones) contain the proline residue which does not have a coordination side chain. The coordination chemistry of the Pro containing oligopeptides, however, is particularly interesting. The nitrogen of Pro is a secondary nitrogen so that, when incorporated within a peptide sequence, it does not possess an ionizable amide proton and cannot form a $Cu-N^-$ bond. It therefore acts as a "break-point" to coordination (Pettit **et al.**, 1991a, 1991b, Livera **et al.**, 1988 and references therein). Pro residue also encourages the presence of β-terns within the peptide chain and, as a result, the N- and C-terminals of short peptides are brought close together allowing the Cu(II) to bridge them. This locks the peptide into a bent conformation with an abnormally large chelate ring. The bent peptide conformations are often critical for the peptide bioactivity and therefore their metal complexes could have significant biological implications (Pettit & Formicka-Kozlowska, 1984).

NATURAL PEPTIDES WITH COORDINATING SIDE CHAINS

Alifatic oxygen donors are rarely involved in the copper ion coordination except the β-carboxylate of Asp residue (Galey **et al.**, 1991a,b, Sovago 1990). The latter residue is effectively involved in the Cu(II) ion coordination when Asp is in any of the first three positions. The binding to $\beta\text{-COO}^-$ is very effective and it can limit the coordination of the consecutive amide nitrogens. Thus, the natural peptides like fibrinopeptide A, (^{2}Asp) thymopoietin (^{3}Asp) or angiotensin II (^{1}Asp) can potentially involve their Asp residue in the metal ion complexation. This may easily happen when locally the peptide concentration increases considerably (**e.g.** fibrinopeptide A near the sites of bodily injury). The major factor that causes the high effectiveness of the $\beta\text{-COO}^-$ donor is the formation of the 6-membered ring involving also the adjacent nitrogen donor(s).

Peptides containing histidyl residue(s) belong to the most powerful among all natural peptide ligands. Gly-His-Lys, a tripeptide present in blood plasma enhances its biological activity in the presence of Cu(II) ions. This is the best known example of the naturally occurring low molecular weight metallo-peptide system. There have been many extensive studies on metal complexes with His containing peptides because the pyridine-like imidazole-N binds effectively to metal ions (especially Cu(II)) to give a large variety of very strong complexes (Pettit **et al.**, 1991a, Sovago **et al.**, 1990).

Usually, the coordination of metal ion (**e.g.** Cu(II)) to peptide ligand starts at the N-terminal nitrogen with other donors bonding after this initial binding. The imidazole-N donor of His is also able to act as an anchor donor for metal ions. The comparative studies on the donor properties of His containing peptides (Pettit **et al.** 1990) indicated that imidazole ring of His residue may be the primary anchoring site for Cu(II) coordination. It is also a primary binding site in the hormones like TRF (Formicka-Kozlowska **et al.**, 1983), LHRH (Gerega **et al.**, 1988) since these contain N-terminal pyroglutamyl residue. In both cases the His residue is second residue and it leads to formation of very stable 3N complexes.

LHRH is a decapeptide amide, pGlu-His-Trp-Ser-Tyr-Gly-Leu-Arg-Pro-Gly-NH_2, and is a main mediator in the neuroregulation of the secretion of gonadotrophins, luteinizing hormone (LH), and the follicle stimulating hormone (FSH). Barnea **et al.**, 1990, have shown that the biology of LHRH may be strongly dependent on copper. The major Cu(II) complexes at pH range above 5.5 are the 3N, ($CuH_{-1}L$ or $CuH_{-2}L$), species involving His and pGlu nitrogens as the binding sites. Since His residue is a dominant residue when bioactivity of LHRH is concerned, it seems to be likely that the metal ion coordination may affect peptide biological functions. The less effective metal ions like Ni(II) or Zn(II) are also bound to LHRH molecule *via* His residue donor set (Gerega **et al.**, 1988, Bal **et al.**, 1989).

The complexation of LHRH by metal ions, (Cu(II), Ni(II) and Zn(II)), affects its basic, ovulation inducing potency in the dose response manner (Kozlowski **et al.**, 1990). The *in vivo* studies with female rats have shown that metal complexes change considerably the ovulation of rats even when injected into a tail vein (Table 2). In such experiments the effect of metal ions is much decreased by the removal of the certain amount of metal ions from LHRH complex in blood by powerful protein ligands. The formation of inert complexes by LHRH or its analogs leads to a much stronger influence of metal ion on hormone potency (Bajusz **et al.** 1989).

The ovulation potency *in vivo* tests suggests that metal ion complexation may affect the release of LH and/or FSH. Our recent work clearly supports this assumption (Kochman **et al.**, 1992). The effect of Cu(II), Ni(II) and Zn(II) and their complexes with LHRH on the release of LH and FSH was estimated *in vivo* experiment with ovariectomized, estradiol and progesterone pretreated rats. The metal-free or complexed LHRH preparations were injected *iv*. A metal alone did not affect gonadotropin release at all. However, the complex of copper(II) with LHRH brought about a high release of LH and even higher release of FSH (Table 3). This indicates that the copper complex is more effective than the metal-free hormone. The nickel complex has shown a similar, although lesser effect. Zinc complex had similar potency as LHRH alone though higher FSH-releasing ability was noticed.

Angiotensin II is a linear octapeptide (**Asp-Arg-Val-Tyr-Ile-His-Pro-Phe**) having very broad range of physiological activities. Several biological functions are enhanced by certain cations although exact mechanism is not clear. This His containing peptide is also very effective ligand for metal ions with very unusual binding pattern (Decock-Le Reverend, **et al.**,1988, Pettit, **et al.**, 1989). The major complex formed at "physiological" pH is the 3N species with Cu(II) ion bound with imidazole-N and two vicinal amide nitrogens of His and Ile residues. It is a very stable complex but increase of pH above 8 leads to formation of the 4N species with metal ion coordinated to N-terminal tetrapeptide fragment. The same coordination pattern was observed for the Ni(II) complexes. The competition between two peptide binding sites is very

Table 2. Induction of ovulation in rat females by LHRH and its complexes. (Kozlowski **et al.**, 1990)

Species	Dose(ng)	Number of animals ovulating /tested	Percentage of animals ovulating	Number of ova (arithmetic mean)
LHRH	200	6/9	66	9.0
	300	8/9	89	11.0
	400	10/10	100	8.8
Cu-LHRH	200	4/8	50	4.6
	300	2/9	22	1.6
	400	9/9	100	10.1
Ni-LHRH	200	2/6	33	11.5
	400	8/10	80	11.6
	600	9/9	100	9.5
Zn-LHRH	200	6/10	60	8.2
	300	6/10	60	8.8
	600	3/8	38	13.0
	1000	2/8	25	5.5
	4000	9/9	100	8.1

Table 3. The LH and FSH release from the pituitary to blood of ovariectomized, estradiol-progesterone pretreated rats, 15 min after *iv* injection of LHRH and its metal complexes.

Enrty	Preparation	LH ng/ml ± SE	FSH ng/ml ± SE
1	saline	1.3 ± 0.29	9.7 ± 2.0
2	LHRH 0.1 μg	5.8 ± 0.40	9.8 ± 0.7
3	LHRH 1.0 μg	9.0 ± 1.00	10.4 ± 0.8
4	CuLHRH 1.0 μg	20.6 ± 5.10	35.3 ± 0.6
5	CuLHRH 5.0 μg	29.3 ± 2.20	29.8 ± 4.7
6	NiLHRH 1.0 μg	14.8 ± 4.20	21.6 ± 3.0
7	NiLHRH 10.0 μg	15.3 ± 1.20	18.4 ± 1.9
8	ZnLHRH 1.0 μg	10.0 ± 1.60	15.9 ± 1.8
9	ZnLHRH 10.0 μg	18.0 ± 2.70	14.3 ± 1.0

hormone levels in serum were determined by specific RIA method, SE standard error; (Kochman **et al.**, 1992)

specific for this particular peptide and it indicates the importance of the anchoring site which decides about the structure and the potential functions of the formed complex species.

CONCLUSIONS

The space limitations have not allowed to put more details into this article but the examples mentioned above clearly indicate that metal ions are critical factors for the oligopeptide structures and their biological activities. The peptides which are very powerful ligands form an infinite variety of complexes with specific conformations and potential biological implications. Even "innocent" peptide sequences may have important impact on the structure and stability of the species fprmed and biological consequences. It is also very likely that besides the strictly biological functions the metallopeptides may be an important group of the drugs and chemotherapeutics (see **e.g.** Bajusz **et al.**, 1989). The concentrations of metal ions are locally very high (**e.g.** copper in the brain) and it is potentially very likely that many natural oligopeptides may be affected by the metal ion coordination in their biological functions.

REFERENCES

Bajusz, S., Janaky, T., Csernus, V.J., Bokser, L., Fekete, M., Strualovis, G., Redding, T.W., and Schally, A.V., (1989), Highly potent metallopeptide analogues of luteinizing hormone-releasing hormone. Proc.Natl.Acad.Sci.USA, 87, 6313- 6317

Bal, W., Kozlowski, H., Kupryszewski, G., Maćkiewicz, Z., Pettit, L.D., and Robbins, R.,(1992a), Interactions of the C-terminal pentapetide of the ANF: Asn-Ser-Phe-Arg-Tyr and its amide with Cu(II): an unexpected gain in stability resulting from intraligand interactions. submitted for publication

Bal, W., Kozlowski, H., Lammek, B., Pettit, L.D., and Rolka, K., (1992b), Potentiometric and spectroscopic studies of the Cu(II) complexes of Ala-Arg^8-vasopressin and oxitocin: two vasopressin-like peptides. J.Inorg. Biochem.in press

Bal, W., Kozlowski, H., Masiukiewicz, E., Rzeszotarska, B., and Sovago, I., (1989), LHRH complexes with Zn(II) ions. J.Inorg.Biochem., 37, 135-139

Barnea, A., Hartter, D.E., Cho, G., Bhasker, K.R., Katz, B.M., and Edwards, M. D., (1990), Further characterization of the process of in *vitro* uptake of radiolabeled copper by the rat brain. J.Inorg.Biochem.,40, 103-110 and refs. therein

Bathena, S.J., Kennedy, B.W., Smith, P.M., Fields, M., and Zamir, N., (1988) Role of atrial natriuretic peptides in cardiac hypertrophy of copper-deficient male and female rats. J.Tr.Elem.Exp.Med.,1, 199-208

Decock-Le Reverend, B., Liman, F., Livera, C., Pettit, L.D., Pyburn, S., and Kozlowski, H., (1988), A potentiometric and spectroscopic study of the interaction of angiotensin II and some of its peptide fragments with Cu(II). J.Chem.Soc.Dalton Trans., 887-894

Formicka-Kozlowska, G., Bezer, M., and Pettit, L.D., (1983), Coordination ability of thyrotropin releasing factor, pGlu-His-Pro-NH_2.III. Cu(II) and Ni(II) complexes with TRF and its di- and tripeptide analogues. J.Inorg. Biochem. 18, 335-347

Galey, J.F., Decock- Le Reverend, B., Lebkiri, A., Pettit, L.D., Pyburn, S., and Kozlowski, H., (1991a), Specific interactions of the β-carboxylate group of the aspartic acid residue in oligopeptides containing one, two or three such residues with copper(II) ions. A potentiometric and spectrsopic study. J.Chem.Soc.Dalton Trans., 2281-2287

Galey, J.F., Kozlowski, H., and Pettit, L.D., (1991b), A potentiometric and spectroscopic study of the proton and copper(II) and zinc(II) complexes formed by fibrinopeptide A. J.Inorg.Biochem., 44, 149-153

Gerega, K., Kozlowski, H., Masiukiewicz, E., Pettit, L.D., Pyburn, S., and Rzeszotarska, B., (1988), Metal complexes of luteinizing hormone-releasing hormone (LHRH). Potentiometric and spectroscopic studies. J.Inorg.Biochem., 33, 11-18

Kochman, K., Gajewska, A., Kozlowski, H., Masiukiewicz, E., and Rzeszotarska, B., (1992) Increased LH and FSH release from the anterior pituitary of ovariectomized rat, *in vivo*, by copper-, nickel-, and zinc-LHRH complexes. J.Inorg.Biochem., in press

Kozlowski, H., Kupryszewski, G., Lammek, B., Livera, C., Pettit, L.D., Pyburn, S., and Radomska, B., (1989), The unusual coordination ability of vasopressin-like peptides; potentiometric and spectroscopic studies of some copper(II) and nickel(II) complexes. J.Chem.Soc.Dalton Trans., 173-177

Kozlowski, H., Masiukiewicz, E., Potargowicz, E., Rzeszotarska, B., and Walczewska-Sumorok, A., (1990), Ovulation-inducing activity of LHRH complexed by copper(II), nickel(II) and zinc(II) ions. J.Inorg.Biochem., 40, 121-125

Livera, C., Pettit, L.D., Bataille, M., Krembel, J., Bal, W., and Kozlowski, H., 1988, Copper(II) complexes with some tetrapeptides containing the "break-point" prolyl residues in third position. J.Chem.Soc.Dalton Trans., 1357-1360

Pettit, L.D., Gregor, J.E., and Kozlowski, H., (1991a), Complex formation between metal ions and peptides. In Perspectives on Bioinorganic Chemistry eds., R.W.Hay, J.R.Dilworth and K.B.Nolan, vol.1., pp.1-41, London: JAI Press

Pettit, L.D., Bal, W., Bataille, M., Cardon, C., Kozlowski, H., Leseine-Delstanche, M., Pyburn, S., Scozzafava, A., (1991b) Thermodynamic and spectroscopic study of the complexes of the undecapeptide substance P, of its N-terminal fragment and of model peptapeptides containing two prolyl residues with copper ions. J.Chem.Soc.Dalton Trans. 1651-1656

Pettit, L.D., and Formicka-Kozlowska, (1984), The suggested role of copper in the biological activity of neuropeptides. Neurosci.Let.50, 53-56

Pettit, L.D., Pyburn, S., Kozlowski, H., Decock-Le Reverend, and Liman, F., (1989), Coordination of Ni(II) ions by angiotensin II and its peptide fragments. a potentiometric, proton NMR and CD spectroscopic study. J.Chem. Soc.Dalton Trans., 1471-1475

Sovago, I., (1990), Metal complexes of peptides and their derivatives. In Biocoordination Chemistry, coordination equilibria in biologically active systems ed.K.Burger, pp.135-184, New York, London: Ellis Horwood

Metal Ions in Biology and Medicine, vol. 2. Eds. J. Anastassopoulou, Ph. Collery, J.C. Etienne, Th. Theophanides. John Libbey Eurotext, Paris © 1992, pp. 10-13

Interaction of copper with proteins : a portrait by FT-IR spectroscopy

R. Anthony Shaw, H. Henry Mantsch

Institute for Biodiagnostics, National Research Council, Winnipeg, Manitoba, R3B 1Y6, Canada

INTRODUCTION

Copper in trace amounts is essential for life, while excess amounts are toxic. One important role of copper is that of a cofactor in a number of the primary oxidases, oxygenases and oxygen carriers in animal cells. Naturally occurring peptide complexes are involved in the transport of copper (Sarkar, 1981), and certain synthetic peptide complexes have been explored as therapeutic agents in cancer treatment (see e.g. Kimoto et al, 1983). Copper also finds use as a complexing agent in the Lowry reaction, which is commonly used in the quantitative determination of proteins (Lowry et al, 1951).

Infrared spectroscopy is playing an increasingly important role in the study of the structure and conformation of biologically important molecules. Modern Fourier transform infrared (FT-IR) spectrometers are capable of providing H_2O and D_2O solution spectra exhibiting very high signal-to-noise ratios. Of particular relevance here is the ability to measure the absorption spectra of proteins and polypeptides in aqueous solution and hence to monitor conformation and conformational changes in an environment that is similar to that found in their natural surroundings. The amide I vibration is particularly useful, as the position of this predominantly C=O stretching mode is both sensitive to the backbone conformation and well removed from other absorptions. For proteins, the region of 1600-1700 cm^{-1} generally exhibits a broad profile representing a superposition of several bands. Features of the secondary structure - i.e. alpha-helical regions, beta-sheet regions, and other contributions to the overall three-dimensional protein structure - may be inferred from the presence and intensities of bands at key positions across this range (Surewicz and Mantsch, 1988). In general these amide I bands are not well resolved from one another. The Fourier self-deconvolution (FSD) technique (Kauppinen et al, 1981) has proven extremely useful in separating these closely spaced features, and is used routinely for this purpose (Mantsch et al, 1988). The software required is standard on the majority of FT-IR instruments. Although straightforward to apply, some care is necessary in optimizing the resolution enhancement while avoiding the introduction of artifacts.

The aim of this article is to provide the reader with a grasp of the strengths and limitations of FT-IR spectroscopy as a probe of metalloprotein structure, taking certain copper containing proteins as illustrative examples.

METALLOPROTEINS

Many proteins require the presence of metal ions either as a means of stabilizing native conformations or as cofactors in fulfilling the catalytic functions of certain enzymes. Ions of the first type include Na^+, K^+, Ca^{2+}, and Mg^{2+}. These are present in relatively high concentrations, and are generally weakly bound to the protein. Ions known to act as cofactors in enzyme activity include iron, zinc, molybdenum, copper, and others. Among these cases we may further distinguish between metalloproteins and metal-activated proteins. The former include certain metal ions as an integral part of their structures, whereas metal-activated proteins lose the metal easily, e.g. through dialysis. While FT-IR cannot easily answer the very difficult question of where and how the metal binds, the infrared spectrum does provide information concerning the role the metal plays in producing and/or stabilizing the conformation required for enzyme activity. These aspects are discussed below.

INFRARED SPECTROSCOPY OF COPPER-CONTAINING PROTEINS AND PEPTIDES

Azurin

Azurin is a blue copper protein of low molecular weight. The FT-IR spectrum has been reported for both *P. fluorescens* azurin and its apo (demetallized) counterpart (Surewicz et al, 1987). FSD of the spectrum in D_2O revealed seven components in the 1600-1700 cm^{-1} range, six of which were assigned as amide I modes. The strongest of these (1636 cm^{-1}) arises from beta structure. Bands at 1663, 1686, and 1696 cm^{-1} were assigned to turns, and those at 1650 and 1657 cm^{-1} to alpha-helical and non-ordered domains respectively (the band at 1657 cm^{-1} appears only in the H_2O solution spectrum). The original spectrum was then curve-fitted using six bands that were fixed in frequency at the values obtained from the deconvolved spectrum and adjusted in intensity to optimize the fit. Having assigned the various absorptions to different components of the overall secondary structure, a quantitative estimate of the relative populations of each form was then derived from the areas under these curves. This estimate was consistent with independent determinations of the secondary structures of related azurins.

These methods are general, and have been used to estimate the secondary structure of a number of proteins. Of greater relevance here are two further aspects of the azurin study, viz infrared studies of the apo form of the protein and of the relative thermal stabilities of the holo (copper-containing) and apo forms. The single copper atom was removed by dialysis against 0.05 M KCN. The infrared spectrum across the amide I region was found to be essentially identical to that of the native protein, demonstrating that the secondary structure is unaffected by the presence (or removal) of copper. The spectra of both species were then measured at intervals between 20°C and 86°C. The native protein exhibited only minor spectral changes up to 76°C. Heating beyond that temperature resulted in dramatic changes, at 86°C leaving a broad unresolvable feature centered at approximately 1643 cm^{-1}. This observation is consistent with an "orderless" structure, and also with earlier differential scanning calorimetry measurements of azurin from *P.aeruginosa* (Engleseth and McMillan, 1986).

Spectra of the apo form were found to show somewhat different variations with temperature. Minor changes were noted at temperatures as low as 55°C, and spectra measured between 55°C and 76°C suggest that the beta structure content is reduced more gradually, and at lower temperatures than is the case for the native protein. The spectrum at 86°C was again indistinguishable from that of the native protein at the same temperature. Upon cooling to 20°C, the spectra of the apo and holo proteins remained similar to one another. Although similar in general appearance the spectra were not identical to those measured prior to the heating cycle, suggesting irreversible although subtle alterations in the secondary structures.

Carbon monoxide as a probe of O_2 binding sites

The substitution of CO for O_2 provides a very powerful infrared probe of respiratory enzymes in particular, due to the exceptional intensity of the CO stretching vibration. This method has been exploited (Alben et al, 1981, Fiamingo et al, 1981,1986) as a means of monitoring the reversible movement of CO between iron and copper in the metalloenzyme cytochrome c oxidase. CO bound to iron in the a3-heme pocket shows two absorptions, with the major band at 1963 cm^{-1} and a weaker one at 1952 cm^{-1} arising from species with an altered a3-heme pocket. Photolysis at low temperature (below 140°K) using visible light leads to photodissociation of the Fe-CO complex and the appearance of two new bands approximately 100 cm^{-1} higher in frequency (2062 cm^{-1} and 2043 cm^{-1}) due to the Cu-CO complex. These changes in the vibrational spectrum indicate that carbon monoxide is bound more strongly at the iron binding site than at the copper site. Differences in the widths of the CO absorptions were also taken as indicating a non-polar, highly ordered environment at the Fe binding site, and a relatively flexible Cu-CO moiety.

Copper(II)-dipeptide complexes

Infrared absorption spectra have been reported for a variety of complexes of di- and polypeptides with copper. (see e.g. Tasumi, 1979). Such studies are important as models of metal-protein interactions. As one example, the origin of the characteristic blue colour associated with the Lowry determination of proteins is not yet clear. The interpretation of these spectra provides challenges of a quite different nature to those outlined above. For example the binding of copper to glycylglycine results in dramatic alterations over the 1550-1700 cm^{-1} range (Fig. 1). At pD 7 the amide I band is shifted to below 1600 cm^{-1} upon complexation with copper; the very low amide frequency results from the displacement of the amide nitrogen by copper. Similar behaviour was found for ten other homo-dipeptides (R.A. Shaw and H.H. Mantsch, unpublished), indicating analogous structures in each case. Earlier reports (Tasumi, 1979) have also suggested that at lower pH (3-5) a complex may form involving the amide oxygen.

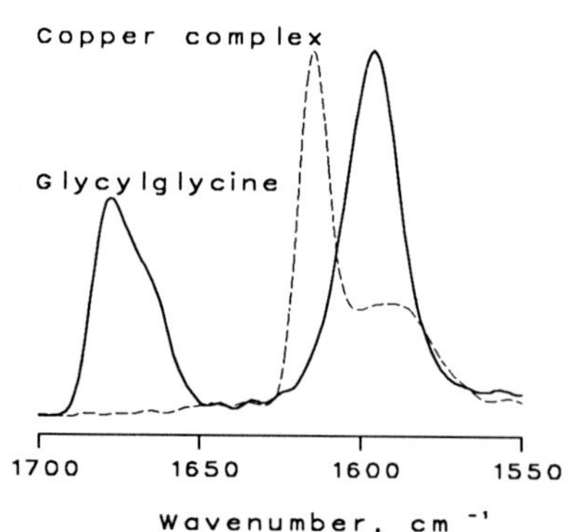

Fig. 1. Deconvolved infrared spectra of glycylglycine (solid line) and its copper(II) complex (D_2O solution, pD=7).

Alben, J.O, Moh, P.P, Fiamingo, F.G. and Altschuld, R.A. (1981): Cytochrome oxidase a3-heme and copper observed by low temperature FT-IR spectroscopy of the CO complex. *Proc. Nat. Acad. Sci. USA.* 78, 234-237.

Engleseth, H.R. & McMillin, D.R. (1986): Studies of thermally induce denaturation of azurin and azurin derivatives by differential scanning calorimetry: evidence for copper selectivity. *Biochemistry* 25, 2448-2455.

Famiango, F.G., Altschuld, R.A., Moh, P.P. and Alben, J.O. (1982): Dynamic interactions of CO with a3Fe and CuB in cytochrome c oxidase in beef heart mitochondria studied by FT-IR spectroscopy at low temperatures. *J. Biological Chemistry* 257, 1639-1650.

Famiango, F.G., Altschuld, R.A., and Alben, J.O. (1986): Alpha and beta forms of cytochrome c oxidase observed in rat heart myocyces by low temperature Fourier transform IR spectroscopy. *J. Biological Chemistry* 261, 12976-12987.

Kauppinen, J.K., Moffatt, D.J., Mantsch, H.H., and Cameron,D.G. (1981): Fourier self-deconvolution: A method for resolving intrinsically overlapped bands. *Applied Spectroscopy* 35, 271-276.

Kimoto, E., Tananaka, H., Gyotoku, J., Morishige, F., and Pauling, C. (1983): Enhancement of antitumor activity of ascorbate against Ehrlich ascites tumor cells by the copper:glycylglycylhistidine complex. *Cancer Res.* 43, 824-828.

Lowry, O.H., Rosebrough, N.J., Farr, A.L., and Randall, R.J. (1951) Protein measurement with the folin phenol reagent. *J. Biological Chemistry* 193, 165-275.

Mantsch, H.H., Moffatt, D.J., and Casal, H.L. (1983): Fourier transform methods for spectral enhancement. *Journal of Molecular Structure* 173, 285-298.

Surewicz, W.K., Szabo, A.G., and Mantsch, H.H. (1987): Conformational properties of azurin in solution as determined from resolution-enhanced Fourier-transform infrared spectroscopy. *European Journal of Biochemistry* 167, 519-523.

Surewicz, W.K. & Mantsch, H.H. (1988): New insight into protein secondary structure from resolution-enhanced infrared spectra. *Biochim. Biophys. Acta.* 952, 115-130.

Sarkar, B. (1981): Transport of copper. In *Metal ions in biological systems. Vol. 12, Properties of copper.* ed. H. Sigel, pp. 233-281, Marcel Dekker Inc., New York.

Tasumi, M. (1979): Interaction of metal ions with peptides in aqueous medium as studied by infrared and Raman spectroscopy. In *Infrared and Raman spectroscopy of biological molecules*, ed. T. Theophanides, pp. 225-240. D. Reidel Publ. Co., Dordrecht, Holland.

Metal Ions in Biology and Medicine, vol. 2. Eds. J. Anastassopoulou, Ph. Collery, J.C. Etienne, Th. Theophanides. John Libbey Eurotext, Paris © 1992, pp. 14-19

^{17}O NMR studies of oxygenated hemoproteins and synthetic model compounds

Ioannis P. Gerothanassis, Michel Momenteau*

*Department of Chemistry, Section of Organic Chemistry and Biochemistry, University of Ioannina, 451 10 Ioannina, Greece and *Institut Curie, Section de Biologie, URA 1387 CNRS, Centre Universitaire, 91405 Orsay, France*

The binding of dioxygen to hemoproteins and model systems has been the subject of extensive research activity and debate for over half a century (Jones et al., 1979). Major emphasis has been placed on elucidating the nature of the iron-oxygen bond and although several X-ray structure determinations are known (Perutz et al., 1987) and numerous spectroscopic techniques have been applied (Stynes, 1981), the detailed electronic structure of the $Fe\text{-}O_2$ moiety still remains controversial. Oxygen-17 NMR spectroscopy appears a promising methodology and in this article we will summarize recent developments in the field (Gerothanassis et al., 1987; 1989; Oldfield et al, 1991).

^{17}O NMR SHIELDING CONSTANTS — THE GEOMETRY OF THE $Fe\text{-}O_2$ MOIETY.

Figure 1 shows the ^{17}O NMR spectrum of the compound "picket fence" porphyrin **1**, of Scheme 1. Two distinct resonances are observed, which are well outside the established oxygen-17 chemical shift scale. This rules out the sideways triangular structure and a rapid flipping of the O-O group between two bent conformers similar to that proposed for $Co(bzacen)(py)(O_2)$ (Melamud et al., 1974). The solution structure, therefore, of the $Fe\text{-}O_2$ linkage is an end-on angular bond first proposed by Pauling (1964).

Differences in nuclear screening constants are usually discussed with respect to contributions from a local paramagnetic term. Velenic and Lynden-Bell (1969) suggested that reasonable estimates of the oxygen-17 shielding constants can be obtained from an extended Hückel method. According to these calculations the nucleus of the oxygen atom O(2) near the iron atom, was found to be more shielded than the nucleus of the terminal oxygen O(1) by about 1400 to 1500 ppm. The difference of the shielding constants between the two nuclei, $\Delta\delta$, is constant and independent of the value of the charge q on the oxygen O(2) and the splitting ΔE of the degenerate π orbitals of the oxygen atoms on complexing. However, the magnitudes of δ_1 and δ_2 strongly depend on both values q and ΔE. For ΔE=1.04 eV and q=0.19 e it was calculated that δ_1=3224 ppm and δ_2=1647 ppm which are in reasonable agreement with the experimental data (Gerothanassis et al., 1987; 1989).

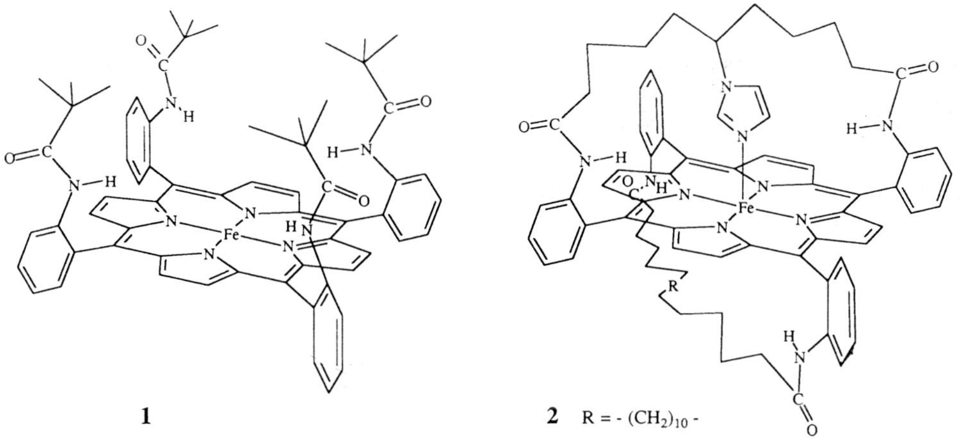

1

2 R = - $(CH_2)_{10}$ -

Scheme 1

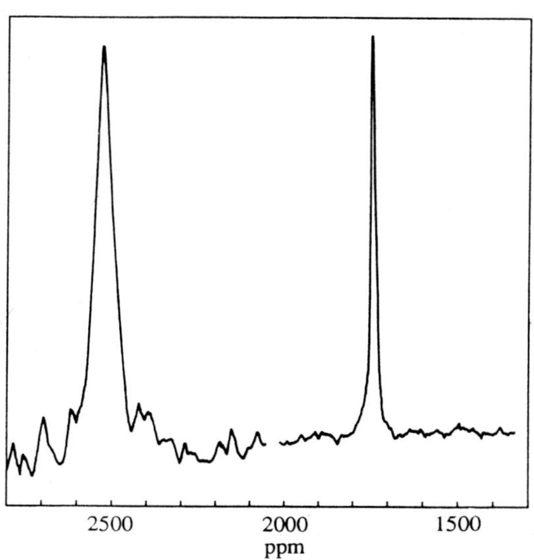

Fig.1. ^{17}O NMR spectrum of compound **1** from use of the normal 90° pulse and recorded in two steps with the carrier frequency on the absorption resonances: concentration ≈1.5×10^{-2} M in CH_2Cl_2; concentration of 1-MeIm 2.5×10^{-1} M; T=273 K; spectral width 71.5 KHz; preacquisition delay time 50 μs; number of scans ≈600000 and 130000 for the high- and low frequency resonances respectively; line-broadening filtering 500 Hz (Gerothanassis et al., 1989).

Oldfield et al. (1991) have studied the model "picket-fence" porphyrin **1** using ^{17}O solid state NMR. The total linewidth breadth of the powder spectrum in ppm was found to be independent of the magnetic field strength. This indicates that the chemical shift anisotropy is the dominant line-broadening interaction. The principal components of the chemical shift tensors for both bridging and terminal oxygens of the Fe-O_2 unit have been determined and the isotropic chemical shifts occur at 1600 and 2017 ppm respectively at 298 K, somewhat shielded from the values in solution state. The solid-state ^{17}O NMR spectra of frozen solutions and polyethylene glycol induced microcrystalline precipitates of oxymyoglobin and oxyhemoglobin indicate a close general similarity between the proteins and the "picket fence" porphyrin. However, the achievable spectral signal to noise ratio does not allow to draw detailed conclusions (Oldfield et al., 1991).

ELECTRON DISTRIBUTION IN FeO_2 LINKAGE-EVIDENCE OF AN OZONE LIKE BONDING.

Considerable controversy has developed in the last decades concerning the electron distribution in the FeO_2 moiety and particularly whether it should be represented as the $Fe(d^6)O_2$ (low spin) or the $Fe(d^5)O_2^-$unit. In the second approach, which was proposed by Weiss (1964) an odd number of electrons is assumed on the coordinated dioxygen and the unpaired spins of $Fe(d^5)$ and O_2^- are reputedly coupled thus resulting in the observed diamagnetism of the Fe-O_2 linkage. According to Huyth et al. (1977) the electronic structure of the FeO_2 linkage can be considered to arise from the interaction of an iron porphyrin moiety and an O_2 molecule with both species in either S=O or S=1 valence states. The latter with populations $Fe\{(x^2-y^2)(yz)^2(xz)^1(z^2)^1\}$ and $O_2\{(\pi_g^s)^1(\pi_g^a)^1\}$ corresponds to an ozone-like bonding, without net charge-transfer $Fe(d^5)O_2^-$ Weiss-type configuration. The analogy between the electronic structure of the FeO_2 moiety and the ozone molecule can be derived from the ^{17}O NMR data. According to Solomon et al. (1968) the bridge oxygen of the ozone molecule absorbs at 1032 ppm, while the terminal oxygens absorb at 1598 ppm. Therefore, the chemical shift difference between the two oxygens is ≈566 ppm in reasonable agreement with the value of 720-770 ppm found for the FeO_2 linkage of the model compounds (Gerothanassis et al., 1987; 1989).

THE QUESTION OF HEMOPROTEIN HYDROPHOBIC POCKET-HYDROGEN BONDING EFFECTS.

The stabilities of oxyhemoglobin and oxymyoglobin have been attributed in part to the steric and nonpolar characteristics on the distal side of the heme. Recently, some investigators have pointed out the significance of hydrogen bond and polar interactions at the distal side (Momenteau, 1986). It was found, for example, that the amide derivatives have an affinity for O_2 an order of magnitude greater than the ether analogs. This was due exclusively to a reduction in O_2 dissociation rate. Further, it was suggested that oxygenation of several model compounds is enhanced by polar solvents. ^{17}O NMR spectroscopy, as a direct probe, can provide a potential approach to exploring hydrogen bond and polarity effects.

With the basket handle porphyrin model **2** a shift of ca. 31 ppm of the resonance of the terminal oxygen atom to lower frequency is observed while the resonance of the oxygen O(1) is shifted to higher frequency by ≈15 ppm. The shift of the terminal oxygen can be attributed to hydrogen bonding interactions with the NH of the distal handle (Momenteau, 1986; Gerothanassis et al., 1989). The high frequency shift of the oxygen

O(2) was attributed to an increase in the metal-oxygen π-bond order (Gerothanassis et al., 1989). It should be emphasized that model compounds in which the superstructures are linked to the macrocycle by ether groups, exhibit chemical shifts similar to those of the picket-fence porphyrin **1**, confirming the absence of hydrogen bonding interactions.

STRUCTURAL DIFFERENCES OF THE $Fe-O_2$ MOIETY OF THE "T" AND "R" STATE HEMOPROTEIN MODELS.

Numerous X-ray and spectroscopic studies have been reported on hemoprotein models with and without axial hindered base since the discovery by Collman et al. (1978) that the proposed tension or strain in the histidine-iron bond in T state Hb can be mimiced in single hemes using 2-MeIm as an axial hindered ligand ("T" state model). The ^{17}O NMR spectra of the "T" state "hybrid" hemoprotein models exhibit two distinct resonances in agreement with the bent end-on geometry (Gerothanassis et al., 1989). The resonance of the oxygen O(2) is shifted by ≈30-39 ppm and that of the terminal oxygen by 50-60 ppm to low frequency in the "T" state relative to that in the "R" state models. The change in the chemical shift of the oxygen atom coordinated to iron could reflect an increase in the Fe-O length (decrease in the Fe-O π-bond order). The shift in the resonance absorption of the terminal oxygen is in the same direction and larger in magnitude to those observed in "hybrid" or "basket handle" porphyrins (a-BHP) bearing NH groups in the handles relative to the ether-BHP (Gerothanassis et al., 1989). It was suggested that this low frequency shift is due to a significant polarization of the O-O bond although the N-H stretching vibrations indicate the absence of conventional hydrogen bonding interactions in the "T" state models (unpublished observations). The high polarizability of the dioxygen moiety in the "T" state models can be interpreted by assuming dipolar interactions at distances longer than conventional hydrogen bonds (see discussion below).

EVIDENCE FOR CONFORMATIONAL EXCITATION: TEMPERATURE DEPENDENCE OF THE ^{17}O LINEWIDTHS IN SOLUTION AND THE ^{17}O SHIELDING TENSORS IN SOLID STATE

The ^{17}O resonance linewidths at half height, $\Delta\nu_{1/2}$, in solution are directly related to the square of the nuclear quadrupole coupling constant, x , and the effective rotational correlation time, τ_c, at the site of the ^{17}O nucleus

$$\Delta\nu_{1/2} = \frac{1}{\pi T_2} = \frac{12\pi^2}{125}\left(1 + \frac{\eta^2}{3}\right) x^2 \tau_c$$

where η is the asymmetry parameter (the motional limit $\omega_0^2\tau^2_c \ll 1$ is assumed, where ω_0 is the nucleus Larmor frequency). A decrease therefore in the linewidths is expected on increasing the temperature due to an increase in the correlation time for molecular tumbling. In the picket-fence porphyrin **1**, the linewidth of the O(2) resonance exhibits a minimum at 273 K and then increases dramatically upon increasing the temperature (Gerothanassis et al., 1989). The linewidth of the O(1) resonance exhibits a minimum around 283 K and increases at higher temperatures. This was interpreted by assuming two conformational pairs which are characterised by a small energy separation and very different electric field gradient tensors at the oxygen sites. According to X-ray structural data of (O_2)FeTpivPP(1-MeIm) the Fe-O-O plane is 4-fold statistically disordered, bisecting the N-Fe-N right angles of the equatorial porphyrin plane. In one orientation, the Fe-O-O plane is approximately parallel to the trans axial base plane and in the other, it is approximately normal to it. The dihedral angle between the alternative orientations of the Fe-O-O plane is 90°. It was suggested (Gerothanassis et al., 1989) that the large changes of the electric field gradient tensors around each oxygen nucleus cannot be primarily due to differences to long-range dipole-dipole interactions which should be expected to affect mainly the terminal oxygen O(1) rather than O(2), contrary to the experimental data. Such a significant change of the electric field gradient tensor at O(2) might result from a difference in the local symmetry due to differences in the Fe-O-O bond angle. Jameson and Drago (1985) noted that in the maximization of the electrostatic attractions between the oxygen molecule and the NH moieties, substantial distortions up to 25° of the Fe-O-O bond angles may occur.

Temperature dependent studies with the "picket-fence" porphyrin in solid state (Oldfield et al., 1991) indicate a small change in the isotropic chemical shift of the terminal oxygen down to 4.2 K while there is an apparent low frequency shift (by $\approx$ 400 ppm) of the bridging oxygen on cooling to 77 K. This indicates the freezing in one of the conformational substates.

OXIDATION MECHANISM OF DIOXYGEN ADDUCTS

The steric encumbrance provided by the protein environment prevents the autoxidation of the oxygenated species by a bimolecular reaction pathway via a μ-peroxo dimer formation. Such a prevention is also obtained in basket-handle porphyrins, **2**, due to the steric hindrance of both faces (Momenteau, 1986). These synthetic model compounds therefore appear as appropriate models to study the oxidation process of iron (II) hemoproteins. During the oxidation process some resonances of oxygen-17 enriched species were detected at low frequencies (Gerothanassis et al., 1989). The resonance at δ=11.1 ppm is characteristic of $H_2{}^{17}O$ and the two resonances at δ=168.5 and173.3 ppm can be assigned to $H_2{}^{17}O_2$. The former absorption is probably due to $H_2{}^{17}O_2$ in microscopic water droplets in suspension which are present in organic solutions. From the presence of the above enriched species formed during the oxidation process, the following reaction scheme was proposed (Gerothanassis et al., 1989).

$$PFe^{II} + {}^*O_2 \rightleftharpoons PFe^{II}-{}^*O_2$$

$$PFe^{II} - {}^*O_2 + H_2O \longrightarrow [PFe^{III} \cdots {}^*O_2^{\bullet -} \cdots HOH]$$

$$[PFe^{III} \cdots {}^*O_2^{\bullet -} \cdots HOH] \longrightarrow PFe^{III} - OH^- + H^*O_2^{\bullet}$$

$$2H^*O_2^{\bullet} \longrightarrow H_2{}^*O_2 + {}^*O_2$$

$$H_2{}^*O_2 \longrightarrow H_2O + \tfrac{1}{2}{}^*O_2$$

Acknowledgements. Finantial support from NATO, the General Secretariat of Research and Technology (Coopération Scientifique Franco-Hellénique), the Research Committee of the University of Ioannina, Greece, and the Centre National de la Recherche Scientifique, France, is gratefully acknowledged.

REFERENCES

Collman, J.P., Gagne, R.R., Reed, C.A., Halbert, T.R., Lang, G. & Robinson, W.T. (1975): "Picket fence porphyrins" Synthetic models for oxygen binding hemoproteins. J. Am. Chem. Soc. 97, 1427-1439.

Collman, J.P., Brauman, J.I.,Rose, E. & Suslick, K.S. (1978): Cooperativity in O_2 binding to iron porphyrins. Proc. Natl. Acad. Sci. U.S.A. 75, 1052-1055.

Gerothanassis, I.P. & Momenteau, M. (1987): ^{17}O NMR spectroscopy as a tool for studying synthetic oxygen carriers related to biological systems: Application to a synthetic single-face hindered iron porphyrin-dioxygen complex in solution. J. Am. Chem. Soc. 109, 6944-6947.

Gerothanassis, I.P., Momenteau, M. & Loock, B.(1989): Hydrogen-bond stabilization of dioxygen, conformation excitation, and autoxidation mechanism in hemoprotein models as revealed by ^{17}O NMR Spectroscopy. J. Am. Chem. Soc. 111, 7006-7012.

Huynh, B.H., Case D.A. & Karplus, M. (1977): Nature of the iron-oxygen bond in oxyhemoglobin. J. Am. Chem. Soc. 99, 6103-6105.

Jameson, G.B. & Drago, R.S.(1985): Role of weak hydrogen bonding in the coordination of dioxygen to hemoproteins and their models. J. Am. Chem. Soc. 107, 3017-3020.

Jones, R.D., Summerville, D.A. & Basolo, F. (1979): Synthetic oxygen carriers related to biological systems. Chem. Rev. 79, 139-179.

Melamud, E., Silver, B.L. & Dori, Z. (1974): Electron paramagnetic resonance of mononuclear cobalt oxygen carriers labelled with oxygen-17. J. Am. Chem. Soc. 96, 4689-4690.

Momenteau, M. (1986): Synthesis and coordination properties of superstructured iron-porphyrins. Pure Appl. Chem. 58, 1493-1502

Oldfield, E., Lee, H.C., Coretsopoulos, C., Adebodun, F., Park, K.O., Yang, S., Chung, J. & Phillips, B. (1991): J. Am. Chem. Soc. 113, 8680-8685.

Pauling, L. (1964): Nature of the iron-oxygen bond in oxyhaemoglobin. Nature (London) 203, 182-183 .

Perutz, M.F., Fermi, G., Luisi, B., Shaanan, B. & Liddington, R.C. (1987) Stereochemistry of cooperativity mechanisms in hemoglobin. Acc. Chem. Res. 20: 309-321.

Solomon, I.J., Keith, J.N., Kacmarek, A.J. & Raney, J.K. (1968): Additional studies concerning the existence of "O_3F_2". J. Am. Chem. Soc. 90, 5408-5411 .

Stynes, D.V. (1981): Probes of proximal and distal effects in hemoglobin and myoglobin. Can. J. Spectrosc. 26, 109-118.

Velenik, A. & Lynden-Bell, R.M. (1969): ^{17}O nuclear magnetic resonance chemical shift in oxyhaemoglobin. Croat. Chem. Acta 41, 205-211 .

Weiss, J.J. (1964): Nature of the iron-oxygen bond in oxyhaemoglobin. Nature (London) 202, 83-84.

Metal Ions in Biology and Medicine, vol. 2. Eds. J. Anastassopoulou, Ph. Collery, J.C. Etienne, Th. Theophanides. John Libbey Eurotext, Paris © 1992, pp. 20-25

Physicochemical behaviour of empty and loaded unilamellar vesicles. Interactions with entrapped chromophores

Rosario Vilaplana, Francisco García, Francisco González-Vílchez

Departamento de Química Inorgánica, Facultad de Química, Universidad de Sevilla, 41071 Sevilla, Spain

INTRODUCTION

Lipidic membranes are essential to the structure and function of living cell, regulating transport of nutrients and toxins, providing a matrix for some enzymatic reactions and as control of other important cellular functions. At the same time, lipidic vesicles are increasingly used nowadays as optimum mediums for the transportation of substances (Mayer *et al.*, 1986) and as excellent substrates for a wide diversity of technical applications (Chang *et al.*, 1990). Many of these functions can be attributed to the ambiphilicity of the lipid molecules, able to create a bilayer with a hydrophobic interior and a charged hydrophilic surface. Furthermore, some lipid behave as liquid crystals, forming in this way supramolecular structures that show biomaterial properties (Ringsdorf *et al.*, 1988).

Trying to progress in the knowledge of the physicochemical properties and behaviour of biomembranes, we have been developing a method for the preparation of large unilamellar vesicles (LUV) as mimicking systems of the natural membranes. Furthermore, we have studied the stability and integrity of the obtained vesicles when loaded with different chromophores such as porphyrins (Tetra-4N-methylpyridylporphine, TMP-4), metalloporphyrins (CuTMP-4) and 2,6-carboxyfluorescein (CF). As known, the concentration dependent self-quenching of CF fluorescence permits possible leakage from loaded liposomes to be monitored continuosly.

EXPERIMENTAL

The lipid palmitoyl-oleoyl-phosphatydilcholine (POPC, Fig. 1) in chloroforrn solution was used because its phase transition temperature is very low and the unsaturated side chains produce an increasing flexibility to the formed membranes. At the same time, this lipid does not show relaxation effects at different wavelengths. The solvent was removed by rotary evaporation at 30°C and the appropriate amount of cholesterol in chloroform solution was added to the lipid film. The mixture was lyophilized and stored until using.

Vesicles were prepared by using the freeze-thaw extrusion method modified as previously reported (Vilaplana *et al.*, 1992). About 50 mg of the lyophilized lipid is mixtured in a cryogenic tube with 1 mL of a porphyrin stock solution which concentration is about 10^{-2} M. A blanck is prepared suspending the lipid in 1 mL of aqueous phosphate buffer. Both samples are further used for preparing LUV. The removing of the non-encapsulated porphyrin is performed by treatment with the ion exchange resin IRC-50. Free CF was removed by passing the vesicles through a Sephadex G-25 column, the resin previously swirled with Hepes buffer also used as solvent of the dye.

$$
\begin{array}{l}
\qquad\qquad\qquad\qquad\qquad CH_3 - (CH_2)_{14} - COO - CH_2 \\
\qquad\qquad\qquad\qquad\qquad\qquad\qquad\qquad\qquad\qquad\quad | \\
CH_3 - (CH_2)_7 - CH = CH - (CH_2)_7 - COO - CH \\
\qquad\qquad\qquad\qquad\qquad\qquad\qquad\qquad\qquad\qquad\quad | \\
\qquad\qquad\qquad\qquad\qquad\qquad\qquad\qquad\qquad\qquad CH_2 - \overset{-}{PO_4} - (CH_2)_2 - \overset{+}{N}(CH_3)_3
\end{array}
$$

Fig. 1
Estructure of the lipid POPC

Temperature-jump studies, and UV-visible and fluorescence spectroscopies were used for the study of the vesicles properties. Quasi scattering light spectroscopy (QELS) was applied for the sizing of the prepared vesicles.

RESULTS AND DISCUSSION

QELS of the loaded vesicles have shown that all the studied samples are homogeneous in size, with the mean diameter of unilamellar vesicles being equal to 130 nm (Fig. 2). The empty vesicles are slightly smaller, it being the mean diameter of about 115 nm.

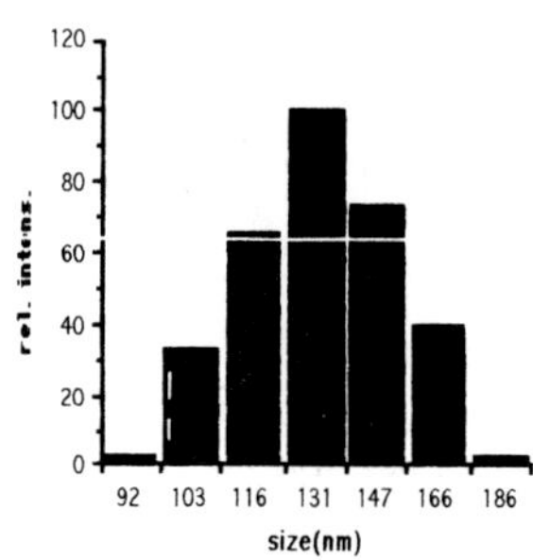

Fig. 2
QELS Analysis of CF-loaded vesicles

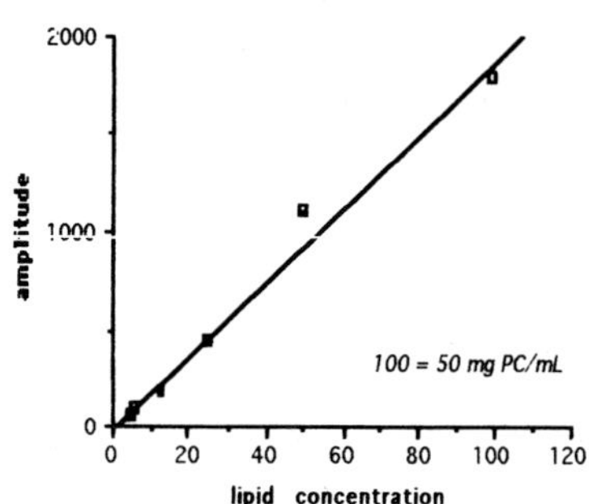

Fig. 3
Variation of TJ amplitude effects with PC concentration

TJ experiments have been performed on empty phosphatydilcholine (PC) and POPC vesicles in order to check the stability, integrity and behaviour of these systems when submitted to electrical discharges. Because we found that PC-LUV show relaxation effects at different conditions, our study has been first carried out at 19°C and at 439 nm, a wavelength at which porphyrins show low absorbance.

As result, increasing of the PC vesicle's concentration leads to the linear increasing of amplitudes (Fig. 3), it being this dependence the best evidence of the sticking's and agglomeration's absence of the vesicles.

On the other hand, higher ionic strenghts lead to lower relaxation effects, specially to much smaller rate constants.

If the same experiments are performed in fluorescence mode, smaller intensity of the kinetic effects are observed. On the other hand, the influence of the applied electric current has been studied, the results indicating that a voltage equal to 25 kV is the most appropriate.

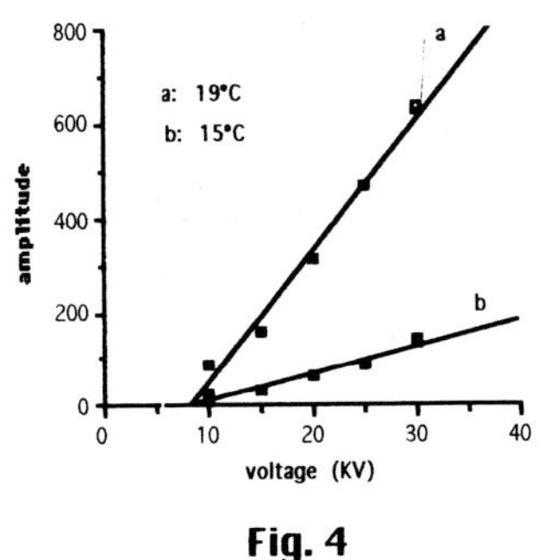

Fig. 4

Amplitude dependence with voltage

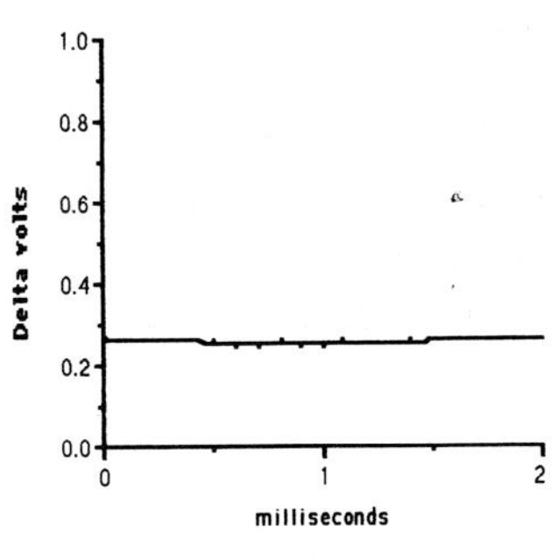

Fig. 5

Laser TJ study of POPC vesicles

Also, the temperature of the experience has been adjusted at 15°C. The comparison of the relaxation effects obtained at the two different temperatures in fluorescence mode shows that the intensity of the named effects drops dramatically at the lower temperature (Fig. 4) while k_e takes a much smaller value {i.e., a = 465.6, k_e = 5300 s^{-1} (19°C); a = 84.4, k_e = 2400 s^{-1} (15°C)}. It can be deduced that TJ experiments carried out on PC vesicles must be performed at temperatures far from the transition phase one (21°C) in order to avoid interferences coming from the own vesicles. In fact, the low values of the relaxation effects measured, permits the performing of TJ experiments on encapsulated substances in PC LUV, carrying out the corresponding corrections after the experiments. TJ experiences performed on POPC vesicles in fluorescence mode have shown the total absence of relaxation effects at the wavelength range 460 nm - 480 nm, although the detected effects are almost negligible between 400 nm and 550 nm. In this way, TJ experiments can be realized on encapsulated substances in POPC LUV without the interferences produced by the own vesicles. This results have been confirmed by Laser TJ experiemnts performed on samples of POPC and POPC-PS (8%) LUV (Fig. 5). Once more, no relaxation effects were observed.

In order to see if the electrical discharges damage or alter the integrity of the vesicles, TJ measurements were performed on liposomes containing TMP-4 and CuTMP-4 in experimental conditions at which the relaxation effects arising from the own vesicles are negligible (a = 88);

before and after carrying out the TJ study, fluorescence spectroscopy was realized to test the possible leaking of the entrapped molecules as result of the membrane alteration.

Kinetic effects are detected when TJ studies are performed on both encapsulated substances (i.e., a = 480, in the case of porphyrin stuffed vesicles). Because the copper complex does not fluoresces, the relaxation effect measured evidences the alteration of the vesicles' membrane as result of the porphyrin interaction.

Emission fluorescence spectra were registered at $\lambda = 439$ nm in fluorescence mode. Table 1shows the wavelengths and relative intensities of the peaks observed.

Table 1

Spectral features (Bands and intensities) observed in the fluorescence spectra of entrapped porphyrin

before TJ		after TJ	
band (nm)	Intensity(cps)	band (nm)	intensity(cps)
653	1.99×10^5	652	1.92×10^5
709	1.47×10^5	709	1.35×10^5

From these experiences we can conclude that loaded TMP-4 vesicles are not opened when targeted with electrical discharges. On the contrary, the porphyrin is delivered only after the addition of a detergent, this fact evidencing that the relaxation effects observed when TJ technique is applied on empty PC vesicles do not arise from the opening of the liposomes.

Fluorescence spectroscopy studies have been realized too on empty and loaded TMP-4 and CuTMP-4 PC vesicles, at 15°C and $\lambda = 500$ nm, a wavelength at which the porphyrins show negligible absorptions. As expected, the copper complex does not show fluorescence, this fact confirming that the relaxation effects detected during the TJ study of this sample can be attributed to the alteration of the membrane caused by the interaction of the entrapped metal complex and the lipid bilayer.

Sorpresively, empty vesicles scatter 4-fold more light at 600 nm that the stuffed vesicles; these last systems behave in the same way respect the incident light independently of the nature of the entrapped substance. This experimental observation demonstrates that vesicles became alter when loaded with porphyrins; the referred behaviour is not followed by vesicles containing a different chromophore, such as CF. Indeed, loaded CF vesicles scatter more light than the empty ones. In this way, the encapsulated porphyrins are the only tested compounds able to change the properties of the lipid bilayer, this fact resulting in the increasing uptaking of the incoming light by the stuffed liposomes. Different interpretations could be in agreement with the observed phenomena. If the photosensitizing character of the porphyrins is playing a role in the absorption of light, new important insights might be deduced by comparison of this system with the natural one responsable for the chlorophylic function.

The authors gratefully acknowledge support of this research from the CICYT of Spain (Grant 519-90).

REFERENCES

Chang, A.C., Pfeiffer, W.F., Guillaume, B., Baral, S. and Fendler, J.H. (1990): *J. Phys. Chem.*, 94, 4284.

Mayer, L.D., Hope, M.J., and Cullis, P.R. (1986): *Biochim. Biophys. Acta*, 858, 161.

Ringsdorf, H., Schlarb, B., and Venzmer, J. (1988): *Angew. Chem. Int. Ed. Engl.*, 27, 113.

Vilaplana, R., Vee Wong, H., and González-Vílchez, F. (1992): *Biochim. Biophys. Acta*, To be published.

Metal Ions in Biology and Medicine, vol. 2. Eds. J. Anastassopoulou, Ph. Collery, J.C. Etienne, Th. Theophanides. John Libbey Eurotext, Paris © 1992, pp. 26-31

Magnesium-nucleic acid interactions in water

J. Anastassopoulou**, M. Polissiou*, M. Manfait***, Th. Theophanides

* *Agricultural University of Athens, Laboratory of General Chemistry, Iera Odos 75, GR 118 55, Athens, Greece. ** National Technical University of Athens, Laboraty of Radiation Chemistry and Biospectroscopy, Zografou Campus, GR 157 73, Athens, Greece. *** Université de Reims, Faculté de Pharmacie, Laboratoire de Pectroscopie Biomoléculaire, 51096 Reims, France*

INTRODUCTION

The importance of cations in the structural stabilization of salts, and in particular, of polynucleotide salts has long been known (1). Since a polynucleotide is a polyanion, it needs cations to be stabilized. The DNA polyanion with its negatively charged phosphate oxygens is neutralized by cations, such as, the hydrated monovalent cations (Na^+, K^+) or the bivalent cations (Mg^{++}, Ca^{++}) or other cationic species. The bivalent magnesium cation, in particular, has long been recognized (2) to be a stabilizing force in tRNA and in DNA by binding to specific backbone phosphate sites, depending on the hydration state of the metal. The two minerals, calcium and magnesium, have considerable correlations with the integrity of the structure of the chromosomes and thus with renal diseases and cancer. Epidemiological evidence is presented that magnesium levels in water, food and air are inversely related to cancer mortality (3).
The hydrated $[Mg(H_2O)_6]^{++}$ ion is always present in water solutions, when there are magnesium salts. The number of waters 6 is the coordination number of magnesium and the salt can be dehydrated by substitution reactions or by temperature (4).

RESULTS AND DISCUSSION

^1H and ^{31}P NMR Data

High resolution proton NMR spectra of the nucleotide, [guanosine 5'-monophosphate-$Mg(H_2O)_5{}^{++}$] complex in water solutions showed significant downfield chemical shifts of H_8 of guanine, in particular at high concentration of Mg^{++}(5). This tendency of downfield shift of proton at C_8, however very weak, suggests that Mg^{++} could be bound to N_7 of guanine forming dynamic and reversible complexes (6).
In the Table 1 are given the coupling constant data of guanosine-5'-monophosphate disodium salt ($G^{5'}p$) in the presence of Mg^{++} ions at various concentrations and temperatures (6). The coupling constant data indicate a perturbation of the equilibrium of the sugar ring, as a consequence of the small reorientation of the purine base with respect to the sugar ring and increase of the ^3E conformer. Temperature elevation shows an increase of the ^3E conformer

indicating a reorientation of the purine base (Fig. 1).As far as, the exocyclic, -$CH_2PO_3^=$ group conformation is concerned the population of the gg, gt, tg, conformers obtained by rotation about the $C_{4'}$-$C_{5'}$ bond (Fig. 1).

TABLE 1. Coupling Constants for Guanosine-5'-Monophosphate disodium salt ($G^{5'}p$) in the Presence of Mg^{++} Ions at Various Concentrations in D_2O Solution and Temperature Effects[1] (6).

$[Mg^{++}]$ M	pD	T°C	J						
			1'2'	2'3'	3'4'	4'5'	4'5''	5'P	5''/P
0	8.3	20	6.1	5.2	3.4	3.7	3.7	4.6	4.6
0.05	7.8	20	5.8	5.3	4.0	3.2	3.7	4.4	4.9
0.20	7.6	20	5.5	5.1	4.2	2.9	3.5	5.1	5.0
0	8.3	80	5.5	5.3	3.8	4.3	4.3	5.5	5.7
0.05	7.8	80	5.2	5.2	4.3	4.0	4.3	5.2	5.5

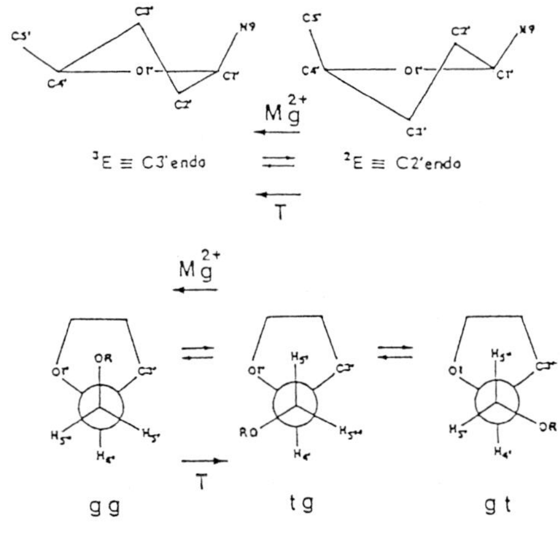

Fig. 1. The temperature and magnesium effects on the sugar-phosphate conformations (6), $R=PO^=_3$

The presence of magnesium ions in aqueous solution favours the gg conformers, whereas an increase of temperature favours the gt, tg conformers. This shows the selective stabilizing effect of magnesium ions upon a particular conformer, in this case the gg conformer. The hydrated magnesium ion rotates the phosphate group and attracts it to itself by hydrogen bonding.
The ^{31}P chemical shifts of $G^{5'}p$ can also give information on the rotation about the $O^{5'}P$ bond and the hydrogen bonding with the coordinated water molecules Mg^{++}-OH_2. It has been found (6) that the ^{31}P resonance of 4.03 ppm for $G^{5'}p$ shifts to 3.80 and 3.70 ppm, respectively for 0.1M and 0.2M $MgCl_2$-$G^{5'}p$ in D_2O solutions downfield from H_3PO_4 as external reference.

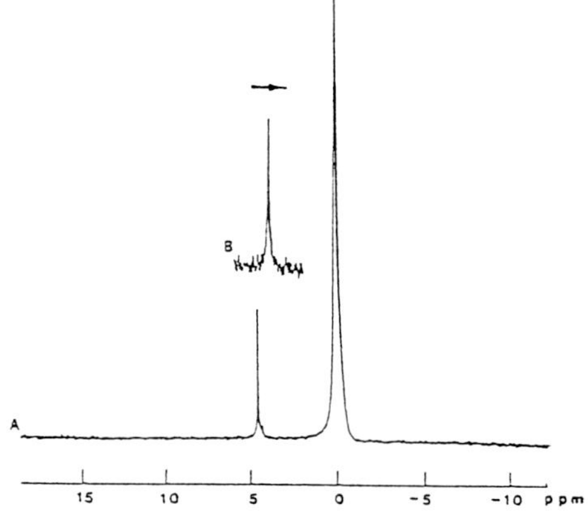

Fig. 2. Proton decoupled (162 MHz) ^{31}P NMR spectra of (A) $G^{5'}p$ 0.1M pH=8.3, and (B) $G^{5'}p$, 0.02M + $MgCl_2$, 0.10M, pH=7.7 both taken in aqueous solution at room temperature and with H_3PO_4 as external reference.

The $G^{5'}p$ concentration was 0.02M. The results show a slight shift to lower ppm which corresponds to a more acidic phosphate group in the presence of Mg^{++} ions. The pH value changes from 8.3 to 7.7 for 0.1M $MgCl_2$ and 7.6 for 0.2M $MgCl_2$ (Fig.2).

Raman and FT-IR Spectra of Nucleic Acid-Magnesium Interactions

Vibrational spectra can also provide information on interaction of Mg^{++} with nucleotides, polynucleotides and nucleic acids. It has been shown previously that Mg^{++} ions may perturb considerably the conformational equilibria of nucleotides. In aqueous media Mg^{++} ions are hydrated, and thus may modify the molecular associations existing in water. The magnesium ions coordinating to water molecules may also control the free water in its surrounding. This in turn may modify the self-association of nucleotides in water.

The vibrational spectra of nucleotides could be studied in water by Raman Spectroscopy and Fourier-Transform Infrared spectroscopy. The Raman spectra of Mg^{++}-$G^{5'}p$ complex in water solutions in the presence of increased concentrations of magnesium ions is given in Figure 3. The increased presence of magnesium ions induces modifications in the relative intensities of bands assigned to the sugar-phosphate vibrations. These bands are located at 810, 865, 980, 1046 and 1088 cm^{-1} (7). It has been proposed previously (8,9) that the 835 cm^{-1} Raman band is characteristic of the B($C_{2'}$-endo) conformation of DNA and disappears in the presence of metal ions which induce the A conformation of DNA ($C_{3'}$-endo). This band shifts to 800 cm^{-1} upon a B to A conformational change and thus the 800 cm^{-1} band is characteristic of $C_{3'}$-endo conformation. Furthermore, in Figure 3 it is also seen that the ratio of intensities of I_{1324} / I_{1368} which increases as the concentration of Mg^{++} ions increases 200 fold. The vibrations at 1324 cm^{-1} and 1368 cm^{-1} are assigned to the imidazole ring specifically to the localized C_8-C_9, N_7-C_8-H and N_9-C_8-H vibrations. This change of intensities is assumed to be due to delocalization of the electronic cloud in the ring upon Mg^{++}- interaction with the N_7 site of guanine. The carbonyl band at 1698 cm^{-1} is shifted to lower frequencies as the concentration of Mg^{++} ions increases in solution. This is attributed to extensive hydrogen bonding of the coordinated water molecules with the carbonyl oxygen. The water vibration at 1640 cm^{-1} attributed to δ_{HOH} is also affected intensity-wise upon increase of Mg^{++} ion concentration. This may be due to the high tendency of Mg^{++} ions to hydrate and take up free water molecules to form a complex hydrated ion $[Mg(H_2O)_6]^{++}$. This may be extremely significant in controlling the water contain within cells and in biological processes, where there are magnesium ions.

The FT-IR spectra of $G^{5'}p$ and $Mg(H_2O)_5^{++}$-G^5p molecules show similar properties (10) as far as the characteristic bands of $G^{5'}p$ are concerned. The FT-IR spectra are shown in Figure 4. In this study the spectrum is given in the region 1000-600 cm^{-1} and is complementary to the Raman spectrum discussed above.

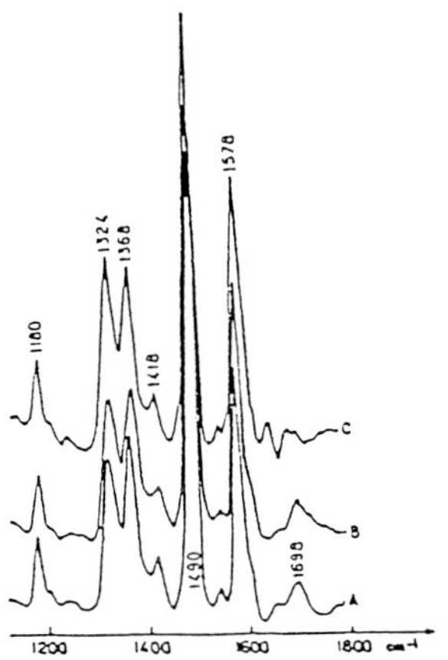

Fig. 3. Raman spectra of complexes of $G^{5'}p$-$Mg(H_2O)_5^{++}$, a) r=0, b) r=2, and c) r=200. The ordinate is normalized in arbitrary units (7).

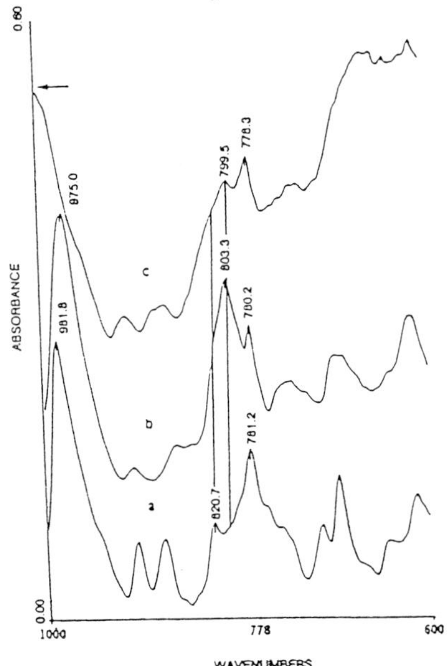

Fig. 4. FT-IR spectra of KCl pellets of a) $G^{5'}p$ commercial, b) $G^{5'}p$ (0.02 M) freeze-dried solution, and c) $G^{5'}p$ (0.02 M) freeze-dried solution with $MgCl_2 \cdot 6H_2O$ (0.05 M) (10).

The characteristic bands of sugar-phosphate at 820.7 cm^{-1} and 803.3 cm^{-1} assigned (10) to $C_{2'}$-endo, anti, and $C_{3'}$-endo, anti, respectively show considerable intensity changes upon freeze-drying the water solutions of $G^{5'}p$ and complex $Mg(H2O)_5^{++}$-$G^{5'}p$.

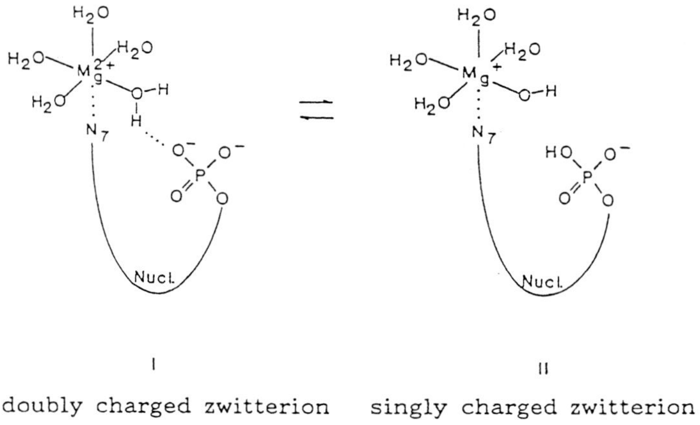

I — doubly charged zwitterion

II — singly charged zwitterion

Fig. 5. Proposed acid hydrolysis of the [$G^{5'}$p-Mg(H_2O)] complex.

The phosphate band at 981.8 cm^{-1} shifts to higher frequencies upon complexation with Mg^{++} ions which is most likely due to the magnesium interaction with the phosphate group through hydrogen bonding with the coordinated water molecules. This interaction could also involve some degree of hydrolysis of phosphate salt through the coordinated water molecules, as is shown in Fig. 5.

In the above equilibrium between I and II the hydrogen bonding through the coordinated water molecule (form I) may cause the transfer of a hydrogen atom to the phosphate group to the acid (form II). This may explain the decrease of pH from 8.3 to 7.7 (0.1M $MgCl_2$), to 7.6 (0.2M $MgCl_2$), and to 4.8 (3.2M $MgCl_2$). The magnesium complex is an interesting pH regulator of biological processes in this range of pH 8.3-7.6 with microconcentrations of $MgCl_2$ up to 0.2M.

Irradiation studies of Magnesium - $G^{5'}$p Water solutions

It was found (11) that irradiation under aerobic conditions shows a decomposition limiting yield G($G^{5'}$p)=0.4 both in the presence and in the absence of [Mg^{++}] (See Fig.6.).

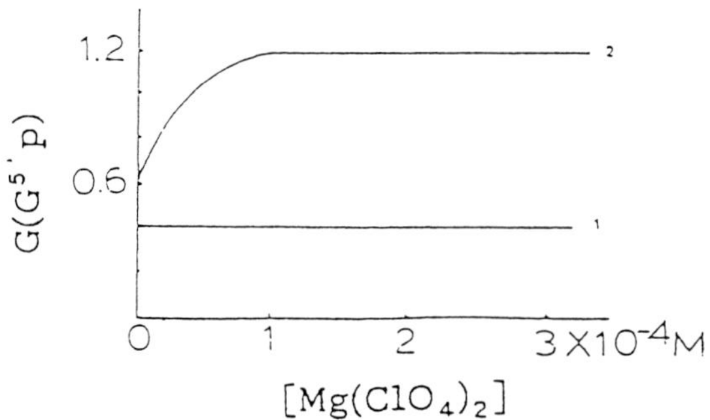

Fig. 6. Variation of the decomposition yield of $G^{5'}$p in aqueous solutions (1) aerated and (2) N_2O-saturated as a function of [$Mg(ClO_4)_2$].

It seems that the competition of oxygen is too strong for the metal to be bound to guanosine N_7 site under these conditions. However, under non aerobic conditions as is shown in curve 2 the decomposition limiting yield $G(G^{5'}p)$ increases from 0.6 to 1.2 as the concentration of Mg^{++} increases to one equivalent ($1X10^{-4}M$). After that value it remains constant. This behaviour suggests that under anaerobic conditions in the presence of magnesium ions the irradiations effect is doubled. This is most likely due to magnesium complexation at the N_7 site of guanosine, in accordance with all the above spectroscopic data.

REFERENCES

1. Theophanides, T. (1984): Metal ions in biological systems. Int. Quant. Chem. XXVI: 933-939.
2. Teeter, M.M., Quigley, G.J. and Rich, A. (1980): Metal ions and transfer RNA. In Nucleic Acid-Metal Ion Interactions Vol.1, Ed. T.G. Spiro, p.p. 145-147, Chichester: John Wiley & Sons.
3. Marier, J.R., Neri, L.C. (1985): Quantifying the role of magnesium in the interrelationship between human mortality/morbidity and water hardness. Magnesium. 4: 53-59.
4. Badilescu, S. and Theophanides, T. (1988): FT-IR-ATR and FAB mass spectrometry studies of magnesium halide hydrate embedded into the surface layer of thalium bromide-iodide single crystal. Appl. Spectrosc. 42: 1118-1124.
5. Theophanides, T. and Polissiou, M. (1981): High resolution proton NMR studies of 5'-GMP and $Mg^{++}$and anticarcinogenic effect of magnesium. Inorg. Chim. Acta. 56: L1-L3 .
6. Polissiou, M. and Theophanides, T. (1981): Conformational flexibility of nucleotides and metal ion interactions. The effect of Mg^{++} ions. Biomolecular Stereodynamics, Vol. II, Ed. R.H. Sarma, pp 487-496. New York: Adenine Press.
7. Manfait, M. and Theophanides, T. (1983): Rôle du Magnésium dans l'interaction Mg^{++}-5'-Guanosine monophosphate. Magnesium. 2: 323- 329.
8. Thomas, G.J. (1989): Water as a bioactivator and probe of DNA structures: investigation by laser Raman spectroscopy. In Spectroscopy of Inorganic Bioactivators, Ed. T. Theophanides, pp. 247-263. Dordrecht: Kluwer Academic Publishers.
9. Theophanides, T. and Anastassopoulou, J. (1988): Metal binding and conformational changes in nucleic acids. In Spectroscopy of Biological Molecules, Eds. E.D. Schmid, FD.W. Schneider, F. Siebert, pp 433-438, John Wiley & Sons.
10. Theophanides, T. and M. Polissiou, (1986): Magnesium-nucleic acid conformation changes and cancer. Magnesium. 5: 221-233.
11. Anastassopoulou, J. (1989): OH radicals bioactivators. In Spectroscopy of inorganic bioactivators, Ed. T. Theophanides, pp. 273-278. Dordrecht: Kluwer Academic Publishers.

Metal Ions in Biology and Medicine, vol. 2. Eds. J. Anastassopoulou, Ph. Collery, J.C. Etienne, Th. Theophanides. John Libbey Eurotext, Paris © pp. 32-36

Biological activity of copper(II) complexes *in vitro*. Species-activity correlation

Giuseppe Arena[a], Mauro Bindone[b], Venera Cardile[b], Enrico Conte[a], Giuseppe Maccarrone[a], Maria Carmela Riello[b], Enrico Rizzaelli[a,c]

(a) *Dipartimento di Scienze Chimiche, Universita'di Catania, Viale A. Doria 6, 95125 Catania, Italy.* (b) *Istituto di Fisiologia, Universita' di Catania, Viale A. Doria 6, 95125 Catania, Italy.* (c) *Istituto per lo Studio delle Sostanze Naturali di Interesse Alimentare e Chimico-farmaceutico, C.N.R., Catania, Italy*

Copper(II) was long ago recognized to be an essential trace element (Hart et al., 1928). It has been shown to be an integral enzyme co-factor in processes such as electron transport, antioxidant protection, connettive tissue biosynthesis, pigment formation, neurotransmitter and hormone production (Ettinger, 1984). However, despite the relevance of copper(II) to the above and other processes (Evans, 1973; Prohaska, 1987), little is known about its cellular metabolism (Palida et al., 1991; Sato et al. 1991).

In the past, copper-containing drugs have been used extensively for the treatment of pathological disorders (Deuschle et al.,1985). Recently, Sorenson (1989) has suggested that the elevated plasma copper levels encountered in a number of diseases such as inflammatory diseases, gastrointestinal ulcers, diabetes, epilepsy, radiation injuries and cancers represent a "physiological" response to the injury. Thus, the use of copper complexes in the treatment of the above pathological conditions would result in mimicking the " physiological" answer (Sorenson, 1989). In contrast with Sorenson's hypothesis, the abnormally high levels of copper occurring in the biological fluids of patients suffering from the above diseases have been interpreted as pathological conditions (Wiesel, 1959; Youssef et al., 1983; Falkman et al.,1987).

Conflicting results concerning the pharmacological activity of copper(II) complexes are found in the literature. In fact, whereas on one hand copper complexes have been shown to possess an anticarcinogenic and antimutagenic activity (Oberley et al.,1982; Sorenson ,1989), on the other hand they have also been reported to be mutagenic (Schaaper et al., 1987) and carcinogenic (Agarwal et al.,1989). Moreover, Copper(II) complexes have been shown to have a superoxidismutase-like activity (Brigelius et al.,1974; De Alvare et al., 1976; Weinstein and Bielski, 1980; Kimura et al., 1983; Sorenson, 1984; Goldstein and Czapski, 1985; Huber et al., 1987; Goldstein et al., 1990). This together with some hypotheses on the role of superoxidismutase in cancer (Oberley and Buettner, 1979; Oberley et al., 1980) has stimulated a number of studies on the cytotoxic and and antitumor activity of copper(II) complexes (Sorenson ,1989).

In our laboratory, some copper(II) complexes have been shown to have a scavenger activity towards oxygen radicals (Costanzo et al. 1989). Thus we have tested a series of copper(II) complexes of small peptides to see whether they have any cytotoxic activity *in vitro*. This series included L-Leu-L-Phe, L-Ala-L-Tyr, L-Leu-L-Leu and *c*-L-His-L-His. These ligands were chosen also because their copper(II) species as well as the stability constants are well established (Bonomo et al. 1986; Arena et al. 1987). When testing the Cu-*c*-L-His-L-His (L) system the conditions were chosen in such a way as to have either the species $[Cu(L)_2]^{2+}$ or the species $[Cu(L)_2H_{-2}]^0$. In addition to small peptides complexes we also tested $CuSO_4$ and Cu-Im-Ac (Im=imidazole; Ac=acetate). Copper sulphate was included because copper(II) inorganic salts have been reported to be uneffective (Sorenson,1989) whereas Cu-Im-Ac was screened because it had been reported to have "strong antitumor activity" against the B16 line, that was one of the lines being investigated in our laboratory. The complexes were tested against the mouse cancer line B16 melanoma, the clone of murine L929, human KB cells and human fibroblasts.

Our goals were to see i) whether these complexes showed any activity *in vitro*; and ii) whether there was any correlation between the activity (if any) and the species administered.

All the tested systems, with the exception of the two *c*-L-His-L-His complexes, inhibited the cell growth of mouse cancer line B16 melanoma, showing roughly the same ID_{50} (10-12γ/ml). Preliminary tests carried out on L929, KB cells as well as human fibroblasts showed that the Cu-*c*-L-His-L-His systems had little cytotoxic activity also against these cells. Thus, these complexes were extensively tested only against the B16 cell line.

The tested systems are not so effective against fibroblasts as they are against tumor cell lines. Interestingly, following the elimination of the test system and re-incubation with the culture medium for 72 hours, B16, L929 and KB cell lines did not show any recovery at all whereas fibroblasts showed a full recovery. This result is of particular relevance in that it indicates that these systems are cytostatic against untransformed cells while they are cytotoxic against tumor cells.

In our *in vitro* experiments as well as in the experiments performed by other Authors (Tamura et al., 1987), the culture medium (MEM) has a large number of potential ligands. In this respect, very often the activity of copper(II) complexes in both *in vitro* and *in vivo* models has been correlated *tout court* with the copper compound administered. However, before doing this one has to prove that:

i) the administered copper(II) complex exists as such in solution;

ii) if it does, it still exists in the conditions used for testing its activity.

Thus, preliminarly, we calculated the concentration of each species taking into account the analytical concentrations of all substances present in the incubation media. To this end a well tested computer program, able to deal with *multi metal-multi ligand* systems, was used (May et al., 1977). The analytical concentrations were chosen in such a way as to reproduce the conditions of the biological tests as close as possible. For the Cu-Im-Ac system, the copper(II) analytical concentration was set to be $3x10^{-5}$ mol dm^{-3} and the concentrations of both imidazole and acetate was set to be $6x10^{-5}$ mol dm^{-3}. The results concerning this system are reported in the Table. The percentage of species is calculated with respect to copper(II); species forming below 1% are not reported in the Table.

Table . Species present in MEM supplemented with $[Cu(Im)_2(Ac)_2]^0$

Species	Percentage
[CuGlnHis]	31
[CuThrHis]	17
$[CuHis_2]$	13
[CuLeuHis]	5
$[CuLysHisH]^+$	4
[CuSerHis]	4
[CuTrpHis]	3
[CuIleHis]	3
[CuValHis]	3
[CuAsnHis]	3
[CuPheHis]	2
[CuMetHis]	1
$[CuAspHis]^-$	1

As shown, Copper(II) turns out to be distributed essentially among histidine containing species, $[Cu(gln)(His)]^0$ being the main species. The $[Cu(Im)_2(Ac)_2]^0$, thought to be responsible for an antitumor activity (Tamura et al.,1987) does not form at all in the experimental conditions used for the biological test. This was easily predictable since such a species could not be detected in water in the pH range of interest (Arena et al. 1992).

One has still to explain why the *c*-L-His-L-His showed little cytotoxic activity and why the inorganic copper(II) sulphate shows a high cytotoxicity. A plot (for the B16 cell line) of cytotoxicity *vs* the amount of copper(II) in each complex, rather than the *vs* amount of complex, shows that all complexes, including the Cu-*c*-L-His-L-His systems, have a cytotoxic activity that is a function of the copper content, within the variability of the biological tests. This indicates that there is a way of action common to all the systems, regardless of the nature of the complex administered. To explain this we calculated the copper(II) distribution among the ligands of a typical MEM upon the addition of copper sulphate. The results of the ECCLES (May et al.,1987) simulation are virtually identical with those obtained for the Cu-Im-Ac system (see Table). In fact i) copper(II) is distributed again among the same complex species and ii) $[Cu(Gln)(His)]^0$ is again the predominant species. The reason for this has to be found in i) the high glutamine content of the culture medium; and ii) the well known affinity of copper(II) for histidine.

The results of this work show that a straightforward correlation of the activity of a copper(II) complex with the complex itself may be erroneous. Preliminarly, it ought to be proved that the complex i) exists in solution and ii) exists in the culture medium employed. Copper(II) complexes are labile and, consequently, the ligands of the culture media may compete with the ligand(s) of the administered complex. The same conclusion can be extended to other metal ions which show cytotoxic activity and form labile complexes. Our results while do not fully explain the mechanism of action of copper(II) complexes are of some relevance. In fact, the cytotoxic and cytostatic activity shown by the tested compounds against tumor and untransformed cells, respectively, together with some literature findings enable us to put forward some hypotheses on the mechanism of action of copper(II) complexes.

REFERENCES

Agarwal, K., Sharma, A., Talukder, G., (1989) *Chem. Biol. Interactions, 69* , 1 and the references therein.

Arena, G., Bonomo R. P., Impellizzeri, G., Izatt, R.M., Lamb, J.D., Rizzarelli, E. (1987) *Inorg. Chem., 26*, 795

Arena, G., Bindone, M., Cardile, V., Maccarrone, G., Riello, M. C.,Rizzarelli, E., Sciuto, S. (1992) *J.Inorg.Biochem.(submitted)*

Bonomo, R.P., Calì, R., Cucinotta, V.,Impellizzeri, G., Rizzarelli, E. (1986) *Inorg. Chem. 25*, 1641

Brigelius, R., Spotti, R., Bors, W., Lengfelder, E., Saran, M. and Weser, U.,(1974) *FEBS Lett., 47*, 72.

De Alvare, L.R., Gada, K.,Kimura, T., (1976) *Biochem. Biophys. Res. Com., 69*, 687.

Deushle, U., Weser, U.,(1985) *Progr.in Clin.Biochem.& Med.,2*, 97 and references therein.

Ettinger, M.J., (1984) in *Copper Proteins and Copper Enzymes,Vol. (III)*, ed R. Lontie, pp 175-229. Boca Raton: CRC.

Ettinger, M.J.,(1991) *J.Biol.Chem., 266* , 4586.

Falkman, R.J., Klagsbrun, M.,(1987) *Science (Washington D.C.)235*, 442.

Goldstein, S. and Czapski,G.,(1985) *Inorg.Chem., 24*, 1087.

Goldstein, S., Czapski, G., Meyerstein, D., *J. Am. Chem. Soc., 112*, 6489

Hart, E.B., Steinbock, H., Waddell, J., Elvehjens, C.A.(1928) *J. Biol. Chem., 77*, 797.

Huber, K.R., Sridhar,R., Griffith, E.H., Amma, E.L., Roberts, J. (1987) *Biochem. Biophys. Acta, 915*, 267

Kimura, E., Yatsunami, A., Watanabe, A., Machida, R., Koide T., Fujioka H., Kuramota,Y., Sumomogi, M., Kunimitsu, K., Yamashita, A. (1983) *Biochem. Biophys. Acta, 745*, 37

May, P., Linder, P.W., Williams, D.R., 1977, *J. Chem. Soc., Dalton Trans*, 588

Oberley, L.W., Leuthauser, S.W.C., Oberley T.D., Sorenson, J.R.J. and Pasternak, R.F.,(1982) in *Inflammatory Diseases and Copper*, ed. J.R.J. Sorenson , pp 423-433, New Jersey: Humana Press.

Palida, F.A., Ettinger, M.J.,(1991) *J.Biol.Chem., 266*, 4586.

Prohaska, J.R.,(1987) *Physiol. Rev., 67* , 858.

Sato, M., Gitlin, J.D.(1991) *J.Biol.Chem., 266* , 5128.

Shaaper, R.M., Koplitz, R.M., Tkeshelashvili, L.K., Loeb, L.A.,(1987) *Mutat. Res., 177* , 179.

Sorenson, J.R.J.,(1984) *J. Med. Chem., 27*, 1747.

Sorenson, J.R.J.,(1989) in *Med. Chem., Vol.26* , eds G.P.Ellis and G.B.West, New York: Elsevier and the references therein.

Tamura, H., Imai, H., Kuwahara, J., Sugiura, Y.,(1987) *J.Am.Chem. Soc., 109*, 6870

Weinstein, J. and Bielski, B.H.J., (1980) *J. Am. Chem. Soc., 102*, 4916

Wiesel, L.L., (1959) *Metabolism, 8* , 256.
Youssef,A.A.R.,Wood B., Baron D.N.,(1983)*J.Clin.Pathol., 36* , 14

Metal Ions in Biology and Medicine, vol. 2. Eds. J. Anastassopoulou, Ph. Collery, J.C. Etienne, Th. Theophanides. John Libbey Eurotext, Paris © 1992, pp. 37-39

The effects of trivalent lanthanide ions on the solution structure of calf-thymus DNA. DNA condensation and structural properties

H.A. Tajmir-Riahi, R. Ahmad, M. Naoui, D.M. Boghai

Centre de recherche en photobiophysique, Université du Québec à Trois-Rivières, 3351, boulevard des Forges, C.P. 500, Trois-Rivières (Québec), G9A 5H7, Canada

Ln^{3+} ions were often used for structural analysis and conformational variations of nucleic acids (Gersanovski *et al.*, 1985). The effects of lanthanide ions on the secondary structures of native and synthetic DNAs have been well elucidated (Klakamp & Horrocks, 1990). It has been suggested that the Tb^{3+} chelation through the guanine N-7 and the backbone PO_2^- groups facilitates DNA B to Z to ψ conformational changes (Gersanovski *et al.*, 1985), whereas Eu^{3+} brings about B to Z structural alterations for poly (dG.dC) poly (dG.dC) and related polynucleotides (Klakamp & Horrocks, 1990). In this work, we have studied the effects of La^{3+}, Eu^{3+} and Tb^{3+} on the solution structure of calf-thymus DNA with respect to metal ion binding mode, DNA condensation and conformational variations, using FTIR spectroscopy. The results were compared with those of divalent metal ions such as Cu^{2+} to determine the status of biopolymer before and after DNA condensation.

A solution of calf-thymus DNA (2% w/w, 0.05 M DNA-P) was treated with metal ion salt solutions ($LaCl_3.6H_2O$, $EuCl_3.6H_2O$ and $TbCl_3.6H_2O$) of different concentrations to have M^{3+}/DNA(P) molar ratios 1/80, 1/40, 1/20, 1/10, 1/4, 1/2 and 1. The spectra were recorded after 2 h of mixing (DNA + salt solution) and the difference spectra were produced by subtracting the spectrum of free DNA from that of the mixtures (DNA + salt)-(DNA) at pH 6-7 and at room temperature. The results are shown in Fig. 1. The IR bands at 1712 cm^{-1} (G,T), 1661 cm^{-1} (T,G,A,C), 1492 cm^{-1} (C,G), 1222 cm^{-1} (PO_2^- antisymmetric stretch) and 836 cm^{-1} (sugar-phosphate backbone) were mostly affected by Ln^{3+} interactions. The difference spectra contain several derivative features at about 1700, 1650, 1480, 1200, 1100, 950, 920, 900 cm^{-1} (Fig. 1). The positive and negative features at 1700, 1650, 1480 are due to the base vibrations, while the features at 1200, 1100, 950, 920 and 900 cm^{-1} are related to the phosphate and the sugar-phosphate backbone (Fig. 1).

At very low metal ion concentration r=1/80, Ln^{3+} ions bind mainly to the PO_2^- groups of the backbone and consequently cause increased base-stacking interaction and duplex stability. Evidence for this comes from major shift of the PO_2^- band at 1222 cm^{-1} towards a higher frequency, which is due to direct metal-PO_2 interaction. The base bands at 1712, 1661 and 1492 cm^{-1} lost intensity and showed no major shifting on Ln ion coordination. The loss of intensity of the base vibrations can be attributed to the increased base-stacking interaction (Fig. 1).

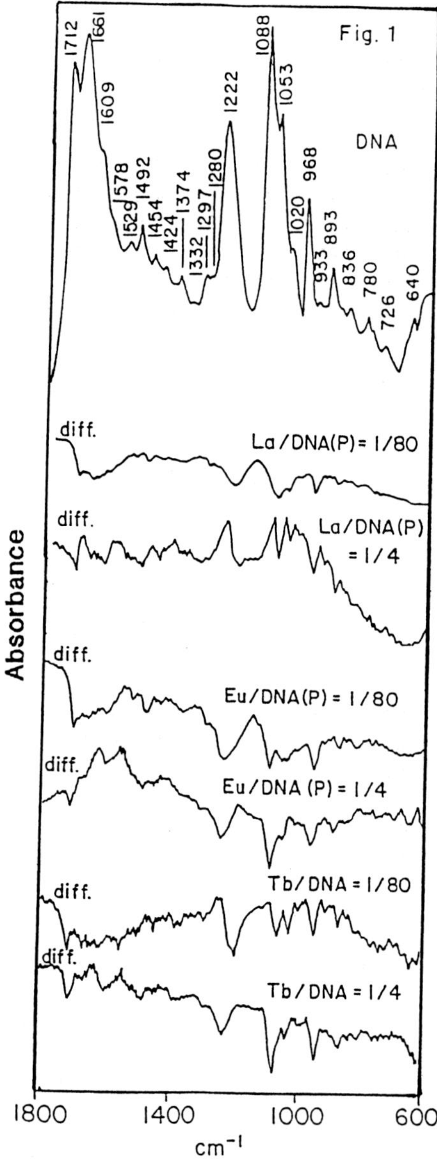

Fig. 1. FTIR spectra and difference spectra [(DNA) + (salt) - (DNA)] of free calf-thymus DNA and its trivalent Ln ions in aqueous solution at pH = 6-7 with different M/DNA-P molar ratios.

At r > 1/40, metal ion binding is through the guanine N-7 site and the PO_2^- group (chelation), which results in destabilizing complexation. Evidence for this comes from the intensity increase of the band at 1712,(G,T) and the displacement of this band towards a lower frequency (Fig. 1). Although the intensity of the band at 1661 cm^{-1} (T,G,A,C) increased, no shifting was observed for this frequency. At r > 1/20, DNA condensation occurs with major reduction of the intensity of the DNA in-plane vibrations at 1712, 1651, 1492 cm^{-1} as well as the PO_2^- band at 1222 cm^{-1}. The reduction in intensity of these vibrations is due to DNA condensation and particle formation, that are accompanied by drastic structural modifications of biopolymer (Wilson & Bloomfield, 1979).

At r > 1/10, helical destabilization was observed, which resulted in increase of intensity of the DNA bands at 1712, 1661, 1492 and 1222 cm^{-1} (Fig. 1). This partial destabilization of helical structure increases the chance of Ln ions to bind to the adenine, thymine and cytosine donor sites that are freed on DNA denaturation. However, a comparison with the IR spectra of Cu-DNA complexes showed that copper denaturation is far more drastic than those of the Ln^{3+} with similar metal/DNA(P) molar ratios. DNA denaturation with copper ion is well known and the affinity of copper ion towards binding to double and single-stranded DNA bases is well demonstrated (Forster et al., 1979).

Although some spectral modifications were observed for the phosphate and sugar-phosphate backbone (Fig. 1), no conformational changes were occurred for DNA in the presence of trivalent Ln ions. The marker IR bands at 1712 cm^{-1} (G, T), 1222 cm^{-1} (PO_2^-) and 836 cm^{-1} (sugar-phosphate) exhibited no major shiftings on Ln ion coordination. If B to A conformational transition takes place, the band at 1712 cm^{-1} shifts towards a lower frequency at about 1708 cm^{-1} and the PO_2^- band at 1222 cm^{-1} shifts towards a higher frequency at 1240 cm^{-1}, while the band at 836 cm^{-1} occurs at about 810 cm^{-1} (Brahms et al., 1974). In B to Z conformational changes, the marker bands appear at 1690, 1215, 830 and 800 cm^{-1} (Alex & Dupuis, 1989). Since there has been no major spectral shiftings of the IR marker bands, DNA remains in the B-family structure before and after condensation in the presence of Ln ions. The observed spectral changes for the bands at 1712, 1222 and sugar-phosphate backbone are attributed to the Ln ion binding to the guanine bases and the PO_2^- groups. In a denaturated DNA by copper ions, the band at 1712 cm^{-1} was observed at about 1700 cm^{-1} in the spectra of Cu-DNA complexes (Tajmir-Riahi *et al.*, 1992). A small shift of this band was observed (1710-1707 cm^{-1}) in the spectra of the Ln-DNA complexes and it can be related to a partial helical destabilization of biopolymer before and after DNA collapse.

REFERENCES

Alex, S. and Dupuis, P. (1989): FT-IR and Raman investigation of cadmium binding to DNA. *Inrog. Chim. Acta, 157*, 271-281.

Brahms, S., Brahms, J. and Pilet, J. (1974): Infrared studies on the backbone conformation of nucleic acids. *Isr. J. Chem., 12*, 153-163.

Forster, W., Bauer, E., Schutz, H., Berg, H., Akimenko, M., Minchenkova, L.E., Evdokimov, Y.M. and Varshavsky, Y.M. (1979): Thermodynamics and kinetics of the interaction of copper (II) ions with native DNA. *Biopolymers, 18*, 625-661.

Gersanovski, D., Colson, P., Houssier, C. and Federicq, E. (1985): Terbium (3+) as probe for nucleic acids structure. Does it alter the DNA conformation in solution. *Biochim. Biophys. Acta, 824*, 313-323.

Klakamp, S.L. and Horrocks, W.D. Jr. (1990): The Eu^{3+} induces conformational transition of poly (dG.dC) poly (dG.dC) and poly (dG.m-5dC) poly (dG.m-5dC) as studies by Eu^{3+} luminescence, U.V. and CD spectroscopy. *Biopolymers, 30*, 33-44.

Tajmir-Riahi, H.A., Ahmad, R. and Naoui, M. (1992): Interaction of calf-thymus DNA with Cu^{2+} and Pb^{2+} in aqueous solution. Denaturation of DNA studied by FTIR spectroscopy. Submitted for publication.

Wilson, R.W. and Bloomfield, V.A. (1979): Counterion-induced condensation of deoxyribonucleic acid. *Biochemistry, 18*, 2192-2196.

Metal Ions in Biology and Medicine, vol. 2. Eds. J. Anastassopoulou, Ph. Collery, J.C. Etienne, Th. Theophanides. John Libbey Eurotext, Paris © 1992, pp. 40-43

Transketolase ternary complex « Application of a new method to identify metal binding site in transketolase »

Bijan Farzami*, Alexender N. Kuimov, German A. Kochetov

* The Department of Biochemistry School of Medicine, Tehran Medical Science University P.O Box 14155-5399, Tehran, Iran
A.N. Belozersky Laboratory of Molecular Biology and Bioorganic Chemistry, Lomonosov State University, Moscow 117234, Russia

Transketolase (TK)obtained from Baker's yeast contains two active sites. Apo-TK is activated to its full capacity by its cofactors, thiamin diphosphate (TDP) and Ca^{2+} or Mg^{2+} ions. Native holo-TK from Baker's yeast contains 2 moles of TDP and two gram atoms of metal ion per mole of protein (1-3). The binding of calcium to one of the subunits has a lower dissociation constant (4). The allosteric charachteristics of the enzyme has been reported recently (5). There are several reports indicating the presence of arginine (6-8), cysteine (9), histidine (10) and tyrosine (11) in the active site of enzyme. These groups are proposed to be involved in coenzyme bindings. and catalysis but there has been no reports, on specificity of binding of metal ions and cofactors or on their coordination schemes.

We tried our previously reported method of ellucidation of the site of binding of metal ions to proteines and enzymes (12). The difference spectra of the apoenzyme that contained the minimal amount of Ca^{2+}. Was used for the solutions of Apo-TK with Ca^{2+} ion as a function of PH. The changes were recorded. 2 Pka's of 6.25 and 7.2 were obtained corresponding to two imidazole groups. In fact each PKa could be assumed to be the average value PKa of two imidazole nitrogens. This results from the fact that the environment of each nitrogens may be different and may cause differences in individual PKa's. Thus we may propose that there are two histidines at the active sites that are responsible in bindings to Ca^{2+} ion as TK cofactors. Previous reports suggest that two histidines are actively involved in binding to cofactors and in catalysis (3). The difference absorption spectra of ApoTK that was modified by histidine modifier, diethypyrocarbonate (DPC) has a maximum absorption at 242 characteristic of ethoxyformyl histidine. The use of DPC (10^{-5}M) in the metal binding site chatacterization studies caused dissapearance of this band and of the minimums in the curves that were assigned to the binding loci of the Ca^{2+} ion to histidine residues. (Fig 1)The specific rate constant for the recombination of metal ion with APO-TK as a function of PH were studied in a time dependent APO-TK reaction with Ca^{2+} ion. Two maximums at PH=6.22 and 7.20 were observed with $k_1=4.2 \times 10^{-2}$ sec^{-1} and $k_2=6.2 \times 10^{-2}$ sec^{-1} respectively.(Fig.2) A 60% inactivation in Apo-TK by DPC reduced the rate constant to a low and a single value of 1.5×10^{-2} sec^{-1} the close correlation between the optimal PH for the direct Ca^{2+} binding to TK and the equilibrium studies of complex formation as a function of PH indicate that the thermodynamic values for the 2 indipendent methods are in close agreement that the 2 optimal PH's are related to the bindings of Immidazol moiety of histidine to Ca^{2+} ion. Furthermore the rate-PH profile substantiated the above observation in that the increase in activity due to PH rise from PH=6 to PH=7.6 had 2 maximums above the regular rise in activity towards the optimal "PH=7.6". These too maximums were at PH=6.25 and PH=7.2 (Fig.3). Inactivation by DPC diminished the two peaks. Although the increasing of activity towards the optimal PH of 7.6 is indicative of other factors that are effective in catalysis, but the binding of Ca^{2+} ion that is most facilitated at the two PH's 6.25 and 7.2 is an evidence to the involvement of 2 immidazol groups in the active sites that are involved in catalysis through binding with Ca^{2+}.

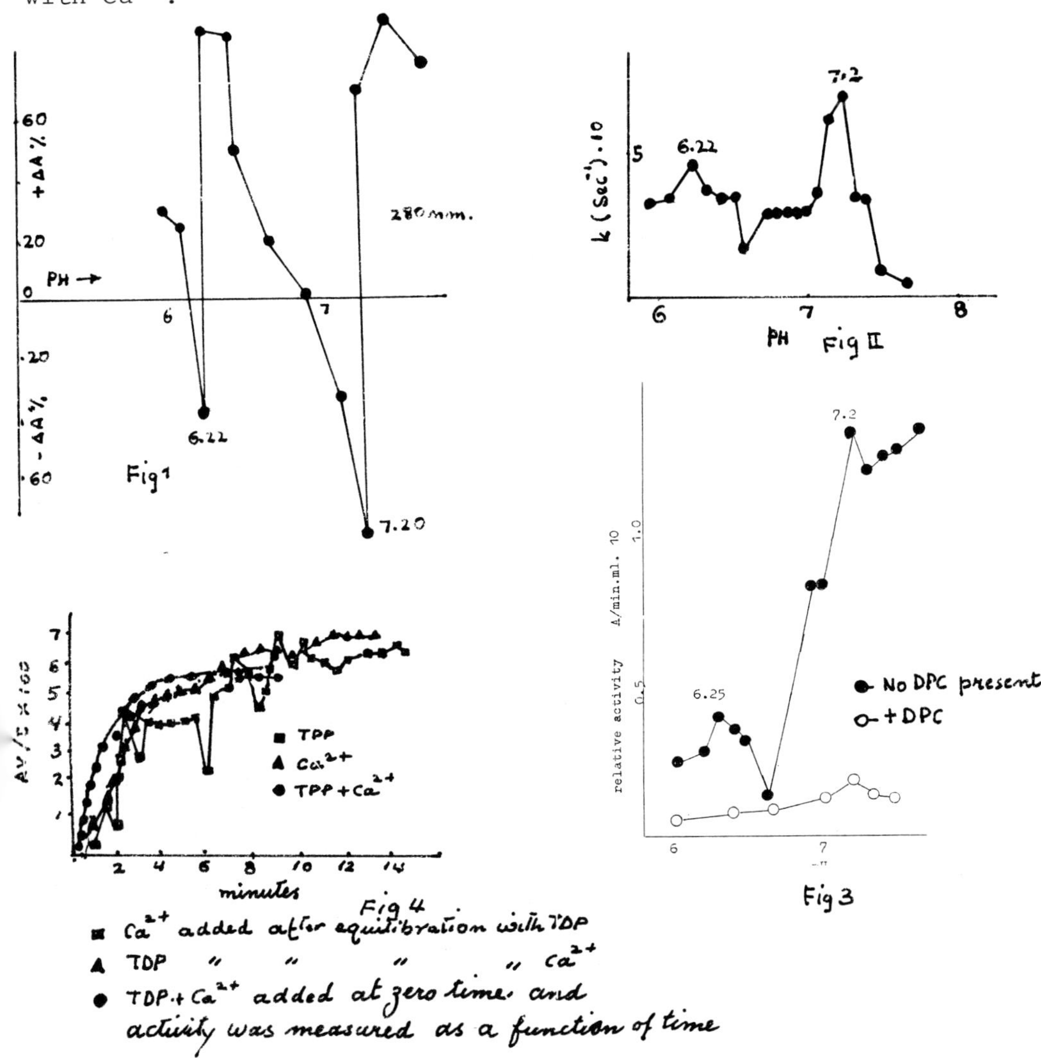

■ Ca^{2+} added after equilibration with TDP
▲ TDP " " " " Ca^{2+}
● TDP + Ca^{2+} added at zero time and activity was measured as a function of time

Previous reports are also indicative of such bindings, for example in our experiments, when thiamin diphosphate (TDP) together with Mg^{2+} or Ca^{2+} ion are reacted with Apo-TK they were completely protected against the action of DPC. The above reports indicate that when the degree of modification of ApoTK is 83%, 6.7 histidine residues are modified in ApoTK, and 5.0 in holo-TK, therefore it could be assumed that there are 2 histidine residues essential for the activity of the enzyme. We studied the mode of TDP binding to the enzyme, both on the model system and on the enzyme. In model studies when thiamin derivatives were subjected to the action of Mg^{2+} ion in solutions the PKa due to (C_4-NH_2) group in pyrimidine was affected by the action of metal ion, solely in thiamin diphosphate. This suggests that the metal ion could interfere in the iozination of (C_4-NH_2) group through bindings with pyrophosphate moiety. Although this interaction can not directly be correlated to the conditions exist at the TK active site, but is indicative of the degree of diffinity between the pyrophoshat moiety and the metal ions in solution. This type of coordination is similar to the binding of Mg^{2+} ion with nucleoside triphosphates in which the metal ion is bound to the pyrophosphate moiety of nucleotide.

Our results with the rate of enzyme activations is suggesting that the TDP binds to the metal that is already bound to the active site of the enzyme. In the experiment, where the coenzyme and the metal ion was reacted at the same initial time with the enzyme the ternary complex formation was completed at 7 minutes, but when the TDP was added first to the enzyme with a residual amount of Ca^{2+} present, the activity was lower and the fluctuations in activity was so high that no exact trend was evidenced. when the TDP was added after the Ca^{2+} was equilibrated with the enzyme, the fluctuations in activity was minimal, but the recombination time was raised to 12 minutes. (Fig.4) The above evidences may suggest that the catalysis is in fact necessitates the existence of the coenzyme-metal complex in solutions. In a separate experiment the inorganic pyrophosphate was used when metal ion was reacted with the enzyme. It was found that the pyrophosphate could protect the enzyme from the reaction with TDP and further deactivation by DPC.

The data and the results cited above may be used as evidences for the existance of a ternary complex of TK-Metal-Coenzyme in which two imidazolium groups at the active sites are the sites of metal bindings.

REFERENCES

1. Kochetov, G.A. Izotova, A.E Philippov, PP. and Tikhomirova, N.K. Biochem. Biophys. Res. Commun. 46 616-620 (1972).

2. Neinrich, C.P., Eyperimenta 15, 1227-1228 (1973).

3. Kochetov, G.A., Annals of the New York Academy of Sciences, 738, 306-311 (1982).

4. Kochetov, G.A. and Belyaeva, R.H., Biochimiya 37, 233-235 (1972).

5. Farzami, B., Iran J. Chem. and Chem. Eng. 10(11) 39 (1988).

6. Saitou, S. Ozawa, T. and Tomita, J., FEBS Lett. 40, 114-118 (1974).

REFERENCES

1. Kochetov, G.A., Izotova, A.E., Philipov, PP. and Tikhamirova, N.K., (1972) Biochem. Biophys. Res. Commun. 46 616-620.

2. Heinrich, C.P. (1973) Experimenta 15, 1227-1228.

3. Kochetov, G.A., (1982) Annals of the New York Academy of Sciences, 738, 306-311.

4. Kochetov, G.A. and Belyaeva, R.H., (1972) Biochimiya 27, 233-235.

5. Farzami, B., (1988) Iran J. Chem. and Chem. Eng. 10(11)39.

6. Saitou, S., Ozawa, T. and Tomita (1974) J. FEBS Lett. 40 114-118.

7. Riordan, J.F. (1979) Mol. and Cell Biochem. 26 P. 71-72.

8. Kremer, A.B., Egan, R.M., and Sable, H.Z., (1980) The J. Biol. Chem. 255(6) 2405-2410.

9. Kochetov G.A. and Lutovinova, G.F. (1966) Dol. Akad. Nauki., USSR. 168 1202-1204.

10. Kochetov, G.A., Kobylyanskaya, K.R. (1970) Biokhymiya 35, 3-12.

11. Kuimov, A.N., Kovina, M.W. and Kochetov, G.A. (1988) Biochemistry International 17(3) 517-521.

12. Farzami, B., Jordan, F., (1990) Metal ions in Biology and Medicine P. Collery, L.A. Poirier, M. Manfait and J.C. Etienne (Eds) 126-128.

Metal Ions in Biology and Medicine, vol. 2. Eds. J. Anastassopoulou, Ph. Collery, J.C. Etienne, Th. Theophanides. John Libbey Eurotext, Paris © 1992, pp. 44-49

Effect of Mg supplement on a biological medium (milk) on ionic transport through a human leaky membrane

C. Pechery*, M. Bara**, A. Guiet-Bara**, J. Durlach***

** Meram Laboratory, avenue de la Libération, 77020 Melun Cedex France. ** Laboratory of Biology of Reproduction, University P.M. Curie, 7, quai Saint-Bernard, BP 10, 75252 Paris Cedex 05, France. *** SDRM, Hôpital Saint-Vincent-de-Paul, 74-82, rue Denfert-Rochereau, 75014 Paris, France*

INTRODUCTION

Bivalent cations have a great importance in various physiological mechanisms and their effects on the ionic transport through the biological membranes have been observed by numerous authors. Among the experiments on biological membranes, many are realized in a survival medium composed of mineral salts dissolved in the water, with a composition frequently identical to those of extracellular fluid. For example, the study of the effects of Mg^{2+} on the ionic conductance through the human amnion (Bara et al., 1990) have shown the importance and the role of Mg^{2+} in the transfer mechanisms. In the organism, the bivalent cations are not only in a free ionized form, but interact with other components. In complex biological systems, there are not only mineral salts, but also lipids, sugars, proteins, and it is very important to know the possible existence of a synergy or an antagonism between mineral salts and these components. For example, albumin is a very sensitive non competitive inhibitor of Mg^{2+} efflux from erythrocytes (Günther and Vormann, 1991).

The aim of this work is to compare the effects of a Mg supplementation in a simple survival medium and in a complex biological medium (milk which has a complex composition) on the ionic transport through a human membrane. The human amniotic membrane, considered as a pharmacological model (Bara et al., 1985; Guiet-Bara et al., 1988) to test the effects of various agents on the ionic transfer, has been chosen because: - it is a human membrane sampling without ethical problem and easily utilizable after delivery, - it is a leaky membrane with a high paracellular component, - it is an asymmetrical membrane with a polarity between the two sides.

MATERIAL AND METHODS

- Membrane preparation: Strips of human amnion, isolated from the placental zone of the amniotic sac, were obtained after normal deliveries at term and immediately transferred into Hanks' solution (37 ± 1°C, pH 7.4). A circular area of the amnion was sampled and placed between two Ussing chambers filled with the studied solution. To improve mixing and to minimize the thickness of the unstirred layers next to the membrane, the saline solution in each chambers was vigorously agitated by magnetically driven stirring bars.

- Electrical parameters: The determination of the ionic transport is based on the measure of two components:

 1- The total transamniotic conductance G_t measured by observing the transepithelial potential difference when a direct current (100 µA) was passed across the whole tissue in the mother to fetus (G_{tM}) and in the fetus to mother (G_{tF}) directions. The potential was recorded with two agar-agar salt bridges placed 1.3-1.5 mm from each side of the tissue, while a current was passed across the tissue by means of Ag/AgCl electrodes and agar salt bridges and was measured on a Schlumberger electrometer.

 2- The ionic fluxes in the mother to fetus (F_1) and in the fetus to mother (F_2) directions were given by the relation:

F_1 or F_2 = Pi z F Um/RT / 1 - exp(-z F Um/RT) with Pi= ionic permeability coefficient, Um = membrane potential, z, F, R, T = usual variables.

- Solutions: In this study two solutions have been used:

 1- Hanks 'solution (mmol/l): NaCl 150, KCl 6, $MgSO_4$ 0.5, $MgCl_2$ 0.5, $CaCl_2$ 1, glucose 5.5, NaH_2PO_4-KH_2PO_4-$NaHCO_3$ 1.

 2- Milk (UHT Saint-Cyr) diluted in Hanks' solution. In the Figure 1, the effects of the milk dilution, on the ionic conductance G_t are observed: dilution rates of 0.05, 0.07, 0.10 have no significant effects ($p= 0.25$) on G_t; at the opposite, dilution rates of 0.2 and 0.5 decrease significantly ($p<0.01$) G_t. The dilution rate of 0.05 has been chosen because, in this case, the Mg supplementation corresponds to physiological and moderate physiopathological concentrations of Mg^{2+}.

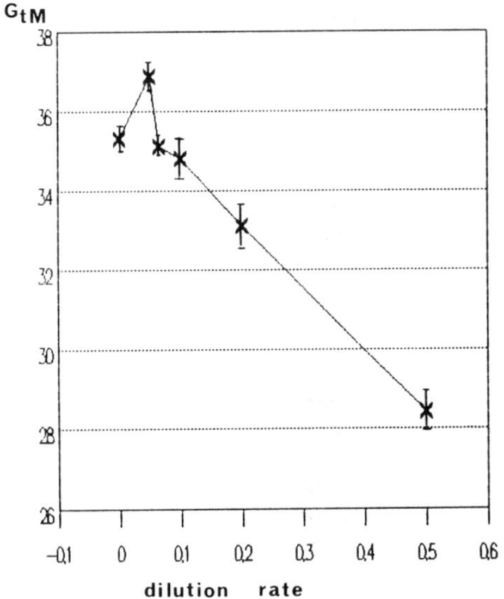

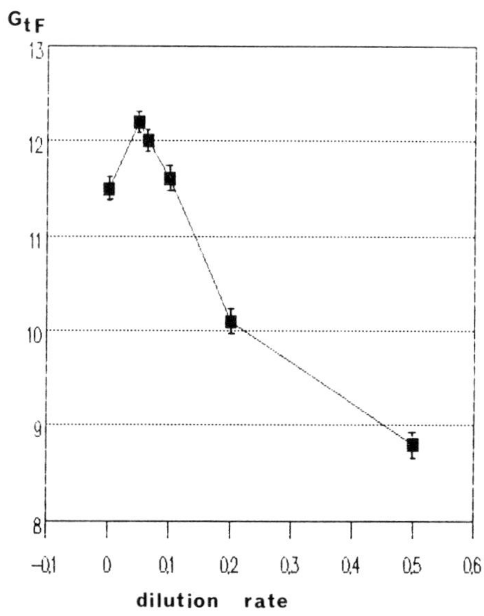

Fig.1. Effects of the dilution rate on the total conductance in the mother to fetus (G_{tM})($mmho/cm^2$) and in the fetus to mother (G_{tF})($mmho/cm^2$) ways.

 3- In the normal cow milk, the molar ratio (MR) Ca/Mg is equal to 6. In the experiments 4 other ratios have been chosen: 0.36, 0.6, 1 and 2. Whatever the MR studied, the Ca concentration remains identical: 1.625 mM. The Mg concentrations have indicated in the following table:

MR(Ca/Mg)	6 (normal milk)	2	1	0.6	0.36
[Mg](mM)	0.267	0.813	1.625	2.675	4.520
[Ca](mM)	1.625	1.625	1.625	1.625	1.625

The Ca concentration and the 5 Mg concentrations would be used in the experiments with Hanks' solution.

RESULTS

1- Effects of Mg supplementation in Hanks' solution: The figure 2 indicates that in the mother to fetus and in the fetus to mother directions, the addition of 1.625 mM Ca and 0.267 mM Mg increases significantly G_t ($p<0.01$) with regard to normal Hanks' solution. The Mg supplementation does not induce a significant difference between the MR 0.36, 0.6, 1 and 2 and the conductance sequence is:

$$G_t(0.36) = G_t(0.6) = G_t(1) = G_t(2) > G_t(6)$$

An identical sequence is obtained with the ionic fluxes F_1 and F_2.

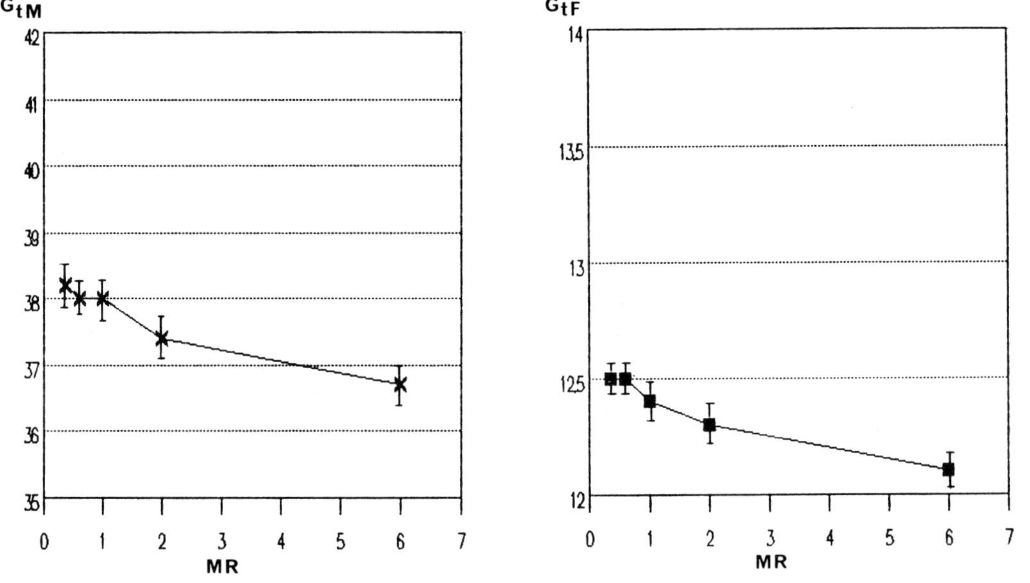

Fig. 2. Effects of different values of the molar ratio (MR) on the total conductance G_{tM} and G_{tF} ($mmho/cm^2$) in Hanks ' solution.

2- Effects of Mg supplementation in milk diluted in Hanks' solution: The figure 3 indicates that in the mother to fetus and in the fetus to mother directions, the addition of milk induces an G_t increase. The Mg supplementation (which reduces the MR value) increases significantly ($p<0.01$) G_t with regard to normal milk in Hanks' solution. There is a significant difference between G_t measured with different studied MR and the conductance sequence is:

$$G_t(0.36) > G_t(0.6) > G_t(1) > G_t(2) > G_t(6)$$

There is a linear correlation between G_t and MR ranged between 6 and 1, then a break and a linear correlation between G_t and MR ranged between 1 and 0.36.

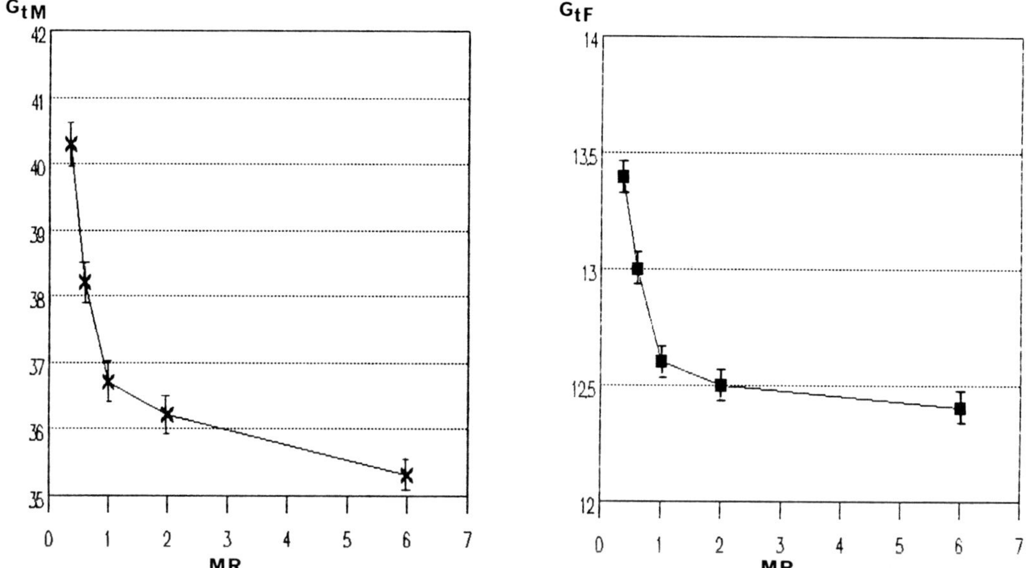

Fig. 3. Effects of different values of the molar ratio (MR) on the total conductance G_{tM} and G_{tF} (mmho/cm^2), in milk diluted in Hanks' solution.

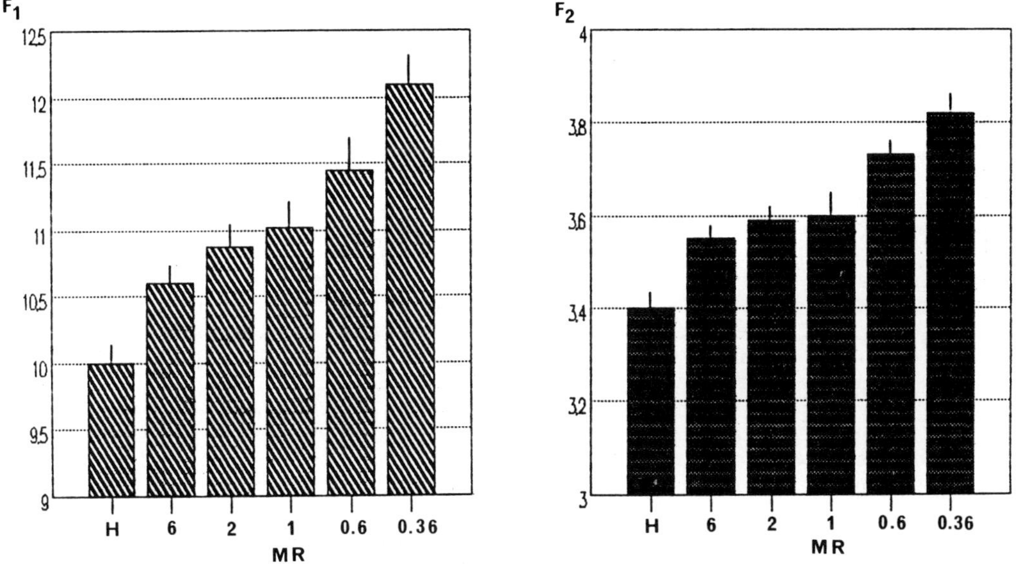

Fig. 4. Effects of different values of the molar ratio (MR), in milk diluted in Hanks' solution, on the ionic fluxes F_1 and F_2 (µM) (H: value in the normal Hanks' solution).

The figure 4 indicates that the ionic fluxes F_1 and F_2 are significantly ($p<0.01$) increased by a Mg supplementation. The fluxes sequences are: F_1: 0.36 > 0.6 > 1 = 2 = 6 > Hanks
F_2: 0.36 > 0.6 > 1 = 2 = 6 > Hanks

The fluxes ratio F_1/F_2 is significantly increased according the same sequence (Figure 5).

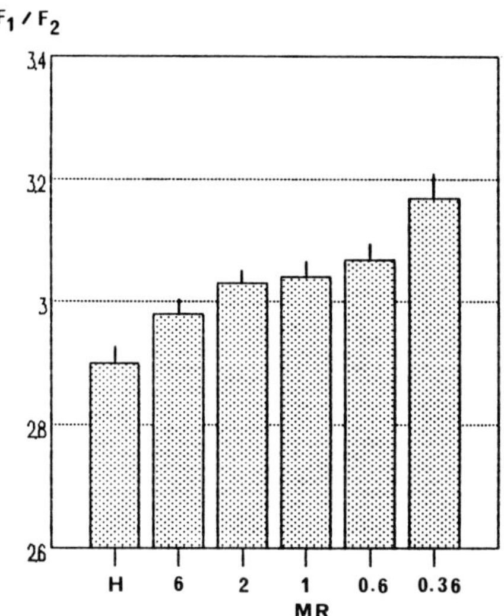

Fig. 5. Effects of different values of MR, in milk diluted in Hanks' solution, on the ionic fluxes ratio F_1/F_2. (H: Hanks' solution).

DISCUSSION

- In Hanks' solution, the addition of Mg and Ca increases G_t with regard to normal Hanks' solution. In the case cf Mg supplementation, there is a linear variation of G_t between MR 6 and 2, then any significant variation between MR 2 and 0.36. This constant action does not agree with the usual effect of Mg addition (Guiet-Bara and Bara, 1978; Bara and Guiet-Bara, 1981). Indeed, when Mg is only added, G_t increases linearily with the Mg concentration comprised between 0.267 and 4.52 mM. The same constatation is observed with Ca only between 1 and 1.625 mM. The simultaneous addition of Mg and Ca does not implicate a linear variation of G_t, but a saturation plateau when the Mg concentration increases. In normal Hanks' solution, there are 1 mM of Ca and 1 mM of Mg, and it is possible that their effects on G_t neutralize each other. With a MR = 6 and 2, G_t is increased because the Ca concentration is largely superior to the Mg concentration. When the MR decreases (2-->0.36), the Mg concentration increases and Mg ions neutralize the effects of Ca ions and reciprocally and G_t is directed towards a saturation plateau. There is a competition between Ca and Mg in the solution and on the surface sites.

- When the milk is added to the Hanks' solution (molar ratio MR = 6, dilution rate 0.05), the conductances G_{tM} and G_{tF} are increased with regard to G_t in Hanks' solution only. This increase is more important that those obtained in Hanks' solution with the same Ca and Mg concentrations. The Mg supplementation induces an increase of G_t with regard to the value obtained in normal milk diluted in Hanks' solution. This increase shows two phases: a linear correlation between G_t and MR ranged between 6 and 1, then an other linear correlation between G_t and MR ranged between 1 and 0.36. There is a break in the curve from MR = 1. This inflexion in the curve (non observed in Hanks' solution) may be due to interactions of Mg with other ions present in the medium or with other components of the milk, and shows a threshold concentration of Mg to obtain an important G_t increase. Among the ions present in the milk, citrates, only, are not in the Hanks' solution. In previous studies (Bara et al., 1988), it has been shown that Mg citrate, at concentrations used in this experiment, decreased G_{tM} and G_{tF}, this effect being inverse comparatively to those observed in the milk diluted in the Hanks' solution. Also, it is possible that the effects of Mg supplementation are due to interactions between Mg and other components of the milk, particularly the proteins. For example, Glick (1990) suggests that Alzheimer's disease involves a defective transport process characterized by both an abnormally low Mg incorporation and an abnormally Al incorporation into brain neurones. The origin of this disturbance rests on an alteration of serum albumin, forming a species which has a greater affinity for Al than for Mg, in contrats to the normal protein which binds Mg better than Al (Durlach, 1990). In the milk, the interactions of Mg with proteins may induce a complex in favour of a great ionic exchange through the amnion. The interactions between Mg and proteins seem the more important, but the interactions Mg-sugars, particularly lactose, and Mg-lipids should not be forgotten, because the complex Mg-lipids, for example, have known effects on the ionic membrane transport.

CONCLUSION

Our constatations and the fact that the blood coagulation is realized by analogous mechanisms to those of milk coagulation may instigate other studies on the milk and its components to give informations to counteract the noxious effects of fibrinogen in cardiovascular pathology.

REFERENCES

Bara, M. & Guiet-Bara, A. (1981): Magnesium effect on the permeability of the amniotic membrane as a whole and of the amniotic epithelial cells. *Magnesium Bull.* 3, 145-150.

Bara, M., Guiet-Bara, A. & Durlach, J. (1985): Monovalent cations transfer through isolated human amnion: a new pharmacological model. *Meth. Find. Exptl. Clin. Pharmacol.* 7, 209-216.

Bara, M., Guiet-Bara, A. & Durlach, J. (1988): Analysis of magnesium membraneous effects: binding and screening. *Magnesium Res.* 1, 29-33.

Durlach, J. (1990): Magnesium depletion and pathogenesis of Alzheimer's disease. *Magnesium Res.* 3, 217-218.

Glick, J.L. (1990): Dementias: the role of magnesium deficiency and an hypothesis concerning the pathogenesis of Alzheimer's disease. *Med. Hypotheses* 31, 211-225.

Guiet-Bara, A. & Bara, M. (1978): Perméabilité de la membrane amniotique humaine isolée aux cations divalents. *C. R. Acad. Sci. Paris* 286, 635-638.

Guiet-Bara, A., Bara, M., Durlach, J. & Pechery, C. (1988): Ethanol effect on the ionic transfer through isolated human amnion. I. Preventive and opposing action of some nutriments and their synthetic congeners. *Alcohol* 5, 63-72.

Guiet-Bara, A., Bara, M. & Durlach, J. (1990): Comparative study of the effects of magnesium and taurine on electrical parameters of natural and artificial membranes. VII. Effects on cellular and paracellular ionic transfer through isolated human amnion. *Magnesium Res.* 3, 249-254.

Günther, T. & Vormann, J. (1991): Inhibition of Mg^{2+} efflux from erythrocytes by serum albumin. *Magnesium Bull.* 13, 82-84.

Metal Ions in Biology and Medicine, vol. 2. Eds. J. Anastassopoulou, Ph. Collery, J.C. Etienne, Th. Theophanides. John Libbey Eurotext, Paris © 1992, pp. 50-53

Damaged axonal transport due to aluminium in uraemia : theoretical and experimental data

G.M. Savazzi, S. Vinci, L. Allegri, S. Orsini, G. Garini

Institute of Clinical Medicine and Nephrology, University of Parma, Parma, Italy

In uraemic population and expecially in dialysed patients cerebral computized axial tomography evidences an unespected high incidence of cerebral atrophy not attributable to senile involution (Cusmano & Savazzi,1986). Computerized psychometric tests also confirm that in the uraemic population performance of superior cortical function gradually diminishes (Savazzi et al, 1988). Discriminant analysis of the possible pathogenic causes suggests that chronic aluminium (Al) intoxication may be strongly implicated (Savazzi et al, 1985) since these patients assume intestinal phosphorus chelating agents to reduce hyperphosphatemia caused by lost renal function. Neurofibrillary pathology has been found particulary in the large cortical neurons of the motor cortex and cingulate gyrus in the subjects on dialysis who have also evidenced high tissue concentrations of Al in the gray matter (Scholtz et al, 1987). It is well known that neurofibrillary pathology is linked to damaged axonal transport: we shall therefore enumerate the theoretical and experimental data that may indicate in Al intoxication a cause of altered axonal transport in uraemia.

AXONAL TRANSPORT AND ALUMINIUM TOXICITY

The following cytoskeletal proteins are synthesized in the perikaryon: tubulin, the main component of neurotubules, actin, the main component of microfilaments, and neurofilamentous proteins for the neurofilaments. Normally these enter the axon and are transported anterogradely to the terminal parts of the axon where the cytoskeleton is disassembled. Normal perikaryon synthesis and axonal transport - slow anterograde component (SC), fast anterograde component (FCa), and fast retrograde component (rFC) allow normal functioning of the axon.

In experimental B-B-iminodipropionitrile intoxication (Griffin et al, 1983) and in Al intoxication (Bizzi et al, 1984), both of which involve damage to SC transport, protein synthesis in the perikaryon continues. Thus neurofilaments continue being synthesized on free polysomes but the abnormalities of slow axonal transport, SC, and the resulting difficulty of translocating the neurofilaments from proximal to distal position on the axon, lead to their accumulation, segregation and disorganization with resulting neurofibrillary degeneration.

In the rabbit $AlCl_3$ intoxication slows or blocks the transport of neurofilaments synthesized and assembled in the cell body and proceeding from it thanks to the SC (Troucoso et al, 1985): neurofibrillary degeneration, a common finding in experimental Al intoxication (Galle et al, 1980) has recently been cultured in human foetal cerebral cortex cells. The neurofibrillary degeneration of cortical neurons observed in patients with acute encephalopathy syndrome is known to be due to Al intoxication (Scholts et al, 1987). The axonal swelling, neurotubular dilatation and reduction of the axonal thickness in uraemia are all morphopathological aspects of Al intoxication also observed in experimental conditions.

Neurotubule function regulated by polymerization of the alpha and beta tubulin constituents is assured by a dynamic equilibrium between the polymerized and depolymerized state (Weisemberg et al, 1976). In vitro and in vivo experiments demonstrate that Al causes neurotubular rearrangement, impeding the polymerization phase (Bonhaus et al, 1980).

Fast axonal transport inevitably suffers too in uraemia, on account of the qualitative and quantitative damage to the cytoskeletal neurotubular component. This is the "rail" of fast transport, and the hypothesis is reinforced by the intra-axonal rearrangement and disorganization of organelles seen in uraemic neuropathy, these organelles being moved along the axon by the FCa.

The aspects of axonopathy with dendritic dying back, loss of dendritic spines, dendritic beading and axonal degeneration found in uraemia are also seen in animals suffering Al intoxication (Savazzi 1987).

The physiological disassembly of the cytoskeleton that partly underlies rFC is impeded in Al intoxication (Marcum et al, 1978). The damage to rFC is linked to the pathophysiology of the distal axonopathies of which uraemic neuropathy is a part with its pattern of slow, insidious, symmetrical dying back symptoms, and related histopathological changes (Savazzi 1987).

Calmodulin, a component of the cytoskeleton, is also a molecular constituent of the microfilaments (Jakobsen et al, 1976) and may be altered by Al accumulation in tissues, inasmuch as there exists strong interaction between Al and calmodulin, which can be explained by the highly solvated nature of Al, with formation of covalent coordinated bonds, and the denaturation of calmodulin (Siegel et al, 1983).

ALTERNATIVE TREATMENTS TO USE OF $AL(OH)_3$ IN UREMIA.

Not much effort has been made to prevent intoxication caused by chronic oral $Al(OH)_3$ in uremia. It has probably lost priority compared to the more pressing clinical need to limit hyperphosphataemia and its harmful vascular effects. Apart from the use of $Al(OH)_3$ as an effective chelating agent for phosphorus (P), therapy of hyperphosphoremia is still a thorny problem, and the main approach is a low-phosphorus diet. This, however, must ensure intake not exceeding 600-800 mg P/day: the resulting lack of palatability causes compliance problems. Removing P more effectively through dialysis would call for longer dialysis times and/or more costly treatment methods and membranes.

Small doses of $CaCO_3$ do not control hyperphosphatemia, and the patient remains exposed to the risk of hypercalcemia if Vit. D is associated to prevent osteodystrophy. Hypercalcemia remains constant when high doses of $CaCO_3$ are given for long periods even if at the same time Ca^{2+} is reduced in the dialysate (Gonnella et al, 1986).

$Mg(OH)_2$ has never caught on in practice, because of its scant effect on phosphoremia, since it frequently induces diarrhoea and the tendency to hyperkaliemia (Guillot et al, 1982). More promise has been held out by the use of $MgCO_3$ concomitantly with Mg-free dialysate to prevent hypermagnesemia. Thus while awaiting the availability of Al-free phosphate binders such as homo-and heteropolyuronic acids, or their derivatives (Scheider et al, 1985), the treatment of hyperphosphoremia without Al binders requires a series of dietary and therapeutic measures, with relative blood tests tailored to the individual patient, that are certainly more complicated than the simple administration of Al $(OH)_3$.

But we can therefore no longer insist that we lack the means to reduce intestinal phosphorus absorption without prescribing Al compounds even though other therapeutic programmes may be more complex than $Al(OH)_3$ administration.

There is in fact no doubt that patients who receive no Al salts have significantly lower serum Al levels. There is thus no excuse for a skeptical, superficial attitude to the experimental and clinical evidence of neuronal damage induced by aluminium intoxication in uraemia.

REFERENCES

Bizzi A., Crane R.C., Autilio-Gambetti L., Gambetti P. (1984): Aluminium effect on slow axonal transport: a novel impairment of neurofilament transport. J. Neurosci. 4: 722-731.

Bonhaus D.W., Mc Cormac K. M., Mayor G. H. Mattson J.C., Hook J.B. (1980): The effect of aluminium on microtubular integrity using in vitro and in vivo models. Toxicol. Letters. 6: 141-147.

Cusmano F., Savazzi G.M. (1986): Cerebral Computed Tomography in Uremic and Hemodialyzed Patients. J. Comp. Ass. Tomography. 10: 567-570.

De Boni V., Seger M., Crapper McLachlan D.R. (1980): Functional consequences of chromatin bound aluminium in cultured human cells. Neurotoxicology. 1: 65-81.

Galle P., Berry J.P., Duckett S. (1980): Electron microprobe ultrastructural localization of aluminium in rat brain. Acta Neuropathol. 49: 245-247.

Gonnella M. Vangelli G., Calabrese G., Pratesi G., Lamon S., Talarico S. (1986): Optimal serum calcium-phosphorus balance by combined high CaCO3 intake and adequate dialysate calcium concentration. In Aluminium and other trace elements in Renal Disease. Taylor A. Ed. 142-146. Bailliere Tindal Eastbourne.

Griffin J.W., Fahnestock K.E., Price D.L., Hoffman P.N. (1983): Microtubule-neurofilament segregation produced by B,B' -iminodipropionitrile: evidence for the association of fast axonal transport with microtubules. J. Neurosci. 3: 557-566.

Guillot A.P., Hood V.L., Rungel P., Gennarif J. (1982): The use of magnesium containing phosphate binders in patients with end stage renal disease on maintenance dialysis. Nephron. 30: 114-117.

Jakobsen J., Sidenius P., Braendgaard H. (1986): A proposal for a classification of neuropathies according to their axonal transport abnormalities. J. Neurol. Neurosurg. Psych. 49: 986-

990.
Marcum J.M., Dedman J.R., Brinkley B.R., Means A.R. (1978): Control of microtubule assembly-disassembly by calcium-dependent regulator protein. Proc. Natl. Acad Sci. USA 75: 3771-3775.
Savazzi G.M., Cusmano F., De Gasperi T. (1985): Cerebral atrophy in patients on long-term regular hemodialysis treatment. Clinical Nephrol. 23: 89-95.
Savazzi G.M. (1987): Features of uremic peripheral polyneuropathy in the light of experience with the short hemodialysis schedule. In Short dialysis. Nijhoff (Ed), The Hague Boston 115-148.
Savazzi G.M., Allegri L., Bocchi B., Borghetti A. (1988): Atrofia cerebrale: una complicanza emergente nel paziente uremico. Annali It. Med. Int. 2: 299-307.
Scheider H., Hulbe K.D., Weber H., Streicher E. (1985): Aluminium-free oral phosphate binder. Clin. Nephrol. 24 (Suppl.1): 98-102.
Scholtz C.L., Swash M., Kogeorgos J., Marsch F. (1987): Neurofibrillary neuronal degeneration in dialysis dementia: a feature of aluminium toxicity. Clin. Neurophathology. 6: 93-97.
Siegel N. Coughin R., Hang A. (1983): A thermodynamic and electron paramagnetic resonance study of structural changes in calmodulin induced by aluminium binding. Biochem. Biophys. Res. Commun. 115:512-517.
Troncoso J.C., Hoffman P. N., Griffin J. W., Hess-Kozlow K. M., Price D. L. (1985): Aluminium intoxication: a disorder of neurofilament transport in motor neurons. Brain Res. 342: 172-175.
Weisenberg R., Deery W., Dickinson P. (1976): Tubulin-nucleotide interactions during the polymerization and depolymerization of microtubules. Biochemistry. 15: 4248-4254.

Metal Ions in Biology and Medicine, vol. 2. Eds. J. Anastassopoulou, Ph. Collery, J.C. Etienne, Th. Theophanides. John Libbey Eurotext, Paris © 1992, pp. 54-58

From platinum nitriles to platinum blues

Giovanni Natile

Dipartimento Farmaco-Chimico, Università di Bari, via G. Amendola 173, 70126 Bari, Italy

The coordination of amides to platinum has fascinated workers ever since the report in 1908 of an intensely blue-coloured compound (Platinblau) obtained by reaction of yellow $[PtCl_2(NCMe)_2]$ with Ag_2SO_4 and formulated as $Pt(NHCOMe)_2{\cdot}H_2O$.[1] Although later revised, its exact structure is still unknown.[2] Interest in this area has been stimulated further by the finding that blue compounds can be prepared by reaction of *cis*-diaminediacquaplatinum(II) complexes with a variety of amides,[3-6] and that these are antitumour agents[7] and useful stains for electron microscopy.[8]

Common characteristics of all blue platinum compounds so far characterized are mixed valency, oligomerization and amidate bridging and were revealed from the first X-ray structure reported from the Lippard's group on a cis-diammineplatinum-α-pyridone blue (PPB).[3a,b] This compound was comprised of a tetranuclear chain of platinum atoms linked through metal-metal bonding interactions, amidate bridges, and hydrogen bonds between ligand substituents; the formal platinum oxidation state was 2.25. PPB and all other blue compounds containing two amines and one amidate anion per platinum atom are cationic polymers of various lengths carrying at least one positive charge per platinum atom and therefore good candidates to bind strongly and cooperatively to polyanionic DNA. However the original complex, termed 'Platinblau' and having a stoichiometry of two amidate anions per platinum atom, cannot carry so many positive charges, moreover it exhibits larger extinction coefficients (1000-1500 M^{-1} cm^{-1})[2b] than diamine-amidate platinum blues (ca. 100 M^{-1} cm^{-1}).[9] Unfortunately the separation and identification of 'Platinblau' and similar species have not always been reliable due to the variety of possible blue products which apparently can be formed. 'Platinblau', for instance, has been claimed to have oxidation states of 2+,3+, and 4+ for platinum; to be monomer or polymer; to be paramagnetic or diamagnetic.

We have been involved in the synthesis of nitrileplatinum(II) complexes[10] and their reactions with amines and alcohols.[11] The investigation has also been extended to hydrolysis reaction which has revealed a surprising and unprecedented behaviour of bisamideplatinum species. Some aspects of their chemistry have been elucidated and are described.

Three different nitrile complexes of platinum have been considered: $[PtCl_3(NCR)]^-$, *cis*-$[PtCl_2(NCR)_2]$, and *trans*-$[PtCl_2(NCR)_2]$ (R = Me, Ph or *t*-Bu) to see the effect of different nitrile to platinum ratios and of geometrical isomerism.

The hydrolysis of platinum-bonded nitriles occurs very readily under basic conditions and leads to the formation of the corresponding amidates. The reaction can be performed either in water (as in the case of saline $K[PtCl_3(NCR)]$) or in chlorinated solvents (as in the case of *cis*- and *trans*-$[PtCl_2(NCR)_2]$).

By acidification of their solution in ice-cold water the corresponding amides ($K[PtCl_3\{HN{=}C(OH)R\}]$, *cis*-$[PtCl_2\{HN{=}C(OH)R\}_2]$ and *trans*-$[PtCl_2\text{-}\{HN{=}C(OH)R\}_2]$ can be formed in quantitative yield. In several cases the isolated compounds might result to be contaminated by a blue material and to require a further purification.

The behaviours of the *cis* and *trans* isomers of $[PtCl_2\{HN{=}C(OH)R\}_2]$ are totally different. For instance the trans isomers are rather stable and monomeric both in the solid state and in solution. On the contrary the cis isomer of $[PtCl_2\{HN=C(OH)t\text{-}Bu\}_2]$ has a great tendency to associate forming a dimer. This has structural features similar to the building blocks of characterized platinum blues with direct intermetallic interactions and hydrogen bonding between ligands, but it does not contain amidate bridges. The dimeric species undergoes oxidation to a platinum(III) dimer which is rather resistant to further oxidation and stable only in the presence of excess oxidant.[12]

The dichlorobis(amidate)platinum(II) complexes are capable to give directly platinum blue species by spontaneous decomposition in water solution. In two cases (R = Ph and *t*-Bu) the blue compounds are scarcely soluble in water and precipitate from solution with a well defined and reproducible stoichiometry corresponding to the formula $[Pt_5\{HN=C(O)R\}_{10}(OH)_2]\cdot 2KCl$. In the case of R = Me the blue compound is soluble in water and must be precipitated by addition of alcohol and ether, the blue solid has the formula $[Pt_4\{HN=C(O)Me\}_7(OH)_2]\cdot 2KCl$. These reactions take place without removal of the chloride ion from the solution and therefore it is not surprising that the blue compounds contain some halide ions which can be either coordinated to platinum or inglobated as alkaline salt. The loss of chloride ion from the starting complex takes place in two steps, the former much faster than the latter. This might explain why other authors have isolated with platinum a blue compound of composition $[Pt\{HN=C(O)Me\}_2Cl]_n$ while with palladium (which usually gives rise to faster reactions) a compound having the same stoichiometry of that prepared by us has been isolated. In principle it would be possible to remove inglobated KCl by crystallization or chromatography, however these processes cause also a change in composition of the blue compounds as already observed by several authors.

Some of these results also clarify the nature of species believed to be a platinum blue of composition $[Pt^{IV}Cl_2(amidate)_2]$ and resulted to be a mixed amide-nitrile complex of composition $[PtCl_2(N{\equiv}CR)\{HN=C(OH)R\}]$.

Acknowledgements

Financial support by the Ministero dell'Università e della Ricerca Scientifica e Tecnologica (MURST) and Consiglio Nazionale delle Ricerche (CNR) and collaboration of Profs R. Cini and L. Maresca and Drs P. Caputo, M. Coluccia and F. P. Intini are gratefully acknowledged.

References

1) K. A. Hofmann and G. Bugge, *Ber.,* **1908**, *41*, 312
2) (a) R. D. Gillard and G. Wilkinson, *J. Chem. Soc.,* **1964**, 2835. (b) D. B. Brown, R. D. Burbank, and M. B. Robin, *J. Am. Chem. Soc.,* **1969**, *91*, 2895. (c) A. K. Johnson and J. D. Miller, *Inorg. Chim. Acta*, **1977**, *22*, 219. (d) J. K. Barton, S. A. Best, S. J. Lippard, R. A. Walton, *J. Am. Chem. Soc.*, **1978**, *100*, 3785. (e) M. P. Laurent, J. Biscoe, H. H. Patterson, *J. Am. Chem. Soc.*, **1980**, *102*, 6576. (f) M. P. Laurent, J. C. Tewksbury, M. B. Krogh-Jespersen, H. Patterson, *Inorg. Chem.*, **1980**, *19*, 1656 (g) J. L. Leffert, K. C. Molloy, J. J. Zuckerman, I. Haiduc, C. Guta, and D. Ruse, *Inorg. Chem*, **1980**, *19*, 1662.
3) (a) J. K. Barton, H. N. Rabinowitz, D. J. Szalda, S. J. Lippard, *J. Am. Chem. Soc.*, **1977**, *99*, 2827. (b) J. K. Barton, D. J. Szalda, H. N. Rabinowitz, J. V. Waszczak, S. J. Lippard, *J. Am. Chem. Soc.*, **1979**, *101*, 1434. (c) T. V. O' Halloran, P. K. Mascharak, I. D. Williams, M. M. Roberts, S. J. Lippard, *Inorg. Chem.*, **1987**, *26*, 1261. (d) L. S. Hollis and S. J. Lippard, *J. Am. Chem. Soc.* **1981**, *22*, 4086. (e) S. Hollis, S. J. Lippard, *Inorg. Chem.*, **1983**, *22*, 2600. (f) L. S. Hollis, S. J. Lippard, *Inorg. Chem.*, **1983**, *22*, 2605. (g) T. V. O' Halloran, M. M. Roberts, S. J. Lippard, *Inorg. Chem.*, **1986**, *25*, 957.
4) (a)B. Lippert, D. Neugebauer, U. Schubert, *Inorg. Chim. Acta*, **1980**, *46*, L11. (b) B. Lippert, H. Shöllhorn, U. Thewalt, *J. Am. Chem. Soc.*, **1986**, *108*, 525. (c) H. Shöllhorn, P. Eisenmann, U. Thewalt, B. Lippert, *Inorg. Chem.* ***1986**, 25,* 3384.
5) J. P. Laurent, P. Lepage, F. Dahan, *J. Am. Chem. Soc.*, **1982**, *104*, 7335. L.
6) (a) K. Matsumoto, H. Takahashi, K. Fuwa, *Inorg. Chem.*, **1983**, *22*, 4086. (b) K. Sakai, K. Matsumoto, *J. Am. Chem. Soc.*, **1989**, *111*, 3074.
7) (a) P. J. Davidson, P. J. Faber, R. G. Fisher, Jr., S. Mansy, H. J. Peresie, B. Rosenberg, L. Van Kamp, *Cancer. Chemother. Rep.*, **1975**, *59*, 287. (b) B. Rosenberg, *Cancer. Chemother. Rep.*, **1975**, *59*, 589. (c) R. J. Speer, H. Ridgeway, L. M. Hall, D. O. Stewart, K. E. Howe, D. Z. Lieberman, A. D. Newman, J. M. Hill, *Cancer. Chemother. Rep.*, **1975**, *59*, 629.

8) W. Bauer, S. J. Gonias, S. K. Kam, K. C. Wu, S. J. Lippard, *Biochemistry,* **1978**, *17*, 1060.

9) J. K. Barton, C. Caravana, S. J. Lippard, *J. Am. Chem. Soc.*, **1979**, *101*, 7269.

10) F. P. Fanizzi, F. P. Intini, L. Maresca, G. Natile, *J. Chem. Soc., Dalton Trans.*, **1990**, 199.

11) (a) L. Maresca, G. Natile, F. P. Intini, F. Gasparrini, A. Tiripicchio, M. Tiripicchio-Camellini, *J. Am. Chem. Soc.*, **1986**, *108*, 1180. (b) F. P. Fanizzi, F. P. Intini, G. Natile, *J. Chem. Soc., Dalton Trans.*, **1989**, 947.

12) R. Cini, F. P. Fanizzi, F. P. Intini, G. Natile, *J. Am. Chem. Soc.*, **1991**, *113*, 7805.

Metal Ions in Biology and Medicine, vol. 2. Eds. J. Anastassopoulou, Ph. Collery, J.C. Etienne, Th. Theophanides. John Libbey Eurotext, Paris © 1992, pp. 59-64

Ternary complexes of *cis*- and *trans*-Pt $(NH_3)_2Cl_2$ with aminoacids and nucleobases. Hydrophobic ligand-ligand interactions

Akis Iakovidis, Vasilis Aletras, Nick Hadjiliadis

Department of Chemistry, University of Ioannina, Laboratory of Inorganic and General Chemistry, Ioannina 45-110, Greece

INTRODUCTION

In an attempt to study the consequences of the formation of ternary complexes of the type DNA-Pt-protein, known to take place with both the antitumor cis- and its inactive isomer trans-$Pt(NH_3)_2Cl_2$ (Banjar etal.,1984; Ciccarelli etal.,1985), we have prepared and studied model complexes of the type cis- and trans-$[(NH_3)_2Pt(Nb)(amac)]^+$ (Iakovidis etal.,1991; Aletras etal.,1992), with Nb=1-Methylcytosine (1-Mec) or 9-Methylguanine (9-MeG) and amacH=glycine (gly), L-alanine (ala), L-2-aminobutyric acid (2-aba), L-valine (val) and L-norvaline (nval).

The aminoacid aliphatic side chains increase regularly from gly to nval and as a consequence, increasing with the same order hydrophobic ligand-ligand interactions can be detected, mainly from ^{1}H-NMR spectra, in solution. The results in solution are compared with the crystal structure of the complexes cis-$[(NH_3)_2Pt(gly)(1\text{-}MeC)]^+$ (Iakovidis etal.,1991) and trans-$[(CH_3NH_2)_2Pt(gly)(1\text{-}MeC)]^+$ (Pesch etal., 1990).

RESULTS AND DISCUSSION

The cis- ternary complexes were prepared according to,

$$\text{cis-}[(NH_3)_2Pt(amac)](NO_3) + Nb \xrightarrow[\text{2-3 days}]{50^{\circ}C} \text{cis-}[(NH_3)_2Pt(amac)(Nb)](NO_3) \quad (1)$$

where amac is the $-NH_2$, $-COO^-$ chelated to Pt^{2+}, aminoacids in the starting complexes, prepared as described (Iakovidis etal., 1989). Both cis- and trans- ternary complexes were also prepared as follows:

$$\text{cis-, trans-}[(NH_3)_2Pt(Nb)Cl](NO_3) \xrightarrow[-AgCl]{+AgNO_3} \text{cis-, trans-}[(NH_3)_2Pt(Nb)(H_2O)](NO_3)_2$$

$$\xrightarrow[\substack{pH=5,\ 30-35\ ^\circ C \\ 2-3\ days}]{amacH_{(excess)}} \text{cis-, trans-}[(NH_3)_2Pt(Nb)(amac)](NO_3) + NO_3^- + H_3O^+ \quad (2)$$

The vibrational spectra (IR-Raman), of the isolated complexes, provide good indications for the $-NH_2$ coordination of the aminoacids and the N(7) and N(3) coordination of the nucleobases 9-MeG and 1-MeC respectively, in the ternary complexes.

The retention of the N(7) and N(3) coordination of the nucleobases is also proved by the ^1H-NMR spectra of the ternary complexes, in both cis- and trans- series.

The difference in the chemical shifts of the terminal methyl group of the aminoacids between their anionic forms and their metal complexes ($\Delta\delta = \delta amac - \delta complex$) has beeen used to indicate the presence of hydrophobic ligand-ligand interactions in other similar systems. Figure 1 represents these results for both the cis- and trans- systems, as a function of the aminoacid.

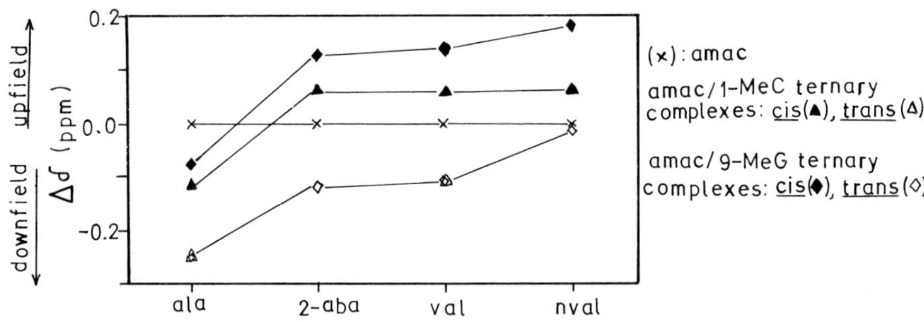

Fig.1 Chem.shift variation of the aminoacid CH_3 from the free anionic form.

It is seen that in the cis- system, the hydrophobic ligand-ligand interactions exist, though weak compared to other similar systems, with 2-aba increasing to nval. In the trans- system on the other hand the difference is always negative, implying the absence of such an interaction. It approaches the zero value however with nval. that has the longest side chain.

The chemical shifts of the various hydrogen atoms of the aminoacids nval in their ternary complexes with 9-MeG and 1-MeC as functions of the difference $\Delta\delta = \delta_{amacH} - \delta_{complex}$ show that the ligand-ligand interactions are larger near the bonding sites (larger $\Delta\delta$) and larger in the cis- than in the trans- systems (Fig. 2).

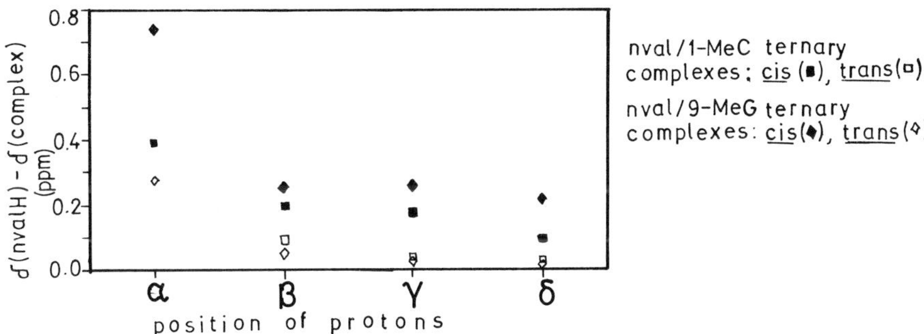

Fig. 2 Chem. shift variation in the ternary nvalH complexes from the free aminoacid.

A comparison of the chemical shifts of the various hydrogen atoms of the aminoacids in nval in their cis- and trans- ternary complexes with 9-MeG, $\Delta\delta = \delta_{trans-[(NH_3)_2Pt(9-MeG)(amac)]^+} - \delta_{cis-[(NH_3)_2Pt(9-MeG)(amac)]^+}$ is done in Table 1. The results show that the $\Delta\delta$'s are always positive, indicating the corresponding smaller upfield shifts (weaker ligand-ligand interactions) in the trans- than the cis- complexes.

Table 1. Chemical shifts (ppm) of the various protons of nval in the series cis- and trans- $[(NH_3)_2Pt(9\text{-}MeG)(nval)](NO_3)$.

Protons	nval zwitterion	cis-complex	trans-complex	$\Delta\delta = \delta_{amac} - \delta_{trans}$	$\Delta\delta = \delta_{trans} - \delta_{cis}$
α	3.734	2.996	3.457	0.277	0.461
β	1.833	1.583	1.784	0.049	0.201
γ	1.395	1.132	1.372	0.023	0.240
δ	0.949	0.732	0.928	0.021	0.196

Table 2 includes the results of the h and t+g percentage calculations around the C_α-C_β bonds of the aminoacids 2-aba and nval and the t and h+g for the val in the ternary complexes, based on ^{1}H-NMR spectra.

Table 2. Vicinal proton coupling constants (Hz) and rotamer distribution in the ternary complexes with 1-MeC

Compound	J_{AB+BC}	J_{BC}	h%	t%	t+g%	h+g%
2-abaH	11.700		37.0		63.0	
cis-$[(NH_3)_2Pt(2\text{-aba})]^+$	10.109		51.3		48.7	
cis-$[(NH_3)_2Pt(2\text{-aba})(1\text{-MeC})]^+$	12.200		32.1		67.9	
trans-$[(NH_3)_2Pt(2\text{-aba})(1\text{-MeC})]^+$	12.400		30.0		70.0	
nvalH	12.200		32.0		68.0	
cis-$[(NH_3)_2Pt(nval)]^+$	10.023		52.1		47.9	
cis-$[(NH_3)_2Pt(nval)(1\text{-MeC})]^+$	12.400		30.3		69.7	
trans-$[(NH_3)_2Pt(nval)(1\text{-MeC})]^+$	13.000		25.0		75.0	
valH		4.400		18.0		82.0
cis-$[(NH_3)_2Pt(val)]^+$		3.370		8.9		91.1
cis-$[(NH_3)_2Pt(val)(1\text{-MeC})]^+$		4.600		20.2		79.8
trans-$[(NH_3)_2Pt(val)(1\text{-MeC})]^+$		4.100		16.0		84.0

In both cis- and trans- series the h conformer decreases in the ternary complexes with 2-aba and nval, while the one of t increases in the complex with val, compared to the chelate complexes cis-$[(NH_3)_2Pt(amac)](NO_3)$ or the free zwitterionic aminoacids. The values with the cis- were higher than with the trans- series reflecting the stronger interactions in the former.

The ^1H-NMR spectra of the cis- ternary complexes, revealed the presence of small amounts of the trans- ternary ones (2.8-13.5%), increasing with temperature.

The crystal structure however, of both complexes cis-$[(NH_3)_2Pt(gly)(1\text{-MeC})](NO_3)$ and trans-$[(CH_3NH_2)_2Pt(gly)(1\text{-MeC})](NO_3)$ show that in the solid state any ligand-ligand interaction is absent, since the $-COO^-$ group of gly points out the pyrimidine plane.

Oxidation finally of the complex cis-$[(NH_3)_2Pt(1\text{-MeC})(N\text{-gly})](NO_3)$ with $S_2O_8^{2-}$, produced the corresponding Pt^{4+} species :

$$2\ \text{cis-}[(NH_3)_2Pt(1\text{-MeC})(N\text{-gly})](NO_3) + 2\ S_2O_8^{2-} + 2\ H_2O \longrightarrow$$

$$\longrightarrow \text{cis-}[(NH_3)_2Pt(1\text{-MeC})(N,O\text{-gly})(H_2O)]_2^{6+} + 4SO_4^{2-} + 2\ NO_3^- \qquad (3)$$

^1H-NMR spectra reveal that in the product, the aminoacid is N,O co-ordinated, while 1-MeC coordination changes from the original N(3) to the rear $-NH_2$ coordination :

$$\text{(Pt complex, N(3)-bound 1-MeC)} \underset{+H_2O}{\overset{-H_2O}{\rightleftharpoons}} \text{(intermediate)}\ H^+ \underset{-H_2O}{\overset{+H_2O}{\rightleftharpoons}} \text{(Pt complex, }-NH\text{-bound 1-MeC, }OH_2\text{)} \qquad (4)$$

CONCLUSION

The importance of hydrophobic aliphatic-aromatic ligand-ligand interactions can not still be completely understood. While ^1H-NMR spectra give some evidence for their existence in solution, the direction of the ligands 1-MeC and gly in both the cis- and trans- complexes, in their crystal structures, show the absence of such interactions in the solid state. Similar direction of both ligands in other similar systems would imply the complete absence of such interactions in the solid state.

Support towards the absence of such interactions in the solid state is also given from the vibrational spectra (IR-Raman) of the binary complexes cis-$[(NH_3)_2Pt(amac)](NO_3)$, where we observe that the $v^a_{COO}-v^s_{COO}$ frequencies increase regularly from gly to val (Iakovidis etal. 1991) and this reflects the degree of stability of the corresponding metal complexes, not implying the presence of a second aromatic ligand for this behavior.

Consequently, the elucidation of such interactions in solution and in the solid state, requires further studies of more complex similar systems (using nucleosides, nucleotides, oligonucleotides and peptides). This is currently among our interests.

REFERNCES

Banjar,J.M., Hnilica,L.S., Briggs,P.C., Stein,J., and Stein,G.(1984) cis- and trans-Diamminedichloroplatinum(II)-Mediated Cross-

Linking of Chromosomal Non-Histone Proteins to DNA in HeLa Cells. Biochemistry,23: 1921-1925.

Ciccarelli,R.B., Solomon,M.J., Varshavsky,A., and Lippard,S.J.(1985) :In Vivo Effects of cis- and trans-Diamminedichloroplatinum (II) on SV40 Chromosomes: Differential Repair, DNA-Protein Cross-Linking, and Inhibition of Replication. Biochemistry 24: 7553-7540.

Iakovidis,A., Hadjiliadis,N., Britten,J.F., Butler,I.S., Schwarz,F., and Lippert,B.(1991):Ternary complexes of cisplatin with aminoacids and nucleobases. The crystal structure of cis-$(NH_3)_2Pt(1\text{-}MeC\text{-}N^3)(gly\text{-}N)$ (NO_3) $2H_2O$. Inorg.Chim.Acta 184 :209-220.

Aletras,V., Hadjiliadis,N., and Lippert,B.(1992):Ternary complexes of trans-$Pt(NH_3)_2Cl_2$ with aminoacids and nucleobases. Polyhedron:Inpress.

Pesch,F.J., Preut,H., and Lippert,B.(1990):Mixed Nucleobase, Amino Acid Complexes of Pt(II). Preparation and X-ray Structure of trans- $(CH_3NH_2)_2Pt(1\text{-}MeC\text{-}N^3)(gly\text{-}N)$ NO_3 $2H_2O$ and its Precursor trans- $(CH_3NH_2)_2Pt(1\text{-}MeC\text{-}N^3)Cl$ Cl H_2O.Inorg.Chim. Acta 169:195-200.

Iakovidis,A., Hadjiliadis,N., Schollhorn,H., Thewalt,U. and Trotscher ,G.(1989):Interaction of cis-$Pt(NH_3)_2Cl_2$ with amino acids. The crystal structures of cis- $Pt(NH_3)_2(gly)$ (NO_3), cis-$Pt(NH_3)_2(ala)$ (NO_3) and cis- $Pt(NH_3)_2(val)$ (NO_3). Inorg. Chim.Acta 164:221-229.

Iakovidis,A., Hadjiliadis,N., and Butler,I.S.(1991):Infrared and Raman spectra in the region below 1800 cm^{-1} of some amino acid chelates of the type cis- $(NH_3)_2Pt(amac)$ (NO_3), where amac=the anions of glycine, l-alanine, L-aminobutyric acid, L-vaLINE AND L-norvaline.Spectrochim.Acta 47A:1567-1574.

Metal Ions in Biology and Medicine, vol. 2. Eds. J. Anastassopoulou, Ph. Collery, J.C. Etienne, Th. Theophanides. John Libbey Eurotext, Paris © 1992, pp. 65-68

Cisplatin and the 5′ -phosphate group of 5′-GMP and 5′-dGMP

Michael Green, David M. Orton

Department of Chemistry, University of York, York, Y01 5DD, UK

The main sites of attack of cisplatin, the anti-cancer drug, are GpG units in DNA (Bruhn *et al*, 1990).

Attack on the first G

The presence of a 5'-phosphate group accelerates reactions of relations of cisplatin with guanosine bases, B, as in (1); note the rise in k_1 (Table): G ≙ 3'-GMP < 5'-GMP < 5'-dGMP. To account for this rise in rates it is proposed that a cyclic intermediate, I, is formed in (1) when a 5'-phosphate group is present. The intermediate is produced more readily in the case of 5'-dGMP compared with 5'-GMP because of the greater flexibility of a deoxyribose ring compared with an (oxy)ribose system.

$$cis\text{-}[Pt(NH_3)_2(OH_2)_2]^{2+} + B \rightarrow cis\text{-}[Pt(NH_3)_2B(OH)_2)]^{x+} + H_2O \qquad (1)$$

Evidence that the 5'-phosphate group can approach the platinum closely is provided by the existence of compounds such as II the existence of which has been shown by ^{31}P-n.m.r. and FAB mass spectrometry (Reily and Marzilli, 1986; Green and Miller, 1987).

Attack on the Second G

Pt^{II}-OH bonds are inert so that reactions such as (2) are very slow (Basolo and Pearson, 1967; Arpalahti and Lehikoinen, 1990). These include those in which G or 3'-GMP are X and Y; k_2 for these systems are at least 20 times smaller than corresponding k_3, see Table. In contrast k_2 when X and Y are

5'-GMP is only half the analogous k_1. It is proposed that the OH^- ligand is activated by formation of a cyclic compound such as III

$$cis\text{-}[Pt(NH_3)_2B(OH)]^{y+} + B \rightarrow cis\text{-}[Pt(NH_3)_2B_2]^{(y-1)+} + OH^- \qquad (2)$$

$$cis\text{-}[Pt(NH_3)_2B(OH_2)]^{z+} + B \rightarrow cis\text{-}[Pt(NH_3)_2B_2]^{z+} + H_2O \qquad (3)$$

Table. Rate Constants ($/M^{-1}\ s^{-1}$) for Reactions (1) to (3) at 25 ^oC (Orton and Green, 1991).

B	k_1	k_2	k_3
G	ca. 0.2	< 0.01	0.16
dG	ca. 0.2		
3'-GMP	ca. 0.35	< 0.01	0.32
5'-GMP	1.44	0.12	0.24
5'-dGMP	16.4		

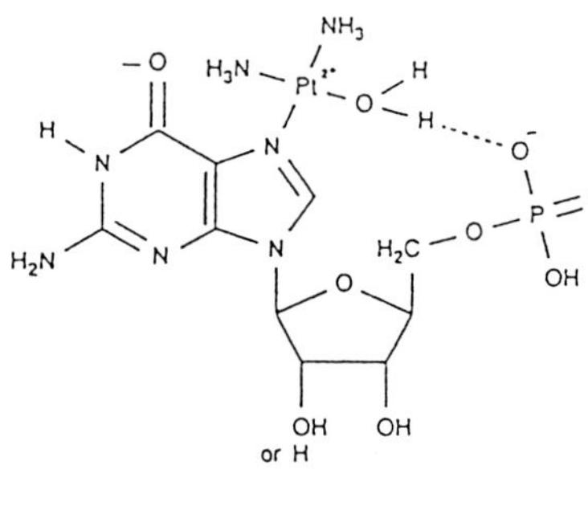

I

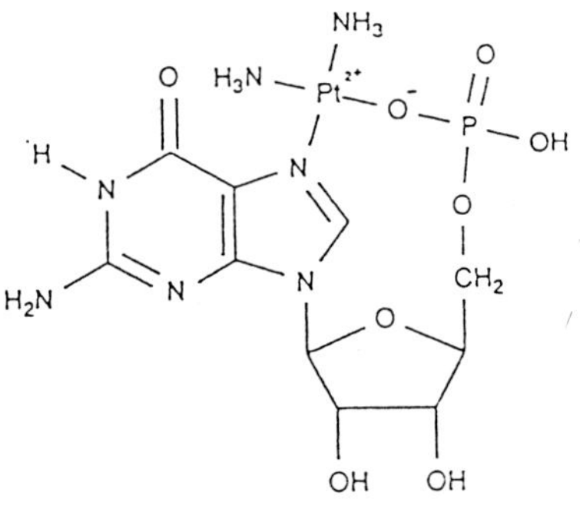

II

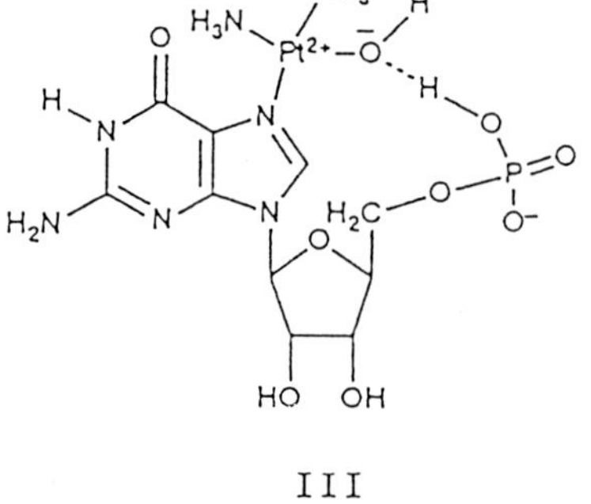

III

Reactive Species in the Cell

The acidity constants of *cis*-$[Pt(NH_3)_2(OH_2)_2]^{2+}$ and, in particular, *cis*-$[Pt(NH_3)_2(OH_2)(OH)]^+$ have been measured at 37°C and found to be 5.0 and 6.9 respectively (Orton and Green, 1992). Taking the pH of a cancerous cell as 7.0 (Tannock and Rotin, 1989), one finds that the predominant forms of cisplatin present are *cis*-$[Pt(NH_3)_2(OH)_2]$, *cis*-$[Pt(NH_3)_2(OH_2)(OH)]^+$ together with some *cis*-$[Pt(NH_3)_2Cl(OH)]$. The first and third of these species are rather inert, but the second is not, nor is *cis*-$[Pt(NH_3)_2(5'\text{-GMP})(OH)]^{y+}$. It therefore seems that the platinum species attack DNA by the following route (*Pt* = *cis*-$Pt(NH_3)_2$):

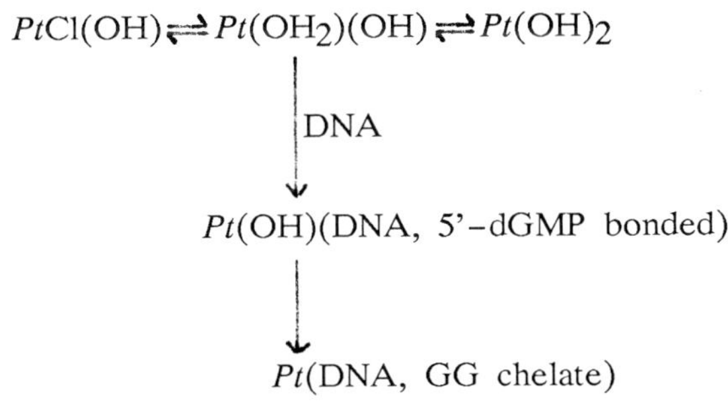

Arpalahti, J. and Lehikoinen, P. (1990): Kinetics of Complexation of Aquated Pt^{II}(dien) with Inosine and 1-Methylinosine as a Function of pH. *Inorg. Chem.* 29, 2564-2567.

Basolo, F. and Pearson, R.G. (1967): *Mechanisms of Inorganic Reactions*, Wiley, New York, 2nd edn., p. 391.

Bruhn, S.L., Toney, J.H. and Lippard, S.J. (1990): Biological Processing of DNA Modified by Platinum Compounds *Progr. Inorg. Chem.*, 38, 477-516.

Green, M. and Miller, J. (1987): A Cyclic Nucleobase Phosphate: Fast Atom Bombardment Studies on a 1:1 Mixture of *cis*-$[Pt(NH_3)_2(OH_2)_2](CF_3SO_3)_2$ and Guanosine 5'-Monophosphoric Acid. *J. Chem. Soc., Chem. Commun.*, 1864-1865.

Orton, D.M. and Green, M. (1991): Acidity Constants and Rates of Reaction of Guanosine Complexes derived from Cisplatin. *J. Chem. Soc., Chem. Commun.*, 1612-1614.

Orton, D.M. and Green, M. (1992): Acidity Constants for *Cis*-diaquadiammineplatinum(II), the aquated form of Cisplatin, *Inorg. Chim. Acta*, in press.

Reily, M.D. and Marzilli, L.G. (1986); Novel, Definitive NMR Evidence for

N(7), α-PO_4 Chelation of 6-Oxopurine Nucleotide Monophosphates of Platinum Anti-cancer Drugs. *J. Am. Chem. Soc.*, 108, 8299-8300.
Tannock, I.F. and Rotin, D. (1989): Acid pH in Tumours and Its Potential for Therapeutic Exploitation. *Cancer Res.* 49, 4373-4384.

Metal Ions in Biology and Medicine, vol. 2. Eds. J. Anastassopoulou, Ph. Collery, J.C. Etienne, Th. Theophanides. John Libbey Eurotext, Paris © 1992, pp. 69-74

Kinetic, spectroscopic and LPLC studies of the interactions of antitumour ruthenium (III) complexes with serum proteins

F. Kratz*, N. Mulinacci***, L. Messori**, I. Bertini**, B.K. Keppler*

** Anorganisch-Chemisches Institut der Universität Heidelberg, Im Neuenheimer Feld 270, 6900 Heidelberg 1, Germany. ** Laboratorio di Chimica Inorganica e Bioinorganica, Università degli Studi di Firenze, Via G. Capponi 7, 50121 Firenze, Italia. *** Departimento di Scienze Farmaceutiche, Università degli Studi di Firenze, Via G. Capponi 5, 50121 Firenze, Italia*

ABSTRACT

The Ru(III) complex *trans*-Indazolium-bisindazole-tetrachlororuthenate(III) [*trans*-HInd($RuInd_2Cl_4$)] holds particular promise as an antitumour agent against colon cancer. Visible spectroscopy and LPLC studies demonstrate that Ru-ind reacts with human serum; the major amount (80 - 90 per cent) is bound to albumin and a much smaller amount to transferrin. A small amount of newly formed unbound Ru(III) species is also present. Bicarbonate is necessary for the above reactions. Ultrafiltration experiments demonstrate that the binding to serum proteins takes place within 2-3 minutes and that molecules below MW 50 000 do not participate in binding.
Albumin can specifically bind 5 moles of Ru-ind and apotransferrin can bind 2 moles according to CD spectroscopy. The Fe(III) binding sites are involved in the binding of Ru-ind to apotransferrin.

INTRODUCTION

A number of Ru(III) complexes exhibit antitumour activity in animal models (Clarke, 1989). We have recently developed two anticancer ruthenium(III) complexes, among others, with the ligands imidazole (Fig.1) and indazole (Fig.2) which are highly active compared to other ruthenium(III) compounds (Keppler et al. 1989). Both of these complexes show excellent antitumour activity in an autochthonous colorectal tumour model in the rat, a model which simulates the colon cancers of humans very well.

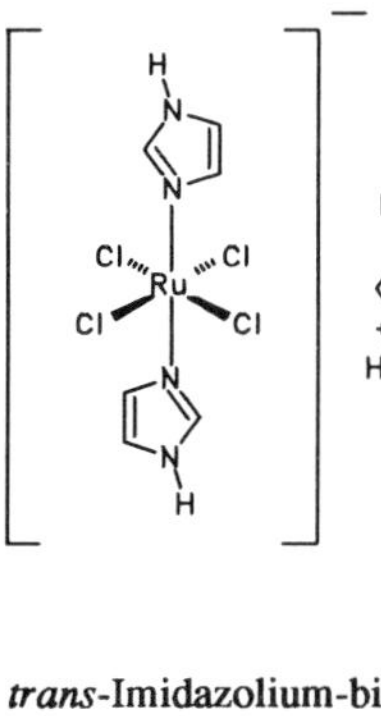

Fig 1: *trans*-Imidazolium-bisimidazole-tetrachlororuthenate(III) [*trans*-HIm($RuIm_2Cl_4$)] (ICR)

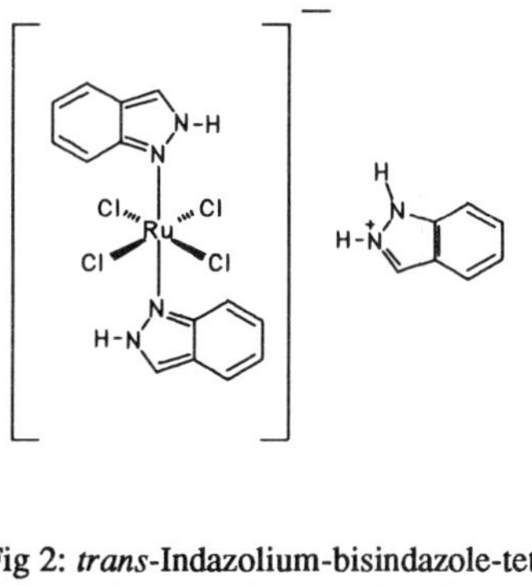

Fig 2: *trans*-Indazolium-bisindazole-tetrachlororuthenate(III) [*trans*-HInd($RuInd_2Cl_4$)]

To obtain an insight of the molecular modes of action of intravenously administered antitumour metal complexes, it is important to study the interactions of these with serum and serum proteins. For example, 3 hours after administration of cisplatin about 95 per cent of the platinum in the blood plasma is bound irreversibly to serum proteins (primarily albumin), and it is believed to be "free" cisplatin which enters cells and then exerts antitumour activity (Cole & Wolf, 1980; Daley-Yates, 1985) because cisplatin bound to albumin has no significant antitumour activity (Takashashi et al., 1985). However, in a patent it was reported that when cisplatin is bound to chemically modified human transferrin, a chemotherapeutic agent is produced which exhibits selective antitumour activity in vitro and also in clinical trials in patients with breast cell cancer (Stjernholm, 1986).

Due to its similarity with iron(III), it has been proposed that antitumour ruthenium(III) complexes could have a high affinity for the plasma protein transferrin (Clarke, 1989). Since neoplastic cells have a high iron requirement and, consequently, a large number of receptors for the iron-transport protein tranferrin, the accumulation of ruthenium(III) complexes in tumours might therefore be mediated by this plasma protein.

To obtain information about the destiny of antitumour ruthenium(III) complexes after they have been injected into the blood, we have investigated the interactions of *trans*-Indazolium-bisindazole-tetrachlororuthenate(III) (Ru-ind) with physiological buffer (pH = 7.4), serum and the human serum proteins apotransferrin and albumin using spectroscopic methods (visible- and CD spectroscopy) and separation techniques (low pressure liquid chromatography [LPLC] and ultrafiltration).

Apotransferrin was chosen for the reasons mentioned above, and albumin was chosen because it is the most common protein in the blood (abundancy of around 55 per cent) which binds a great number of therapeutic drugs, such as penicillins, sulfonamides or aspirine and also metal ions, such as copper(II) or zinc(II).

EXPERIMENTAL

Crystalline human serum albumin (MW 66 500) and apotransferrin (MW 80 000) were purchased from Serva, Heidelberg and human serum from Sigma. The Ru(III) complexes were synthezised as described earlier (Keppler et al., 1989). In all experiments Ru-ind was added from a standard 5 x 10^{-4} M aqueous solution.

The physiological buffer was: 0.1 M NaCl, 0.004 M NaH_2PO_4, 0.025 M $NaHCO_3$ - pH = 7.4.

Visible spectra were recorded with a Cary 17D spectrophotometer and the CD spectra with a JASCO 200D.

Ultrafiltration experiments were carried out by centrifugal ultrafiltration at 6000 U/min with a MPS-1 Kit from Amicon at a MW 30 000 or MW 50 000 cut-off.

HPLC and LPLC studies were performed with a Perkin Elmer Series 410 LC pump and a LC-95 UV/Visible spectrophotometer detector. The columns were:

1.) a 5 ml Econo-Pac anion exchange cartridge (Macro-Prep 50 Q) from Bio-rad. The buffers were - buffer A: 50 mmol Tris-HCl (pH = 8.6), buffer B: 50 mmol Tris-HCl + 0.5 M NaCl (pH = 8.6). The gradient was 0 -25 % A-B in 30 minutes and 25 - 100 % in 5 minutes and then 100 % B in 5 minutes..

2.) Nucleosil (300-7 μ) diole column (250mm x 8mm). Mobile phase: 70% CH_3CN and 30% of 0.005 mol KH_2PO_4 in bidest. water.

RESULTS AND DISCUSSION

When Ru-ind, a light brown complex, is added to serum at T = 37 °C, a reaction takes place within two hours which can be followed spectrophotometrically by the appearance of a d-d transition at around λ = 585 nm (blue-green) in the visible region. This transition is not present in the original complex because it has a centre of symmetry thus forbidding d-d transition in accordance with the Laporte selection rule.

A reaction also takes place when Ru-ind is added to a physiological buffer, where no proteins are present, but this time a blue-green precipitate is formed after 10-15 minutes. If a few drops of ethanol are added, the visible spectrum again shows a d-d transition at λ = 585 nm, which is 4 times as intense as that of the reaction with serum at the same concentrations of Ru-ind. HPLC of the

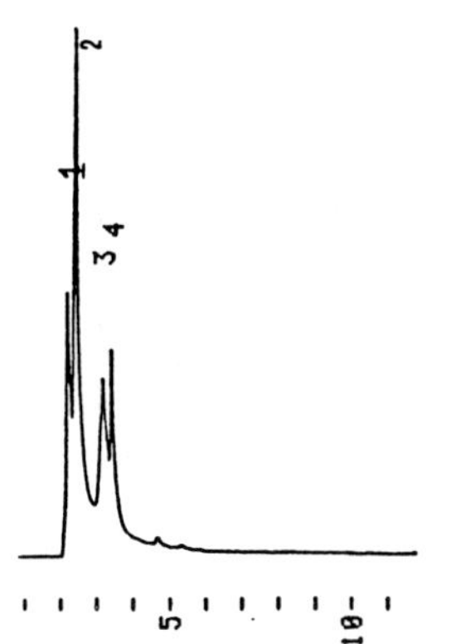

Fig.3: HPLC of the precipitate formed from Ru-ind in physiological buffer at 280nm

precipitate using a diole phase shows 4 signals (Fig.3). These species are (when analysing the mixture by microanalysis) not simply hydrolysis species where water or hydroxide replaces the chloride. The reaction, when followed by HPLC, is quite complex: three signals appear after the first minutes which then disappear and are replaced by the 4 signals mentioned above. Unfortunately, we have not been able to isolate these 4 species. It is also important to note that the above reaction is not solely dependent on the pH-value but on the amount of *bicarbonate* present. In the absence of bicarbonate at pH = 7.4 or even higher pH-values the 4 products are not seen with HPLC. A bicarbonate buffer alone is sufficient to produce the above reaction.

Apotransferrin and albumin react with Ru-ind producing the identical d-d transition of similar intensity as with serum, but *no* precipitation occurs indicating that the resulting products bind to the proteins. After ultrafiltration of serum at a cut-off of MW 30 000 and MW 50 000 Ru-ind reacts with the ultrafiltrate producing insoluble products, which are, when analysed by HPLC, identical to those formed in the physiological buffer alone. This demonstrates that low molecular species in the ultrafiltrate do not react significantly with Ru-ind

The benefit of such a band at 585 nm in the visible region is that we can use it to follow the destiny of the complex in human serum in separation studies, such as LPLC.

<u>LPLC studies with an anion exchange column</u>

Figure 4 shows a comparison of the chromatograms for the reactions of Ru-ind with serum and for a mixture of albumin and apotransferrin at a ratio of 10:1 (detected at 585 nm) after 3 hours; the chromatogram of Ru-ind with serum at 280 nm is also shown.

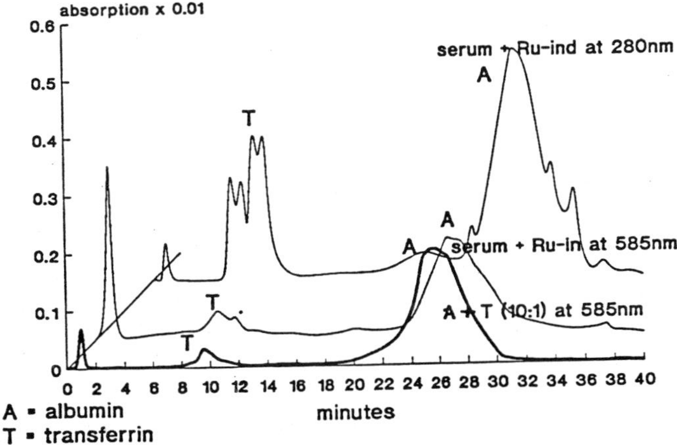

Fig.4: Chromatograms of Ru-ind reacted with albumin : apotransferrin = 10:1, with serum (both at 585 nm) and with serum (at 280 nm) after 3 hours. c(Ru-ind) = 5×10^{-4} M, c(albumin) = 5×10^{-4} M and c(apotransferrin) = 5×10^{-5}M

Comparing the chromatograms gives a rough approximation to which proteins binding has taken place. Most of the Ru-ind is bound to albumin in serum (about 80-90 %). This is not that surprising when one not only considers the amount present in *serum* (approximately 42 weight per cent of solutes), but also the size of albumin compared to other serum proteins (Fig.5). Both size and abundancy explain the fact that so many many drugs are bound to albumin in the blood, and it is likely that the major amount of antitumour metal complexes with hydrolyzable groups will nearly always be bound by this protein. A small amount of Ru-ind is bound to transferrin as can be seen from LPLC, but some binding also occurs to proteins with a similar retention time compared to transferrin. These could be α- or β-lipoglobulins. In addition, there is an initial sharp peak present in the chromatograms of serum and albumin and transferrin at 585 nm (1.0 min). This is likely to be a small amount of the newly formed unbound Ru(III) species because the intensity is very high and it appears in the chromatogram of albumin and transferrin. Additionally, we had already demonstrated that Ru-ind does not react with low molecular species (below MW 50 000) of serum.

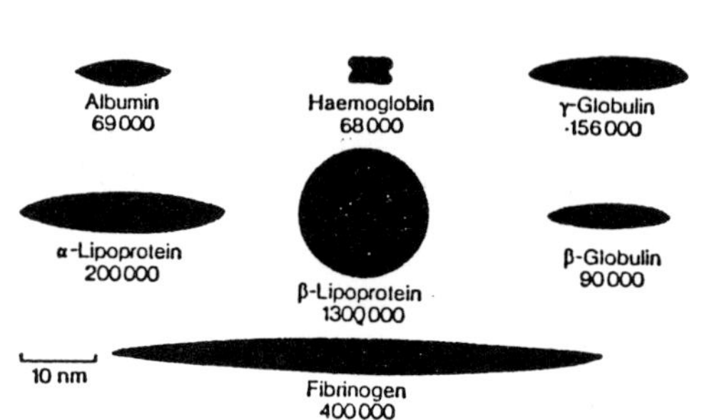

Fig.5: Schematic presentation of the relative sizes of the major plasma proteins

At present, we are trying to improve the resolution of the serum proteins using different columns.

Kinetics

When Ru-ind is let to react with albumin, apotransferrin, or serum at a molar ratio of Ru-ind : albumin, apotransferrin, or serum (in respect to the albumin concentration in serum) = 1:1 or 2:1, no ruthenium species could be detected with UV/visible spectroscopy in the ultrafiltrate even after 2-3 minutes. This indicates that the interaction with biomolecules larger than MW 50 000 occurs very rapidly.

The kinetics of the reaction of Ru-ind in physiological buffer and with apotransferrin, albumin and serum at T = 37 °C (ratio of 2:1 as above) were also studied using the increase of the d-d transition at 585 nm as an indication of the reaction rate. The results are shown in Fig.6.

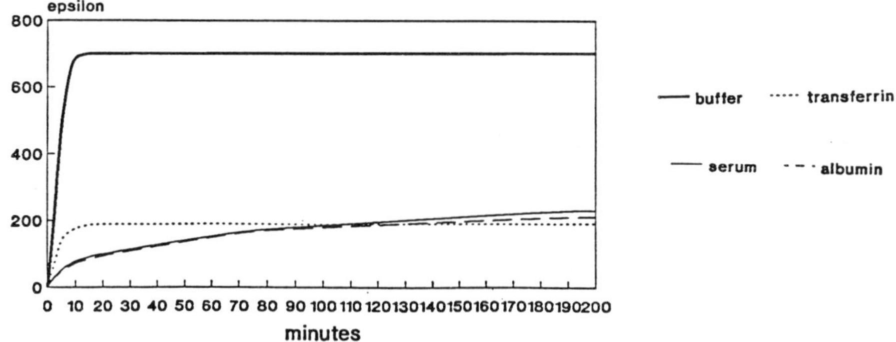

Fig.6: Appearance of the maximum ε-value at 585 nm with time for Ru-ind reacted in physiological buffer, serum, apotransferrin and albumin. c(Ru-ind) = 2×10^{-4} M.

We should be aware, however, that interpreting the increase in intensity of the d-d transition is not necessarily a direct measure of binding. In fact, the intensity of the transition solely reveals information on the change of the surroundings of Ru-ind but not on the kind of molecular reaction or binding taking place. Apotranferrin reacts with Ru-ind within 14 minutes which is on the same time-scale as the reaction in the physiological buffer. Complete reaction of Ru-ind with serum and albumin takes longer, about 2 hours, although 50 per cent intensity of the ε-value is seen after approximately 35 minutes.

<u>CD spectroscopy</u>

The interaction of Ru-ind with albumin and apotransferrin was studied with CD (circular dichroism) spectroscopy. CD-spectra demonstrate that apotransferrin specifically binds 2 equivalents of Ru-ind and albumin binds 5 equivalents (Fig. 7 and 8).

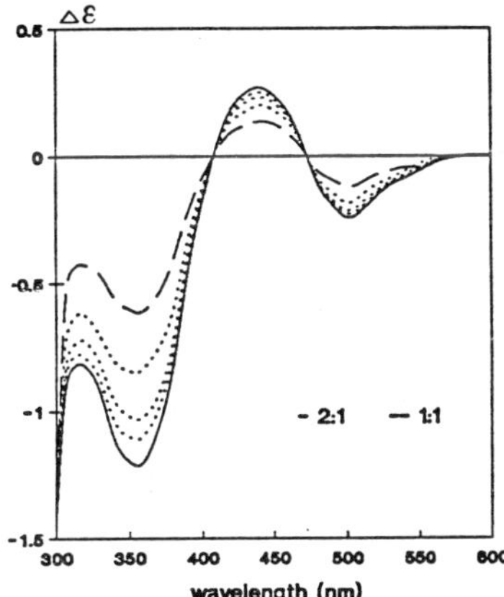

Fig 7: CD spectra showing the stepwise titration of apotransferrin (1 x 10^{-4} M) with Ru-ind

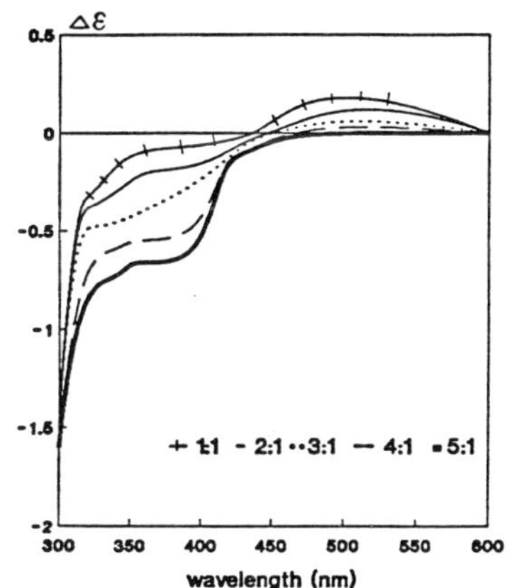

Fig.8: CD spectra showing the stepwise titration of albumin (1 x 10^{-4} M) with Ru-ind

Further additions do not produce changes in the CD-spectra, but the intensity of the d-d transition increases steadily in the visible spectra (data not shown) showing that further binding does not change the structure of the proteins. Both albumin and transferrin can bind at least 10 moles of Ru-ind according to the UV/vis data, although such great amounts are unlikely to be bound in chemotherapeutical application.

To find out whether the two binding sites for Fe(III) in transferrin are relevant for the binding of the first 2 equivalents of Ru-ind, we blocked these sites with Al(III), added Ru-ind and recorded the CD-spectra. The former spectra was not observed demonstrating that the iron binding sites in transferrin are important for the specific binding of the first 2 moles of Ru-ind to apotransferrin.

The CD spectrum of Ru-ind bound to transferrin differs substantially from the respective spectrum for Ru(III) bound transferrin. Two equivalents of Ru(III) react specifically with apotransferrin with binding taking place at the two Fe(III) sites (Kratz and Messori, 1992). Two equivalents of Ru-ind also react with apotransferrin around the Fe(III) sites but the indazole ligand seems to remain bound to Ru(III).

At present, we are carrying out comparative animal experiments to assess the antitumour activity of Ru-ind bound to apotransferrin or albumin, of the newly formed Ru(III) species and of the original Ru(III) complex *trans*-Indazolium-bisindazole-tetrachlororuthenate(III) (Ru-ind).

CONCLUSIONS

Ru-ind reacts with serum and new Ru(III) species are formed which react rapidly with serum proteins. The major amount of Ru-ind is bound to albumin and a small amount is bound to transferrin. A small amount of the newly formed free Ru(III) species is also present. The protein binding of Ru-ind seems to occur very rapidly (3 minutes), and these reactions are not only dependent on the pH-value but also on the amount of bicarbonate present.

As the binding of Ru-ind to serum proteins is so much faster in comparison to cisplatin (it takes 3 hours for cisplatin to bind irreversibly to serum proteins), the Ru-ind bound to albumin or tranferrin might be responsible for antitumour activity. Alternatively, the newly formed "free" Ru(III) species could also play a part.

Finally, when comparing the antitumour activity of *trans*-Indazolium-bisindazole-tetrachlororuthenate(III) (Ru-ind) with *trans*-Imidazolium-bisimidazole-tetrachlororuthenate(III) (ICR) in the colorectal tumour model, the former was shown to exhibit a slightly higher activity but also a reduced toxicity (Keppler et al., 1989).

Preliminary investigations of ICR with serum show that this complex also reacts with serum but binding to proteins is slower (several hours). This difference between the two complexes might explain the reduced toxicity of Ru-ind, but it is surprising that Ru-ind exhibits a higher antitumour activity than ICR suggesting that Ru-ind bound to serum proteins might be important for antitumour activity.

Animal experiments are under way to test the above mentioned hypotheses.

Acknowledgements: The support of the Mildred-Scheel Stiftung der Deutschen Krebshilfe, FRG, is gratefully acknowledged.

REFERENCES

Clarke, Michael, J., (1989): Ruthenium chemistry pertaining to the design of anticancer agents, *Progress in Clinical Biochemistry and Medicine*, Vol. 10, Springer-Verlag Berlin Heidelberg, 25-39.

Cole W.C. and Wolf W., (1980): Preparation and metabolism of a cisplatin/serum protein complex, *Chem.-Biol.Interactions 30*, 223-235.

Daley-Yates, P.T., (1985): The metabolites of platinum antitumour drugs and their biological significance, from *Biochemical Mechanisms of Platinum Antitumour Drugs*, Ed. by D.C.H. McBrien and T.F. Slater, IRL Press Limited, Oxford, England, 121-146.

Keppler B.K., Henn, M., Juhl, U.M., Berger, M.R., Niebl, R., and Wagner,F.E., (1989): New Ruthenium complexes for the treatment of cancer, *Progress in Clinical Biochemistry and Medicine*, Vol.10, SpringerVerlag Berlin, 41-69.

Kratz, F. and Messori, L., (1992), Spectral characterization of Ru(III) transferrin, *J. Inorg. Biochemistry*, submitted for publication February 1992.

Stjernholm, R.L., US patent 4590001 A 20, May 1986.

Takahashi K., Seki,T., Nishikawa, K., Minamide, S., Iwabuchi, M., Ono, M., Nagamine, S., and Horinishi, H., (1985): Antitumour activity and toxicity of serum protein bound platinum formed cisplatin, *Jpn.J.Cancer Res.(Gann)* 76, 68-74.

Metal Ions in Biology and Medicine, vol. 2. Eds. J. Anastassopoulou, Ph. Collery, J.C. Etienne, Th. Theophanides. John Libbey Eurotext, Paris © 1992, pp. 75-79

Alkali metal ion catalysis in nucleophilic displacement reactions at phosphorus centres

E. Buncel*, E.J. Dunn**, R. Nagelkerke*

* *Department of chemistry, Queen's University, Kingston, ON K7L 3N6 Canada.*
** *Department of Laboratory Medicine, St. Joseph's Hospital, Hamilton, ON L8N 4A6 Canada*

Among the most important biochemical reactions is the phosphoryl transfer reaction. The breakdown of adenosine triphosphate (ATP) provides the energy which allows the processes of synthesis, active transport, muscle action and nerve function to occur. Many of these reactions are catalysed by metal ions. For example, flavokinase catalyses the transfer of the gamma-phosphoryl group of ATP to riboflavin during the biosynthesis of the flavocoenzyme, FMN. The enzyme prefers Zn^{2+} for activity, likely using a bidentate Zn-ATP complex as substrate (1). Na, K-ATPase is a membrane-bound enzyme which catalyses the hydrolysis of ATP coupled to the transport of Na^{+} out of the cell and K^{+} into the cell. Phosphorylation of the enzyme by ATP occurs as an intermediate step and requires intracellular Mg^{2+} and Na^{+}. The dephosphorylation of the enzyme is accelerated by K^{+} (2). Similarly, (Ca^{2+}/Mg^{2+})-ATPase of the sarcoplasmic reticulum vesicles catalyses the hydrolysis of ATP couple to Ca^{2+} transport across membranes. The enzyme catalyses the hydrolysis of acetylphosphate in the presence of Mg^{2+} and is stimulated in the presence of Ca^{2+}. Addition of 20% DMSO to the reaction doubles the rate and addition of KCl increases the rate further (3).

The above examples show how important both mono- and divalent metal ions are in certain biochemical reactions. However, the mechanisms for catalysis of phosphoryl transfer reactions and the role that metal ions play in this catalysis are still not well understood.

Mechanistically, nucleophilic displacement reactions at a phosphoryl centre in compounds of the general structure 1, in which R_1 is an organic moiety much as alkyl (aryl) or alkoxy (aryloxy), R_2 may be an alkyl (aryl), alkoxy (aryloxy) or hydroxy, while X is a potential leaving group, can be classified as proceeding by either association or dissociative processes.

$$R_1-\overset{\overset{\displaystyle O}{\|}}{\underset{\underset{\displaystyle R_2}{|}}{P}}-X$$

1

The dissociative pathway is the elimination-addition or SN1(P) mechanism. For phosphates (2), the dissociative mechanism involves a monomeric metaphosphate intermediate (3) which then adds a nucleophile Y^- to give the products:

$$R-P(=O)(OH)-X \xrightarrow{-X^-,\ H^+} R-PO_2 \xrightarrow{+Y^-,\ H^+} R-P(=O)(OH)-Y \quad (1)$$

2 **3**

The associative pathway can involve a concerted displacement of X^- by Y^- SN2(P), or an addition-elimination mechanism with a discrete intermediate being formed:

$$R-P(=O)(R)-X \xrightarrow{Y^-} \left[Y\text{--}P(O)(R)(R)\text{--}X \right]^- \xrightarrow{-X^-} R-P(=O)(R)-Y \quad (2)$$

4 **5**

Catalysis by metal ions could occur by several different mechanisms. These include the metal ion acting as a strong Lewis acid which coordinates to and polarises the phosphoryl group, thus enhancing its reactivity. Hydrolysis of phosphate diesters is catalysed by Zn^{2+} and Mg^{2+} ions. This effect was explained as originating by polarization of the phosphoryl moiety making it more reactive towards nucleophilic attack. The catalysis is said to arise from stabilisation of the transition state leading to formation of a penta-coordinated intermediate (4). Complexation of metal ions with potential leaving groups was also proposed to explain the accelerated methanolysis of trialkylphosphates by Zn^{2+}, Hg^{2+}, Mg^{2+} and Pb^{2+} metal ions (5). Alternatively, the metal ion may, through coordination at a suitable centre in the substrate, promote the ionisation of the base, thereby increasing its nucleophilicity. As an example of metal ion promoted ionization of the base, the hydrolysis of phosphorylated pyridines is accelerated by Mg^{2+}, reportedly due to complexation of the substrate with Mg^{2+} and the greater nucleophilicity of $Mg(OH)^+$ compared to water (6).

Reported instances of catalysis of substitution reactions at phosphoryl centres by monovalent cations are much less common. We have been investigating alkali metal ion catalysis in nucleophilic displacement reactions at carbon, phosphorus and sulfur centres (7-14). Among these studies, we have reported catalysis by alkali metal ions of the nucleophilic displacement reaction of p-nitrophenyl diphenylphosphinate 6 with ethoxide ion (7,8) and phenoxide ion (9) in ethanol and tetraglyme (10) at 25°C, while similar studies with p-nitrophenyl diphenylphosphate, 7, are in progress.

$$Ph-P(=O)(Ph)-O-C_6H_4-NO_2 \qquad PhO-P(=O)(OPh)-O-C_6H_4-NO_2$$

6 **7**

The kinetic data for the reaction of 6 with lithium ethoxide (LiOEt), sodium ethoxide (NaOEt), potassium ethoxide (KOEt), and LiOEt and KOEt in the presence of metal ion complexing agents, in ethanol are presented in Figure 1. Qualitatively similar results have been obtain for the reaction of 7.

In ethanol there will be an equilibrium established between alkali metal ethoxide ion pairs and the dissociated ions (eq. 3). The cryptand and crown ether complexing agents complex the metal ions completely, separating the metal ion from the nucleophile and giving rise to what may be called "free" ethoxide ion (EtO^-). The data show that all of the metal ion ethoxides are more reactive than the free ethoxide ion, with the order of reactivity being LiOEt > NaOEt > KOEt > EtO^-.

$$MOEt \rightleftharpoons M^+ + EtO^- \qquad (3)$$

Figure 2 presents the kinetic data for the reaction of 6 with lithium phenoxide (LiOPh), sodium phenoxide (NaOPh), potassium phenoxide (KOPh), and benzyltrimethylammonium phenoxide (BTMAOPh) in ethanol at 25°C. The large benzyltrimethylammonium ion does not associate well with the phenoxide ion and does not catalyse the reaction. Lithium, however, is a more effective catalyst than either sodium or potassium. The downward curvature in these plots arises from a combination of phenoxide and ethoxide ion reactions (9).

The greater reactivity of the metal ion ethoxides and phenoxides relative to the reactivity of the nucleophile in the absence of metal ions, or in the presence of metal ion complexing agents, indicates participation of the metal ion in lowering the free energy of activation of the rate determining step. This participation could occur in several ways and these interactions are illustrated in Figure 3. Pre-equilibrium association of the metal ion with the substrate could make the substrate more susceptible to attack by the nucleophile, or facilitate the cleavage of the leaving group. It can be seen from Figure 3B, path b, that pre-association of the substrate with the metal ion may enhance the electrophilicity of the phosphoryl group by complexation of the P=O group by M^+ leading to a transition state ($AM^{\neq}$) which is stabilised relative to the uncatalysed reaction (path a).

Alternatively, the metal ion could associate with the nucleophile in such a way as to increase its reactivity. This would appear unlikely since pairing with the metal ion will lower the ground state energy of the nucleophile making it less reactive. However, association of the metal ion with the transition state of the reaction will also tend to lower the energy of the transition state and could account for the catalytic effect of the metal ion. Figure 3A, path b, illustrates that, providing the stabilisation of the transition state is greater than the stabilisation of the nucleophile ground state, catalysis could occur as a result of an overall lowering of the free energy of activation.

Table 1. Equilibrium constants for the association of alkali metal ion with ethoxide ion (K_a) and transition states (K'_a) for reactions of phosphorus enters 6 and 7

Metal ion	K_a M^{-1}	$K'_a(6)$ M^{-1}	$K'_a(7)$ M^{-1}
Li^+	212	5188	3071
Na^+	102	1207	1122
K^+	90	347	816

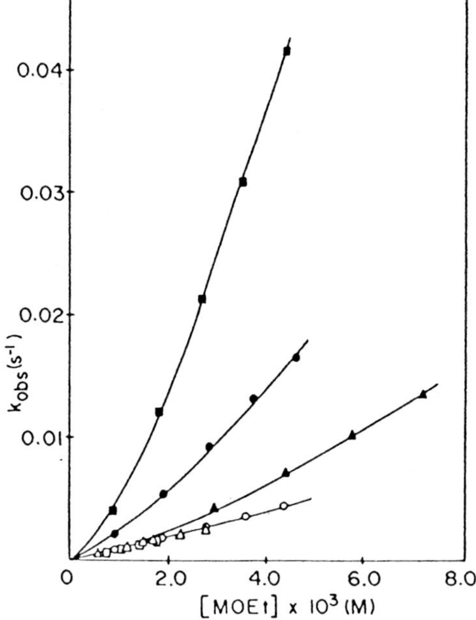

FIG. 1. Reaction of *p*-nitrophenyl diphenylphosphinate (6) with LiOEt (■), NaOEt (●), KOEt (▲); LiOEt plus excess [2.1.1]cryptand (□); NaOEt plus excess [2.2.2]cryptand (○); and with KOEt plus excess [2.2.2]cryptand (△), in EtOH at 25°C.

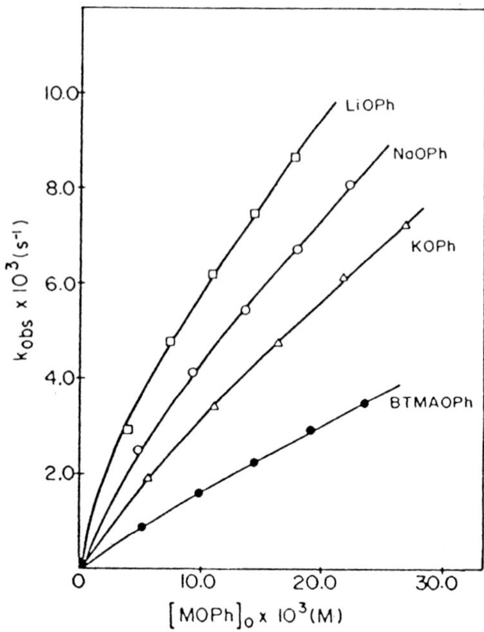

FIG. 2. Reaction of *p*-nitrophenyl diphenylphosphinate (6) with LiOPh (□), NaOPh (○), KOPh (△), and BTMAOPh (●) in EtOH at 25°C.

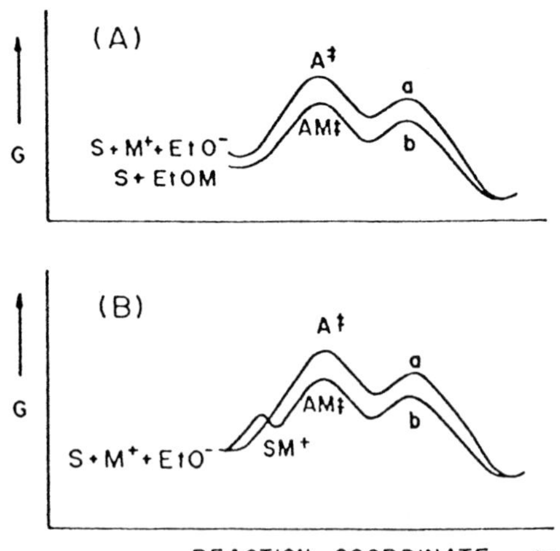

FIG. 3. (A) Path *a* illustrates the uncatalysed reaction of substrate (S) with EtO^-, while path *b* shows the lowering of both ground state and transition state free energies for the reaction of metal-alkoxide ion pairs due to association with M^+. (B) Catalysis by preassociation of M^+ with S is shown in path *b* while path *a* represents again the uncatalysed reaction.

Equilibrium constants for association of alkali metal ions with ethoxide ion and the transition states can be calculated from the experimental data (8). These data are presented in Table 1. The calculated equilibrium constants for the association of the alkali metal ions with the transition state are greater than the corresponding equilibrium constants for the association of the metals ions with the ethoxide ion. Thus, the tighter association of the transition state with the metal ion relative to the ground state, will result in catalysis of the reaction. The reasons for the strong interaction of the metal ion in the transition state are still unclear. It may, however, result from increased charge localisation in the transition state or by chelation of the metal ion by multiple charged centres in the transition state (8,9). We are currently engaged in theoretical studies in order to try to shed light on these questions.

Acknowledgement

We thank the Natural Sciences and Engineering Research Council of Canada for financial support of this research.

REFERENCES

1. Nakano, H., & McCormick, D.B. (1991): J. Biol. Chem., 266,22125.

2. Berberian, G., & Beauge, L. (1991): Biochim. Biophys Acta., 1063, 217.

3. Chini, E.N.; Montero-Lomeli, M., & de Meis, L. (1990): Biochim. Biophys. Acta. 1030, 152.

4. Steffens, J.J.; Sampson, E.J.; Siewers, I.J., & Benkovic, S.J. (1973): J. Am. Chem. Soc., 95, 936.

5. Wadsworth Jr., W.S. (1981): J. Org. Chem., 46, 4080.

6. Herschlag, D., & Jencks, W.P. (1990): Biochemistry, 29, 5172.

7. Buncel, E.; Dunn, E.J.; Bannard, R.A.B, & Purdon, J.G. (1984): J. Chem. Soc. Chem. Commun. 162.

8. Dunn, E.J., & Buncel, E. (1989): Can. J. Chem. 67, 1440.

9. Dunn, E.J.; Moir, R.Y.; Buncel, E.; Purdon, J.G. & Bannard, R.A.B. (1990): Can. J. Chem. 68, 1837.

10. Buncel, E.; Dunn, E.J.; Truong, Ng. van; Bannard, R.A.B., & Purdon, J.G. (1990): Tetrahedron Lett. 31, 6513.

11. Buncel, E., & Pregel, M.J. (1989): J. Chem. Soc. Chem.Commun. 1566.

12. Pregel, M.J.; Dunn, E.J., & Buncel, E. (1990): Can. J. Chem. 68, 1846.

13. Pregel, M.J.; Dunn, E.J., & Buncel, E. (1991): J.Am.Chem. Soc. 113, 3545.

14 Pregel, M.J., & Buncel, E. (1991). J.Org.Chem. 56, 5583.

Metal Ions in Biology and Medicine, vol. 2. Eds. J. Anastassopoulou, Ph. Collery, J.C. Etienne, Th. Theophanides. John Libbey Eurotext, Paris © 1992, pp. 80-83

Electrochemical and structural studies of manganese complexes different oxidation state as a model for photosystem II

László Nagy, Tamás Gajda, Toshio Yamaguchi, Kálmán Burger

Department of Inorganic and Analytical Chemistry, A. József University, H-6701 Szeged, P.O. Box 440, Hungary

Introduction

Manganese plays a significant role in biological systems of vital importance e.g. in photosystem II, superoxide dismutase. The biocatalytic behaviour of such macromolecules is mainly attributed to the presence of manganese in different oxidation states (+2, +3, +4) and its participation in the electron transfer processes. Although it is known that photosystem II contains four manganese ions, there are currently debates over whether the active center of water oxidation consists of a binuclear, trinuclear, or tetranuclear cluster of manganese ions.

If a dark-adapted sample of photosystem II is illuminated by short. intense flashes of light, so that a single charge separation takes place in each reaction center per flash, the yield of O_2 is found to be maximal on the third flash and to oscillate with a periodicity of four thereafter. To account for this result, Kok and co-workers proposed that photosystem II cycles through five states during flash illumination. Magers reported (Magers et. al. 1978) that the manganese(III)-catechol system reversibly binds molecular oxygen in non-aqueous media. This system seems to imitate the thermal step of the oxygen evolution model suggested by Kok et. al. for photosystem II. Our aim was to find a model of similar behaviour in aqueous solutions. We have started therefore the systematic electrochemical and structural studies of manganese complexes in different oxidation state formed with sugar type ligands.

Experimental

Manganese complexes of maltitol (4-O-α-glycopyranosyl-D-sorbitol), lactobionic acid and saccharose have been studied in aqueous alkaline solution by polarographic, potentiometric, pH-metric, spectrophotometric and ESR methods. Several complexes were prepared in solid state. Their composition was determined by standard analytical methods. The local structure of complexes was measured by EXAFS

(Extended X-ray Absorption Fine Stucture) method. EXAFS and XANES spectra were recorded in transmission mode using BL7C station at the Photon Factory in the National Laboratory for High Energy Physics (Japan).

Results and Discussion

The polarographic characteristics of manganese complexes studied together with the results of controlled-potential electrolysis data performed to assist the assignment of the polarographic waves to the corresponding electron transfer processes, are presented in Table 1.

Table 1
Polarographic characteristics of manganese complexes

Electrode processes	$E_{1/2}$ V vs. SCE for					
	lactobionate		saccharose		maltitol	
	complexes	n		n		n
Mn(II) — Mn(III)	-0.613	0.98	-0.477	1.02	-0.625	1.05
Mn(III) — Mn(IV)	-0.315		-		-0.347	
Mn(II) — Mn(0)	-0.670	1.97	-1.732	2.10	-1.715	1.90
Mn(IV) — Mn(III)	-0.320		-		-0.382	
Mn(III) — Mn(II)	-0.630		-0.474	0.99	-0.690	
Mn(II) - Mn(III) Mn(III) - Mn(III)	-		-0.493		-	

n = electron number changes obtained by conrolled potential electrolysis

The polarogram of manganese(II) in the presence of excess lactobionic acid (Nagy et al. 1985) or maltitol (Nagy et al. 1989) in alkaline media and in inert atmosphere exhibits two anodic and one cathodic wave. In analogous investigations with saccharose (Nagy et al. 1986) only one anodic and cathodic wave was observed. According to the controlled potential electrolysis data and some chemical evidences the cathodic waves can be assigned to the reduction of manganese(II) to manganese(0) and the anodic waves to the stepwise oxidation of manganese(II) to manganese(III) and manganese(IV). In alkaline media the manganese(II) complexes can also be oxidized by dioxygen, hydrogen-peroxide or potassium-ferri-cyanide to the corresponding manganese(III) and manganese(IV) complexes.

In the manganese-saccharose system a dimeric manganese(II,III) complex containing manganese in mixed oxidation state is also formed. This mixed valence complex could be oxidized gradually by the addition of dioxygen to the manganese(III). Storing the solution, containing the manganese(III) complex in an oxygen-free nitrogen atmosphere for 24 hours, the complex spontaneously reduced to the parent mixed valence complex. The whole procedure proved to be completly reversible and was repeated several times. Further investigations are planned to determine the mechanism of these processes. The main question is that whether the ligand reduced the manganese(III) complex or latter oxidised the water leading to the formation of dioxygen.

In the case of reversible electrode processes, polarography can be used to determine the composition of the complexes (metal:ligand::OH^- ratio) by measuring the half-wave potencial shift of the corresponding polarographic wave due to the complex formation process as a function of the hydroxide ion and the organic ligand concentrations. Knowing the composition of the complexes as well as the total concentrations of manganese, ligands and EDTA used as auxiliary ligand and the stability constants of the manganese(X)-EDTA complex (X = II or III) the corresponding conditional stability constants were determined by competition reaction. This method is based on the fact that all manganese EDTA complexes are polarographically inactive and the limiting current of the reduction wave of the complexes increases linearly according to the Ilkovic equation with manganese concentration.

The composition of the complexes and the correspondig conditional stability constants obtained by methods discussed above are summarized in Table 2.

Table 2

Overall conditional formation equilibrium constants (β complex products) of the manganese complexes

Composition of the complexes	logβ
$[Mn^{II}L(OH)_2]^{2-}$	13.0
$[Mn^{II}S(OH)_2Mn^{III}S(OH)_4]^-$	37.0
$[Mn^{III}S_2(OH)_8]^{2-}$	51.9
$[Mn_2^{II}M_3(OH)_4]^{6-}$	27.2
$[Mn_2^{III}M_3(OH)_6]^{6-}$	52.0

where L, S and M represented the lactobionate, saccharose and maltitol ligand respectively.

EPR and UV spectroscopic data indicated the dimerization of the manganese(II)-saccharose and maltitol complexes in slightly alkaline media. The EPR spectrum of the aqueous solution of manganese(II) and ligands (pH 6) showed 6 lines of almoust the same intensity which corresponds to the 5/2 nuclear spin of manganese. Increasing the pH of this solution by adding sodium hydroxide in an inert atmosphere did not cause any change in the pattern of the spectrum till pH$\sim$10; only its intensity decreased. The further increase of pH resulted, however, in significant changes. At pH 10,4 the intensity of the six-line pattern decreased further then started to be transformed into a broad curve. The latter increased in intensity with increasing pH of the solution, becoming dominant in strongly alkaline media where the six line pattern completly disappeared.

This change in the EPR signal indicated that due to the increase of the pH in the solution, the manganese(II) complex dimerized, resulting in a decrease in the number of unpaired electrons.

The solid complexes were prepared according to the basic prescriptions presented in (Nagy et al. 1989). The EXAFS data collection and the data reduction procedure is described in the same literature. The EXAFS and XANES spectra supported the distorted octahedral structure of both manganese(III)- and manganese(IV)-carbohydrate complexes with a mean Mn(III)-O and Mn(IV)-O distances 207 and 209 pm respectively irrespective of the conformation of ligands. All of the complexes are dimeric. The Mn-Mn distance is of about 280 pm, which is in good agreement with numerous structurally characterized di-μ-oxo-bridged binuclear and tetranuclear manganese complexes (Brudvig, et al. 1989), as well as with Mn-Mn distance (270 pm) in both the S_1 and S_2 states of photosystem II measured by EXAFS (Brudvig et al. 1989).

References

Brudvig, G.W., and Crabtree, R.H. (1989): Bioinorganic Chemistry of Manganese Related to Photosynthetic oxygen evolution: in Progress in Inorganic Chemistry Vol. 37. Ed. S.J. Lippart pp. 100-142. John Wiley and Sons.

Magers, K.D., Smith, C.G., and Sawyer, D.T. (1978): Reversible binding of dioxygen by Tris(3,5-di-terc-butylcatecholato)manganese(III) in dimethyl sulfoxide. J. Am. Chem. Soc., 100, 989-991.

Nagy, L., Horváth, I., and Burger, K. (1985): The electrochemical investigation of the manganese complexes of lactobionic acid. Inorg. Chim Acta, 107, 179-185.

Nagy, L., Gajda, T., Páli, T., and Burger, K. (1986): Saccharose complexes of manganese in different oxidation states. Inorg. Chim. Acta, 123, 35-40.

Nagy, L., Gajda, T., Páli, T., and Burger, K. (1988): Electrochemical and spectroscopic study of the maltitol complexes of manganese in different oxidation states. Acta Chim. Hung., 125, 403-414.

Nagy, L., Yamaguchi, T., Nomura, M., and Ohtaki, H. (1989): EXAFS and XANES studies of iron(III) complexes of sugar--type ligands. Inorg. Chim. Acta, 159, 201-209.

Nagy, L., Yamashita, S. Nomura, M., Yamaguchi, T. and Wakita, H. (1992): EXAFS and XANES studies of manganese(III) and manganese(IV) complexes of sugar-type ligands. To be published in J. Chem. Soc. Dalton Trans.

Metal Ions in Biology and Medicine, vol. 2. Eds. J. Anastassopoulou, Ph. Collery, J.C. Etienne, Th. Theophanides. John Libbey Eurotext, Paris © 1992, pp. 84-85

Famotidine, antiulcerogenic agent and a potent ligand for metal ions

Henryk Kozlowski*, Teresa Kowalik-Jankowska*, Jolanta Swiatek**, Jan Spychala**, Abdellah Anouar***, Patrick Decock***, Maria-Luisa Ganadu****

** Institute of Chemistry, University of Wroclaw, F. Joliot-Curie 14, 50383 Wroclaw, Poland. ** Dept. of Basic Medical Sciences, Medical Academy of Wroclaw, Wroclaw, Poland. *** Université de Lille I, 59655 Villeneuve d'Ascq, France. **** Dipt. di Chimica, Universita di Sassari, 07100 Sassari, Italy*

Famotidine (1) is known as an anti-ulcer drug having excellent histamine H_2

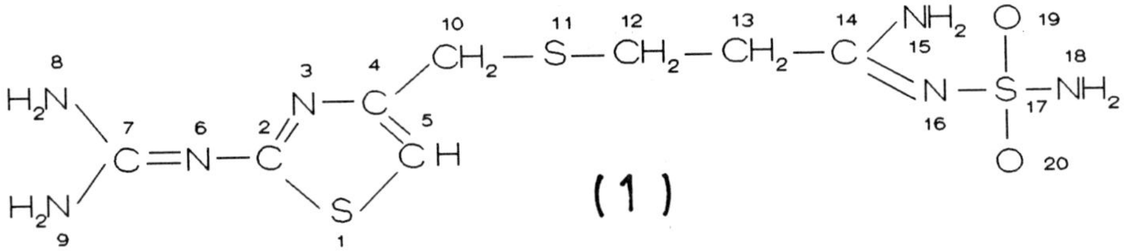

(1)

receptor blocking effect similar to that of cimetidine. The latter drug was shown to interfere with metal ions, especially with copper, although the computer-simulated distributions of the involved complexes did not show any important impact of this drug on the bioavailability of essential metal ions (Freijanes & Berthon, 1986). Recent work of Kimura et al. (1986) has shown that Cu-cimetidine complexes exhibit unusually high superoxide dismutase activity. Even if the co-ordination ability of cimetidine are not very potent the biological implications of the metal drug complexation may be quite important although still unknown.

Famotidine, recent analog of cimetidine, contains potentially more effective donor sets including sulfamide moiety with two nitrogen atoms and guanidine group with very effective basic nitrogen donors.

Potentiometric data indicate that famotidine (HL) contains one dissociable proton with pK = 6.86 which corresponds to the protonation of the thiazole ring nitrogen. this value is close to that found for imidazole ring of cimetidine (pK = 6.70, Akrivos et al., 1984).

According to spectroscopic, potentiometric and polarographic results the binding of cupric ions with famotidine starts already at pH below 2. The stability constants (Table 1) are much higher than those of the cimetidine complexes suggesting very different binding modes served by both drugs (Kozlowski et al., 1992). The thermodynamic and spetroscopic data allow to suggest that the metal ion co-ordination begins at the sulfamide terminal ($\{N^{15},N^{18}\}$), then it involves thiazole ring nitrogen and vicinal thioether sulfur ({N^{15},N^3,S}), and at high pH also the guanidine nitrogen ({N^{15},N^3,N^8}), respectively. This co-ordination pattern involving three different donor sets at different pH ranges causes that famotidine is very effective chelating agent for cupric ions at any medium and it can compete with so powerful low molecular wieght ligands as histine or histamine.

In order to check this possibility we have performed also the studies on the ternary systems: Cu(II)-famotidine-histidine and Cu(II)-famotidine-histamine. The obtained results collected in Table 1 clearly indicate that the only complexes formed at pH above 4 are the ternary systems. Histamine or even histidine are not able to remove famotidine from the co-ordination sphere of metal ion at any pH range. The formed ternary complexes are very stable and it is very likely that the presence of famotidine in biological systems may affect considerably the behavior of Cu(II) ions in physiological fluids.

Table 1. Stability constants (logβ) for binary and ternary Cu(II) complexes with famotidine. Standard deviations are given in parentheses. L = famotidine, L'= histidine.

binary species M L H	logβ	ternary species M L L'H	logβ
0 1 1	6.86(0.01)		
1 1 0	7.27(0.02) 7.37(0.02)*	1 1 1 0	17.46(0.03)
1 2 0	14.03(0.01) 13.95(0.02)*	1 1 1-1	18.90(0.06)
1 2-1	7.79(0.01)	1 1 1-2	3.34(0.06)
1 2-2	0.90(0.01)		
1 2-3	-6.92(0.01)		

* stability obtained from polarographic data

REFERENCES

Akrivos, F., Blais, M.J., Hoffelt, J., and Berthon, G.,(1984), An assessment of the physiological significance of cimetidine interactions with copper and zinc in biofluids as based on the computer-simulated distribution of the involved complexes at therapeutic levels of the drug. Agents Actions,15 649-659

Freijanes, E., and Berthon, G., (1986), Biological significance of cimetidine sulfoxide complexes with copper(II) and zinc(II) ions during cimetidine treatment. Inorg.Chim.Acta, 124, 141-147

Kimura, E., Koike, T., Shimuzu, Y., and Kodama, M., (1986) Complexes of histamine H_2 antagonist cimetidine with divalent and monovalent copper ions. Inorg.Chem. 25, 2242-2246

Kozlowski, H., Kowalik-Jankowska, T., Anouar, A., Decock, P., Spychala, J., Swiatek, J., and Ganadu, M-L., (1992): Famotidine, the new antiulcerogenic agent, a potent ligand for metal ions., J.Inorg.Biochem. in press

Metal Ions in Biology and Medicine, vol. 2. Eds. J. Anastassopoulou, Ph. Collery, J.C. Etienne, Th. Theophanides. John Libbey Eurotext, Paris © 1992, p. 86

Labcatal and the research on trace elements

Laboratoire LABCATAL, 7, rue Roger-Salengro, B.P. 305,
92541 Montrouge Cedex, France

The concept of catalytic oligotherapy at moderate doses was introduced by **LABCATAL** 40 years ago with the range of its specialties : the OLIGOSOLS®. It is now developing a metallotherapy based on pharmacological doses such as lithium in psychiatry (NEUROLITHIUM®), zinc in dermatology (RUBOZINC®), and a combination of copper and manganese for topical use (OLIGODERM®) that has just been marketed.

LABCATAL has four priorities : collaboration with hospitals and universities, communication with the physicians who prescribe its medicines, dialogue at international level and fundamental research.

An important part of **LABCATAL** turnover is devoted to research on trace elements : pharmacological and clinical trials, epidemiological and nutritional studies.

Among other things **LABCATAL** has shown the interest of zinc in inflammatory acne, and is now widening its field of interest for this metal : immunity of the elderly with Professor PRASAD (Detroit), allergology with Professor ABDULLA (New-Delhi), and rhumatology with Professors NEVE and PERETZ (Brussels).

LABCATAL has recently created 'ARIZE', an association of hospital pediatricians, whose aim is to promote and award research work in biological and clinical aspects of zinc in child and adolescent pathology.

Encouraging research on trace elements and developing irreproachable pharmaceutical specialties are the challenge of **LABCATAL.**

Metal Ions in Biology and Medicine, vol. 2. Eds. J. Anastassopoulou, Ph. Collery, J.C. Etienne, Th. Theophanides. John Libbey Eurotext, Paris © 1992, pp. 87-88

Polymorphonuclear neutrophils aggregation induced by endothelin in presence and in absence of Ca and Mg

Manuel Guerra, Jesús F. Escanero, Jesús Villanueva, Jesús Egido*

*Departemento de Fisiología. Facultad de Medicina, Universidad de Zaragoza, 50009 Zaragoza, Spain. * Servicio de Nefrología, Fundación Jiménez Diaz, 2840 Madrid, Spain*

Introduction. Endothelin (ET) is a newly described polipeptide that has been isolated in the culture of porcine aortic endothelial cells (Yanagisawa et al., 1988). The effects of human-porcine ET (ET-1) on the polymorphonuclear neutrophils (PMN) are unexplored. We have now studied the activity of ET-1 from PMN of volunteer healthy and we tested the "in vitro" effects of this polipeptide on PMN aggregation.

Materials and methods. Endothelin was obtained from Peninsula labs. (U.K.), verapamil from Koll labs., platelet activating factor (PAF), 8-(n,n-diethylamino)-octyl-3,4,5-trimethoxybenzoate hydrochloride (TMB-8), and neomicyn were from Sigma Chemical Co. Polymorphonuclear neutrophils were obtained from fresh venous blood of healthy adults donors, anticoagulated wiht EDTA 0.2 M. They were separated from mononuclear cells and residual erythrocytes through Monopoly Resolving Medium (Flow lab.). Blood was centrifuged at 300 x g for 30 minutes. Polymorphonuclear neutrophils were drased and used at 10^7 cel/ml for aggregation. Buffers used were: without Ca^{++} and Mg^{++}, 10 mM N-2-hydroxyethyl piperazine-N-2-ethanesulfonic acid (Hepes), pH 7.4; and with Ca^{++} and Mg^{++}, Kreb's Ringer phosphate (KRP), pH 7.4. Both buffers contained 0.25 g/dl bovine serum albumin (BSA). Aggregation was performed in a 2 Kanal-aggregometer Labor, 100 mvolt. The PMNs were stirred at 800 rpm during all experiment. The results were expressed in percentage of transmission, calculated respect to KRP (100 %). As positive control for aggregation was used PAF 10^{-7} and 10^{-8} M final concentration (FC). Negative control was the basal aggregation without inducers. Endothelin was used at doses 10^{-7}, 10^{-8}, 10^{-9}, 10^{-10} and 10^{-11} M (FC). In order to investigate the action mechanism of ET, it was tried to block the aggregation of PMN with neomicyn 200 μM (FC), an aminoglycoside antibiotic that strongly binds polyphosphoinositides and inhibits the phospholipase C, and to analyze the variations of the PMN aggregation with verapamil 10^{-4} M (FC), a Ca++ channel antagonist and TMB8 65 μM (FC), an inhibitor of Ca^{++} releasing from the intracellular store sites.

Results. The aggregation induced by ET-1 was dose-related reaching the plateau at 10^{-8} M. The aggregation was already observed at 30 sec, increasing until the 3rd min; between the 3rd and the 10th min the increase was only of 2 %.

basal	ET^{-7} M	ET^{-8} M	ET^{-9} M	ET^{-10} M	ET^{-11} M
11.8 ± 2	22.3 ± 2 *	40.8 ± 3 *	19 ± 2 *	15.5 ± 1	12.6 ± 2
PAF 10^{-7} M control: 76 ± 5*			PAF 10^{-8} M control: 48.3 ± 5*		

Table 1. Percentaje of human PMN aggregation after 10 min of the beginning of the experiment in a Ca^{++} buffer and different concentration of ET-1. Data are mean ± SEM, n = 3 to 20. * = p<0.05 with respect to baseline values.

	Ca free	TMB8	TMB8 Ca free	Verapamil	Neomicyn
PAF^{-8} M	28 ± 2 *	31 ± 13	19 ± 11 *		31 ± 9
ET^{-8} M	27 ± 3 *	24 ± 8 *	16 ± 3 *	26 ± 1 *	32 ± 4 **

Table 2. Percentaje of human PMN aggregation after 10 min of the beginning of the experiment in a Ca^{++} free buffer, TMB8 with and without Ca^{++}, Verapamil and Neomicyn. Data are mean ± SEM, n = 3 to 7. * = $p<0.05$, ** = $p<0.1$ with respect to calcium values.

Discussion. The percentage of PMN aggregation in the groups with ET at dose of 10^{-7}, 10^{-8} and 10^{-9} M with Ca^{++} and with ET at dose of 10^{-8} M without Ca^{++} show a significant ($p<0.05$) increase in relation to the basal values. On the same way there is also a significant ($p<0.05$) increase between the basal group and the groups PAF $10^{-7}/10^{-8}$ M with Ca^{++} and PAF 10^{-8} M without Ca^{++}. The effect described is produced in a similar range of concentration that the required by other effects (Hirata et al., 1988).

The mechanism of action of this vasoconstrictor is at present controversial. Based on its homology with a group of calcium channel agonists, and the observation that endothelin-induced contraction was inhibited by removal of extracellular Ca^{++}, ET was proposed to induce contraction by stimulating Ca^{++} influx trough voltage-dependent ion channels (Yanagisawa et al. 1988). Auget et al. have reported that the ET response have two components, one dependent and the other independent of Ca^{++} influx (Auget et al., 1988). Others authors (Muldoon et al., 1989; Griendling et al., 1989) have shown that ET induced stimulation of phosphatidilinositol turnover, producing inositoltriphosphate, which has been show to promote mobilization of Ca^{++} from intracellular stores. The study of ET action mechanims showed that the absence of Ca^{++} in the medium and/or the addition of TMB8 produced a significant decrease of the PMN aggregation in groups with Ca^{++} and ET 10^{-8} ($p<0.05$). The addition of verapamil decrease the percentage of aggregation ($p<0.05$), and there is not significative difference between the basal group and groups with verapamil and ET 10^{-8} without Ca^{++}, TMB8 and ET 10^{-8} without Ca^{++} and basal TMB8.

The addition of neomicyn decrease the platelet aggregation in groups with Ca^{++} and ET ($p<0.01$) and this group shows significative differences in relation to the basal ($p<0.05$). We observe a partial inhibition of ET-1 aggregation produced by neomicyn, suggesting a possible implication of phospholipase C in these mechanisms.

Acknowledgments. This work has been supported by the grant nº 91/1231 from Fondo de Investigaciones Sanitarias de la Seguridad Social (FISss).

References.

Auguet, M., Delaflotte, S., Chabrier, P.E., Pirotzky, E., Clostre, F. and Braquet, P. (1988): Endothelin and Ca^{++} agonist bay K 8644: Different vasoconstrictive properties. *Biochem. Biophys. Res. Commun.* 156, 186-192.

Griendling, K.K., Tsuda, T. and Alexander, R.W. (1989): Endothelin stimulates diacylglycerol accumulation and activates protein kinase C in cultured vascular smooth muscle cells. *J. Biol. Chem.* 246, 8237-8240.

Hirata, Y., Yoshimi, H., Takata, S., Watanabe, T.X., Kumagai, S., Nakajima, K. and Sakakibara, S. (1988): Cellular mechanism of action by a novel vasoconstrictor endothelin in cultured rat vascular smooth muscle cells. *Biochem. Biophys. Res. Commun.* 154, 868-875.

Muldoon, L.L., Rodlan, K.D., Forsythe, M.L. and Magun, B.E. (1989): Stimulation of phosphatidylinositol hydrolysis, diacylglycerol release, and gene expression in response to endothelin, a potent new agonist for fibroblasts and smooth muscle cells. *J. Biol. Chem.* 264, 8529-8536.

Yanagisawa, M., Kurihara, H., Kimura, S., Tomobe, Y., Kobayashi, M., Mitsui, Y., Yazaki, Y., Goto, K. and Masaki, T. (1988): A novel potent vasoconstrictor peptide produced by vascular endothelial cells. *Nature.* 232, 411-415.

Metal Ions in Biology and Medicine, vol. 2. Eds. J. Anastassopoulou, Ph. Collery, J.C. Etienne, Th. Theophanides. John Libbey Eurotext, Paris © 1992, pp. 89-90

Zinc exchange between erythrocytes and a medium with and without albumin at different temperatures

Mercedes Gálvez, Luis M. Elósegui, Manuel Guerra*, Jose A. Moreno, Jesús F. Escanero

*Departamento de Bioquímica Clínica, Hospital Clínico Universitario, Avenida San Juan Bosco, s/n, 50 009 Zaragoza, Spain. * Facultad de Medicina, Calle Domingo Miral, s/n, 50 009 Zaragoza, Spain*

Introduction. Albumin is the protein with higher levels in serum or plasma. It has several functions concerning with the maintenance of the osmotic pressure, protein storage or carrier of different, exogenous and endogenous, ligands (Kragh-Hansen, 1981). The ligand hypothesis postulates that the biological activity of the ligand "in vivo" may be predicted by measuring the concentration of free ligand "in vitro" (Recant and Riggs, 1952). This paper intends to analyze the zinc (Zn) exchange between erythrocytes and a medium with and without albumin at different temperatures with the aim of examining the rol of the albumin in this exchange.

Material and methods. Human erythrocytes washed 5 times with NaCl 0.9 % and with leucocytes concentrations less than 1.100/µl were used in his experiment. Aliquots of two ml of erythrocytes were incubated with eigth ml of the different media used (hematocrit about 14-16 %). Before the experiment the erythrocytes were preincubated for 15 minutes and determinations were performed 15 minutes and 1, 2, 4 and 6 hours after the beginning of the experiment. The buffer was MOPS-TRIZMA (10 mM), pH 7.4, with $MgCl_2$ 75 mM, glucose 10 mM, sacarose 85 mM. Osmolarity ranged in all solutions at physiological level. Some aliquots were added with bovine serum albumin (BSA) 0.2 mg/dl. The final media, with and without BSA, contained 100, 500 or 1000 µg/dl of Zn ($ZnCl_2$). The experiments were performed at three different temperatures: 4, 20 and 37º C. The Zn levels were determined by atomic absorption spectrophotometry (Thermo Jharrell Ash) and the ultrafiltrable (UF) element were performed by serum centrifugation in ultrafiltrable cones (centricon 30 -Amicon-). The SIGMA programme by the statistical treatment was used in a compatible computer.

Results. The results obtained in the times indicated (1000 µg/dl of Zn and 37ºC) are shown in the table 1 and the variations for the different temperatures studied (1000 µg/dl and 4 hours) are reported in table 2.

Medium (1000 µg/dl)	Zinc uptake by erythrocytes 15 min.	1 h	2 h	4 h	6 h
With BSA	7.1	28.0	44.0	57.0	64.6
Without BSA	21.6	61.0	78.0	90.6	94.5
% of Zn uptaked*	34	133	209.5	271.5	308.7

* Percentage of UF element is taken as 100%.

Table 1. Percentage (mean) of Zn uptake by erythrocytes at 37ºC in the indicated times (n = 3 to 5). In the lower part of the table is represented the percentage of Zn transfered to the erythrocytes in relation with the UF element.

Medium (1000 µg/dl)	Temperature (º C) 4	25	37
With BSA	10.6	36.1	56.8
Without BSA	20.6	67.0	90.6
....			
% of ZnUF	16.0	-	20.9

Table 1. Percentage (mean) of Zn transfer by erythrocytes at the indicated temperatures (n = 3 to 5) 4 hours after the beginning of the experiment. In the lower part of the table is represented the percentage of Zn UF.

Discussion. For several decades it has been thought that the binding of different substances to the albumin provoked a decrese in their cellular uptake, lastly it has been observed that the fatty acids, steroids hormones, dyes, etc. bound to the albumin are transported much more efficiently than could be expected by a simple transport model constructed on the traditional teaching that only spontaneously dissociated ligand is available for uptake (Weisiger et al., 1989; Pardridge, 1987; Forker and Luxon, 1985). Our experiments show that the albumin difficults the Zn uptake by erythrocytes when the media, with and without albumin, of equimolar concentration are compared; but when only the percentage of UF element is considered, the total of Zn transfered to the erythrocytes is higher than the total existent of the UF element. By the other hand the temperature increases the Zn uptake by the erythrocytes more efficiently in the medium without albumin. Finally, as it is well known, the temperature increases the percentage of UF element, but these increases are less than the increases of the transfer of Zn induced by the temperature.

Acknowledgments. This work has been supported by the grant nº 90/211-04 from Universidad de Zaragoza.

REFERENCES.

Forker, E.L. and Luxon B.A. (1985): Effects of unstirred Disse fluid, nonequilibrium binding, and surface-mediated dissociation on hepatic removal of albumin-bound organic anions. Am. J. Physiol. 248, G709-G717.

Kragh-Hansen, U. (1981): Molecular aspects of ligand bindig to serum albumin. Pharmacol. Rev. 33, 17-54.

Pardridge, W.M. (1987): Plasma protein-mediated transport of steroid and thyroid hormones. Am. J. Physiol. 252, E157-E164.

Recant, T.L.and Riggs, D.S. (1952): Thyroid function in nephrosis. J. Clin. Invest. 31, 789-797.

Weisiger, R.A., Pond, S.M. and Bass, L. (1989): Albumin enhances unidirectional fluxes of fatty acid across a lipid-water interface: theory and experiments. Am. J. Physiol. 257, G904-G916.

Metal Ions in Biology and Medicine, vol. 2. Eds. J. Anastassopoulou, Ph. Collery, J.C. Etienne, Th. Theophanides. John Libbey Eurotext, Paris © 1992, p. 91

Cu (II) complexes with functionalized β-cyclodextrins having sod-like activity

R.F. Bonomo*, E. Conte**, E. Rizzarelli**, G. Vecchio*

** Dipartimento di Scienze Chimiche, Universita' di Catania, viale Andrea Doria 8 CT 95125, Italy. ** Istituto per lo Studio delle Sostanze Naturali di Interesse Alimentare e Chimico-Farmaceutico, CNR, via Reclusorio del Lume 8 Valverde (CT), Italy*

There is a growing interest about synthetic compounds wich are able to mimick some natural enzymes present in biological systems.

In this context the functionalization of cyclodextrins with moieties able to coordinate metal ions is a very useful approach aiming at mimicking metallo-enzymes (1).

Accordingly, we have synthesized ß-cyclodextrins with one or two coordinanting residues (2,3) and have also investigated their copper(II) complexes, a potential SOD-mimiking systems.

The copper(II) complexes of ß-cyclodextrins, functionalized in the 6 position with 1,4,10,13-tetraoxo-7,16-diazacyclooctadecane (cyclam) or with N,N di-n-propyl-L-Phenylalanyl (PheNN$_3$), have been characterized by e.p.r. spectroscopy.

We have also studied the Cu(II) complexes of some ß-cyclodextrins having in position 6 either two histamines or two 2-picolylamine or two cyclo-histidyl-histidyl. For each system the three possible isomers (A,B; A,C; A,D) have been characterized.

SOD activity has been determined by the indirect method originally developed by Beauchamp and Fridovicth (4).

Our results suggest a correlation between the structure of the complexes in solution and SOD activity, and point a synergistic effect due the contemporary presence of cyclodextrin hydrophobic cavity and the coordinanting moieties.

REFERENCES.

1.R. Breslow,(1986) *Adv. Enzymol. Related. Areas Mol. Biol. 58,1.*
2.R. F. Bonomo, V. Cucinotta, F. D'Alessandro, G. Maccarrone, G. Impellizzeri, G. Vecchio, E. Rizzarelli (1991) *Inorg. Chem, 31, 2708.*
3.V. Cucinotta, F. D'Alessandro, G. Impellizzeri, G. Pappalardo, E. Rizzarelli and G. Vecchio, (1991) *J. Chem. Commun. 293.*
4.C. Beauchamp and I.Fridovich, (1971) *Analytical Biochemistry, 44, 276*

Metal Ions in Biology and Medicine, vol. 2. Eds. J. Anastassopoulou, Ph. Collery, J.C. Etienne, Th. Theophanides. John Libbey Eurotext, Paris © 1992, pp. 92-93

Laser raman spectroscopic study of the growth-modulating tripeptide glycil-L-histidyl-L-lysine free and bound to copper (II) - ion

Christine Pujol*, Maurice Berjot*'**, Françoise Charton*, Jean Marx**, Alain J.P. Alix*'**

*Laboratoire de Spectroscopies et Structures Biomoléculaires. * INSERM U. 314, CHR Maison Blanche, 45, rue Cognacq Jay, 51092 Reims Cedex. ** Faculté des Sciences, B.P. 347, 51062 Reims Cedex, France*

Human plasma contains approximatively 1 µg / ml of Cu(II). Growth-modulating peptides that bind transition metals as Cu(II) are relatively small peptides. Moreover, it is possible that families of chelating peptides exist.

A synthetic tripeptide Glycyl-L-histidyl-L-lysine (GHK), which is analogous in composition to the growth-promoting peptide contained in the plasma, possesses bioactivities which are comparable to those of the human serum factor.

Bioactivity associated with GHK may be due to the complex formed, before interaction with cells, with Cu(II) :

- GHK can remove Cu(II) from the Cu(II) - Albumin complex very effectively at neutral pH ;
- it acts as a Copper transport factor and enhanced the uptake of the metal into cultivated cells.
- glycyl and histidyl residues function as Cu(II) chelators whereas lysine seems to be only involved in bioactivity (recognition process).

The X-ray study of the solid crystal of GHK showed the existence of a tridentate bonding structure involving the imidazole group, the α - amino group, the peptide nitrogen atom and two oxygen bridges in a square pyramidal distorted polyhedron Copper(II) coordination site and an helical polymeric form.

Aqueous solutions of the binary system GHK / Cu(II) are strongly pH-dependent structures (multiple species distribution; monomeric, mononuclear Cu(II) complexes). At medium pH range, Cu(II) is described as to be ligated to the tripeptide through one oxygen atom and three nitogens atoms coordinating to the central Cu(II) ion in a square planar configuration.

In view of the broad potential physiological role of GHK, with and without the presence of the Cu(II) ion the one hand, and the ambiguous description of its molecular structure, as it exists in aqueous solution at a given pH range, on the other, LASER Visible RAMAN spectrocopic studies were undertaken in order

- to obtain the structural characterization of the free or bound GHK in the solid state and in aqueous solutions (in particular: importance of histidyl residues as Cu(II) ion binding site),
- to precise structure - function (activity) relationships.

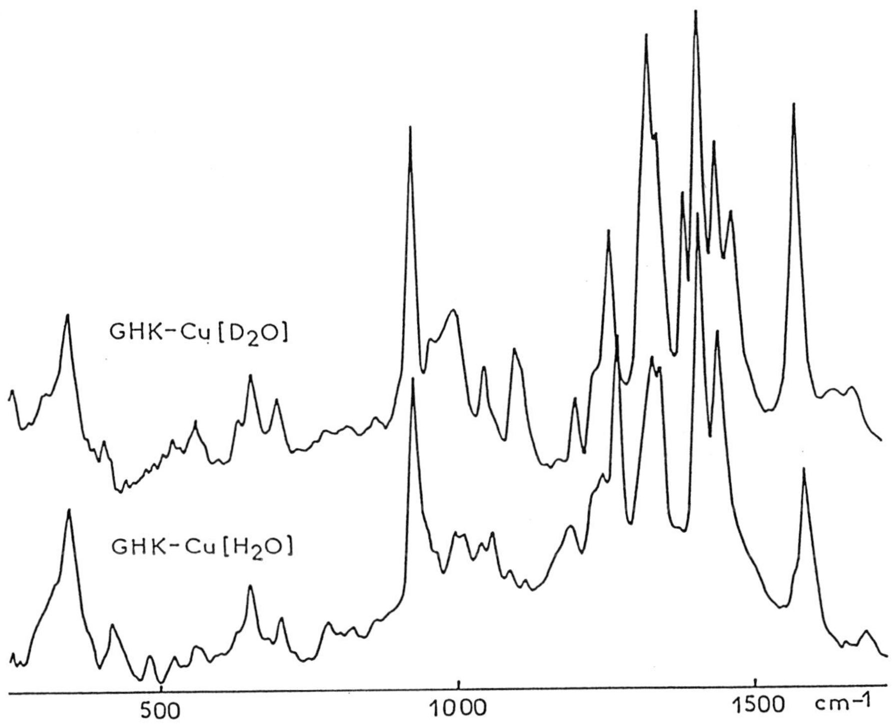

Fig. 1. Laser-visible Raman spectra of the tripeptide GHK bound to Cu(II) in solution in ultra pure H_2O (pH ≈ 5.5) and D_2O in the range 300 - 1700 cm^{-1} with the spectrum of the solvent subtracted and the base line corrected. Excitation line 457.9 nm, power 500 mW slit width 6 cm-1; room temperature; time averaging is over 8 scans (steps of 2 cm^{-1}, counting time 2 s per step).

So we recorded the first LASER - Visible - RAMAN spectra of the tripeptide GHK, free and bound to Cu(II), in the solid state (powder) and in H_2O and D_2O solutions respectively (see Fig. 1.).

Thus, spectroscopic structural informations are discussed in details :

(i) comparison of solid and solution spectra of the free tripeptide shows no characteristic difference regarding the conformation of the peptide;

(ii) comparison of solid spectra of the free and bound tripeptide reveals some new characteristic bands assigned to the binding of the copper ion; these spectroscopic data are consistent with the crystal structure as determined by X-ray crystallography;

(iii) comparison of solid and aqueous solution (H_2O and/or D_2O) spectra of the tripeptide bound to Cu(II) reveals large differen ces in the low frequency range (200 - 450 cm^{-1}); this clearly indicates different types of binding of the ion to the peptide; a first semi - quantitative analysis of our Raman spectroscopic data is consistent with a planar O - Cu - N_3 configuration.

Thanks are due to Pr BOREL and Pr MACQUART from Université de REIMS for their generous gifts of GHK and GHK-copper(II)-hydrate. C.P. is recipient of a Bourse Région Champagne-Ardennes.

Metal Ions in Biology and Medicine, vol. 2. Eds. J. Anastassopoulou, Ph. Collery, J.C. Etienne, Th. Theophanides. John Libbey Eurotext, Paris © 1992, pp. 94-95

Raman spectra of copper complexes with long chain diamines

J.D. Anastassopoulou*, A.J.P. Alix**, M. Berjot, J. Marx**, C.M. Paleos***, Th. Theophanides*

** National Technical University of Athens, Laboratory of Radiation Chemistry-Biospectroscopy, Zografou Campus, Zografou 157 73, Athens, Greece. ** UFR des Sciences Exactes et Naturelles de Reims, B.P. 347, 51062 Reims Cedex. *** Nuclear Center « Demokritos », Agia Paraskevi, 153 10 Athens, Greece*

Metal ion complexes of long chain methylene diamines of the formula $CuL_2(H_2O)_22NO_3$ with $L=NH_2-(CH_2)_n-NH_2$, where n=10,12 are interesting to study as a probe to conformational changes induced to the chain by complexation of the terminal amine groups with the metal. The compounds were studied by Raman spectroscopy. Conformational information concerns the $-CH_2-$ chain geometry (Levin). The structures of the complexes may be a polymeric network (Paleos), where the copper ions link several diamines together (Fig.1).

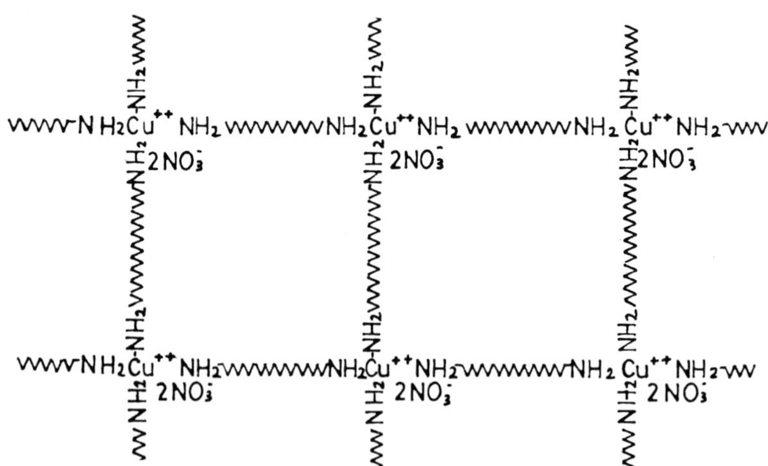

Fig.1. Proposed structure of the copper complexes.

The Raman spectra of the complexes show considerable intensity changes in the 3100-800 cm^{-1} region. The intensity variations of the $-CH_2-$ symmetric and antisymmetric stretching give information on packing and conformational details of the $-CH_2$-groups. Decomposition of the $\nu(CH_2)$ band gives several peaks due to order/disorder packing properties of the new materials. These properties are obtained by the intensity ratios I(2930)/I(2884) and I(2850)/I(2884). The total intensity of the ν(CH) band could be obtained by at least 6 or 7 components or strong peaks. The same components have been also found for the C12-diamine. The region of interest is the 1700-900 cm^{-1}, where the ν(C-C) bands are observed (Fig. 2&3). The two strong Raman

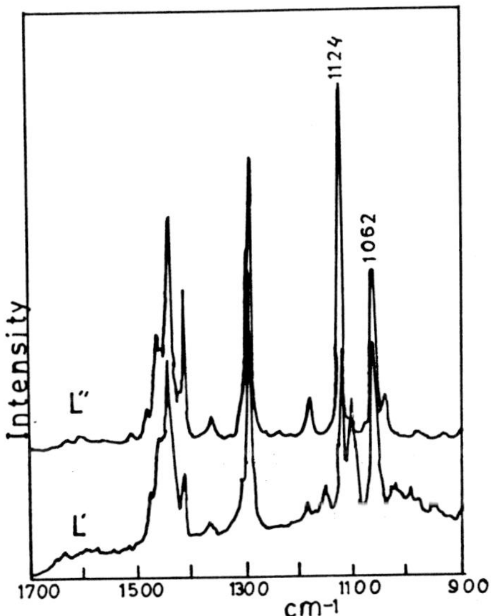

Fig.2. Raman spectra of diamines, L':$NH_2(CH_2)_{10}NH_2$, L":$NH_2(CH_2)_{12}NH_2$

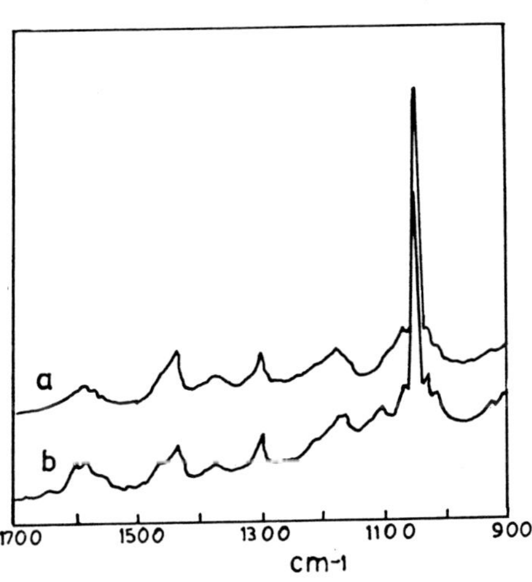

Fig.3.Raman spectra of the complexes a: $CuL'_2 2(H_2O)$, b: CuL''_2 $2(H_2O)$

bands at 1122 and 1062 cm^{-1} of the free diamines have been assigned to the ν_s(C-C) and ν_a(C-C) skeletal vibrations (Tasumi). However, the copper-complexes here show only one strong band at 1042 cm^{-1}, in this region which should be assigned to the ν_s(C-C). However, this assignment implies that the previous assignment of the free ligand should be inverted i.e., ν_s(C-C)=1062 cm^{-1} and ν_a(C-C)=1122 cm^{-1}, in agreement with the original assignment (Ling).

The copper metal ion, thus introduces a polarizing effect to the molecules by coordinating to the $-NH_2$ groups and induces interesting intensity variations in the Raman bands of the diamines.

REFERENCES

Levin I.W., Keihn E. and Harris C., (1985), A Raman spectroscopic study on the effect of cholesterol on lipid packing in diether phos phatidylcholine bilayer dispersions, Biochim. et Biophys. Acta 820: 40-47.

Ling C.Y., Krimm S. and Sutterland G.B.B.M.,(1956), Infrared Spectra of High Polymers. I. Experimental Methods and General Theory, J. Chem. Phys.25: 543

Paleos C., Tsiurvas D., Malliaris A., Anastassopoulou J. and Theophanides T., (1992) Physicochemical Characterization of Novel Polymeric Copper Complexes with Long-chain aliphatic Diamines, Metal ligand complxes, eds., Salahoub D. and Russos N., in press.

Tasumi M.,Shimanouchi T. and Miyazawa T.,(1962),Normal Vibrations and Force Constants of Polymethylene Chain, J. Mol. Spectrosc.,9: 261

Metal Ions in Biology and Medicine, vol. 2. Eds. J. Anastassopoulou, Ph. Collery, J.C. Etienne, Th. Theophanides. John Libbey Eurotext, Paris © 1992, pp. 96-97

Drug-metal interaction and metal-ions antagonism

D.P. Kessissoglou, G.E. Manoussakis, A.G. Hatzidimitriou, C. Dendrinou-Samara, C.P. Raptopoulou

Department of General and Inorganic Chemistry, Faculty of Chemistry, Aristotle University of Thessaloniki, P.O.B. 135, Thessaloniki 54006, Greece

Introduction : It is well known that coordination compounds can be used in medicine. Four areas could be distinguished of the use of transition metal ions. (a) The use of metal-based drugs to treat disease. (b) The use of linkage agents to treat metabolic dysfunction. (c) The use of ligands to remove heavy metals from the body.(d) The use of coordination complexes to transport metals to specific sites in the body to aid in imaging.

We have initiated studies on the coordination chemistry of sulphonylurea hypoglycemic drugs with Zn^{2+}, Cd^{2+}, Hg^{2+}, Cu^{2+}, and Au^{3+} and of Cu^{2+} with the antiinflamatory drugs tolmetin, ibuprofen and naproxen, as well as Cu^{2+} and Mo^{6+}complexes with schiff-bases. The first class of compounds deals with whether and how drug-metal interaction may affect drug delivery to target cells. The second class refers to metal ion antagonism and how heavy metal ions could be blocked.

DRUG-METAL INTERACTION

Synthesis : The sulfonylurea compounds have been prepared according to the reactions:

$$RSO_2NHCONHR' + M^IOH \xrightarrow{EtOH} [RSO_2NCONHR']M^I + H_2O$$

$$M^{II}(CH_3COO)_2 + m[RSO_2NCONHR']M^I \rightarrow (M^I)_{m-2}[M^{II}(RSO_2NCONHR')_m] + 2CH_3COOM^I$$

$M^I = Na^+, K^+$; $M^{II} = Zn^{2+}, Cd^{2+}, Hg^{2+}, Cu^{2+}$; $R = CH_3C_6H_4, ClC_6H_4$; $R' = n\text{-}C_4H_9, n\text{-}C_3H_7$; $m = 2$ or 3.

The synthesis of the antiinflammatory binuclear and mononuclear complexes have been achieved via the reaction of $CuCl_2$ with the sodium salts of the ligands.

Spectroscopy . The major characteristic of the sulfonylurea complexes IR spectra is the position of the C=O stretching vibration. The energy of this band depends upon the coordination mode of the sulphonylurea ligands (Kessissoglou, et al., 1987). In $[ZnL_3]^-$, $[CdL_3]^-$, $[CuL_3]^-$ complexes the v(CO) band occurs at a lower frequency, ca. 1590 cm^{-1}, than that of mercury analog (1650 cm^{-1}) and the C=N stretching frequency of the $-SO_2N=C-$ fragment occurs at a higher frequency, about 1545 cm^{-1} (1525 cm^{-1} for the mercury complexes). The energies of these bands suggest bidentate mode of coordination for Zn^{2+},Cd^{2+},Cu^{2+} and monodentate mode for Hg^{2+} compounds. The crystal stuctures of $K[Cd(ClC_6H_4SO_2NCONHC_3H_7)_3]$ and $Hg(CH_3C_6H_4SO_2NCONHC_4H_9)_2$ reveals the two types of coordination.

For the antiinflammatory complexes the X-band ESR spectra of mononuclear complexes consist of well resolved super-hyperfine splitting lines with a splitting of $\approx 14 \times 10^{-4}$ cm^{-1} characteristic of in-plane bonded nitrogen atoms. The binuclear complexes (Fig. 1) are strongly antiferromagnetically coupled, with a singlet-triplet splitting of the order of $2J > -300$ cm^{-1}. The positions of the lines lead to the spin-Hamiltonian parameters of $g_{||} = 2.28 - 2.35$ $g_{\perp} = 2.07 - 2.08$ and $D = 0.380 - 0.395$ cm^{-1} (Dendrinou, et al., 1990).

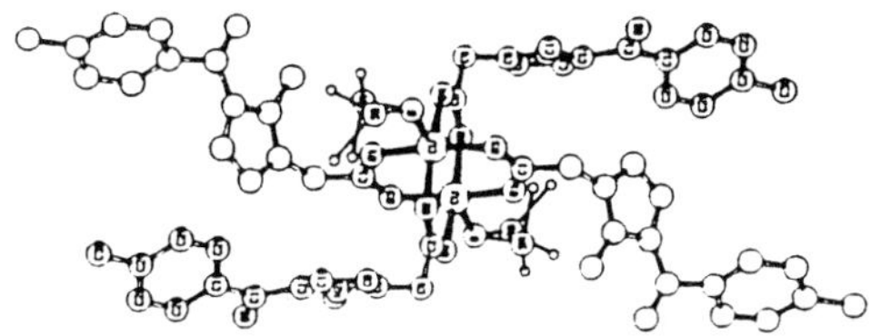

Figure 1. The crystal structure of $Cu_2(TOLMETIN)_4(DMSO)_2$

The electronic spectra of all the antiinflammatory complexes prepared, show two types of spectra which are defined by the choice of solvent. In DMSO and DMF both $[Cu^{II}Cu^{II}]$ and $[Cu^{II}]$ contain one broad absorption (band I) at ≈720 nm, a shoulder (band II) at ≈370 nm and a strong band (III) at ≈310 nm.

Molecular Modelling of $K[Zn(ClC_6H_4SO_2NCONHC_3H_7)_3]$. We found that Zn-tolbutamide and Zn-chlorpropamide complexes have a better action as hypoglycemic agents than the ligands themselves. Using the MMX89 program, we propose a model (Hatzidimitriou, et al., 1990) for $K[Zn(ClC_6H_4SO_2NCONHC_3H_7)_3]$ compound.

Solution behavior: All the limited molar conductances indicate that all the complexes are 1:1 electrolytes. The pH* values of the solutions where protonation of the ligands occurs, is in the range 4.2 to 5.6. This shows clearly that the zinc complexes at pH=7.34 have the form $[ZnL_3]^-$ and this form should act as hypoglycemic agent.

Biological study. The results showed that the used zinc-sulphonylurea complexes reduced glycemia to a statistically significant degree compared either to the corresponding ligand or to the liquid vehicle.

Mo-Cu ANTAGONISM

The well known antagonistic function of molybdenum ion against copper in ruminants has raised the interest in the interaction of Cu ions with ligated molybdenum species. A cubane like core of the formula $Cu_2Mo_2O_4$ has not been reported in the literature.

The crystal structure of the $[(saladhp)MoO_2CuCuO_2Mo(saladhp)]$ compound(I) (saladhp=2-salicyliden-iminato-1,3-dihydroxy-2-methyl-propane) shown below revealed the existence of a cubane-type core of $[Mo_2Cu_2O_4]$. The O(3) atom of the Mo=O moiety has a contact to the neighboring cubane through the Cu(2) atom giving an infinite chain arrangement.

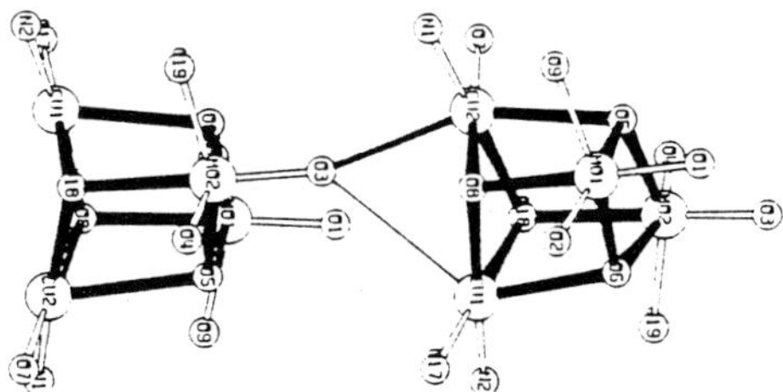

The EPR spectra show that the oxidation state of Cu is +2 and the paramagnetism comes formally from the copper atoms.

References

Dendrinou-Samara, C., Kessissoglou, D.P., Manoussakis, G.E., Mentzafos, D., and Terzis, A. (1990) : Copper(II) complexes with antiiflammatory drugs as ligands. *J. Chem. Soc. Dalton Trans.*, 959-965.

Hatzidimitriou, A.G., Kessissoglou, D.P., Manoussakis, G.E., Kourounakis, P.N., and Economidis, G., (1990) : Solid and solution behavior of sulphonylurea complexes with ions of IIA group metals. *J. Inorg. Biochem.* 39, 263-276.

Kessissoglou, D.P., Manoussakis, G.E., Hatzidimitriou, A.G., and, Kanatzidis, M.G. (1987) : Synthesis and characterization of sulphonylureacomplexes with Cd^{2+}, Hg^{2+} and Ag^{+}. *Inorg. Chem.* 26, 1395-1402.

Metal Ions in Biology and Medicine, vol. 2. Eds. J. Anastassopoulou, Ph. Collery, J.C. Etienne, Th. Theophanides. John Libbey Eurotext, Paris © 1992, pp. 98-101

A comparative study of calf-thymus DNA binding trivalent A1, Ga, Cr and Fe ions in aqueous solution

H.A. Tajmir-Riahi, M. Naoui, R. Ahmad

Centre de recherche en photobiophysique, Université du Québec à Trois Rivières 3351, boulevard des Forges, Trois-Rivières (Québec), G9A 5H7 Canada

Although the interaction of DNA with divalent metal ions has been known for a long time (Eichhron, 1962), such interaction with trivalent metal cations has been less investigated (Snow & Xu, 1991 & Karlik *et al.*, 1980). However, in recent years, the important role of trivalent metal ions in biology and medicine is well recognized. The involvement of $A1^{3+}$ in a variety of neurological disorders such as Alzheimers's disease, the carcinogenic properties of Cr^{3+}, the antitumor activity of Ga^{3+} and the biological importance of other trivalent cations have been reviewed (Collery *et al.*, 1990). In this communication, we have studied the interaction of calf-thymus DNA with trivalent A1, Ga, Cr and Fe ions in aqueous solution at various pHs, using FTIR spectroscopy. Correlations between metal ion binding, DNA condensation and helical destabilization as well as conformational features were established.

Different metal ion concentrations (trivalent metal-chloride salts) were reacted with calf-thymus DNA solution (2% w/w, 0.05 mol DNA-P) to obtain M^{3+}/DNA-P molar ratios 1/80, 1/40, 1/20, 1/10, 1/4, 1/2 and 1. The spectra were recorded after 2 h of initial mixing (DNA + salt) at pH 4-6 at room temperature. The difference spectra were produced by subtracting the free DNA from that of metal-DNA complex (DNA + salt) - (DNA) and the results are shown in Fig. 1. The difference spectra contain several negative and positive derivative features around 1700, 1655, 1485, 1210, 1100, 960, 930, 920 and 800 cm^{-1} (Fig. 1). The features at 1700, 1655 and 1485 cm^{-1} are coming from DNA in-plane vibrations, whereas other features at 1210, 1100, 960, 930, 920 and 800 cm^{-1} are arising from phosphate and sugar-phosphate vibrations (Fig. 1). The general idea of metal ions can mainly bind to the PO_2^- groups of the backbone or to the DNA bases or to both phosphate and the bases donor groups can be also applied to trivalent metal ions.

At pH = 4.5 - 5.5 the interaction of $A1^{3+}$ leads to the formation of more than one type of A1-DNA complexes. A1 binds to the PO_2^- groups up to the r = 1/40, with increased base-stacking interaction and helical stability. The reduction in intensity of the DNA bands at 1712 cm^{-1} (G,T), 1661 cm^{-1} (T,G,C,A) and 1492 cm^{-1} (C,G) and the increase in intensity of the PO_2^- antisymmetric band at 1222 cm^{-1} are indicative of a direct A1-PO_2 binding with no metal-base interaction (Fig. 1). At r > 1/40, A1-base binding begins with major increase in intensity of the bands at 1712, 1661, 1492 and 1222 cm^{-1}. The binding involves the guanine-N-7 and adenine N-7 sites as well as phosphate groups. However, at r > 1/20, DNA condensation occurs in the presence of the A1 ions, which associated with reduction of intensity of the

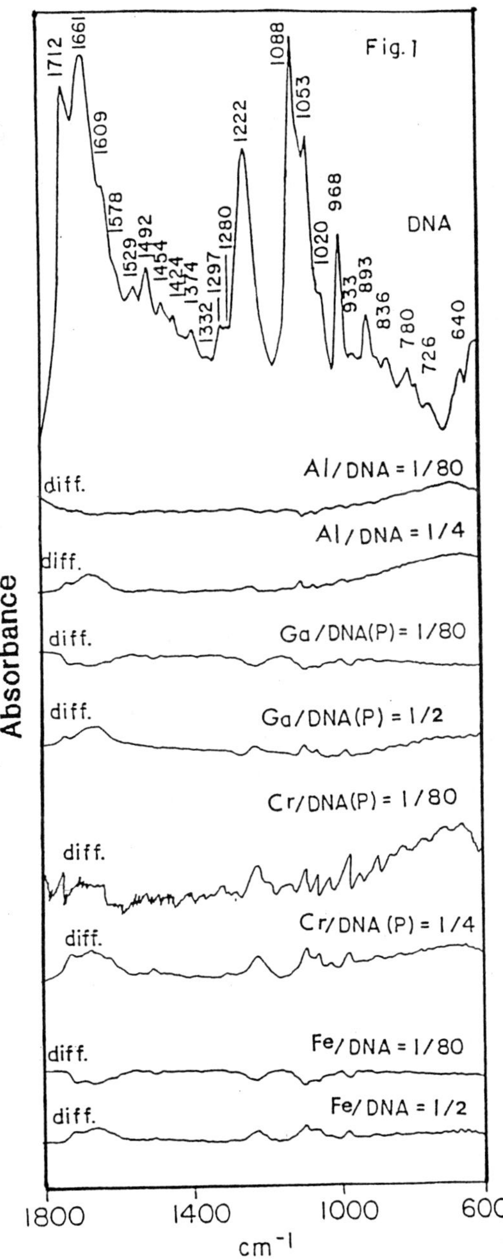

Fig. 1. FTIR spectra and difference spectra [(DNA + salt) - (DNA)] of free calf-thymus DNA and its trivalent A1, Ga (pH = 4-5), Cr and Fe (pH = 5-6) in aqueous solution and different M/DNA-P molar ratios.

bands at 1712, 1661, 1492 and 1222 cm^{-1}. At r > 1/10, metal ion complexation causes a partial helical destabilization, which accompanied with major increase in intensity of the DNA in-plane and the PO_2^- vibrations. At this stage metal ion binds to the bases donor sites (A,G,T or C) that are available on DNA destabilization. At r = 1/2 and 1, solid gel A1-DNA complexes are formed and the IR spectra of such complexes can not be recorded as solution.

At pH = 4-5, and at a very low metal ion concentration r = 1/80, the Ga^{3+} ion binds to the PO_2^- group of the backbone with no metal-base interaction (stabilizing complex formation). Evidence for this comes from major reduction of the intensity of the base bands at 1712, 1661, 1492 cm^{-1} and an increase in intensity of the PO_2^- band at 1222 cm^{-1} (Fig. 1). At r = 1/40, major intensity increase of the base and the phosphate band was observed, which is due to direct Ga-base and Ga-PO_2 bindings (destabilizing complexation) (Fig. 1). At r > 1/40, DNA condensation was observed in the presence of Ga ions, which accompanied with major loss of intensity of the bands at 1712, 1651, 1492 and 1222 cm^{-1} (Fig. 1). The loss of intensity of these vibrations is a result of sudden DNA collapse and particle formation, which is coming from drastic structural modifications of biopolymer in the presence of Ga ions (Wilson & Bloomfield, 1979). At r > 1/20, major metal-base <u>via</u> guanine and adenine bases was observed, while at r > 1/10, a partial destabilization of the helical structure was occurred with major increase in intensity of DNA in-plane vibrations and the phosphate group (Fig. 1). This increases the chances of Ga ions to bind to cytosine and thymine as well as guanine and adenine sites that are freed upon DNA helical destabilization.

At pH = 5-6 and at r = 1/80, the Cr^{3+} ion binding is mainly to the PO_2^- groups of the DNA backbone with no major metal-base interaction (stabilizing complexation). A major increase in intensity of the PO_2^- antisymmetric band at 1222 cm^{-1} with considerable loss of intensity of DNA in-plane vibrations at 1712 cm^{-1} (G,G), 1661 cm^{-1} (T,G,C,A) and 1492 cm^{-1} (C,G) lend support for such complex formation (Fig. 1). However, at r = 1/40, major intensity increases of the base bands and phosphate stretching were observed, that are indicative of strong metal-base and metal-PO_2 interactions (chelation) (Fig. 1). At r > 1/40, biopolymer condensation occurs in the presence of Cr ions. The collapse of DNA is associated with reduction in the intensity of the bands at 1712, 1661, 1492 and 1222 cm^{-1} that arises from major structural alterations on DNA collapse (Osterberg *et al.*, 1984). At r > 1/20, metal cation binding causes destabilization of helical structure and this accompanied by metal ion binding to more binding sites on G,A,C,T that are available upon a partial helical destabilization. At r > 1/4, solid gel Cr-DNA complexes are formed and this makes it difficult to record the infrared spectra as solution.

At pH 4.5 - 6.2, the Fe^{3+} ion binds mainly to the phosphate groups of the backbone and causes duplex stability (stable complex formation). Drastic decrease of intensity of the base bands at 1712, 1661, 1492 cm^{-1} and the intensity increase of the PO_2^- band at 1222 cm^{-1} are the results of stable complexation (Fig. 1). At r > 1/40, strong metal-base and metal-PO_2 bindings occur, with major gain in intensity of several base bands and the PO_2^- vibrations (Fig. 1). Metal-base binding is possible through the guanine N-7 and adenine N-7 sites. At r > 1/20, the Fe^{3+} ion interaction causes DNA condensation and brings about major reduction in the intensity of the bands at 1712, 1661, 1492 and 1222 cm^{-1} (Fig. 1). At r = /10, iron ion binding results in a partial helical destabilization and causes major gain in intensity of the DNA in-plane vibrations (Fig. 1). This event increases the chance of Fe ions to bind to other sites such as cytosine, thymine and adenine donor groups that are freed on partial destabilization. Strong metal-base binding continues up to r = 1/2 and for r = 1, solid gel complexes are formed.

Eventhough major structural alterations were observed before and after DNA collapse, no major conformational changes were observed from B-family structure in the presence of these trivalent metal cations. No major spectral changes were observed for IR marker bands at 1712 cm^{-1} (G,T), 1222 cm^{-1} (PO_2^- antisymmetric stretch) and 836 cm^{-1} (sugar-phosphate backbone), upon trivalent metal ions interactions. When B to A conformational changes occur, the marker band at 1712 cm^{-1} shifts to 1710-1708 cm^{-1}, the PO_2 band at 1222 cm^{-1} appears at 1240 cm^{-1} and the sugar-phosphate band at 836 cm^{-1} shifts to 810 cm^{-1} (Brahms et al., 1974). For the Z conformation, the marker bands are shifted to 1690, 1215, 830 and 800 cm^{-1}. No such spectral changes were observed for DNA in the presence of these trivalent metal ions and thus, DNA remains in the B-conformation before and after biopolymer condensation.

In conclusion, trivalent metal ions A1, Ga, Cr and Fe bind to the PO_2^- groups of the backbone at low metal ion concentrations. At high metal ion concentration, metal-base and metal-PO_2 binding (chelation) predominates. These metal cations cause DNA condensation at moderate metal ion concentrations. High metal ion concentrations result in a partial helical destabilization. DNA remains in the B-family structure before and after condensation.

REFERENCES

Brahms, S., Brahms, J. and Pilet, J. (1974): Infrared studies on the backbone conformation of nucleic acids. *Isr. J. Chem., 12,* 153-163.

Collery, Ph., Poirier, L.A., Manfait, M. and Etienne, J.C. (eds.) (1990); Metal ions in biology and medicine, John Libbey, Paris.

Eichhorn G.L. (1962): Interaction of metal ions with polynucleotides and related compounds. *Nature, 194,* 474-475.

Karlik, S.J., Eichhorn, G.L., Lewis, P.N. and Crapper, D.R. (1980): Interaction of aluminum species with deoxyribonucleic acid. *Biochemistry, 19,* 5991-5998.

Osterberg, R., Persson, D. and Bjursell, G. (1984): The condensation of DNA by Chromium (III) ions. *J. Biomol. Struct. Dyn. 2,* 285-290.

Snow, E.T. and Xu, L.-S. (1991): Chromium (III) bound to DNA templates promotes polymerase processivity and decreased fidelity during replication in vitro. *Biochemistry, 30,* 11238-11245.

Wilson, R.W. and Bloomfield, V.A. (1979): Counterion-induced condensation of deoxyribonucleic acid. *Biochemistry, 18,* 2192-2196.

Metal Ions in Biology and Medicine, vol. 2. Eds. J. Anastassopoulou, Ph. Collery, J.C. Etienne, Th. Theophanides. John Libbey Eurotext, Paris © 1992, pp. 102-107

Mg^{2+} ion binding to thiamin diphosphate in aqueous solutions A novel spectroscopic method in detection of metal-coenzyme conformation in solutions

Bijan Farzami

Department of Biochemistry School of Medicine, Teheran University of Medical Sciences P.O. Box 14155-5399 Tehran, Iran

Our present work deals with a method by which the PKa's of some ionizable groups as a substituent to a chromophore could be estimated. The interactions of metal ion with the molecule could result in spectral changes that are revealing as to the location of metal bindings. The assumption for such studies stemed from the fact that a substituants to a chromophore such as an aromatic ring could induce shifts and changes in intensities of absorption due to deprotonation or protonation of the group. The relationship exists between the degree of electronic transition and the electron density in the excited state (1,2). In a more complex system where two or more ionizable groups afffect the π structure of the ring, each group may in turn affect the transitions. Nevertheless the total optical density of the absorptive specie, may change its trend at the PKa of the group in question.

In present work several thiamin derivatives were studied. The formation of ionized species due to PH changes, in all the derivatives showed gradual changes in the total optical density of the absorptive ring in such a way that the changes were reversed at the PKa of the ionizable groups. This fact was substantiated by considering that an ionizable group can induce electronic changes in the chromophore attached to, therefore the changes will obey a logarithmic trend similar to Henderson-Hasselback equation. In fact the plot of $(\log(A^+ - A\pm)/(A^+ - A)$ and $(\log(A^- - A)/(A^- - A\pm)$ against the PH gave two linear lines on the 2 sides of PH scale for Thiamin (Fig. 1,2) the lines had a common intercept at PH=PKa for the group in question. Some of the results were substantiated where microtitration techniques could be used.

On the basis of the above evidence, the PKa's of some active groups in proteins and enzymes that are specifically bind to metal ions were also estimated using metal ions as probes (3).

The importance of pyrimidine ring and more specifically, the $(C_4\text{-}NH_2)$ group of TDP in enzyme catalysis was first proposed by schellenberger and coworkers, for the enzyme, pyruvate decarboxylase (4). They proposed that the $(C_4\text{-}NH_2)$ group of pyrimidine ring is functional as an acid base catalyst in the stability of the intermediate and the release of final product of acetaldehyde (4). The mechanism of enzyme action on pyruvate as substrate was delineated by Breslow (5), as follows;

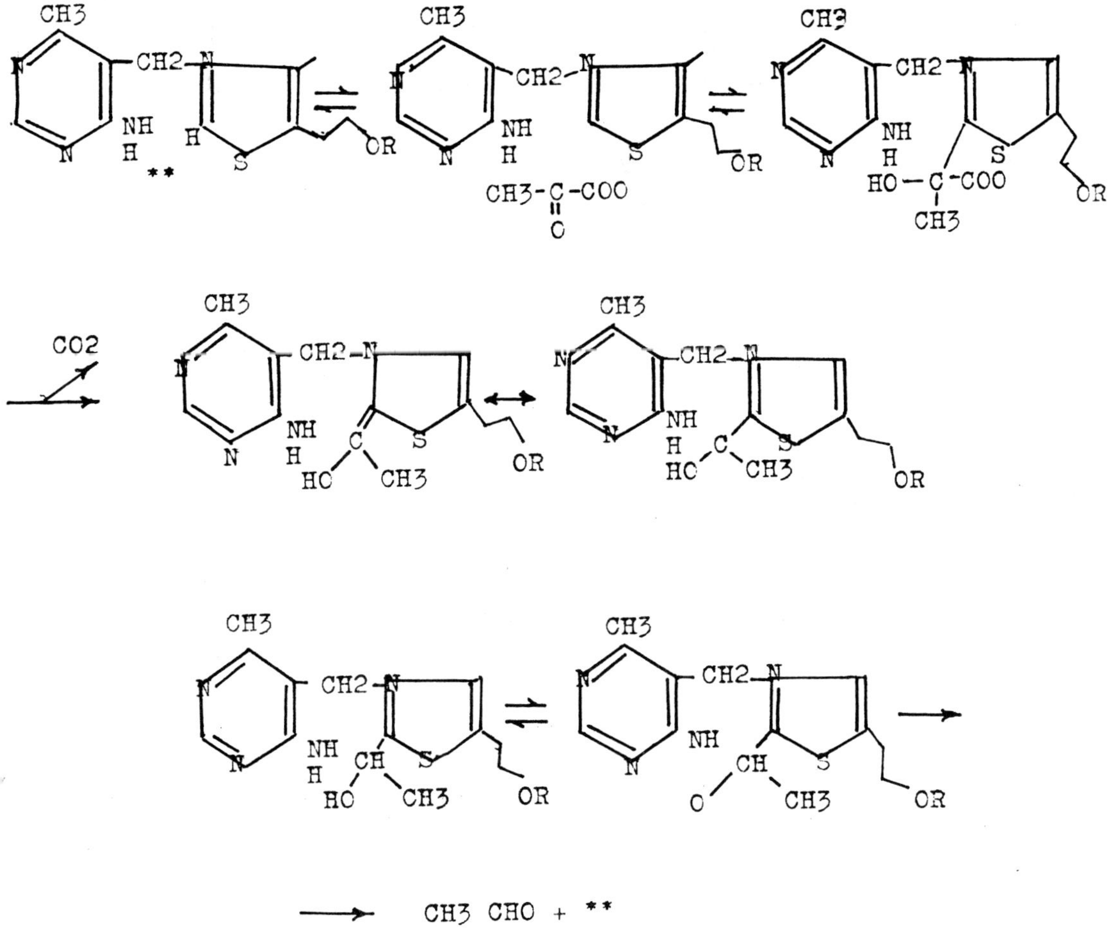

$\longrightarrow$ CH_3CHO + **

The role of 4'-amino group in stabilizing the intermediate in TDP has been proposed by schellenberger as follows.(6)

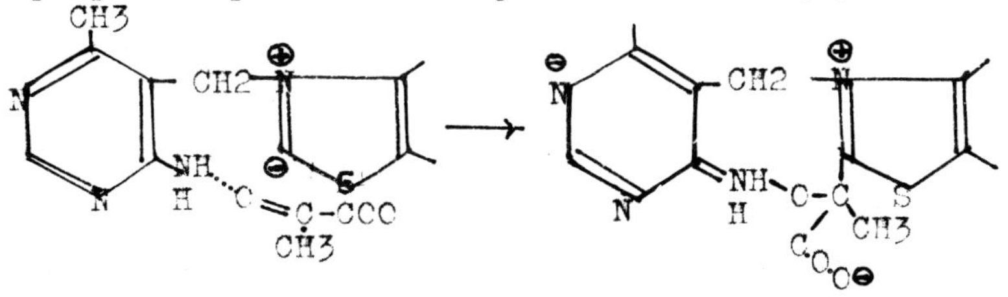

This mechanism was depicted using thiamin diphosphate derivatives in enzme reactions. The presence of some substituent groups on the pyrimidine ring that sterically hindered the conformation where the C_4-NH_2 nitrogen forced away from (C_2) of thiazol ring, decreased the rate of the reaction to the extent of one order of magnitude (6).

On the basis of the above information. This survery is mostly directed to thiamin conformational studies in solution using Mg^{2+} ion as a probe to study the binding locus of the metal ion on thiamin and its derivatives. Some thiamin derivatives were synthesized in our laboratory are shown below

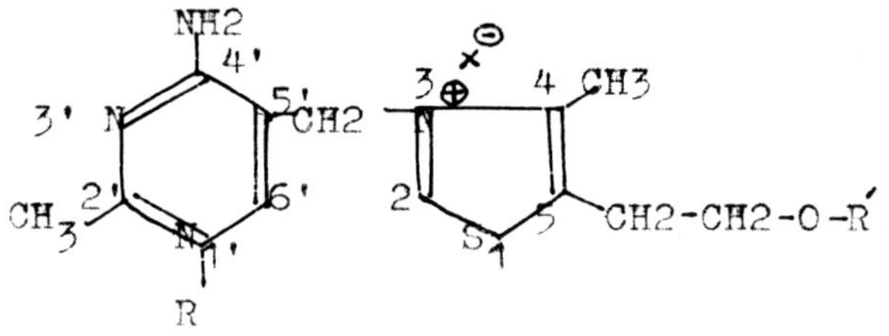

Ia	R=H	R'=H	X=Cl
Ib	R=CH_3	R'=H	X=Cl
Ic	R=H	R'=$P_2O_6^{2-}$	X=Cl
Id	R=H	R'=H	X=No_2

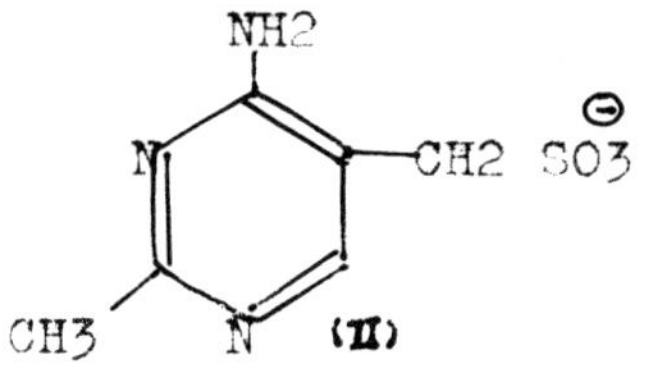

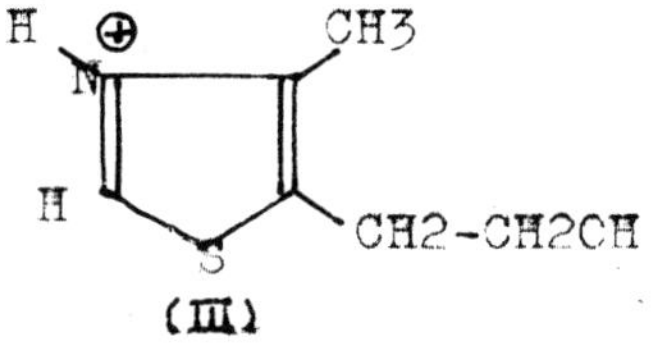

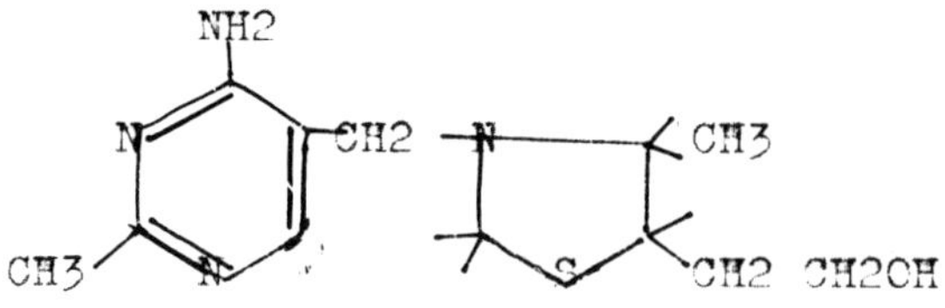

The spectral studies with (IC) showed that there were two changes in the direction of curves corresponding to two PKa's (Fig.3,4)

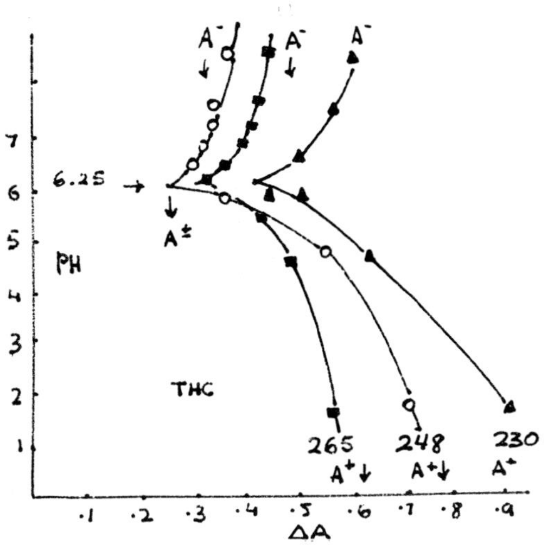

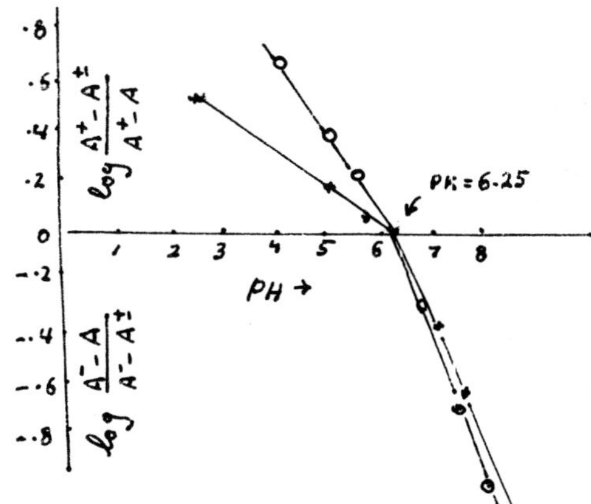

Fig (1,2) difference spectra and the logarithmic plots for Thiamine hydrochloride as a function of pH.

The pKa's of some thiamin derivatives were determined from these plots. Some of these pKa's could be obtained by microtitration using pH stat with microtitration assembly. As it is evident from. (Tab.1) Thiamine and the derivatives portray at least two pKa's. The lower pKa was assigned to "N'_1 " of the pyrimidine ring and the second pKa to (C_4-NH_2). The assignment of the first pKa was established through the use of "Ib" since the respective pKa was totally abolished with N'_1 methyl sustitated compound. The second pKa was assigned to (C_4-NH_2) since in using (II) the changes due to ionization, could only be from that of (N'_1) group. Compound (III) gave a pKa=3.3 for "N_3" of thiazol ring, since the ionization was vanished when the compound with pyrimidyl moiety as substituant to thiazol was used.

The effect of other side groups on pKa's are important. For example when (Ib) was used the positive charge on "N'_1" and the resulting electron withdrawing effect on the pyrimidyl ring caused a decrease in pKa from 6.34 in "1a" to 5.75 in "1b". Conversely when "II" was used pKa of (C_4-NH_2) was raised from 6.34 in "1a" to 6.5 and N'_1 pKa from 3.48 to 3.75. This increase was also evidenced in IV.

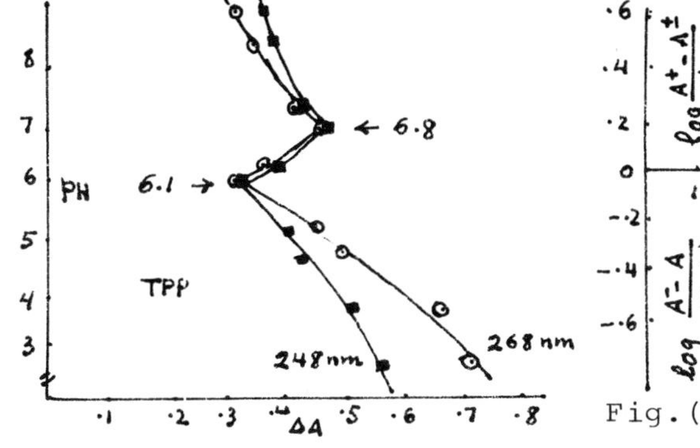

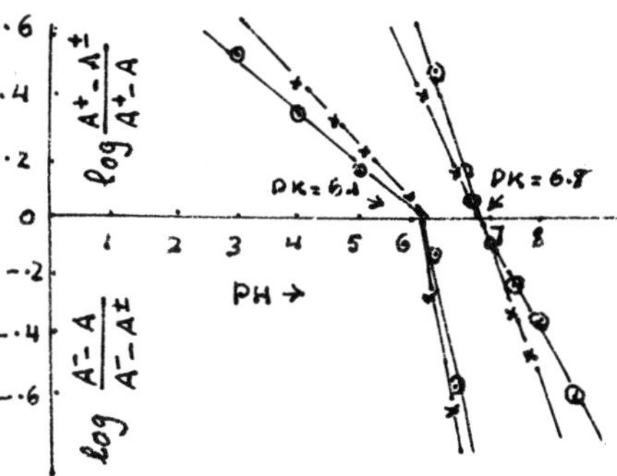

Fig.(3,4) difference spectra and the logarithmic plots for TDP.

The increase of N'_1 pKa to 3.6 in (IV) compared to that in "la" signifies the role of quaternary amino group with the positive charge that is eliminated in IV. In thiamin diphosphate (TDP), two pKa's were assigned to (C_4-NH_2);' pKa=6.1 and pKa=6.8. These pKa's were collectively seen as one in microtitration method and was equal to pKa=6.47, the effect of pyrophosphate on (C_4-NH_2) may be through the induction and stabilization of 2 structures that are produced in the process of ionization (Fig.5). "Ib" showed two (C_2-NH_2) pKa's that were the result of positive charge induced by "N'_1" methylation. pKa's of (C_4-NH_2) and N'_1 has been reported previously using NMR techniques (PKa(C_4-NH_2)=7.5-7.8 and pKa (N'_1)=4.3-3.54 (7, 8)

The use of Mg^{2+} with the reaction mixtures of several thiamin analogues signified the effect of metal ion as a probe to investigate the enviornment of groups that are affected by metal bindings. Among the thiamin derivatives only "lc" showed this effect. The pKa's of (C_4) amino group were enhanced to 6.25 and 7.05 from 6.1 and 6.8 due to the binding of Mg^{2+} ion. It could be assumed that the Mg^{2+} ion binds to pyrophosphate destabilizing the ionizing structures.

It has been previously reported that the hydrogen bonds between the (C_4-NH_2) and the intermediate acetaldehyde in enzymatic reaction could lead to the stability of inter-mediate as well as the access to the release of the product. (8) Therefore the conformation that facilitates this mechanism is proposed to be when C_4-NH_2 is adjacent to (C_2) carbon of thiazolium ring , where the attack on the carbonyl group of substrate takes place. We suggest that the conformation presented above may be stabilized by H-bonding effect of the pyrophosphate moiety of thiamin diphosphate with (C_4-NH_2) of pyrimidine ring and is in accordance with the conformation that is most suitable for the catalysis in the enzyme reaction.

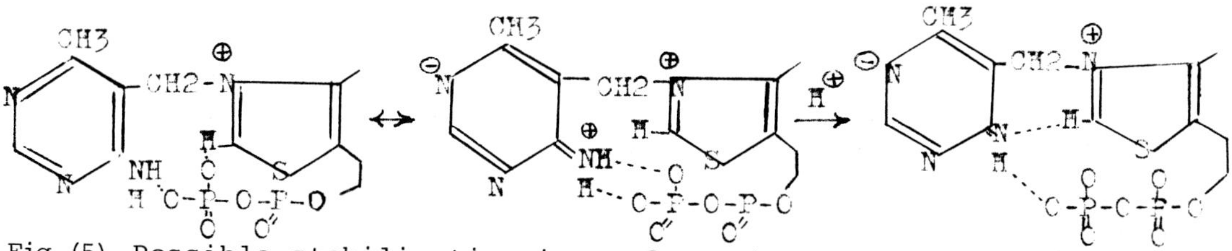

Fig.(5) Possible stabilization in conformation of pyrimidyl group due to pyrophosphate.

Compound	pK (N_1') microtitration	pK(4'-NH_2) microtitration	pK_1(4'-NH_2) spectrophoto meteric	pK_2(4'-NH_2) spect.	pK thiazol (N_3)
TPP(Ic)	3.48	6.47	6.1	6.8	-
TPP+Mg^{2+}	3.50	6.36	6.25	7.05	-
THc(Ia)	3.48	6.34	6.25	-	-
THc+Mg^{2+}	3.48	6.34	6.25	-	-
TMN(Id)	3.40	6.30	6.25	-	-
TMN+Mg^{2+}	3.40	6.31	6.25	-	-
N_1'-CH_3(Ib)	-	5.75	5.54	5.8	-
ADPS(II)	3.75	6.5	-	-	-
THT(IV)	3.60	6.3	-	-	-
5-Hyd-ethyl 4-methyl - thiazol (III)	-	-	-	3.3

REFERENCES:

1. Pavia, D.L.,Lampman, G.M. and Kriz, G.S.(1976) Introduction to spectroscopy, W.B.Saunders Company, New York.

2. Dyer,R.T. (1965) Application of absorption spectroscopy of organic compounds Prentice Hall. Inc., Englewood Cliffs, N.J.

3. Farzami, B., Jordan, F., Metal ions in Biology and Medicine, P. Collery,L.A., Poirier, M., Manfait, J.C. Etienne (Eds), Paris, 126-128.

4. Schellenberger, A. (1967) Angew. Chem., Int. Ed., 6, 1024.

5. (a) Breslow, R., (1959) J.AM Chem. Soc., 80, 3719;(b) Breslow and McNellis, (1959), Ibid, 81, 3080.

6. Schellenberger, A.(1982) Annals of the New York Academy of Sciences, V. 378 p. 51.

7. Hopmann, R.F., Brugnoni ,G.P. (1973) Nature New Biology, Vol. 246, No. 153 pp. 157-158.

8. Jordan, F., (1982) J. Org. Chem. 2748, 47.

Metal Ions in Biology and Medicine, vol. 2. Eds. J. Anastassopoulou, Ph. Collery, J.C. Etienne, Th. Theophanides. John Libbey Eurotext, Paris © 1992, pp. 108-110

The effect of cadmium(II) ions on the association behavior of guanosine 5'-monophosphate

M. De la Fuente, A. Hernanz, R. Navarro, Th. Theophanides*

*Departamento de Química Física, Facultad de Ciencias, UNED, Senda del Rey, s/n, 28040-Madrid, Spain. * National Technical University of Athens, Chemical Engineering Department, Radiation Chemistry-Biospectroscopy, Polytechnioupoli, Zografou 157 73, Athens, Greece*

INTRODUCTION

Interaction of nucleotides with the metals that have been found to be essential in living systems has been the subject of numerous studies due to the importance of the metal ions role in a large variety of biological processes. Spectroscopic techniques and X-ray crystallography studies are revealing the potential coordination sites of mononucleotides with respect to these metals. We have studied the interaction of cadmium(II) with guanosine 5'-monophosphate based on the important role of cadmium as an enviromental pollutant and its toxic activity in quite small quantities. It is known that the main coordination site of 5'-GMP with Cd(II) is the N(7) of the guanine molecule (Aoki, 1976). Previous infrared studies, 1800-400 cm^{-1}, on Cd(II)-5'-GMP complex in solid phase have been done (Tajmir and Theophanides, 1983, 1984). Now we have consider a wider spectral range, 4000-75 cm^{-1}, and we have tried to study the complex in aqeous solution aproaching physiological conditions.

EXPERIMENTAL

The disodium salt of guanosine-5'-monophosphate was purchased from Boehringer Mannheim GmbH, and the cadmium nitrate tetrahydrate (99.999%) was from Aldrich Chemical Co. Both compounds have been used without further purification. The Cd(II)-5'-GMP complex was prepared adding a 0.5M aqueous solution of disodium salt of guanosine 5'-phosphate to the same volume of a 0.5M solution of cadmium nitrate tetrahydrate at room temperature and pH=7, a white precipitate was obtained.

Solutions containing 0.05M of 5'-GMP and concentrations of Cd(II) ranging from 10^{-6} to 10^{-3}M were prepared. At higher Cd(II) concentrations a precipitate of the complex appears. Time evolution of the solution containing 10^{-3}M of Cd(II) have been studied. The FTIR spectra of the complex in solid phase have been recorded from 4000 to 500 cm^{-1} in a BOMEM MB-100 spectrometer coadding 200 scans at a resolution of 2 cm^{-1}. Far infrared spectra of the solid from 650 to 74 cm^{-1} have been recorded with a NICOLET 20F spectrometer using the same conditions. Spectra of the solutions from 4000 to 750 cm^{-1} have been obtained with a BOMEM DA3 spectrometer coadding 4000 scans with a resolution of 2 cm^{-1} and a Ca_2F cell of 40μm pathlength.

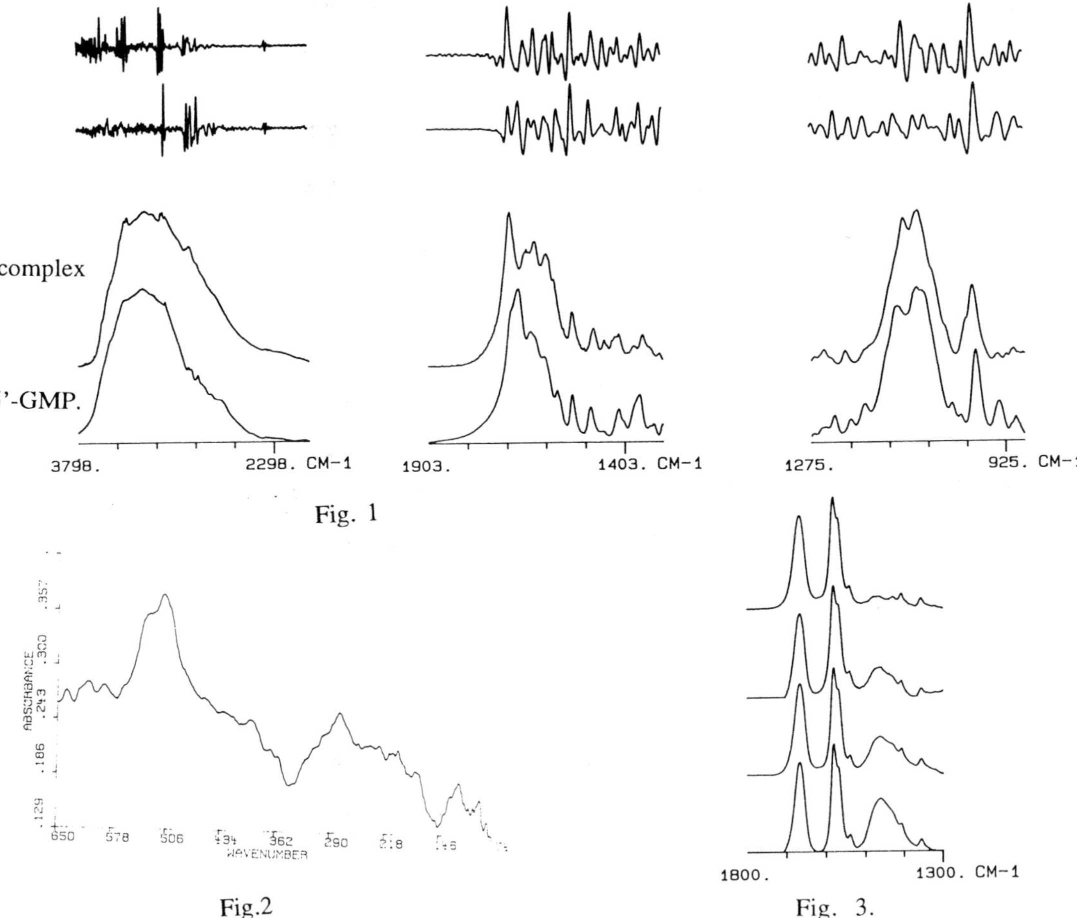

Fig. 1

Fig.2

Fig. 3.

The spectra of the complex in solid phase are clearly different from the spectra recorded for polycrystalline 5'-GMP. On the second derivative of these spectra (with sign changed) these differences are more evident, see Fig. 1. In the spectra of the complex a new component appears on the broad band a 3400 cm^{-1}, the component at 1672 cm^{-1} almost vanishes, the symmetric stretching of the phosphate group (de la Fuente *et al.*, 1992) is shifted to 984 cm^{-1} and a shoulder is detected especially in the second derivative plots. Two weak bands appear in the far infrared region at 608 and 513 cm^{-1} and the intensity of the band at 279 cm^{-1} increases considerably,Fig.2 Changes of the 5'-GMP 0.01M spectra are not detected when Cd(II) ions are added within the indicated concentration interval 10^{-6}-10^{-3}M in which there is no precipitation of the complex, see Fig. 3. Significant changes with time are not detected also when the Cd(II) concentration is in their interval.

REFERENCES

Aoki, K. (1976): Crystallographic Studies of Interactions between Nucleotides and Metal Ions. II. The Crystal and Molecular Structure of the 1:1 Complex of Cadmium(II) with Guanosine 5'-Phosphate. *Acta Cryst.* B32, 1454-1459.

de la Fuente, M., Navarro, R., Hernanz, A. and Theophanides, Th. (1992): Normal coordinate analysis of the 1:1 complex of cadmium(II) with 5'-GMP. In this book.

Tajmir-Riahi, H.A. and Theophanides, Th. (1983): Platinum(II) nucleotide complexes. Sinthesis, FT-ir spectra and structural properties. *Can. J. Chem.* 61, 1813-1822.

Tajmir-Riahi, H.A. and Theophanides, Th. (1984): A Fourier transform infrared study of the electrophilic attack at the N7-site of guanosine-5'-monophosphate. *Can. J. Chem.* 62, 266-272.

Metal Ions in Biology and Medicine, vol. 2. Eds. J. Anastassopoulou, Ph. Collery, J.C. Etienne, Th. Theophanides. John Libbey Eurotext, Paris © 1992, pp. 111-112

Normal coordinate analysis of the 1:1 complex of cadmium (II) with 5' -GMP

M. De la Fuente, R. Navarro, A. Hernanz, Th. Theophanides*

*Departamento de Química Física, Facultad de Ciencias, UNED, Senda del Rey, s/n, 28040-Madrid, Spain. * National Technical University of Athens, Chemical Engineering Department, Radiation Chemistry-Biospectroscopy, Polytechnioupoli, Zografou 15773, Athens, Greece*

Force constant calculations and normal coordinate analysis of nucleic acid components are a valuable help for the assignment of the vibrational spectra of these compounds (Ghomi and Taillandier, 1985; Majoube, 1985; Tsuboi *et al.*, 1987; Vergoten *et al.*, 1991). A normal coordinate analysis of 5'-GMP was previously done (Escribano *et al.*, 1991), and now this analysis has been applied to the 1:1 complex of cadmium(II) with 5'-GMP. Detailed FT-infrared studies on different metal-5'-GMP complexes in solid phase have been performed and an assignment of the observed infrared bands in the region of 1800-400 cm^{-1} has been proposed (Tajmir and Theophanides, 1983, 1984). On the basis of the FTIR spectrum of the Cd(II)-5'-GMP complex in the region of 4000-74 cm^{-1} (de la Fuente *et al.*, 1992) and considering the force field previously tested for 5'-GMP (Escribano *et al.*, 1991) an assignment of the infrared bands has been inferred in the present work.

The normal coordinate analysis has been done applying the Wilson GF method. The G matrix is written in internal coordinate representation, using an extended basis of 126 internal coordinates, which includes 21 redundancies. Through diagonalization of G we get rid of these redundancies whose corresponding eigenvalues are zero, plus the non-null eigenvalues *G*. The eigenvectors of G provide a "symmetry" coordinate basis, which is then applied to the F matrix in internal coordinates, to yield a "symmetrized" *F* matrix. The product *GF* gives rise to the usual secular equation, whose eigenvalues are the harmonic vibration wavenumbers. The analysis has been performed using computer programmes developed in our group (Escribano *et al.*, 1991). The valence force field has been transferred from the one used for 5'-GMP. Geometrical data for the 1:1 Cd(II) - 5'-GMP complex are taken from the crystallographic study of the complex by X-ray diffraction (Aoki, 1976), data for the two H atoms bonded to the amino nitrogen atom N(2) of the 5'-GMP molecule have been taken from X-ray patterns of disodium guanosine 5'-phosphate heptahydrate, molecule A, (Katty *et al.*, 1981).

The results obtained show that fundamentals predicted for the complex in the range 3300-2700 cm^{-1} correspond to the same normal modes computed for 5'-GMP (molecules A and B)in this range. But at lower wavenumbers this correspondence is not so evident, normal modes for the complex and the mononucleotide are not usually the same. A force field refinement considering Cd-N(7) stretching constant has not a relevant effect on the computed frequencies due to the low contribution of this internal coordinate to the normal modes of the complex. The change of mononucleotide geometry from 5'-GMP to its Cd(II) complex affects mainly to fundamentals appearing at wavenumbers lower than 2700 cm^{-1}.

Table 1.- Some of the stronger bands of the FTIR spectrum of polycrystalline 1:1 complex of Cd(II) with 5'-GMP. The potential energy distribution, PED, for the normal modes is also included.

ν(obs.)/cm^{-1}	ν(calc.)/cm^{-1}	Assignments (PED of the main contributions)
3417	3304	(49)ν(N2H)-(48)ν(N2H')
3271	3199	(48)ν(N2H)+(49)ν(N2H')
3151	[3149,3149]	[(99)ν(O2'H), (99)ν(O3'H)]
2944	2925	(70)ν(C1'H)+(22)ν(C4'H)
1695	1694	(37)δ(C2N1H)-(27)δ(C6N1H)-(20)δ(HC5'H') ...
1653	1647	(13)δ(C5C4N9)+(10)δ(C4C5C6)+(9)δ(C4N9C1')-(2)ν(C6O) ...
1632	1623	(22)δ(N9C8H)-(9)δ(N7C8H)+(7)δ(C2N1H) ...
1602	1593	(48)δ(C5'C4'H)-(27)δ(C3'C4'H) ...
1108	1101	(23)ν(PO12)-(9)ν(PO13)-(8)δ(PO5'C5') ...
1084	1089	(26)ν(PO11)-(22)τ(O11,O12,O13 PO5'C5')-(18)ν(PO13) ...
984	994	(27)δ(O5'C5'H)-(17)ν(PO5')+(8)ν(PO13)+(7)ν(PO11)+(5)ν(PO12)
799	803	(41)τ(O11,O12,O13 PO5'C5')+(15)δ(C4'C5'H)+(10)δ(O5'C5'H) ...
531	542	(13)τ(C1'N9C8C4)-(8)τ(O11,O12,O13 PO5'C5') ...
511	500	(63)τ(HN1C6N2)+(6)δ(C2N1H) ...
279	283	(30)τ(O11,O12,O13 PO5'C5')+(14)τ(C3'C2'O2'H) ...
120	113	(24)τ(C3'C2'O2'H)+(15)τ(N9C4C5N1)+(14)τ(C4N9C1'O4') ...
91	95	(37)τ(O11,O12,O13 PO5'C5')+(11)τ(N9C4C5N1)-(10)τ(N7C5C6C4)

REFERENCES

Aoki, K. (1976): Crystallographic Studies of Interactions between Nucleotides and Metal Ions. II. The Crystal and Molecular Structure of the 1:1 Complex of Cadmium(II) with Guanosine 5'-Phosphate. *Acta Cryst.* B32, 1454-1459.

Escribano, R., Navarro, R., and Hernanz. A. (1991): Normal coordinate analysis of 5'-GMP. Application to the assignment of its vibrational spectra in aqueous solutions. In *Spectroscopy of Biological Molecules*, ed. R.E. Hester and R.B. Girling, pp. 397-398. Cambridge: The Royal Society of Chemistry.

de la Fuente, M., Hernanz, A., R. Navarro and Theophanides, Th. (1992): The effect of cadmium(II) ions on the association behaviour of guanosine 5'-monophosphate. In this book.

Ghomi, M., and Taillandier, E. (1985): Normal coordinate analysis of 5'-dGMP and its deuterated derivatives. *Eur. Biophys. J.* 12, 153-162.

Katti, S.K., Seshadri, T.P., and Viswamitra, M.A. (1981): Structure of Disodium Guanosine 5'-Phosphate Heptahydrate. *Acta Cryst.* B37, 1825-1831.

Majoube, M. (1985): Guanine Residue: A Normal-Coordinate Analysis of the Vibrational Spectra. *Biopolymers* 24, 1075-1087.

Majoube, M. (1985): Vibrational Spectra of Adenine and Deuterium-Substituted Analogues. *J. Raman Spectrosc.* 16, 98-110.

Socrates, G.(1980): *Infrared Characteristic Group Frequencies*, p. 146. New York: John Wiley.

Tajmir-Riahi, H.A., and Theophanides, T. (1983): Platinum(II) nucleotide complexes. Synthesis, FT-ir spectra, and structural properties. *Can. J. Chem.* 61, 1813-1822.

Tajmir-Riahi, H.A., and Theophanides, T. (1984): A Fourier transform infrared study of the electrophilic attack at the N7-site of guanosine-5'-monophosphate. *Can. J. Chem.* 62, 266-272.

Tsuboi, M., Nishimura, Y., Hirakawa, A.Y., and Peticolas, W.L. (1987): Resonance Raman Spectroscopy and Normal Modes of the Nucleic Acid Bases. In *Biological Applications of Raman Spectroscopy*, ed. T.G. Spiro, pp. 109-179 and refs. therein. New York: John Wiley.

Vergoten, G. *et al.*(1991): On the Use of Ultraviolet Resonance Raman Intensities to Refine Molecular Force Fields: Application to Nucleic Acid Bases. In *Spectroscopy of Biological Biological Molecules*, ed. R.E. Hester and R.B. Girling, pp. 35-36. Cambridge: The Royal Society of Chemistry.

Metal Ions in Biology and Medicine, vol. 2. Eds. J. Anastassopoulou, Ph. Collery, J.C. Etienne, Th. Theophanides. John Libbey Eurotext, Paris © 1992, pp. 113-114

Study of $Rh_2(CF_3CO_2)_4$ complexes with adenosine and 5′ -AMP by NMR spectroscopy

Aglaia Koutsodimou, Chariclia I. Stasinopoulou Nikos Katsaros*

*NCSR « Demokritos », Inst. of * Physical Chemistry and Biology, 15310 Ag. Paraskevi Attikis, Greece*

The biological reactions of adenine nucleosides and nucleotides are generally mediated by metal ions. Nuclear magnetic resonance is one of the powerful techniques used in the determination of metal binding sites and the nature of the complexes in these systems.

Interactions of $Rh_2(CH_3CO_2)_4$ with adenine derivatives (Pneumatikakis & Hadjiliadis, 1979) showed that both N(1) and N(7) sites are bonded to Rh(II)with few exceptions. For better understanding the chemistry of such systems and in order to obtain complexes with other than adenine nucleotides and nucleosides, we used $Rh_2(CF_3CO_2)_4$ (RT), instead of the acetate derivative. We report here complexes of RT with adenosine (Ado) and adenosine -5′-monophosphate (HAMPNa) which were isolated from aqueous solutions and studied by elemental analysis, magnetic susceptibility measurements, infrared and nuclear magnetic resonance spectroscopies. The formation of the HAMPNa complex, was also followed by NMR at different ratios, r, of nucleotide/metal. Both complexes are diamagnetic and have the following formulas: RT.Ado.$2H_2O$ and RT.$(HAMPNa)_2$.$10H_2O$. The IR spectra for both complexes show non-involvement in bonding of the amine-group at position 6 whose stretchings remain unchanged on complex formation. The ^1H NMR spectra reveal that the aforesaid adenine derivatives are bonded through both their N(1) and N(7) sites to Rh^{II}. The assignments are given in Tables 1 and 2.

Table 1. Adenosine ^1H and ^{13}C-NMR chemical shifts (ppm downfield from TMS)

Compound	H(8)	H(2)	H(1′)	Solvent	C(6)	C(2)	C(4)	C(8)	C(5)	C(1′)
Ado	8.35	8.14	5.88^{d}	$(CD_3)_2SO$	156.2	152.4	149.1	140.0	119.4	88.0
RT-Ado	8.36	8.14	5.88^{d}	$(CD_3)_2SO$						
RT-Ado	9.55	8.99	6.54	$(CD_3)_2CO$	158.3	155.9	150.8	146.2		92.0
Ado	8.30	8.17	5.96^{d}	CD_3OD		155.2		143.7		
RT-Ado										
fresh	9.00^{sh}	8.77^{br}	6.33	CD_3OD						92.0
3d old	9.00^{sh}	8.77^{br}	6.33			147.7		144.2		91.8
	9.61	8.05	6.20^{sh}			163.2				
		8.17^{sh}	5.90^{sh}							
14d old	9.61	8.82	6.23^{d}			147.7		144.1	123.8	91.7
	8.75	8.03	6.19^{d}			156.1		146.3		91.2
	8.73	8.18	5.99^{d}			148.1		143.4		93.2
	8.70		5.86^{d}							92.1

From the above NMR data it can be concluded that the behaviour of the adenosine complex varies in different deuterated solvents. DMSO being a drastic solvent, it replaces adenosine, so the ^{1}H-NMR spectrum of the complex in DMSO shows no proton shift for adenosine protons. In acetone, H(8) and H(2) shift by 1.20 and 0.85 ppm downfield compared to free adenosine diluted in DMSO and this indicates that both the N(1) and N(7) sites co-ordinate to Rh(II); this is also verified by the ^{13}C-NMR spectra, where C(6), C(2) and C(8) shift by 2.1, 3.5 and 6.2 ppm downfield whereas C(5) disappears (Lim and Bruce Martin, 1976).
Methanol-d_4 seems to be the most interesting solvent, where more than one complexes appear their concentrations being time dependent. When the solution is fresh H(8) and H(2) shift by 0.70 and 0.60 ppm downfield compared to the free ligand in methanol, impliciting that adenosine interacts via N(1) and N(7) with Rh(II). After 3 days in solution we have new peaks at 9.61, 8.05 and 6.20ppm, in which adenosine appears as corresponding to H(8), H(2) and H(1′) of a new complex interacting with Rh(II) only through N(7). A small quantity of free ligand exists also in exchange with the complexed one, whose peaks appear as shoulders at 8.17 and 5.90ppm for H(2) and H(1′). The solution reaches equilibrium after some days and the NMR spectrum after 14 days remains unchanged even when recorded 3 months later. In 14 days time the H(1′) and the ribose carbons show that 4 different complexes exist in solution as 4 peaks correspond to each one of them.

Table 2. HAMPNa ^{1}H-NMR chemical shifts (ppm downfield from DSS) in $D_2O/(CD_3)_2CO=9:2$

HAMPNa/RT	H(8)	H(2)	H(1′)	H(2′)	H(3′)	H(4′)	H(5′)	Temper.(°C)
1:0	8.53	8.20	6.11^d	4.75^{tr}	4.52^q	4.39^m	4.15^q	20
1:0	8.52	8.24	6.12^d	4.75^{tr}	4.52^q	4.38^m	4.14^q	45
3:1	8.52	8.27	6.16^d		4.55^{tr}	4.42	4.17^{tr}	20
	8.88^{br}	8.75^{br}	6.40^{br}					
3:1	8.61	8.35	6.20	4.81		4.42	4.18	45
	8.88^{br}	8.75^{br}	6.40^{br}					
2:1	8.61	8.29	6.18^d		4.56^{tr}	4.43	4.17	20
	8.90^{br}	8.74^{br}	6.40^{br}					
2:1	8.61	8.31	6.19^d		4.56	4.43	4.17	30
	8.92	8.71	6.41					
1:1	8.95	8.72	6.42		4.56	4.46	4.15	20

The complexation of HAMPNa with RT leads to downfield shifts for both H(8) and H(2) by 0.42 and 0.52ppm at 20°C and for r=1:1, Table 2, indicating interaction of the metal with both N(1) and N(7). This complex is formed at lower ratios too, with its bands appearing broadened at the same region. For r=3 and 2 also the peaks corresponding to uncomplexed HAMPNa appear; the ratios of uncomplexed/complexed HAMPNa are 3:1 and 1:1 respectively. The ^{13}C-NMR of the solution with r=1:1 shows downfield shifts for C(2) and C(8) by 4.1 and 3.6ppm, also impliciting co-ordination via N(1) and N(7).

REFERENCES

Lim, M.C., and Bruce Martin, R. (1976) Coordination of uridine and adenosine to Pd(II) and Pt(II) complexes. J.Inorg. Nucl. Chem. 38: 1915-1918.

Pneumatikakis, G., and Hadjiliadis, N. (1979) Interactions of Tetrakis-μ-acetato-dirhodium(II) with Adenine Nucleosides and Nucleotides. J.C.S. Dalton Trans. 596-599.

Metal Ions in Biology and Medicine, vol. 2. Eds. J. Anastassopoulou, Ph. Collery, J.C. Etienne, Th. Theophanides. John Libbey Eurotext, Paris © 1992, pp. 115-116

Complex formation of transition metals with β-alanyl-histamine

Tamàs Gajda, Bernard Henry, Jean-Jacques Delpuech

Laboratoire d'Étude des Solutions Organiques et Colloïdales, LESOC, URA CNRS n° 406, Université de Nancy I, BP 239 F-54506 Vandœuvre-les-Nancy Cedex, France

Carcinine (β-alanyl-histamine) was discovered in cardiac tissue of the crustacean Carcinus maenas (Arnould & Frentz,1975), and has been since showed that carcinine exists in multiple tissues of rats , guniea pigs , mice and man , in levels as high as or higher than those reported for the related imidazole compounds : carnosine (β-alanyl-histidine) , histidine and histamine . Furthermore , the incorporation - within minutes - of ^3H from ^3H-labelled histidine into carcinine , carnosine and histamine in the rat , is consistent with a metabolic link among these compounds (Flancbaum et al., 1990) . It has been also found that carcinine might play role(s) in both mammalian cardiac physiology and cardiovascular response to stress , based on both its positive inotropic effect and its presence in mammalian cardiac tissue , but also on its structural similarity and metabolic link to histamine (Brotman et al., 1990).

The present investigations aroused from the biological interest of carcinine , with the additional interest of allowing comparisons with the histidine containing peptides , to understand their coordination behaviours .

The copper(II), nickel(II), cobalt(II) and zinc(II) complexes of carcinine and BOC-carcinine have been studied by potentiometric , visible spectrophotometric , EPR and NMR methods . In nickel(II)-, cobalt(II)- and zinc(II)-carcinine systems - before the formation of metal-hydroxyd precipitation - MLH, ML, ML_2 and for nickel(II) the additional ML_2H_{-1} complexes are formed (charges omitted) . In case of nickel(II) and zinc(II) above pH=11 - accompanying with a further base consuming process - the precipitate redissolves , forming mono- and oligomeric species , just as in the case of copper(II)-carcinine system (see below). The formation constants determined for carcinine , comparing with carnosine , show the lack of carboxyl group (and its further stabilyzing effect) in the former cases .

The BOC-carcinine - as its terminal amino group is protected - forms CuL_n-type complexes (n=1-4) with copper(II) . In the copper(II)-carcinine system at acidic pH the CuLH complex forms with monodentate coordination of carcinine via N(3)-nitrogen of imidazole . Increasing the pH the CuL complex forms with the metal promoted deprotonation of terminal amino group . At higher pH the deprotonation of peptide nitrogen takes place with the formation of $CuLH_{-1}$ complex involved 3N-coordination of copper(II) . The pK for the peptide deprotonation (pK=7.27) is clearly greater than the same value for carnosine (pK=5.60) and this difference one can assigne to the further stabilyzing effect of carboxylate group in the latter case . The comparison with glycyl-histidine (pK= 4.26) shows an additional stability due to the more stable (5,6)-chelates againts the (6,6)-chelates formed in former cases . Due to this limited coordination ability of peptide nitrogen , at excess of ligand ([L]/[Cu] > 2/1) a very unusual CuL_4H_2 complex also forms , as the potentiometric and wideranging spectrophotometric measurements are showed . In this species the four ligands bind to copper(II) in plane via N(3)-nitrogen of imidazoles . These results clearly demonstrate that imidazole N(3)-nitrogens themself can compete with the chelated 3N-coordination (in $CuLH_{-1}$) , helping to understand the unfrequent occurence of metal-amide bond in the case of proteins under biological conditions . In alkaline solution (pH=10-12) there is an equilibrium between a mono- and oligonuclear species depending on the total concentrations . In dilute solution the further base consuming process should be assigned to the deprotonation of H_2O to OH^- in the fourth coordination site of the monomeric complex , forming the $CuLH_{-2}$ species . The significant blue shift in concentrated solution strongly suggests 4N-coordination of copper(II) in the polymeric complex $(CuLH_{-2})_n$. The fourth nitrogen donor in carcinine should be the deprotonated N(1)-pyrrolic nitrogen of imidazole . The N(1)- and N(3)-nitrogens of one imidazole ring however cannot be coordinated to the same copper(II) on steric grounds . The only way for that if the hydroxide ion in $CuLH_{-2}$ is replaced by a N(1)-pyrrolic nitrogen from another - bridging - imidazole ring . Following earlier suggestions in the literature for copper(II) complexes of glycyl-histidine and its derivatives , a tetrameric species is preferred to any other on steric grounds , accounting for a planar coordination around the copper(II) ions without any bond distortion .

REFERENCES

Arnould J.-M. , Frentz R. (1975) : Mise en evidence , isolement et structure chimique d'une substance caracteristique du coeur de Carcinus Maenas (L): laß-alanyl-histamine. Comp. Biochem. Physiol. 50:59

Brotman D.N. , Flancbaum L. , Y.-H. Kang , G.F. Merrill and Fisher H. (1990) : Positive inotropic effect of carcinine in the isolated perfused guinea pig heart. Crit. Care. Med. 18:317

Flancbaum L., Brotman D.N., Fitzpatrick J.C., Van Es J., Kasziba E., Fisher F. (1990) : Existence of carcinine , a histamine-related compound , in mammalian tissues. Life Sciences 47:1587

2 ANALYSIS

Metal Ions in Biology and Medicine, vol. 2. Eds. J. Anastassopoulou, Ph. Collery, J.C. Etienne, Th. Theophanides. John Libbey Eurotext, Paris © 1992, pp. 119-124

Bioaccumulation of aluminium in the brain of several teleost fish as a consequence of environmental pollution. A structural, ultrastructural and microanalytical study

Colette Chassard-Bouchaud*, Michelle Hubert*, Pierre Boumati**, Françoise Escaig**, Christian Galle**, Evelyne Lopez-Rabereau***

** Laboratoire de Biologie et Physiologie des Organismes marins, Université P. et M. Curie, 4, place Jussieu, 75252 Paris Cedex 05. ** Centre de Microanalyse appliquée à la Biologie du CNRS et de l'INSERM (SC 27), Faculté de Médecine de Créteil, 6, rue du Général-Sarrail, 94000 Créteil. *** Laboratoire de Physiologie Générale et Comparée, CNRS URA 90, Museum National d'Histoire Naturelle, 7, rue Cuvier, 75005 Paris, France*

Aluminium toxicity has been implicated in children and adults receiving total parenteral nutrition and in various neurodegenerative diseases. In patients who took up Al from contaminated dialysis fluids, during haemodialysis treatment, anaemia, osteomalacia and encephalopathy were observed: a general review on this subject has been published (P.Galle,1986).

Fish represent the largest and most diverse group of vertebrates. Their evolutionary position relative to other vertebrates and their ability to adapt to a wide variety of factors make them ideal for studying various areas such as environmental biology and neurobiology (Powers, 1989).Fish are particularly useful for the assessment of water-borne and sediment-deposited pollutants where they may provide advanced warning of the potential danger of new chemicals and the possibility of environmental pollution.

Falling rains are precipitation process that transfer pollutants and their acidic product on to the surface of the land and the waters: they are called " acid rains" and induce, in particular, an increase in the levels of Al ions leached from soil-rock systems.

The availability of Al in natural waters being established, it is a matter of interest to investigate Al bioaccumulation in freshwater fish used as model systems to elucidate the array of mechanisms that they use to cope with the Al environmental pollution.

Two sets of fish as model systems were chosen.The first set consisted of the brown trout *Salmo trutta fario*. Aluminium contaminated samples were collected from acidified rivers of eastern France (Vosges mountains): Grand Clos (pH 6, Al level: 40 $\mu g/L^{-1}$) and Xoulces (pH 5,6, Al level: 194 $\mu g/L^{-1}$). Control samples were collected from non acidified waters of central France near Clermont-Ferrand (pH 7,6) and were shown to be aluminium free. The second set consisted of the bream *Abramis brama* collected from an acidified lake (Ile de France).

Among the available technical approaches which may be considered to identify the elements and in particular aluminium, several may be used. However,two of them appear to be particularly suitable: on the one hand, the secondary ion mass spectrometry (SIMS), using the ion microscope and the ion microprobe and on the other hand, the wavelength dispersive X-ray microanalysis using the electron microprobe (EMP). Both of them have already been shown to be of unlimited value in the field of ecotoxicological investigations at the cellular and subcellular levels (Chassard-Bouchaud, 1991).Moreover, SIMS is associated with an image processing system using a highly sensitive television camera connected to an image computer. Polychromatic images are obtained, allowing to establish the cellular distribution

of metal contaminants.
In previous investigations performed on *S.trutta fario* collected from acidic waters, we were able to detect Al in gills and kidneys (C.Galle et al.,1990). Then, brain of this species and the one of *A.brama* were investigated in order to detect a possible Al bioaccumulation within the nervous tissue. Brains were dissected and underwent several treatments depending on the microanalytical technique to be used .They were prepared according to classical techniques of photon or electron microscopy.Preparation of specimens has been described elsewhere (Chassard-Bouchaud, 1991). Quantitative data were obtained using neutron activation analysis.

	Control samples	Contaminated samples	
		Grand Clos river	Xoulces river
Water pH	7.6	6	5.6
Water Al conc.($\mu g/L^{-1}$)	7	36-40	110 - 194
Brain (dry weight) ($\mu g/G^{-1}$)	0.92$\pm$0.21	13.2$\pm$1.6	41.6$\pm$ 1.3

Table 1. Salmo trutta fario. Brain. Neutron Activation analysis.Al concentration.

They are presented in table 1: the highest Al levels in waters corresponded to the lowest pH and the highest Al levels was detected from trout brains collected from the highest Al level contaminated waters.

Aluminium	Phosphorus	Sulfur	Calcium
416 $\pm$ 66	328 $\pm$ 62	108 $\pm$ 38	160 $\pm$ 50

Table 2. Salmo trutta fario (Xoulces river). Brain. Electron probe X ray microanalysis. Element contents (100 s.counts) obtained from lysosomes.

Results at the structural level were obtained using SIMS as this technique allowed the detection, imaging and precise localization of mineral elements in tissue sections with a very high sensitivity. Ion images showed tiny spots of a high Al emission located within the tissue (Fig.1 and 2).Other ion images showed large Al deposits (up to 100 µm in length) in areas where the cerebral tissue has been destroyed (Fig.3 and 4), in *S.trutta fario*. Similar images were obtained from *A.brama*, in the brain of which a high Al emission was observed from tiny spots located within the tissue, from the meninge (Fig.7 and 8) and from larger Al deposits observed in areas where the nervous tissue has been destroyed (Fig.9 and 10).
Results at the ultrastructural level were obtained using the electron microprobe associated with a conventional transmission electron microscope. This technique allowed to determine elemental composition of organelles. The electron micrographs of *S.trutta fario* (Fig.5 and 6) demonstrated the presence of lysosomes corresponding to the Al ion emissive spots; they contained electron dense precipitates which were analysed with the electron microprobe. Table 2 presents data on elemental contents obtained from these lysosomes: aluminium, phosphorus, sulfur and calcium. No silicium was detected in association with Al, thus eliminating the possibility of artefacts due to silicoaluminates contamination of an exogenous origin. Thus, in the fish brain, Al was precipitated in the form of phosphate in lysosomes. The mechanism of this reaction has been extensively described (Berry et al, 1982): Al penetrates by simple diffusion into lysosomes and is then precipitated in the form of an unsoluble phosphate due to the activity of an intralysosomal enzyme acid phosphatase. This intralysosomal precipitation is therefore a very common mechanism which prevents the cell from injuries due to the metal contami-

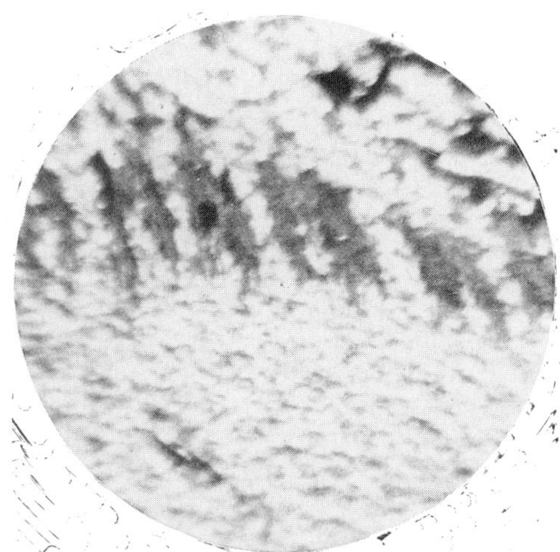

Fig.1.*Salmo trutta fario*.Brain.
40 Ca + ion image showing the topography of the section . X 500.

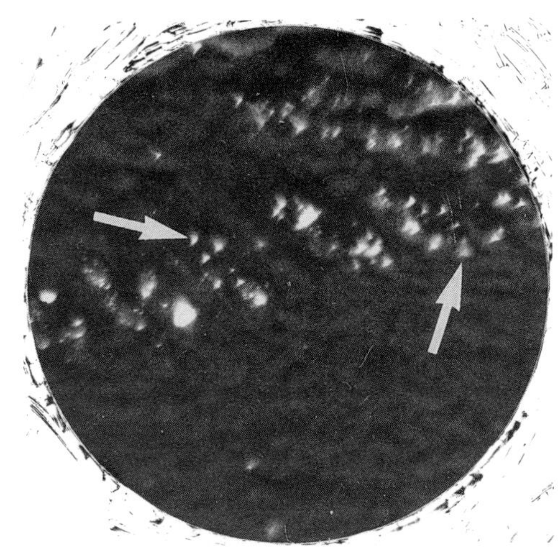

Fig.2.*Salmo trutta fario*. Brain.
27 Al + ion image obtained from the same area as (1)showing the high Al emission from bright points which correspond to lysosomes (arrows).X 500.

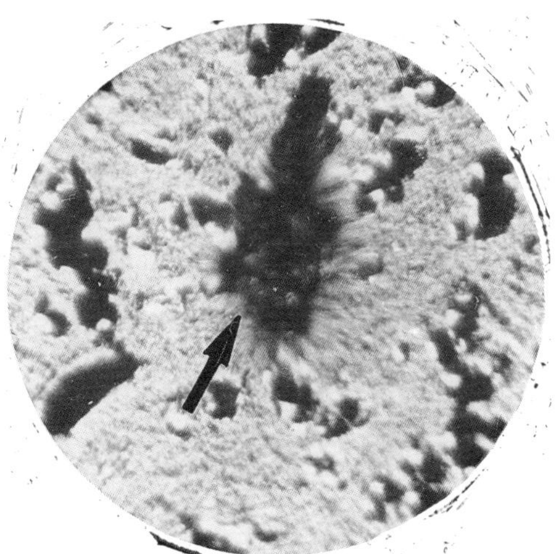

Fig.3.*Salmo trutta fario*. Brain.
40 Ca + ion image showing the topography of the section and the area where nervous tissue has been destroyed (arrow). X 500.

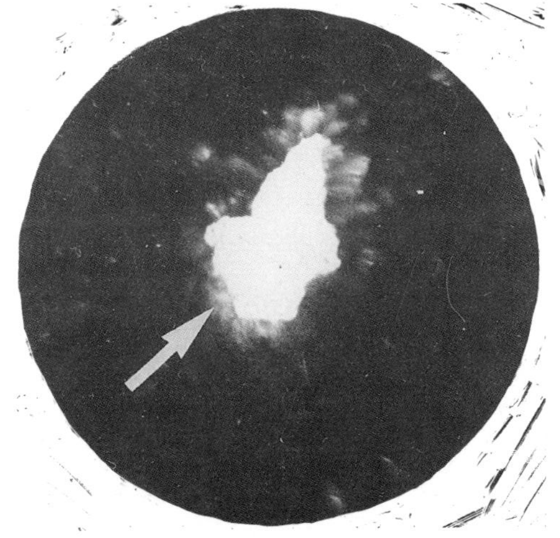

Fig.4.*Salmo trutta fario*. Brain.
27 Al + ion image obtained from the same area as (3) showing a high level Al emission from the large deposit (arrow) located in the area where tissue has been destroyed . X 500.

nant. But, as brain is a very sensitive organ which cannot eliminate, it retains Al within its cells. Consequently, larger deposits may be formed progressively, thus inducing tissue damage and destruction.

Many previous studies have shown that Al ions are toxic to fish (Stogheim and Rosseland, 1986). But the cellular and subcellular mechanisms had not yet been completely elucidated. Thus, our investigations carried out on brains of Al contaminated Teleost fish lead to the following conclusions:

Fig.5. Salmo trutta fario. Brain. Transmission electron micrograph (osmicated and unstained material). Lysosomes (L) at different stages of formation can be observed: 1, 2 and 3.
M: mitochondria
N: neurotubules
R: rough endoplasmic reticulum.
X 32.000.

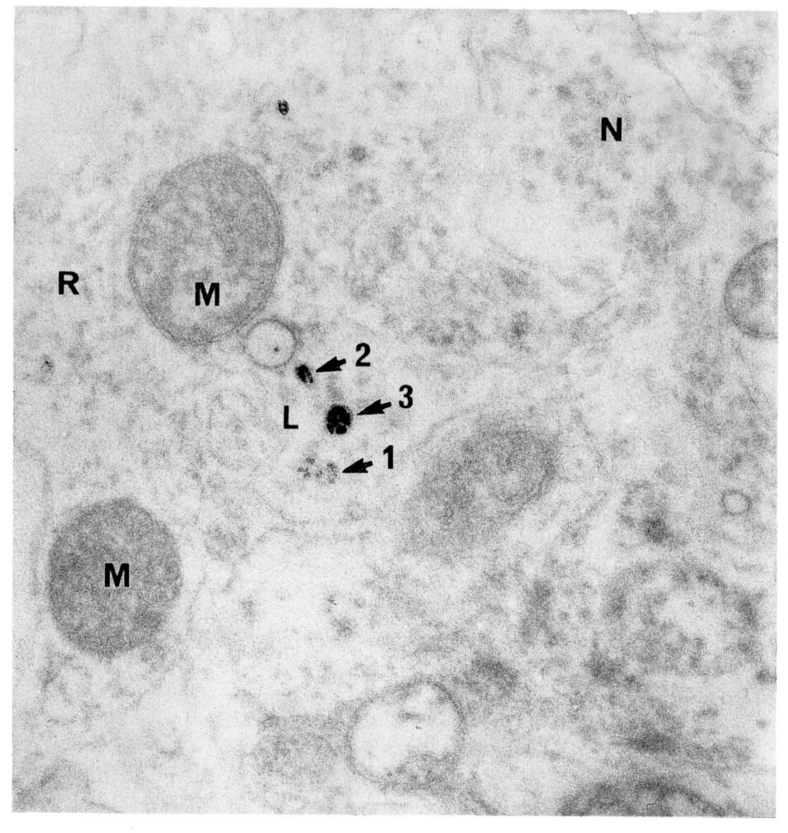

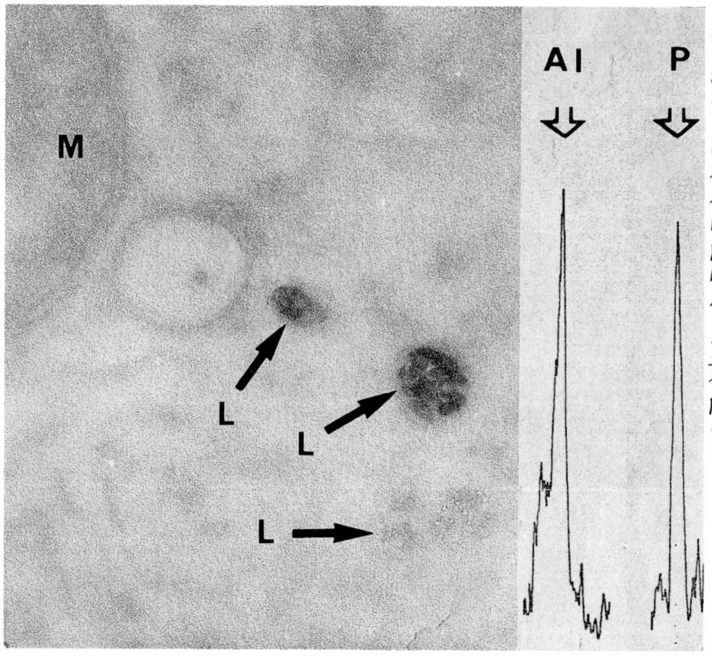

Fig.6. Salmo trutta fario. Transmission electron micrograph (osmicated and unstained material). Part of Fig.5 seen at a higher magnification showing lysosomes (L) with dense precipitates of aluminium associated with phosphorus.
M: mitochondria
X 90.000.

Inset: X ray emission spectra af aluminium (Al) and phosphorus (P) obtained from the largest lysosome. (Kα lines).

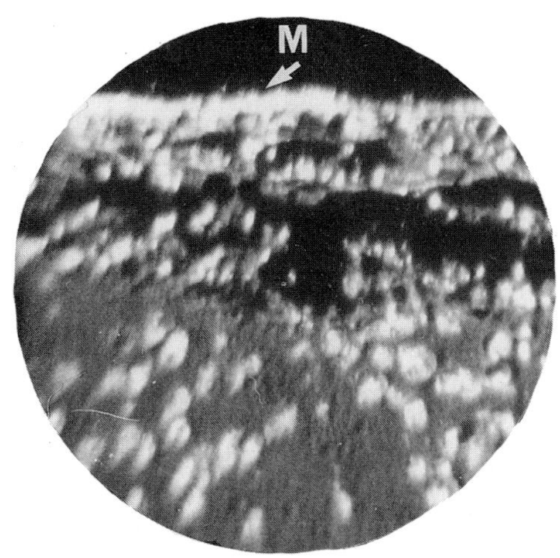

Fig.7. *Abramis brama*. Brain.
40 Ca + ion image showing the topography of the section. M:meninge . X 500.

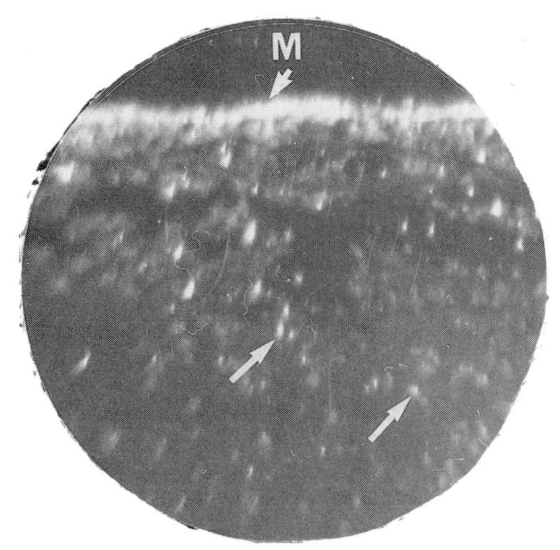

Fig.8. *Abramis brama*. Brain.
27 Al + ion image obtained from the same area as (7) showing the high Al emission from the meninge (M) and from small bright points which correspond to lysosomes (arrows). X 500.

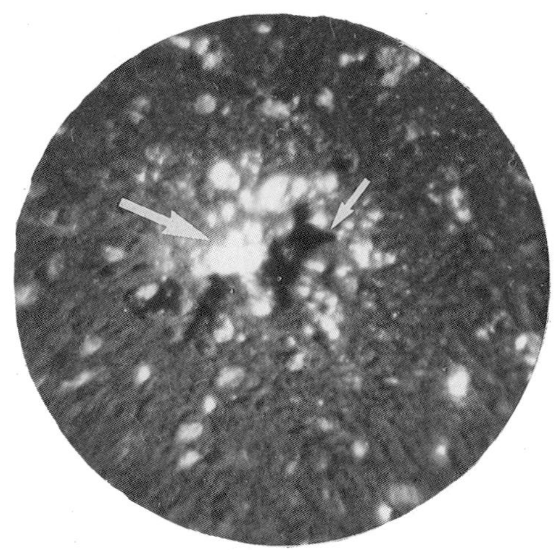

Fig.9. *Abramis brama*. Brain.
40 Ca + ion image showing the topography of the section with large Ca depos its (large arrow) and the area where nervous tissue has been destroyed (small arrow). X 500.

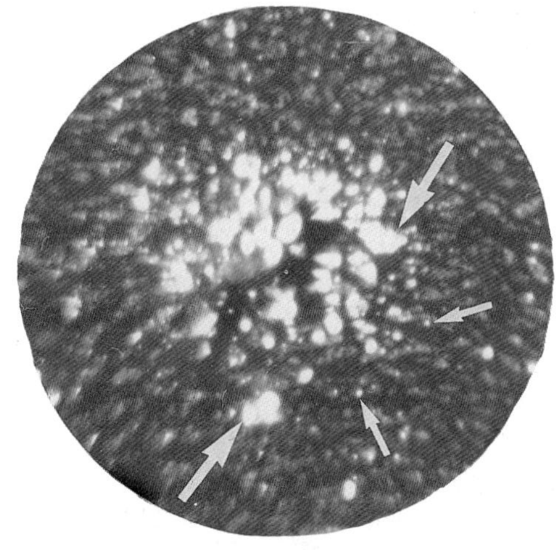

Fig.10. *Abramis brama*. Brain.
27 Al + ion image obtained from the same area as (9) showing a high level Al emission from large deposits (large arrows). Small bright points correspond to lysosomes (small arrows). X 500.

- Al concentrations in brains of fish, obtained from bulk samples were directly proportional to the water Al content which was itself directly proportional to its acidity.

- Intracellular bioaccumulation of Al in the fish brains of *S.trutta fario* and of *A.brama* was demonstrated using Ion microscope at the cellular level and electron microprobe associated with a conventional transmission electron microscope, at the subcellular level. Lysosomes appeared as the target organelles of Al concentration: an insolubilisation of Al phosphate within lysosomes, due to an enzymatic activity was observed.

- An Al overloading of the cerebral tissue which is not able to eliminate and thereby to detoxicate, led to the formation of large Al deposits inducing pro gressive neurological disease and tissue necrosis; it is well known that nervous tissue cannot regenerate. This brain damage suggests a correlation between Al contamination and fish disappearance from the acid rivers of eastern France.

- Present data obtained from Al contaminated fish, on the cellular and sub cellular mechanisms of Al bioaccumulation in the brain, are in complete agreement with observations carried out on encephalopathy and related data obtained from patients suffering from renal failure and who took up Al from contaminated dialysis fluid. Our results point out a typical instance where fish, used as model systems, may play an important role in specific disciplines such as ecotoxicology and neurobiology. Research on fish may pave the way for an understanding approach of various human neurodegenerative disorders including Parkinsonism - dementia and Alzheimer disease.

ACKNOWLEDGMENTS.
This work was financially supported by CNRS, INSERM and DRIR (Direction Régionale de l'Industrie et de la Recherche).We thank J.C.Massabuau for providing us with contaminated trouts (CNRS,Laboratoire de Neurologie et Physiologie comparées).

REFERENCES

Berry,J.P.,Hourdry,J.,Sternberberg,M.,Galle,P. (1982): Aluminium phosphate visualization of acid phosphatase activity. A biochemical and X-ray microanalysis study.J.Histochem.Cytochem. 30:86-90.

Chassard-Bouchaud,C.(1991): Microanalytical techniques in toxicological investigations.In Ecotoxicology and the Marine Environment, eds P.D.Abel and V. Axiak: Ellis Horwood, New-York,pp.176-200.

Galle,C.,Chassard-Bouchaud,C.,Massabuau,J.C.,Escaig,F.,Boumati,P.,Bourges M.,Pépin,D. (1990): Localisation subcellulaire de l'aluminium véhiculé par les pluies acides dans les reins et les branchies des truites des Vosges.Données préliminaires.C.R.Acad.Sc.Paris,311,série III:301-307.

Galle,P. (1986): La toxicité de l'aluminium. La Recherche,178, 17: 766-775.

Powers, D.A.(1989): Fish as Model Systems. Science, 246: 352-358.

Skogheim,O.K.,Rosseland, B.O. (1986): Mortality of smolt of atlantic salmon Salmo salar L at low levels of aluminium in acidic softwater. Bull. Environ. Contam. Toxicol.,37: 258-265.

Metal Ions in Biology and Medicine, vol. 2. Eds. J. Anastassopoulou, Ph. Collery, J.C. Etienne, Th. Theophanides. John Libbey Eurotext, Paris © 1992, pp. 125-130

PIXE microanalysis of intracellular platinum on IGROV1 human ovarian cancer cell line, after cisplatin exposure

Ph. Moretto*, R. Ortega*, M. Simonoff*, Y. Llabador*, G. Simonoff*, J. Robert**, J. Benard***

** Centre d'Études Nucléaires de Bordeaux Gradignan, 33175 Gradignan Cedex, France. ** Fondation Bergonié et Université de Bordeaux II, 180, rue de Saint-Genès, 33076 Bordeaux Cedex, France. *** Laboratoire de Pharmacologie Clinique et Modéculaire, Institut Gustave Roussy, 94800 Villejuif, France*

INTRODUCTION

To survey the diffusion of cytotoxic drugs through the various cell compartments is one of the major experimental difficulties encountered in cellular pharmacology. For some chemotherapeutic agents, the lack of simple marker prevents the direct probing of the drug within the cell. Fortunately, in some cases, the presence of exogenous metal in the molecule under investigation or natural fluorescence properties can be exploited for intracellular measurement. The capabilities of X-ray fluorescence techniques to reveal heavy metals were early used by electronic microprobes (Berry et al., 1983). New sensitive methods of microanalysis, taking advantage of the latter molecular characteristics, have been developed during the last decade. Microspectrofluorometry founded upon fluorescence emission has been applied for the measurement of intranuclear anthracyclines (Gigli et al., 1989). Quantitative mapping of 4'-iododeoxyrubicin by secondary ion mass spectrometry (SIMS), a microanalysis technique making use of the presence of iodine in the molecule, was lastly reported (Fragu et al., 1992).
Recent technological improvements in the focalization of ion beams allow now to carry out the PIXE fluorescence method at the cellular scale, providing thus an attractive multielemental technique of quantitative microanalysis. One of these so called nuclear microprobe has been developed at the Gradignan Nuclear Center. Applied to cellular pharmacology studies, this instrument enables us to map the intracellular distribution of cytotoxic drugs with a minimum detection limit of the μg/g.
The aim of this paper is to present the first results of intracellular platinum measurement, obtained with such a device, on isolated cultured cells following *in vitro* exposure to cisplatin. This important antineoplastic drug, used for testicular and ovarian cancer treatment, is generally classified with the antitumor alkylating agents because it forms bidentate adducts with DNA. It induces DNA cross-linking which seems to be the lethal lesion explaining its cytotoxic action. This DNA-cisplatin chemical interaction has been extensively studied since the discovery of its biological activity by Rosenberg in 1965 (Reedijk, 1987). Futhermore, the cellular drug uptake is now well defined in *in vitro* and *in vivo* models following numerous studies with macroanalytical techniques .
However, the frequent emergence of tumor cell resistance to cisplatin is a great limitation of clinical usefulness of this drug. Investigations in that field of research led to the establishment of experimental tumor cell lines with selected drug resistant subpopulations. This study is part of a research program intending to compare cisplatin intracellular distribution in sensitive and resistant cell lines using micro-PIXE. In this report, we describe an original experimental procedure of cell culture on thin polymer films compatible with the nuclear analysis requirements. In addition, first results of platinum distribution in sensitive human ovarian carcinoma cells and quantitative data will be presented. Particular emphasis will be placed on the capabilities of this new method.

MATERIALS AND METHODS

Cell culture. The human ovarian carcinoma cell line, IGROV1, was kindly provided by Dr Bénard (Institut Gustave Roussy, Villejuif, France). The characterization process of this line was already described (Bénard et al., 1985). These cells grew as a monolayer in RPMI 1640 medium supplemented with 10 % (v/v) fetal calf serum (Seromed) and antibiotics (penicillin 100 units/ml and streptomycin 100 μg/ml). Growth conditions were at 37°C in a humidified atmosphere of 5% (v/v) carbon dioxyde in air. The medium was changed three times a week, the cells were passaged each week after they reached confluence.

Substrate preparation. Thin Formvar[R] films were prepared on fresh distilled water and used as substrate for the cell culture in order to support the cells during the beam exposure. The films of about 15 $\mu g/cm^2$ were then stretched on the final microprobe target holders over a 5 mm diameter orifice drilled in the center of these frames. As the cells had to be cultured directly on these supports, the preparation described previously had to be carried out under aseptic conditions.
Those sterile holders were individually placed in 20 cm^2 Petri dishes and air dried overnight. In order to ensure the cell growth they were precoated with collagen type I (Sigma), an attachment factor. A sterile solution of 0.01% (w/v) collagen in 0.1 M acetic acid was used to coat the surface of the film at about 2 $\mu g/cm^2$ during 5 minutes at 37°C. After rinsing with sterile water the frames were stored in Petri dishes and air dried overnight.
IGROV1 cells were seeded in these dishes with 5 ml of medium, keeping the support frames entirely immersed. After three days, confluence was achieved on the film providing a well-organized monolayer of polygonal cells.

Drug exposure. Cisplatin was obtained from Laboratoire Roger Bellon (Neuilly-sur-Seine, France) and drug solutions were prepared just before use. When cells became confluent, the medium was substituted by fresh medium containing various increasing concentrations of cisplatin in the range 10-200 μg/ml. The incubation was performed for 2 hours at 37°C.

Sample processing. To be analysed, the sample had to be placed under vacuum in the irradiating chamber. In order to preserve the biological structure under these conditions, specific techniques were required, related to those developed by SEM users.
Cryofixation and freeze-drying of cells were obtained as follows:
- samples were carefully washed with cold PBS (Sigma) in order to remove extracellular compounds. The remaining traces of minerals resulting from the buffer were quickly washed out with fresh distilled water.
- the excess liquid was drained off with a filter paper and the holder was dipped quickly into liquid nitrogen. Then it was rapidly transfered in a cryostat at - 25°C. After a couple of hours, freeze-drying was obtained.
- samples were stored in a dessicator over silica-gel before analysis.

The nuclear microprobe. The microbeam line settled close to the Van de Graaff particle accelerator of the CENBG was described elsewhere (Llabador et al., 1990). On this experimental device, several methods of analysis founded upon the nuclear and atomic interaction of a particle beam with material, can be carried out:
- the particle induced X-ray emission (PIXE), method well-known in the field of trace-element research for its sensitivity in the detection of metal ions in living tissues.
- the Rutherford backscattering spectrometry (RBS) which allows, by detecting the scattered particles of the beam, to measure the main constituents of the organic matrix : carbon, nitrogen and oxygen. In this manner, the mass of the irradiated sample can be assessed.

When the two techniques are used simultaneously, a large panel of quantitatives results can be derived :
- the absolute amount of the element under investigation in the irradiated part of the specimen.
- the mass of the analysed volume of sample.
- the corresponding concentration (in μg per unit of dry weight) achieved with the ratio of the two latter values.

The main features of PIXE and micro-PIXE were depicted in excellent reviews by Mahenhaut (Mahenhaut, 1990) and Lindh (Lindh, 1990).

Beam exposure. The analysis were effected using two different approaches. For the single cell analysis, a 2.5 MeV proton beam focalized down to a probe diameter of about 2 μm provided a current of 100 pA on the target. This beam was scanned for twelve hours on a 35x35 μm square area centered on the isolated cell.

For the drug uptake measurement, larger scanning areas of 150x150 μm were selected over homogeneous parts of the cellular monolayer. A broader beam of 5 μm section, with a current of 500 pA, permitted us to reduce the analysis time to three hours.
A 80 mm^2 energy dispersive Link Si(Li) X-ray detector was located 25 mm away from the target and coated with a 100 mg/cm^2 carbon absorber to reduce the low energy count rate. The backscattered particles were detected with a 20 mm^2 Si solid state detector placed at a scattering angle of 135°.

Elemental mapping. All the emitted radiations were computer processed. Each detected event, particle or X-ray, was labelled with its energy and the coordinates of the emitting point of the scanned area. All these datas were sieved, according to the energy, to construct the X-ray and particle spectra with the object of achieving quantitative results. They were also sieved according to the spatial coordinates, to build 128x128 pixels maps of the elements disclosed in the sample. Taking advantage of the multielemental capabilities of the method, any one of the X-ray lines could be used to map the related spatial distribution. Potassium, calcium, iron, copper, zinc and platinum were thus mapped following the same run. The carbon distribution pattern, resulting from RBS analysis, gave us a useful topographic representation of the matrix density in the sample. The distributions were plotted either with colored scale maps or three dimensional representations.

Quantitative results. The X-ray emission yields and detection efficiency were determined on reference targets calibrated to $\pm$ 5% obtained from MicroMatter Inc (USA).
As depicted previously, total X-ray spectra derived from the whole scanned areas were used, after conventional fitting of X-ray lines, to calculate the absolute amount of elements in mass per unit of surface of the specimens ($\mu g/cm^2$). The corresponding RBS spectra enabled us to monitor the beam current and to normalize the previous quantitative results in term of concentration per unit of mass of the dry samples (in μg/g of dry weight). This calculation scheme was applied for the uptake measurement on groups of about forty cells.
For individual cell measurement, the location and boundaries of cells were first disclosed by carbon mapping. Afterwards, a very tight window including only one isolated cell was chosen on the original map by off-line computer processing. Local X-ray and RBS spectra were then extracted from this subsurface region of the primary scanned area. Quantification was achieved in such precisely defined structure.
With this treatment of data, a complete set of units was available for cellular platinum: the absolute amount per cell, the dry mass of this cell and consequently the concentration (in μg per g of dry mass).

RESULTS

The cells were cultured and exposed to the drug as depicted in the latter section. One of the frames, exposed to a cisplatin concentration of 200 μg/ml was chosen after dehydration, for single cell analysis, according to the structural preservation of the adherent cell monolayer. On this substrate, three cells, named IGROV1a, b, c, were successively analysed under the experimental conditions already reported. The spatial distributions within the cells were obtained using K_α X-ray lines for K, Ca, Fe, Zn and (L_α+L_β) lines for Pt. Concentration measurements of metals in the three cells were obtained with local spectra. The values appeare in Table 1. The spectra and maps connected to the cell IGROV1c are presented in Fig. 1, 2 and 3.

Cells	Pt (µg/g)	Zn (µg/g)	Cu (µg/g)	Fe (µg/g)
IGROV1a	913.4	191.4	27.6	97.2
IGROV1b	1070.7	221.9	19.4	134.1
IGROV1c	1106.1	201.9	8.8	164.3

Table 1: Single cell analysis of platinum and metals following 2 hours incubation at 200 μg cisplatin per ml of medium.

To check the availability of our quantitative results, a drug uptake essay was performed. Four frames treated with the respective cisplatin concentrations of 10, 50, 100 and 200 μg/ml were selected.
Areas containing about forty cells on 150x150 μm surfaces were scanned. Results are displayed in Table 2.

Cisplatin (μg/ml)	Pt (μg/g)	Zn (μg/g)	Cu (μg/g)	Fe (μg/g)
10	81.4	492.3	38.1	314.6
50	414.2	350.5	21.1	179.1
	279.9	288.4	14.7	118.5
100	553.5	192.2	10.7	99.5
200	1339.7	219.3	31.3	139.6

Table 2: Effect of various concentrations of cisplatin on intracellular platinum and metal content. Incubations were performed during 2h.

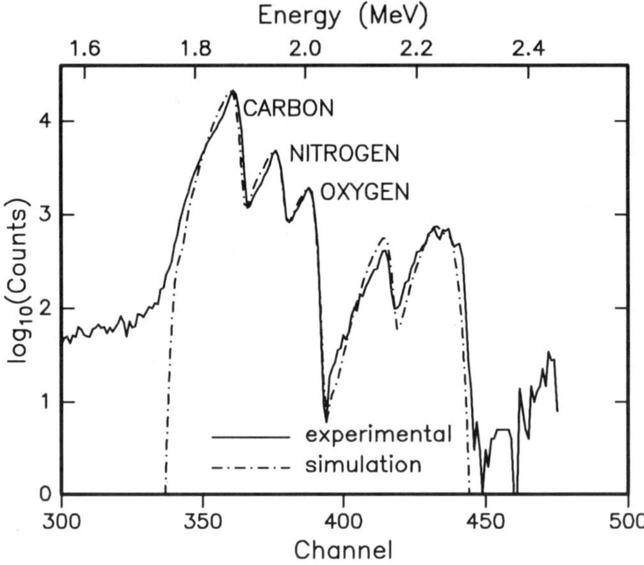

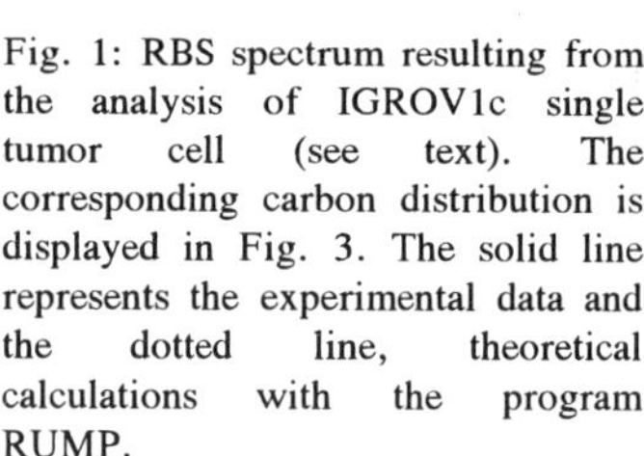
Fig. 1: RBS spectrum resulting from the analysis of IGROV1c single tumor cell (see text). The corresponding carbon distribution is displayed in Fig. 3. The solid line represents the experimental data and the dotted line, theoretical calculations with the program RUMP.

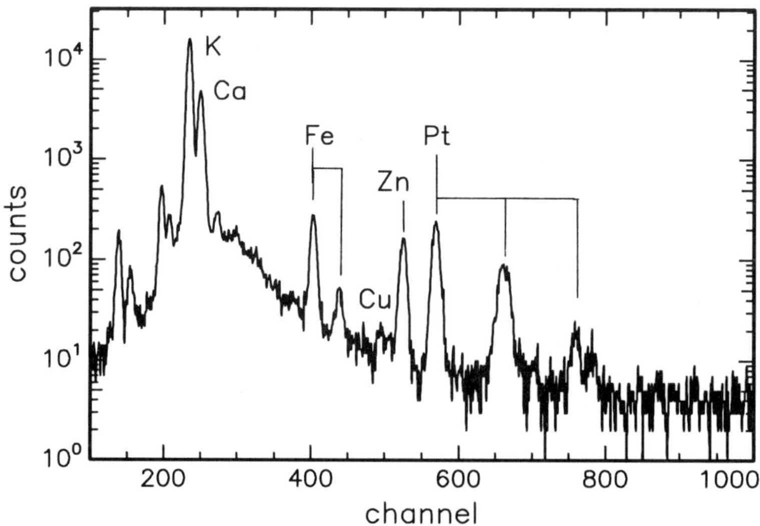

Fig. 2: X-ray spectrum following PIXE analysis of the IGROV1c cell mapped in Fig. 3.

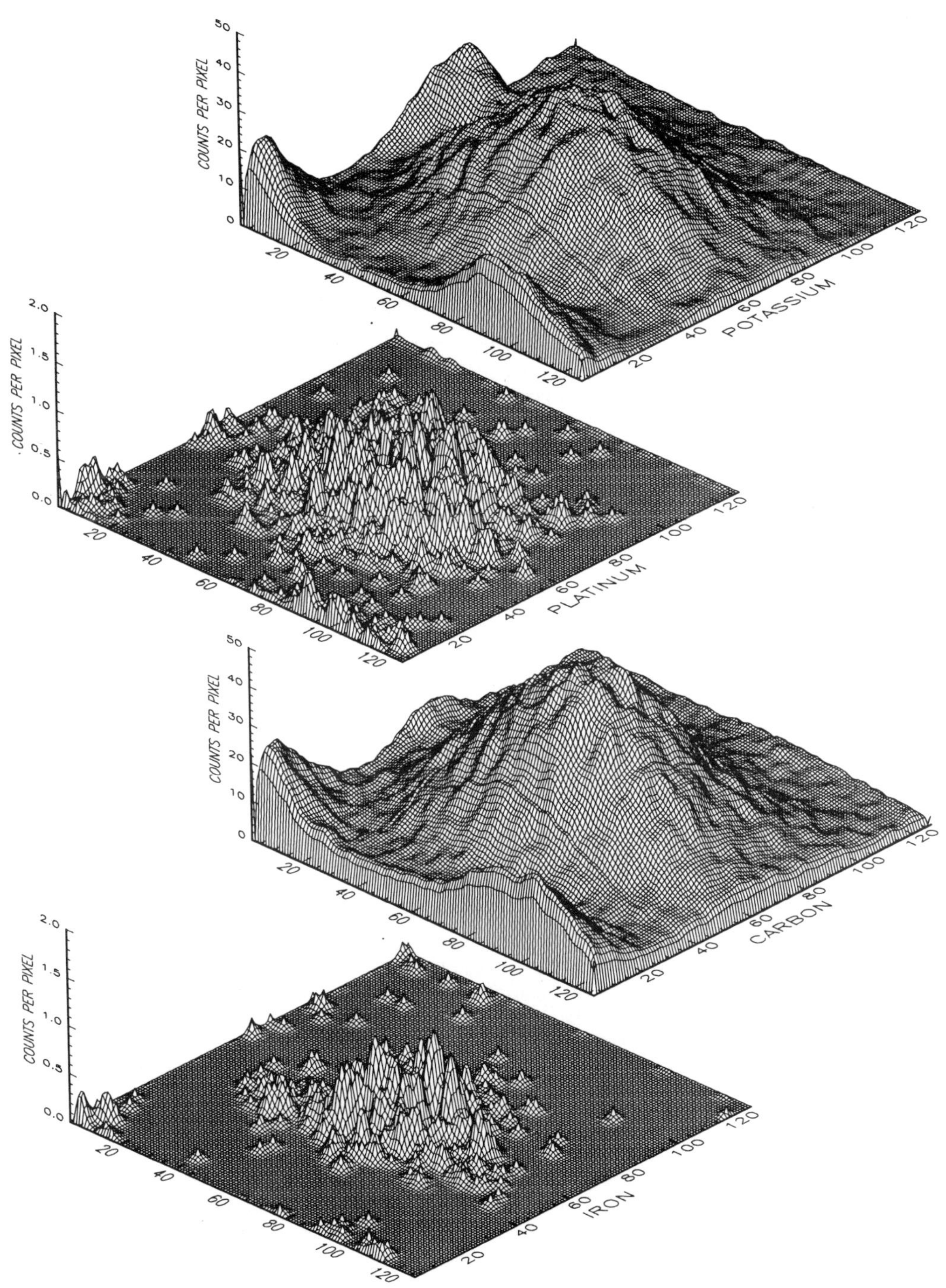

Fig. 3: Three dimensional plotting of carbon, potassium, iron and platinum distributions in the same IGROV1c cell after cisplatin exposure. The scan size is 35x35 μm and the vertical axis represents the X-ray and RBS counts per matrix pixel.

DISCUSSION

It is soon to draw conclusions about cisplatin uptake after so few measurements. It was not the purpose of this pilot study even though it is always instructive to cross-check experimental values with different methods. We can however notice that the order of magnitude of the results presented in Table 2 seems to be in good agreement with the values of cisplatin uptake already reported (Eichholtz-Wirth & Hietel, 1986).
Fig. 3 shows that the carbon distribution, and consequently the sample thickness, roughly describes the cellular shape. This distribution is strongly correlated with that of potassium. The preservation of the natural gradient of this intracellular cation indicates that the cryofixation prevents spatial redistribution at a scale consistent with the resolution of the beam. The iron map exhibits a preferential localization in a narrow region of the center of the cell.
Platinum seems to be homogeneously distributed in the whole cell. The smooth gradient which appeares on the map of Fig. 3 can undoubtedly be explained by a larger thickness of the matrix in the nuclear region, i.e. the center of the cell. These observations agree with the fact that cisplatin binds to numerous cellular ligands such as cytosolic proteins or nucleic acids.
However, this technique is suffering from the lack of topographic reference on the analysed cells. The determination of cellular ultrastructure and especially, the precise localization of the nucleus would be of primary interest in that study. But this cannot be achieved as simply as in a tissue section. The carbon distribution does not display a sharp increase of density in the proximity of the nucleus when the natural markers such as intracellular minerals are only suitable to find out the cellular boundaries. To delineate the nuclear region, compounds with a strong affinity for nucleic acids can be used as markers. Bromodeoxyuridine labelling is now under investigation.
The cellular pharmacology field of research can take advantage of interesting features of the nuclear microanalysis:
- its multielemental capability which allows to disclose possible correlations in the elemental distribution of trace metals and why not to study simultaneously multidrug exposure.
- the unique possibility to achieve quantitative results normalized in term of cellular mass or absolute amount per cell. This allows comparison and cross-check with values obtained with reference methods of macroanalysis.
- its ability to extract quantification in irradiated areas up to 2x2 mm as well as in subcellular structures. This last field of investigation will be surely developed in the future, the spatial resolution of microbeams beeing permanently improved. A limit of 0.5 μm was recently achieved. However, this latter characteristic will not be fully exploited without a precise identification of cell ultrastructure.
To conclude, we can remark that the versatility could be a major advantage for the development of this technique. The characterization of the biological activity of new metal compounds under investigation could provide potential applications.

Aknowledgements- This work was supported by a grant from la ligue française de lutte contre le cancer.

REFERENCES

Bénard J., Da Silva J., De Blois M.C., Boyer P., Duvillard P., Chiric E., Riou G. (1985): Characterization of human ovarian adenocarcinoma line, IGROV1, in tissue culture and in nude mice. Cancer Research 45, 4970-4979.

Berry J.P., Galle P., Viron A., Kacerovská H., Macieira-Coelho A. (1983): Preferential nucleolar localization of cis-DDP in human fibroblasts. *Biomed. & Pharmacother.* 37, 125-129.

Eichholtz-Wirth H., Hietel B. (1986): The relationship between cisplatin sensitivity and drug uptake into mammallian cells *in vitro*. *Br. J. Cancer* 54, 239-243.

Fragu P., Klijanienko J., Gandia D., Halpern S., Armand J.P. (1992): Quantitative Mapping of 4'-iododeoxyrubicin in metastasic squamous cell carcinoma by Secondary Ion Mass Spectrometry (SIMS) microscopy. *Cancer Research* 52, 974-977.

Gigli M., Rasoanaivo T.W.D., Millot J.M., Jeannesson P., Rizzo V., Jardillier J.C., Arcamone F., Manfait M. (1989): Correlation between growth inhibition and intranuclear doxorubicin and 4'-deoxy-4'-iododoxorubicin quantitated in living K562 cells by microspectrofluorometry. *Cancer Research* 49, 560-564.

Lindh U. (1990) : Micron and submicron probes in biomedecine. *Nucl. Instr. and Meth.* B49,451-464.

Llabador Y., Bertault D., Gouillaud J.C., Moretto Ph.(1990):Advantages of high speed scanning for microprobe analysis of biological samples. *Nucl. Instr. and Meth.* B49, 435-440.

Maenhaut W. (1990) : Recent advances in nuclear and atomic spectrometric techniques for trace element analysis. A new look at the position of PIXE. *Nucl. Instr. and Meth.* B49, 518-532.

Reedijk J. (1987): The mechanism of action of platinum anti-tumor drugs. *Pure & Appl. Chem.* 59, 181-192.

Metal Ions in Biology and Medicine, vol. 2. Eds. J. Anastassopoulou, Ph. Collery, J.C. Etienne, Th. Theophanides. John Libbey Eurotext, Paris © 1992, pp. 131-136

Evaluation of the XRF analytical method as a tool for medical and biological sciences

Themis Paradellis

Institute of Nuclear Physics, NCSR « Demokritos »
GR-153 10 Aghia Paraskevi, Greece

In the last ten years, X-ray fluorescence analytical techniques have received much attention by scientists working in medicine and biology. These methods are based on our ability to excite and to monitor the characteristic X-rays of the elements present in a given sample. Thus these multielement techniques are extremely useful in determining concentrations of naturally occuring trace elements as well as their changes due to pathological conditions.

In this article we intend to give a short description of the method, discusse the achievable sensitivities and give examples of applications. The reader who is interested in a more detailed presentation of the subject is referred to the excellent article by Feller et al, 1985.

PRINCIPLES OF X-RAY FLUORESCENCE

The phenomenon of fluorescence is produced when an ionizing radiation penetrates matter. Since an element with an atomic number Z is surrounded by a negatively charged cloud of Z electrons, their interaction with the ionizing radiation will result in the ejection of an atomic electron as long as the energy supplied by the radiation is in excess of the binding energy of the atomic electron.

The vacancy created by the ejected electron is filled by a less tightly bound electron from the same atom. This internal rearrangement of electrons will be followed by the emission of a photon which is called a characteristic X-ray.

The detection of this characteristic X-ray provides the qualitative information needed for the identification of a given element. Thus a requirement for the qualitative analysis of a sample is the ability to measure and resolve characteristic X-rays of adjacent elements. This is accomplished today with modern X-ray detectors namely either Si(Li) or Ge(Li) solid state detectors.

In Fig. 1 a spectrum obtained using a Si(Li) detector is shown. Here a penetrating radiation of 22 keV X-rays is bombarding a sample which contains atoms of Ti, Fe, Cu, Se and Mo. The impinging radiation excites the characteristic $K\alpha$ and $K\beta$ X-rays of each element which are registered by the detector. The electronic processing of the detector signals results in the spectrum shown in Fig. 1. All characteristic X-rays are simultaneously displayed a fact which allows for a direct identification of all the elements present in the sample in a single measurement.

Quantitative information

During the process of fluorescence the number I_i of emitted characteristic X-ray photons from a given element is proportional to the flux of the exciting photons and the number of atoms of the element i present in the sample

$$I_i = K_i \bullet \Phi \bullet N_i \tag{1}$$

where Φ is the flux of the exciting radiation, N_i is the number of atoms of element i present per cm^2 and K_i is a proportionality constant which is specific for each element.

The number of photons per second R_i of the characteristic X-rays of element i which is register by the detector is proportional to $I_i \bullet \Omega$ where Ω takes into account the geometry of detection and is a constant. It is easily shown that eq. 1 may be written

$$R_i = K_i' \bullet \Phi \bullet \xi_i \tag{2}$$

where ξi is the thickness of the sample in $\mu g/cm^2$. The number of photons per second Ri can be estimated from the accumulated spectra like the one in Fig. 1. By measuring the total number Ai of events registered under each X-ray peak after a counting interval of t seconds and using the relation R_i = Ai/t we obtain

$$\xi_i = (K_i'\Phi)^{-1} \bullet R_i = \widetilde{K}_i R_i \tag{3}$$

This relation is correct only when the samples used are very thin and thus no matrix corrections are needed. Matrix corrections are necessary when samples are thick enough to cause self absorption on the emitted X-rays. In this case eq. (3) is written

$$\xi_i = \widetilde{K}_i \bullet R_i \bullet f(\xi_i, \xi_t) \tag{4}$$

where the correction function f depends on the energy of the exciting radiation, the energy of the characteristic X-ray, the geometry of the system and the total thickness ξ_t of the sample.

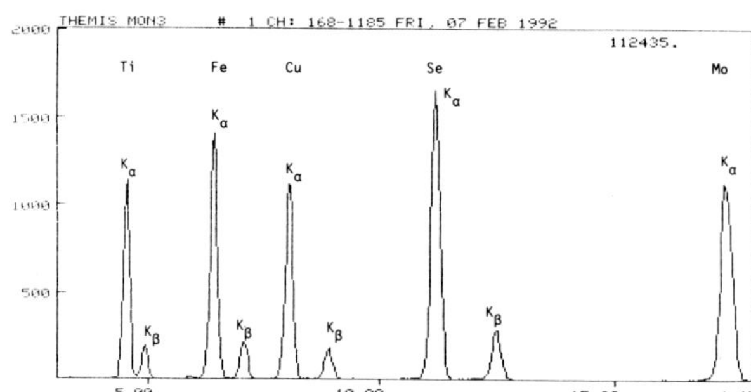

Fig.1 XRF spectrum obtained with a Si(Li) detector. The sample consist of atoms of Ti, Fe, Cu, Se, Mo and the exciting source is a ^{109}Cd radioactive source.

The correction functions are relatively easy to establish, especially for samples of interest to biology and medicine. Due to the fact that elements are present only in small quantities the so called secondary excitation effects are small and the correction function can be calculated from the X-ray attenuation coefficients of the matrix through the use of simple relations. More details may be found in Feller et al, 1985; Alenius et al, 1977; Paradellis, 1977.

The constants K_i are determined from both thin standards of well known thickness and from thick pure elements, where the proper corrections are made for absorption of the X-rays. The thin standards are made in our lab by evaporation of pure elements on mylard or kapton foils and their thickness is monitored either by microbalances and/or using the nuclear technique which is called Rutheford back scattering.

The complete analytical system

A complete analytical system includes (1) a source which provides the ionizing radiation (2) one X-ray detector (3) The electronic processing system (4) The computer through which data is accumulated and exploited.

The X-ray exciting source may be either an X-ray tube or a radioactive source. X-ray tubes provide high photon fluxes, however this is in the form of bremsstrahlung continuum spectrum. Using

X-ray tubes to excite a secondary fluorescer target whose characteristic X-rays are just above the binding energy of the elements we need to analyse, is a much better choise. In such a geometry photon output will be reduced but the spectra will be cleaner and more easy to treat.

Radioactive sources are much more easy to handle and cheaper but provide less photon fluxes. The radionuclides used decay mostly by electron capture providing thus with a flux of characteristic X-rays of the daughter element. The most useful of the available sources is ^{109}Cd. This isotope decays by electron capture with a half life of 453 days and emit the characteristic X-rays of the daugther element which is silver. (E=22 and 25 keV for Ag, $K\alpha$ and $K\beta$). These sources are usualy readily available in capsules with an annular ring geometry (Feller et al, 1985) and are placed directly on top of the detector. The recommendable nominal strength of the source at purchase time is about 20 mCi.

The detectors used are either Si(Li) or Ge(Li) solid state detectors, with resolution ranging from 165 to 185 eV at the 6.4 keV Fe, $K\alpha$ peak. Since these detectors must be cooled in liquid N_2 temperatures, they are placed in a vacuum which is isolated from the rest of the system with a thin Be window. This Be window will absorb of course some of the weakest X-rays emitted from the sample under investigation. Thus a lower cut off is introduced in the range of elements which can be analysed. A good quality Be window will allow the observation of all elements from Sulfur and up. (Z=16).

Modern amplifiers, analog to digital converters coupled with PC's permit for a rapid accumulation and process of data.

THE ANALYSIS OF MEDICAL AND BIOLOGICAL SAMPLES

At this point a system which employ a ^{109}Cd radioactive source is adopted to describe in more details the analysis of biomedical samples. The range of element which can be analysed with this source is from S to Mo using $K\alpha,\beta$ lines and from Cd to U using the $L\alpha,\beta$ lines.

Minimum detection limits

A major factor which affects the detection limits in all measurements is the background. In all spectra even if there are no characteristic X-rays, background photons which are due to scattering from the supporting materials as well as the matrix of the sample, will be present. Thus is order to be able to achieve the observation of a peak of a given element, the area under it must exceed the background area. Statistically this is defined by the statement that the minimum detectable area of a characteristic peak should exceed 3 times the square root of background. Assuming a constant background rate R_B then $B=R_B \bullet t$ and $A_{min} \geq 3 \sqrt{R_B t}$. Hence, eq. 3 will be written

$$\xi_{min} \leq 3 \bullet K \sqrt{R_B} / \sqrt{t} \qquad (5)$$

Thus the length of the measurement is explicitly introduced into the definition of the Minimum Detection Limit. MDL will decrease as Z increases since excitation is more efficient. For organic samples which contain a minimal amount of water (presence of water increases background) MDL ranges from 100 ppm for elements like K, Ca to about 0.8 ppm for elements like Se, Br and Sr, for measuring intervals of about t = 1000 s with a ^{109}Cd source of 20 mCi strength.

Sample preparation

Any form of sample is acceptable for analysis by XRF. From a piece of bone to a liquid solution, an analysis can be performed directly. However, whenever possible, water should be removed from samples to increase MDL. The removal of water decreases the amount of scattering material and acts as a natural preconcentration process.

Serum sample preparation followed in our lab is such an example. A volume of 1 ml of serum is doped with 0,1 ml of solution containing 15 μg/ml of Y. After mixing, 0,5 ml of the solution is deposited as a large drop on a frame covered with a 0,8 mg/cm^2 Kapton foil and allow to dry gently under an infrared lamp (fast heating may result in a loss of Se). The final sample will have an area of 1cm^2 and a mass of about 20 mg/cm^2. Since the initial mass was about 0,5 gr a preconcentration factor of 25 is achieved. The sample manipulation is minimal and chances for contamination are negligible.

Figures 2 and 3 show a spectrum obtained from such a sample. The achievable MDL for the dried organic serum matrix is about 10^{-6} which due to preconcentration is equivalent to about $4 \cdot 10^{-8}$ μg/ml of serum for a counting interval of 1500 s with a 20 mCi ^{109}Cd source.

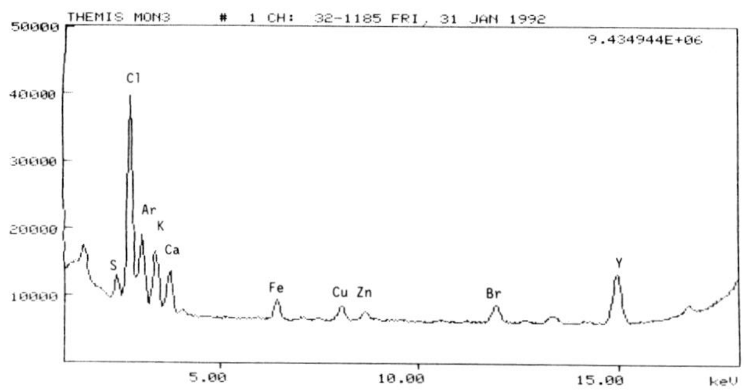

Fig.2 XRF spectrum of a serum sample obtained with a ^{109}Cd source. The sample is doped with Y.

The elements which can be detected in serum are S, Cl, K, Ca, Fe, Cu, Zn, Se, Pb, Br, Rb, Sr. Only Mn, Ni and Mo are below detection limit and need special preconcentration techniques.

Similar techniques may be used for all liquid samples. Blood is treated in the same manner. By measuring both whole blood and serum and using the hematocrit value, concentration in trace elements of erythrocytes can be extracted. Urine and bile may be treated the same way but special preconcentration techniques are necessary for measuring certain elements.

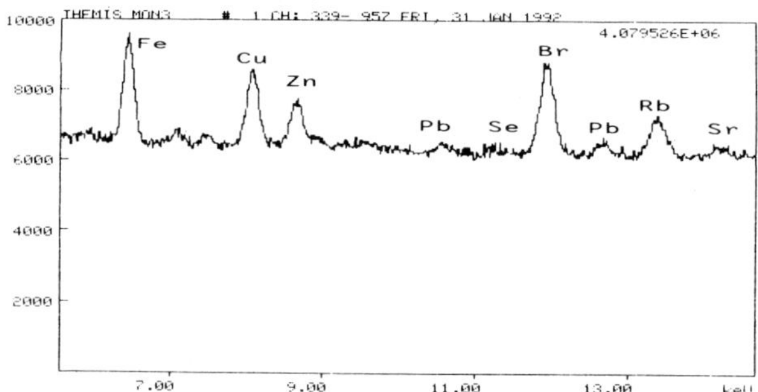

Fig.3 An expansion of the spectrum of Fig.2 in the region 5-15 keV

The doping of the solutions with Y increases the accuracy of the measurements and avoids problems which may be caused by inhomogenuities in the samples.

Samples of tissues may be either ashed in a temperature of 450^0C or freeze dried at LN_2 temperatures. The resulting residue may be grinded and pressed into a pellet which can be directly analysed.

Examples

The method described is suitable for the determination of the normal range of concentration for a number of elements in sera and other fluids of biological importance as well as for the study of their variations in a number of pathological situations. Studies of the postoperative variations in serum copper has been reported by Gregoriadis et al, 1982 and of serum bromine by Gregoriadis et al, 1985. A long list of references with studies of this nature is reported by Feller et al, 1985.

The measured concentration for a number of elements in sera and erythrocytes in Greek population is given in Table 1. This study is ongoing for several years and is a collaboration of our analytical lab with the first propaedeutic surgical clinic of the Medical School of Athens University. Additional measurements of concentration of elements in urine of healthy people combined with the determination of the same elements in the average greek diet, is providing valuable information on the metabolic balance of these elements in the average Greek subject. This same study has been extended to the investigation of the changes induced on the metabolism of these elements in patients with end stage renal failure and patients treated with continuous ambulatory peritoneal dialysis.

The high precision and accuracy of the method permits the extraction of very reliable and reproducible results. In Fig. 4 the distribution of measured serum Cu values in 19 healthy males and 16 healthy females is shown. The data shown are taken from one of our earlier work (Gregoriadis et al, 1982).

The results of the work supported the conclusion that females had a higher average serum copper concentration of 1,20 μg/ml than males whose average was 1,06μg/ml. This difference is statistically significant to p<0,01. These averages (see Table 1) have not changed after the addition of 17 more recent samples. At this moment with 25 female samples and 27 males the corresponding averages are 1,2 μg/ml for females and 1,04 μg/ml for males.

Table 1

Measured concentration of elements in sera and erythrocytes of healthy Greek subjects (n is the number of samples)

Element	n	Serum (μg/ml)	n	Erythrocytes (μg/g)
S	17	915 ± 125	17	2018 ± 590
Cl	52	3557 ± 276	–	–
K	52	165 ± 21	17	3051 ± 557
Ca	52	95.8 ± 7.6	–	–
Fe	51	1.39 ± 0.36	17	1077 ± 116
Cu*	52	1.12 ± 0.18	17	0.62 ± 0.30
Zn	52	0.98 ± 0.14	17	11.6 ± 1.9
Se	17	0.09 ± 0.01	17	0.133 ± 0.035
Br	52	4.52 ± 1.11	17	0.63 ± 0.50
Rb	52	0.20 ± 0.036	17	3.41 ± 0.72
Sr	51	0.030 ± 0.007	–	–

*This value for males (n=27) is 1.04 ± 0.16 μg/ml and for females (n=25) is 1.20 ± 0.15. The difference is significant at p<0.01.

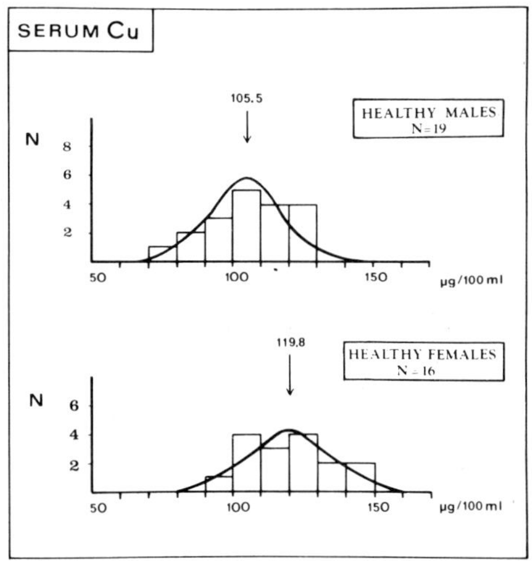

Fig. 4 Measured distribution of serum copper in male and female healthy subjects

Examples of a study of elemental distributions and their comparison in normal and cancerous colorectal tissues may be found in Gregoriadis et al, 1983. In this study a consistent picture of well established differences in elemental concentrations between healthy and cancerous tissues emerged but the interpretation of these changes was inconclusive.

In Fig. 5 the spectrum obtained from a healthy liver tissue is compared with the spectrum of a nearby cancerous tissue. The cancerous tissue has been classified as metastatic from a primary rectum cancer. In the bottom a tissue spectrum obtained from the removed rectum cancer is also shown. All three tissues have been removed at a single operation from one patient.

On the elemental level, liver tissues differentiate from other body tissues in the sense that they contain Mo and Mn at about 1,3 μg/g as well as excessive Zn which amounts to 56 μg/g. In contrast colorectal tissues contain about 15 μg/g of Zn and no Mo and Mn.

Comparing the three spectra it becomes evident that the elemental structure of the metastatic tissue is similar to the cancerous rectum tissue, having the same amount of trace elements and a lack of Mn and Mo. In addition the metastatic tissue contains large calcium quantities indicating calcification, fact which was supported by the histological report. More information on this case report may be found in Apostolidis et al, 1987.

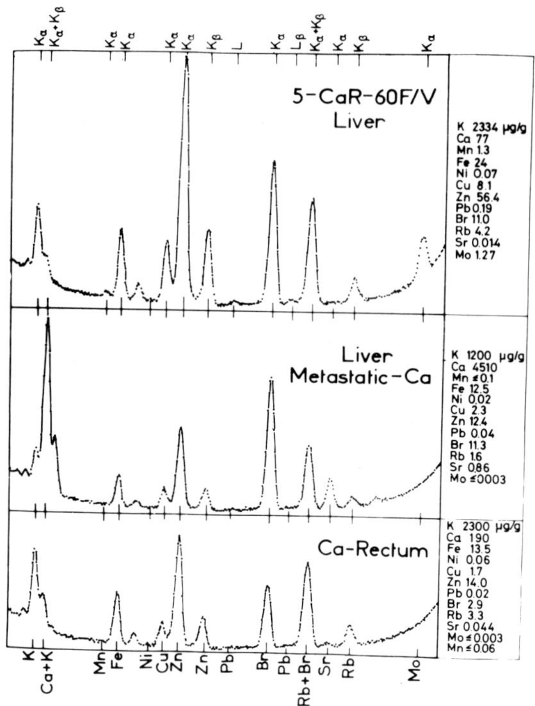

Fig. 5 Top: Spectrum from healthy liver tissue. Middle: Spectrum from a near to healthy metastatic cancerous tissue. Bottom : Spectrum from the primary tumoral focus

CONCLUSIONS

The X-ray fluorescence method is a relatively cheap, reliable, accurate and easy to perform technique for the elemental analysis of biological and medical samples. It needs no bulky instruments, can be operated on a continuous 24 hours basis and provides the researcher with an easy, fast, multielemental information which is hard to obtain with other analytical techniques.

REFERENCES

Alenius, G., Riedl, H., Rindby, A. , Selin, E. , and Standzenieks, P. (1977): Trace element analysis in thick organic speciments by photon excited X-ray fluorescence. Physica Scripta 15: 220-224.

Apostolidis, N.S., Gregoriades, G.S., Manouras, A.J., Paradellis, T.P. (1987): A case of trace elements identification in primary tumoral focus and metastasis: Hell. Arm Forces Med. Review 21: 119-122

Feller, P.A., Kereiakes, J.G., and Thomas , S.R. (1985): Medical applications of elemental analysis using fluorescence techniques. In Progress in Medical Radiation Physics, Volume 2, ed. G. Orton, pp. 139-180. New York and London, Plenum Press.

Gregoriadis, G.S., Apostolidis, N.S., Romanos, A.N., Paradellis, T.P. (1982): Postoperative changes in serum copper value. Surgery G & O 154: 1-5.

Gregoriadis, G.S., Apostolidis, N.S., Romanos, A.N., Paradellis T.P. (1983): A comparative study of trace elements in normal and cancerous colorectal tissues: (1983). Cancer 52: 508-519.

Gregoriadis G.S., Apostolidis, N.S., Romanos, A.N., Paradellis, T.P. (1985) : Postoperative changes in serum bromine value. Surgery G & O 160: 243-249.

Paradellis, T.P. (1977): Thin target thickness measurement by photon induced X-ray fluorescence. Nucl. Inst. Meth.: 205-209.

Metal Ions in Biology and Medicine, vol. 2. Eds. J. Anastassopoulou, Ph. Collery, J.C. Etienne, Th. Theophanides. John Libbey Eurotext, Paris © 1992, pp. 137-138

Ultrastructural localisation of aluminium in the tegument of trouts taken in Vosges from acidified streams

C. Galle*, C. Chassard Bouchaud**

** Laboratoire de Biophysique, SC 27 de l'INSERM, Faculté de Médecine de Créteil, 94010 Créteil Cedex, France. ** Laboratoire de biologie et physiologie des organismes marins, Université Pierre et Marie Curie, 4, place Jussieu 75005 Paris, France*

The intracellular concentration of aluminium in tegument has been studied in trouts "Salmo trutta fario" taken from acidified streams of Cornimont (Vosges,France) in june 1988. This area is exposed to acid rain. As a result, the acidified stream contain aluminium at a concentration from 76 to 194 mg/l (after filtration through 0,02µ filter).

In this work,we present the results obtained using electron microscopy and two microanalytical methods : Secondary ion mass microanalysis (Ion Microscopy) ; and electron probe X ray Microanalysis with an instrument equiped with a transmission electron microscope (CAMEBAX).

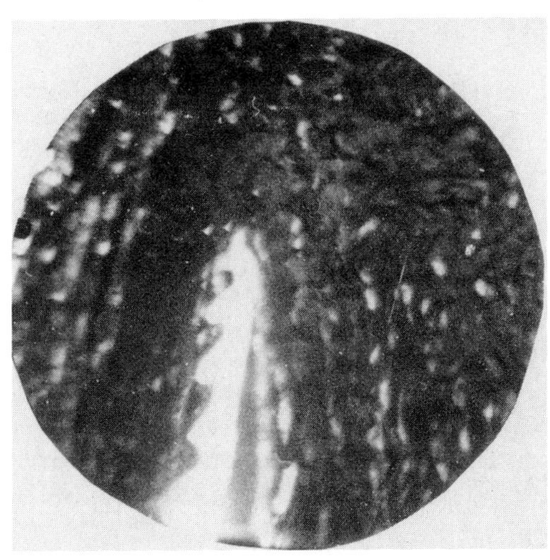

$^{40}Ca^{+}$

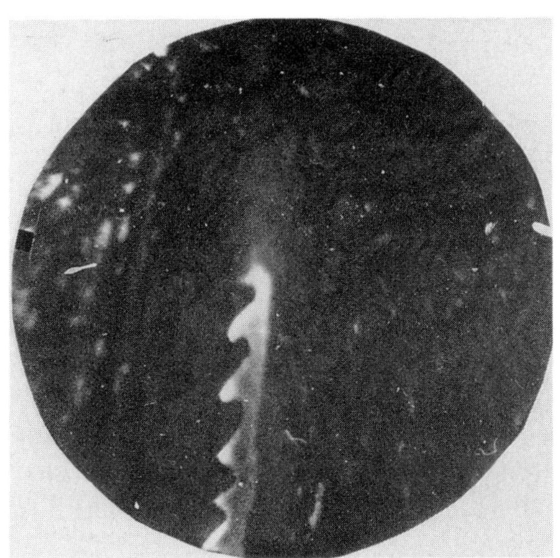

$^{27}Al^{+}$

Fig. 1. Ion images from the same area. $^{40}Ca^{+}$ image shows the scale in tegument and $^{27}Al^{+}$ image shows an emission of aluminium precisely from the creetes of scales and from the root.(X250).

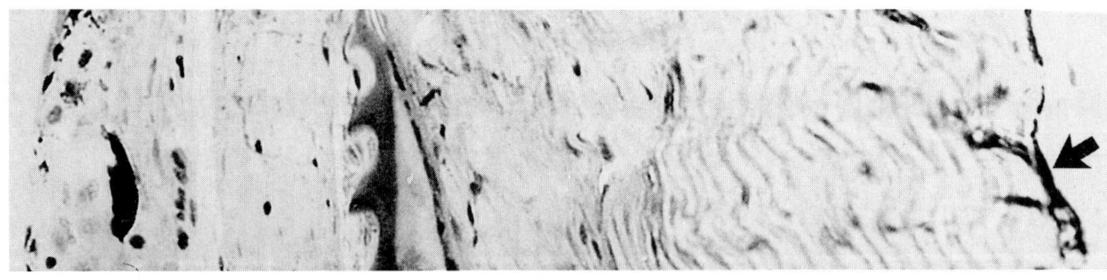

.A.

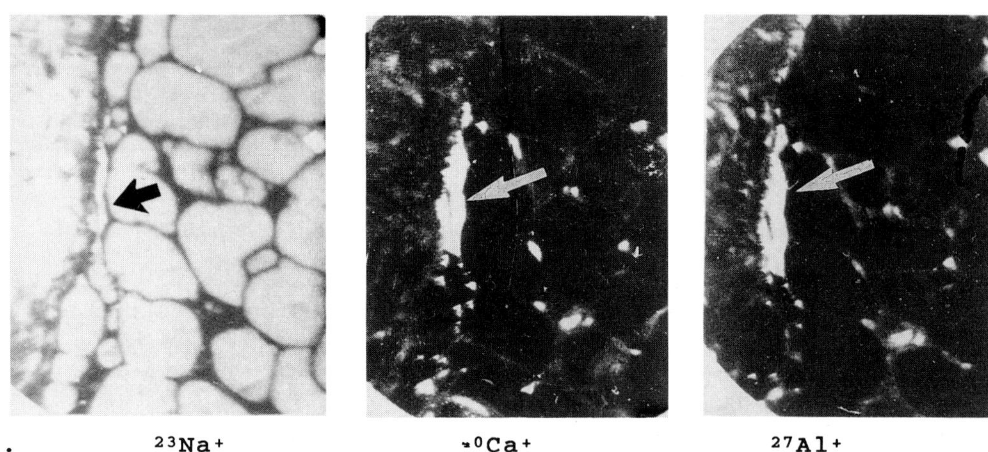

Fig.2. **A.** Histologic image of tegument from the epidermis (left) to the muscle (right). (X 400).

B. Ion images on mass 23, 40 and 27 in the derm revealing a concentration of aluminium in a layer between derm and muscle corresponding to a melanocytes layer (arrow). we can see this melanocytes layer on the histologic image on the top (arrow) (X270).

Electron Probe X Ray microanalysis confirms the informations given by ion microscopy. We detected aluminium localized in the creetes of scales, with increasing concentration as we go up from the old part to the root of the scale in the derm.

CONCLUSION

Melanin grains concentrate aluminium in all the studied organs of trouts where these organites can be found (liver, kidneys, gills and tegument).But in the tegument, we can also see aluminium concentration at the surface of the scale. This accumulation on calcified tissue is known on men (Galle P., 1981).

Beside gills and kidneys, tegument appears to be a tissue representative of an aluminium poisoning in fish.

GALLE P. (1986): La toxicité de l'Aluminium. _La recherche. 178,_ 766-775

Metal Ions in Biology and Medicine, vol. 2. Eds. J. Anastassopoulou, Ph. Collery, J.C. Etienne, Th. Theophanides. John Libbey Eurotext, Paris © 1992, pp. 139-140

Development and optimization of a radioimmunoassay for metallothionein

Jaume Folch, M. Teresa Colomina, Domenech Sánchez, José L. Paternain

Unit of Biochemistry, School of Medicine, University of Barcelona, 43201 Reus, Spain

Metallothionein (MT) is a low molecular weight, cysteine-rich protein, with a characteristic high metal content (Kägi & Schäfter, 1988). MT is believed to play physiological roles in essential metal-content regulation (Zn, Cu) and heavy metal detoxification(Cd, Hg) (Bremner & Beattie, 1990).

The quantification of MT observes different methods based, most of them, in their capacity to bind metals such as cadmium (Eaton & Toal, 1982), mercury (Piotrowski et al., 1973) or silver (Scheuhammer & Cherian, 1986). All these metal saturation methods have the problem of its low specificity. The specific and sensitive quantification of MT is possible using a inmunoassay method (RIA; ELISA, etc...), although the low size and structural homology of the mammalian MT minimize their immunogenic capacity. Antisera with constant high titers of antibodies against MT are not routinely avalable.

We report the development of a radioimmunoassay (RIA) for quantification of MT using a rabbit antiserum against MT. The immunization method consisted of repeated intradermal injections in New Zealand rabbits of glutaraldehide polimerized horse comercial MT with bovine IgG and emulsioned with Freund's adjuvants. The content of anti-MT antibodies in the sera of treated rabbits was tested by binding of ^{125}I-MT and by dot-blot technique.

The RIA was developed using the sera with highest titer values. To 200 μl of standard or sample in a buffer 0.05M Tris-HCl, 0,25% gelatine, 0,02% sodium azide, pH 8.0, we added 100 μl of antiserum in a final dilution of 1:6000 and with a capacity to bind of 52% of tracer when no cold ligand was present. The standard used was the same type as the one used as tracer, MT-I or MT-II of rabbit in a range from 0.1 to 100 ng/tube. We added as tracer 100 μl of ^{125}I-MT (5000 cpm) labeled by Bolton-Hunter reagent (3.8 MBq/μg MT). After incubation for 18 h at 4°C we separated the antibody-MT complex from free tracer by addition of 100 μl of anti-rabbit antisera (goat) at 1:50 and 10% polyethylene glycol 6000 in buffer. After 2 h at room temperature the reaction mixture was centrifuged, the supernatant was discared and the sediments were counted in a gamma counter.

As shown in Fig. 1 a lineal response was obtained from the standard curve between 0.2 and 20 ng MT/tube. The assay showed a high specific and sensitive response for MT with a detection limit about 0.07μg/l.

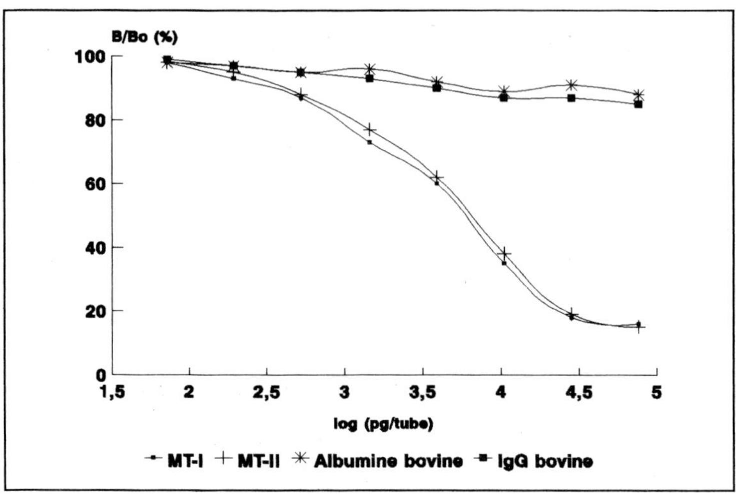

Fig. 1. Standard curves for different types of MT and other proteins.

The intra- and interassay coefficient of variation of the RIA at working concentrations were 4.5 and 11.5 % respectively. Analytical recorvery of known dilutions of added MT ranged from 95 to 110% (average value = 102%). The antiserum cross-reacts with MT from different mammalian species tested (rabbit, rat and human). The serial dilutions of tested samples followed the same curve as standard.

REFERENCES:

Bremner I., and Beattie J.H. (1990): Metallothionein and the trace minerals. *Annu. Rev. Nutr. 10:* 63-83.

Eaton D.L., and Toal B.F. (1982): Evaluation of the Cd/hemoglobin affinity assay for the rapid determination of metallothionein in biological tissues. *Toxicol.Appl.Pharmacol. 66:* 134-142.

Kägi J.H.R., and Schäffer A.(1988): Biochemistry of metallothionein. Biochemistry 27 (23): 8509-8515.

Piotrowski J.K., Bolanowska W., and Sapota A. (1973): Evaluation of metallothionein content in animal tissues. *Acta Biochim.Pol. 20:* 207-215.

Scheuhammer A.M., and Cherian M.G. (1986): Quantification of metallothioneins by a silver-saturation method. *Toxicol.Appl.Pharmacol. 82:* 417-425.

*This work was supported by CICYT, Spain trough project SAL 90-0998.

Metal Ions in Biology and Medicine, vol. 2. Eds. J. Anastassopoulou, Ph. Collery, J.C. Etienne, Th. Theophanides. John Libbey Eurotext, Paris © 1992, pp. 141-142

Subcellular concentration of neptunium 237

H. Boulahdour*, J.L. Poncy**, P. Galle*

** Laboratoire de Biophysique, INSERM SC 27 Faculté de Médecine, 94010 Créteil Cedex, France. ** CEA/DSV/DPTE/LRT, Bruyères Le Chatel, France*

Neptunium, an actinide of atomic number 93 is the first transuranic element. The isotope 237 of neptunium has to be considered with a particular attention because of its very long half life (2.14 10^6 years).
In this work, the microscopic distribution of neptunium 237 in two mammallian tissues (liver and kidney tissues) has been studied by analytical microscopy. Neptunium is both a chemotoxic and a radiotoxic after injection as a soluble form. This element is concentrated in the bones, the liver, the kidneys and the suprarenal glands(5). However, this radionuclide emits alpha tracts of short length and its subcellular distribution remains to be determined.

A solution of neptunium 237 nitrate (valence V, ph 3.5) has been injected in the peritoneum cavity of 12 male rats at the rate of 0.1 mg of neptunium per injection and per day, during two months corresponding to a total administered dose of 6 mg. Rats have been sacrified the day following the last injection. Liver and kidney tissues have been prepared according to the conventional methods used in electron microscopy: glutaraldehyde fixation, osmium post fixation, deshydratation with alcool and embedding in epon.
Ultrathin tissues section deposited on titanium grids have been studied with a Philips EM 300 electron microscope and electron probe microanalysis has been performed on the same sections using a Camebax electron microprobe equipped with a conventional transmission electron microscope and 4 wavelenght dispersive X-ray spectrometers of high resolving power.

In the liver, abnormal structures have been observed by electron microscopy in the nuclei of hepatocytes (Fig.1) and the same structures have also been observed in the nuclei of the proximal tubules cells of the kidneys (Fig.2). These structures are formed of clusters of very small and dense particles, several nanometer in diameter. The clusters are localised in the central part of the nuclei and they are separated from nucleoli and heterochomatin. Electron probe X-ray analysis of these clusters has showned that they contain neptunium associated with phosphorus. Severe ultrastructures lesions such a picnotic nuclei and degenerative states of the cytoplasm are observed in some of the cells containing intranuclear neptunium.These alterations are induced probably by chemical toxicity of neptunium since one desintegration is produced every 6 months corresponding to a mass of 10^{-15} g neptunium into the nuclei.The specific concentration of a mineral element in the cell nuclei is very rare .Intranuclear inclusions have been observed after lead(1) and bismuth(2) intoxication in the same varieties of cells. However, in these cases, the intranuclear inclusions are not of the same ultrastructure.

Concerning other actinides, only two of them, uranium(3) and thorium (4) have already been studied by microanalytical methods and their subcellular localisation determined. These elements are specifically concentrated in the cytoplasm and more precisely in lysosomes.
The explanation of this particular localisation of neptunium remains unknown.

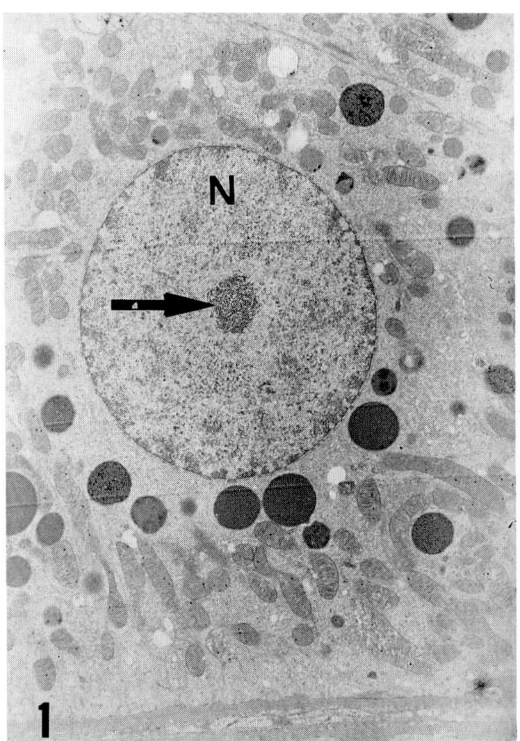

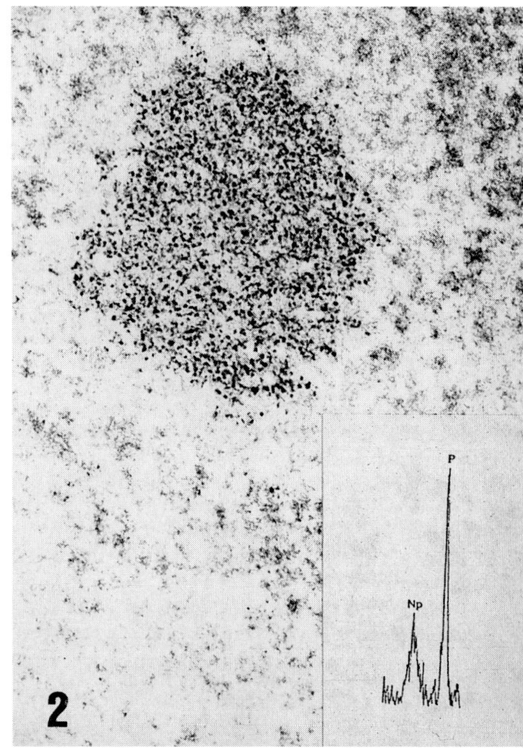

Figure 1. Electron microscopy of the kidney section of a rat after neptunium intoxication.A dark and round inclusion (arrow) is observed in the center of the nucleus.(N:nucleus).(M x 5000).
Figure 2. Higher magnification of figure 1.The inclusion is formed of a cluster of small and dense granulations,about 30 nm in diameter.On the right, caracteristics rays of neptunium (M alpha ray) and phosphorus (K alpha ray) obtained by electron probe X ray microanalysis of the dark inclusion presented above.(M X 29000).

REFERENCES

1- Beaver, D.L. (1961): The ultrastructure of the kidney in lead intoxication with particular reference to intranuclear inclusions. Amer. J. Path. 39: 195-208.
2- Beaver, D.L., and Burr, R.E. (1963): Electron microscopy of bismuth inclusions. Amer. J. Path. 42: 609-618.
3- Galle, P. (1974): Rôle des lysosomes et des mitochondries dans les phénomènes de concentration et d'élimination d'éléments minéraux (uranium et or) par le rein. J. Microscopie. 19: 17-24.
4- Hallegot, Ph. and Galle, P. (1988): Microanalytical study of thorium 232 deposits in bone marrow and liver. Radiat. Environ. Biophys. 27: 67-78.
5- Thompson, R.C. (1982): Neptunium-the Neglected Actinide: A Review of the biological and Environmental Literature. Rad. Res. 90: 1-32.

3 CANCER

Metal Ions in Biology and Medicine, vol. 2. Eds. J. Anastassopoulou, Ph. Collery, J.C. Etienne, Th. Theophanides. John Libbey Eurotext, Paris © 1992, pp. 145-150

Hemin uptake and detection of hemin binding proteins (HeBP) in human leukemia K562 cells

Athina I. Tsamadou*, Willie Wong **, Asterios S. Tsiftsoglou*

** Laboratory of Pharmacology, Department of Pharmaceutical Sciences, Aristote University of Thessaloniki, 54006, Greece and ** Department of Medicine, Beth Israel Hospital and Harvard Medical School, Boston, MA 02215, USA*

It has been established over the past years that treatment of human leukemic K562 cells with hemin (ferric protoporphyrin IX, the oxidized form of heme) stimulates production of both embryonic (Gower I, Portland) and fetal hemoglobins (HbF, Barts) in substantial quantities by activating expression of globin genes (Rutherford et al, 1979, Charney and Maniatis, 1983, Dean et al,1983, Tsiftsoglou et al, 1989). Hemin treatment, however , does not induce terminal erythroid maturation of K562 cells and synthesis of adult- type hemoglobins (HbA_1, HbA_2), although hemin does so cooperatively with aclacinomycin (Tsiftsoglou et al, 1991). The lack of production of adult globin is not due to apparent deletion of β-globin gene but rather to incomplete termination of transcription of these DNA sequences (Tsiftsoglou et al, 1989). In addition, hemin enhances self renewal capacity of primitive erythroid progenitors (BFU-Es, CFU-Es) (Monette and Holden, 1982), activates protein biosynthesis, regulates iron uptake and heme biosynthesis and causes various other biological effects recently reviewed (Sassa, 1988). How hemin is transported in K562 cells and activates transcription of globin genes is still entirely unknown.

In this study, we have attempted to investigate the mode of hemin uptake in K562 cells with the use of radiolabelled hemin ([^{59}Fe]- or [^{14}C]-labelled) and to demonstrate whether K562 cells contain proteins that bind selectively to hemin.

MATERIALS AND METHODS

Hemin (ferric protoporphyrin IX) (Fig. 1) was purchased from Eastman Kodak, Rochester, NY. [^{59}Fe]-labelled hemin was synthesised by non enzymatic incorporation of 1.0 mCi [^{59}Fe]Cl_2 (New England Nuclear, Boston MA; specific activity 2-40 Ci/gr)into 1.2 mgr of protoporphyrin IX (Protoporphyrin Products, Utah) according to a method described by Galbraith et al (1985). [^{14}C]-labelled heme was prepared from $3x10^{10}$/10 ml rabbit reticulocytes that were incubated with [2-^{14}C]-glycine (80μCi) (specific activity 41mCi/ nmole) in RPMI-1640 culture medium containing 10% FCS and 400mg of ferrous citrate.

---

*To whom correspondence should be addressed

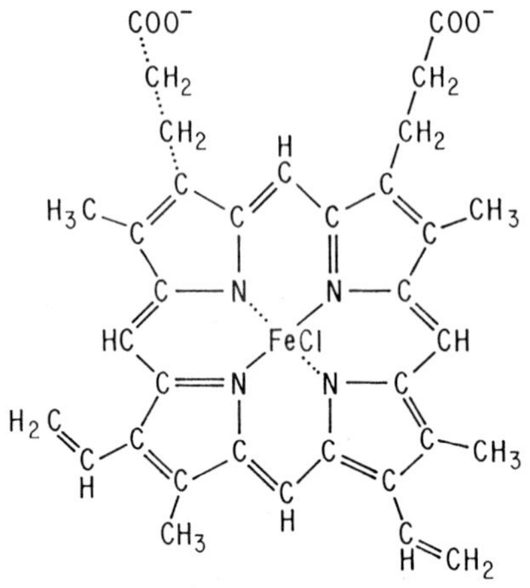

Fig 1. Structure of hemin (ferric-protoporphyrin IX)

[^{14}C]-labelled heme was extracted from hemoglobin released from reticulocytes which were lysed under hypotonic conditions. Radiochemical purity of radiolabelled hemin ([^{14}C]- or [^{59}Fe]-labelled) was tested by TLC chromatography using 2, 4- lutidine saturated with ammonia vapors. Agarose bearing heme residues covalently attached was purchased from Sigma Chemicals Co. MO, USA

Cell Cultures Human leukemia K562 cells originally developed by Lozzio and Lozzio (1975) were used throughout this study and maintained in culture as described earlier (Tsiftsoglou et al. 1989)

Assessment of uptake and intracellular distribution of radiolabelled hemin in K562 cells K562 cells were seeded in culture medium with 10% FCS and antibiotics at a concentration of 1x 10^6 cells / ml and labelled with [^{14}C]-hemin (2.5 x 10^5 cpm/ml) (spec. activity 5.3x 10^3 cpm/µg hemin). At various times following incubation duplicate aliquots (0.4 ml) of cell suspension were removed, layered over an ice cold 24% sucrose Na^+ Ringer solution and centrifuged at 13000x g for 3min. Pellets were lysed with 200µl 1% SDS and counted for radioactivity. To determine intracellular distribution of radiolabelled hemin, cells (harvested by centrifugation throughout the sucrose solution) were fractionated into cytoplasm and nuclei with the use of lysis buffer (0.14 M NaCl, 1.5mM $MgCl_2$, 10mM Tris-HCl pH 8.6, 1%NP-40). Radioactivity associated with each fraction was measured in a liquid scintillation counter.

Heme-Agarose affinity Chromatography of cytoplasmic proteins Soluble cytoplasmic extracts (5-7 mg) prepared from cultured K562 cells by lysis with buffer A (10 mM Tris-HCl pH 7.4, 1mM $CaCl_2$, 7% sucrose in 0.9% NaCl, 1mM PMSF, and 1% NP-40) and subsequent removal of the nuclei by centrifugation at 13000 rpm for 30 min at 4°C were analysed by hemin agarose affinity chromatography column prepared in a Pasteur pipete (0.75 ml) according to Tsutsui and Mueller (1982). Proteins bound to heme-agarose were eluted with 8M urea.In some occa sions proteins were eluted from column stepwise with NE buffer (0.5M NaCl and 10mM Na_3PO_4) containing increasing concentrations of NaCl (0.01M- 0.1M) at slightly alkaline conditions pH 8.2 prior to final elution with 8M Urea.

Gel filtration of protein complexes and SDS- PAGE electrophoresis of hemin binding proteins Proteins purified by hemin agarose affinity column chromatography were tested for their capacity to form putative proteins complexes with [^{59}Fe]-hemin by gel filtration on Sephadex G-150 column (50cm high, 1mm diameter) and subsequently analysed by SDS-PAGE electrophoresis as described by Laemmli (1970).

RESULTS

The uptake of radiolabelled hemin in K562 is a time and concentration dependent process.

Incubation of K562 cells with [^{14}C]- hemin in culture medium with 10% FCS

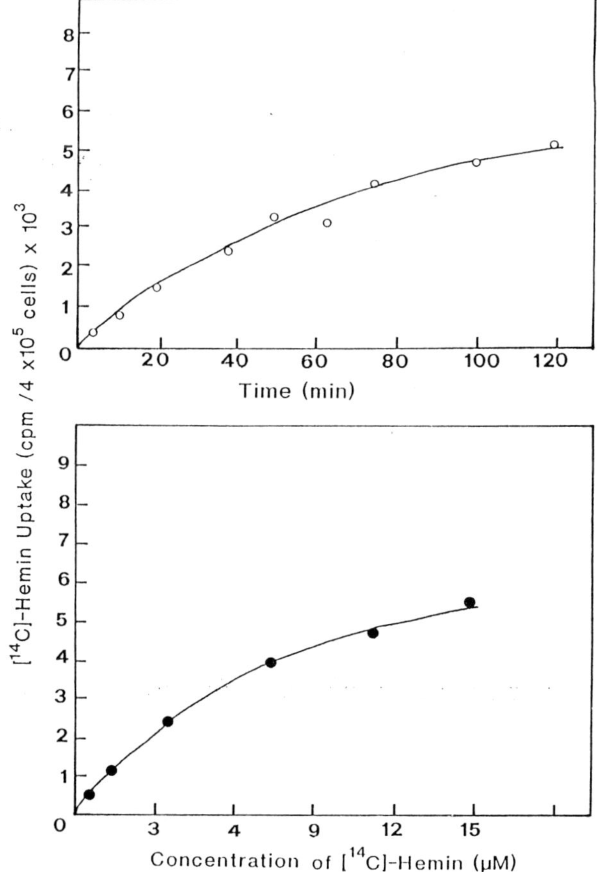

Fig 2. Uptake of [^{14}C]-hemin by cultured K562 cells as a function of time and concentration of labelled hemin added in the medium.
K562 cells (1 x 10^6 cells/ml) were incubated in culture with a known amount of [^{14}C]-hemin (2.5 x 10^5 cpm/ml). At time points indicated, cells were removed from culture and hemin uptake was measured (upper panel). In a different experiment, K562 cells were incubated with varying concentrations of labelled hemin and hemin uptake was determined after 60 min incubation (lower panel).

indicated that the intracellular level of [^{14}C]- hemin approached a steady state (plateau) value within 60-80 min. (Fig.2 upper panel). These data indicate that hemin uptake is time dependent. Incubation of K562 cells with increasing concentrations of [^{14}C]-hemin and assessment of hemin uptake revealed that hemin uptake is also concentration dependent process that exhibits saturation kinetics at relatively high concentations of hemin added in medium (15μM) (Fig. 2. lower pannel). Exogenously added hemin (15μM) reduced uptake of labelled hemin in a dose dependent manner presumably due to competition and / or displacement of labelled hemin from cellular bindings sites (data not shown). In addition, hemin uptake was reduced by 20-30% in cells pretreated with trypsin that modulates cell surface architecture and possible hemin-receptor sites located at the level of plasma membrane. Analysis of intracellular distribution of [^{14}C]-labelled hemin as a function of time indicated that hemin at first appears into cytosol and then accumulates into the cell nucleus (data not shown) at substantially quantities.

K562 cells contain several hemin binding proteins

Hemin agarose affinity chromatography of cytoplasmic proteins prepared from K562 cells, solubilized with the non-ionic detergent NP-40, loaded on a column and subsequently eluted with 8M Urea indicated that a substantial proportion of the proteins (8-12 %) were bound to heme covalently attached to agarose. (Fig. 3)

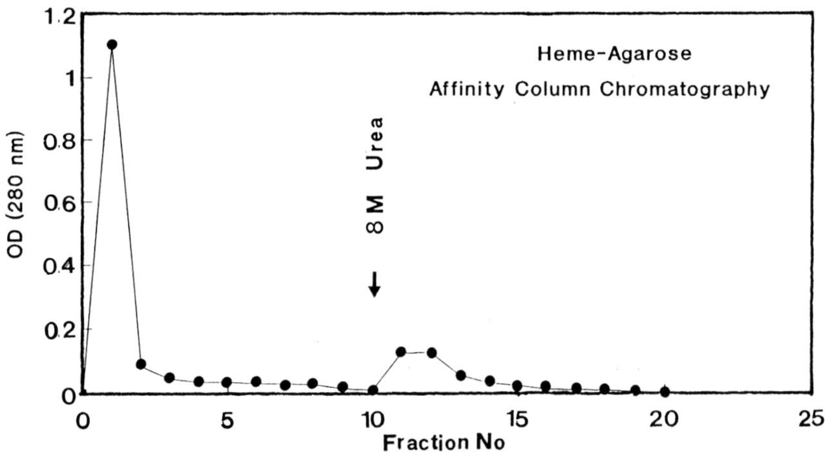

Fig 3. Hemin -agarose affinity column chromatography of soluble cytoplasmic proteins prepared from K562 cells.
Soluble proteins extracted from K562 cells were loaded on a hemin-agarose affinity chromatography column and eluted by 8M Urea as described under "Material and Methods".

When the eluted proteins were dialysed to remove urea and then analysed by SDS-PAGE electrophoresis, a restricted number of peptides of different molecular weights appeared (data not shown). The majority of these proteins were different from those eluted in the run off fraction without binding to hemin affinity column. When such hemin binding proteins were eluted first with NE buffer at slightly alkaline buffer pH (8.2) prior to elution with 8M urea, only a few proteins were eluted.Proteins eluted from heme-agarose column incubated with [^{59}Fe]-labelled hemin as shown by gel filtration formed protein complexes (Tsamadou, unpublished observations). These data indicate that cytoplasmic proteins bound to hemin agarose differ not only in molecular weight but also in affinity and physicochemical properties which are under current investigation.

DISCUSSION

Hemin, the oxidised form of heme is produced during hemoglobin degradation following red blood cell death, is a relatively lipophilic agent that is well dissolved in slightly alkaline environment but aggregates at high concentration in aqueous media. This agent in addition to cause a lot of interesting biological effects (see Sassa, 1988) has been used as hemin arginate for treating acute porphyrias and other hematological disorders quite effectively (Mustajoki, 1989,). These findings suggest that hemin may play a wider regulatory role in many cells than was earlier anticipated. This observation implies that plasma hemin is distributed to various tissues and must enter the cells in order to exert its pleiotropic effects(Muller-Eberhard and Nikkila, 1989, Smith and Morgan, 1987). Evidence exists to indicate that in liver cells hemin is transported via hemopexin, a plasma protein just like iron delivered by transferrin (van Renswoude et al, 1982,). This represents, however, a minor pathway of transport, since only a small fraction of hemin enters the cells this way. A large portion of hemin is bound to albumin and the rest (unbound hemin) enters the cells via an unknown process .
Hemin uptake was examined (with the use of radiolabelled hemin) as a function of time and concentration of hemin added in the culture medium. Hemin distribution in different intracellular compartment was also examined as a function of time. These data indicate that hemin uptake exhibits saturation transport kinetics; labelled hemin first interacts with cell membrane and appears in the cytosol and then accumulates in the cell nucleus.
The findings that hemin uptake is reduced by trypsin treatment of K562 cells or by nonlabelled exogenously added hemin tend to indicate that hemin may be transported via a carrier mediated transport system located at the level of cell membrane of K562 cells. Although this hypothesis needs further verification is in agreement with the observations of Galbraith et al (1985) that hemin is transported via a receptor mediated process in murine erythroleukemia cells (MEL) , a cell line that is also induced by hemin to produce hemoglobins (Ross and Sautner, 1976).
These observations prompted us to investigate whether K562 cells contain proteins that selectively interact with hemin. Previous studies indicating that major tetrapyrroles like hemin interact with cytosolic proteins Z and glutathione-S-transferrases (GST) (Muller-Eberhard and Nikkila, 1989) led additional support to our search for hemin binding proteins. We chosen to use hemin agarose affinity column chromatography rather than gel filtration, for detection, isolation and characterisation of such proteins from K562 cells since we experienced nonspecific absorption of free [^{14}C]-labelled hemin to sepharose beads during gel filtration of cytoplasmic proteins that had been incubated with free [^{14}C]-hemin. Hemin-agarose affinity chromatography would

be more successful in circumventing the nonspecific stickness of free hemin to proteins. By applying similar experimental conditions as Tsutsui and Muller (1985), we were able to detect cytoplasmic proteins that selectively bind to heme -agarose, and form protein complexes upon incubation with radiolabelled [^{59}Fe]-hemin. The question whether intracellular hemin binding proteins (HeBPs) play an important regulatory role in distribution of hemin in different intracellular compartments or in hemin-induced activation of transcription of globin genes is under current investigation in our laboratory.

REFERENCES

Charney P. and Maniatis T. (1983): Transcriptional regulation of globin gene expression in the human erythroid cell line K562 Science 220: 1281-1283.

Dean A., Ley T., Humphries R., Fordis M., Schechter A. (1983): Inducible transcription of five globin genes in K562 human leukemic cells Proc. Natl. Acad. Sci. USA 80: 5515-5519.

Galbraith R.F., Sassa S., Kappas A. (1985): Heme binding to murine erythroleukemia cells. Evidence for a heme receptor. J. of Biol. Chem. 260: 12198-12202.

Laemmli U.K. (1970): Cleavage of structural proteins during the of the assembly of the head of Bacteriophage T_4 Nature (London) 227: 680-685.

Lozzio C.B., Lozzio B.B. (1975): Human chronic myelogenous leukemia cell line with positive Philadelphia chromosome Blood 45: 321-334.

Monette F.C. and Holden S.A. (1982): Hemin enhances the in vitro growth of primitive erythroid progenitor cells Blood 60: 527-530.

Muller-Eberhard U. and Nikkila H. (1989): Transport of tetrapyrroles by proteins Semin. in Hematol. 26: 86-104.

Mustajoki P., Tenhunen R., Pierach C. and Volin L. (1989): Heme in the treatment of porphyrias and hematological disorders Semin. in Hematol. 26(1): 1-9.

Ross J., Sautner D. (1976): Induction of globin mRNA accumulation by hemin in cultured erythroleukemic cells. Cell 8: 513-520.

Rutherford T.R., Clegg J.B., Weatherall D.J. (1979): K562 human leukemic cells synthesize embryonic hemoglobin in response to hemin Nature (London) 280: 164-165.

Sassa S. (1988): Heme stimulation of cellular growth and differentiation Semin. in Hematol. 25: 312-320.

Smith A. and Morgan W.T. (1981): Hemopexin -mediated transport of heme into isolated rat hepatocytes J. Biol. Chem. 256: 10902-10909.

Tsiftsoglou A.S., Wong W., Robinson S.H., Hensold J. (1989): Hemin increases production of β-like globin RNA transcripts in human erythroleukemia K562 cells Develop. Gen. 10: 311- 317.

Tsiftsoglou A.S., Wong W., Tsamadou A.I., Robinson S.H. (1991): Cooperative effects of hemin and anthracyclines in promoting terminal erythroid maturation in K562 human erythroleukemia cells Exp. Hematol. 19: 928-933.

Tsutsui K., Mueller G.C. (1982): Affinity Chromatography of heme binding proteins: An improved method for the synthesis of hemin-agarose Anal. Biochem. 121: 244-250.

van Renswoude J., Brigdes K.R., Harfold J.B. and Klausner R.C. (1982): Receptor-mediated endocytosis of transferrin and the uptake of Fe in K562 cells: Identification of a nonlysosomal acidic compartment Proc. Natl. Acad. Sci. USA 79: 6189-6190.

Metal Ions in Biology and Medicine, vol. 2. Eds. J. Anastassopoulou, Ph. Collery, J.C. Etienne, Th. Theophanides. John Libbey Eurotext, Paris © 1992, pp. 151-156

Induction of differentiation in neoplastic cells by selenium

Shu-Yu Yu, Xian-Ping Lu

Department of Biochemistry, Cancer Institute, Chinese Academy of Medical Sciences. 100021, Beijing, P.R. China

Selenium (Se) is an essential dietary trace element. Considerable epidemiological data indicate that Se serves as a naturally occurring anticancer-agent (Shamberger and Willis, 1971; Schrauzer et al., 1977; Yu et al.,1985). Se is also found in lower concentrations in the blood of many cancer patients, and patients with Se concentration approaching or exceeding the mean value of all cancer patients had tumors that remained confined to the region of origin, developed less distant metastasis, had a decreased frequency of recurrences. (Broghamer et al.,1976). In animals, dietary Se inhibits the development of carcinogen-and virus-induced tumors (Clayton and Baumann, 1949; Thompson and Becci, 1980; Schrauzer et al., 1976; Yu, et al., 1988). Furthermore, evidence in both tumor-bearing animals and human tumor cells in culture have confirmed an antitumor effect of Se and potential clinical benefit (Milner and Hsu, 1981; Ao et al., 1987; Nano et al.,1989). The mechanism of selenium's antitumor effect is not yet well explained. Evidence suggests that Se may be acting to enhance immune response (Spallholz, 1981; Hu and Zhang, 1990), inhibit the metabolic activation of carcinogen (Schilaci et al., 1982), or stimulate detoxification and excretion of car cinogens (Jacobs,1983). Other studies show that Se influences neoplastic cells directly (Medina and Obora, 1981; Lewko and McConnell, 1982). Recently our interest in the mode of action of Se has focused attention on its effects on differentiation of established tumor cells. In the present study an evidence was carried out to show the role of Se on the induction of hepatoma's carbamyl phosphate synthetase I (CPS- I), a tissue-specific enzyme associated with the differentiation of liver cells.

MATERIAL AND METHODS

Tumor cells and treatments 10^6 of viable hepatoma ascites cells (AH-22) were inoculated into the peritoneal cavity of male Kunming mice (20 ~25g). Four days after tumor injection Na_2SeO_3 at a dose of 1 µg/g body weight of the host (1 µg/g b.w.) was administered i.p. for consecutive 4 days. Control mice received daily injections of physiologic saline. The ascites cells were collected and washed twice with saline, then destructed by sonipreparation (15 sec×7 amplitude micronce×5 times with 1 min. interval) in distilled water. Homogenate were centrifuged and supernatants were assayed for CPS- I activity as described by Li et al.(1977).

Immunotitration CPS-I antisera was prepared as described by Huang et al., (1982). A definite amount of CPS-I extracts (3.5~8.5 units CPS-I) from 4-day's Se-treated hepatoma cells was incubated with various amount of CPS-I antisera in 2 µl of buffer solution (50 mM gly. gly buffer, pH 7.3, 0.14 M NaOH, 10 mM DTT) at 37 °C for 1 hr.. After standing overnight at 0 ~ 4° C, centrifuged at 4° C, 4000g for 30 min. the residual activity of CPS-I in supernatants was analyzed.

[^{3}H] Leucine incorporation Mice fasted overnight were injected i.p. with [^{3}H] leucine (2 µCi/g.b.w.) 50 min. before decapitation. The hepatoma cells were collected and destructed by sonipreparation in 9 vol of buffer I (20 mM Tris.Cl, PH 8.0, 20% glycerol, 10 mM β-mercaptoethanol) at 0- 4 ° C. The homogenates were centrifuged at 4° C, 15,000g for 20 min. and the supernatants were precipitated with 20 mM $MgCL_2$ and 10 mM DTT at 37° C for 30 min., centrifuged at 4° C, 4,000g for 10 min.. 25 µl and 200 µl supernatants was taken for assay of CPS-I activity and total cpm counts by TCA precipitation respectively. Another 150 µl supernatants were reacted with CPS-I antisera or normal rabbit IgG respectively in buffer II (0.4 M gly. gly buffer, PH 7.5, 1.12 M NaCL)at 37 ° C for 60 min., and stored overnight at 4° C. The CPS-I antibody precipitates were centrifuged in 1 M sucrose gradient at 4° C, 15,000g for 20 min., rinsed with cold saline for three times,dissolved in 0.3 ml 88% formate and counted cpm by liquid scintillation. The amount of protein was measured by the method of Lowry et al (1951) using serum bovine albumin as standard. Absolute amounts of incorporation were expressed as counts/minute/mg protein (cpm/mg pr.)

Dot blot and Northern blot analysis The method of white (1982) and Thomas (1980) were adopted. CPS-I cDNA probe of 0.8 kb was prepared as described by Wu et al (1987). ^{32} P-Probe was obtained by nick translation (specific activity: 1-2 X 10^8 cpm/ug DNA). Total RNA was extracted by NP-40 and phenol -chloroform, the mRNA was purified through oligo(dT)-cellulose.

RESULTS:

Table 1. demonstrates the differential effects of selenium on the CPS-I activity of hepatoma ascites cells and normal liver cells. It was shown that in hepatoma cells, compared with normal liver cells, the CPS-I activity decreased significantly (1.36±0.82 Vs undetectable). Intraperitoneal injection of Na_2SeO_3 (1 µg/g b.w./day) into hepatoma-bearing mice for consecutive 4 days led to a pronounced increase in CPS-I activety to 8.08± 2.83. By contrast, under the same condition, there was no stimulation of CPS-I activity in normal liver of mice treated by Se.

Teble 1. Effect of Se on the activity of CPS-I in hepatoma and normal liver cells.

Group	CPS-I activity (µmoles/mg pr./hr.)
Normal liver	1.360 ± 0.816 (10)[a]
Hepatoma	Undetectable (15)[b]
Normal liver+Se	1.115 ± 0.517 (10)[c]
Hepatoma+Se	8.020 ± 2.831 (12)[d]

The results are expressed as mean ±S.E (number of mice).
P value by t-test: a:b P<0.001, b:d P<0.001, a:c P>0.5.

Immunotitration experiment was carried out to determine whether the incrased CPS-I activety induced by Se in hepatoma cells is due to the increase of enzyme protein. The result showed that CPS-I activity was decreased with increasing of antisera added (Fig.1). It suggests that the increased CPS-I activity in hepatoma cells by Se-treatment was due to the increase of CPS-I protein.

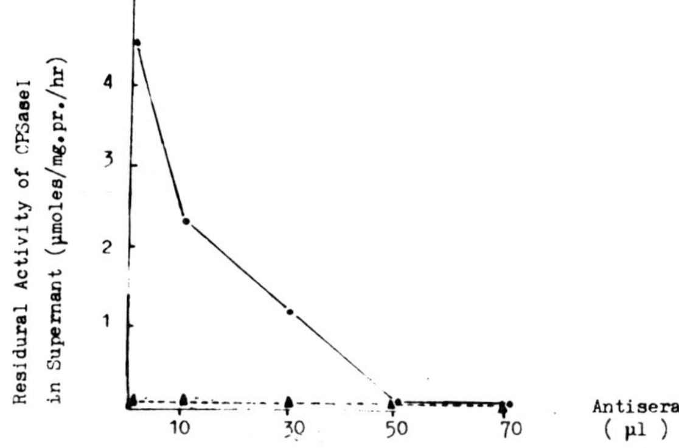

Fig.1. The immunotitration of CPS-I by antisera.
●--● Hepatoma+Se; ▲--▲ Hepatoma

The further experiment examined the effect of Se on the biosynthesis of CPS-I in hepatoma ascites cells *in vivo* by [^{3} H] leucine incorporation. The results showed that the cpm per mg of enzyme protein in hepatoma cells was undetectable, while that in Se-treated group was significantly high (Table 2). It suggests that the biosynthesis of CPS-I enzyme in hepatoma cells is increased by Se-treatment.

Table 2. Effect of Na SeO_3 on the biosynthesis of CPS-I in hepatoma ascites cells in vivo.

Group	CPS-I activity μmoles/mg pr./hr.	Total cpm per mg protein (a)	Cpm per mg enzyme protein (b)	Relative rate of synthesis (b/a %)
Hepatoma	Undetectable	1474.7±180.9	Undetectable	Undetectable
Hepatoma+Se	5.4±4.06	1693.6±392.1	215.4 ±98.1	12.0±3.0

In order to explore the mechanism of CPS-I increased in hepatoma of tumor-bearing mice treated with Se, Dot blot and Northern blot hybridization of RNA extracted from hepatoma was conducted with^{32}P-labeled CPS-I cDNA probe. The results demonstrated that only a small amount of CPS-Im RNA was found in control hepatoma cells, it appeared increasingly after administration of Se for 3 days and increased significantly by 4-day's Se treatment.

By Northern blot analysis it was shown that the molecular weight of CPS-I mRNA is about 29s which is the same as reported by Nyunoya (1985).The change pattern of CPS-I mRNA in groups of hepatoma ascites cells, 3-day's Se-treated and 4-day's Se-treated hepatoma ascites cells were same as obtained by Dot blot analysis (Fig.2). These findings were in accordance with those observed in changes of CPS-I activity by Se treatment.Thus it would indicate that increase in CPS-I content in hepatoma cells by Se treatment might be associated with changes in gene expression of CPS-I.

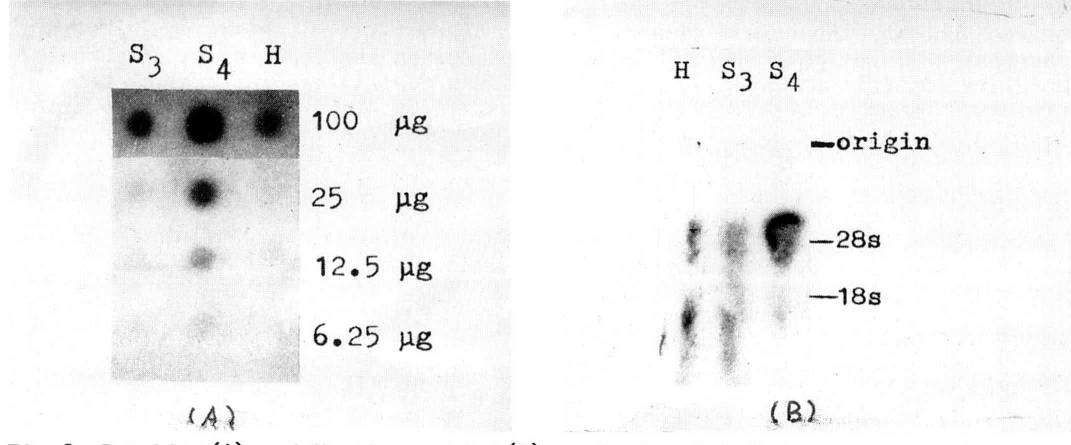

Fig.2. Dot blot(A) and Northern blot(B) analysis of CPS-I gene expression H, Hepatoma ascites cells. S_3 ,3-day's Se-treated hepatoma ascites cells. S_4 , 4-day's Se-treated hepatoma ascites cells.

Discussion:

CPS-I is a tissue-specific enzyme for liver cell differentiation. The enzyme activity is low in fetal liver and increases rapidly after birth. (Murakami, et al. 1983). During hepatocarcinogenesis it is decreased and its decrement is correlated with the degree of malignancy of hepatoma cells (Li et al. 1977). The present study demonstrated that the CPS-I was undetectable in transplantable hepatoma ascites cells,it increased significantly in hepatoma ascites cells from host injected i.p. with Na_2SeO_3 (1 µg/g b.w.) for consecutive 4 days. By immunochemical analysis and [^{3}H]leucine incorporation assay, it indicated that the increased activity of CPS-I in Se-treated hepatoma cells was caused by increased biosynthesis of CPS-I protein rather than stimulating the enzyme activity only.The coincidence of the appearance and increment of mRNA for CPS-I with those of enzyne itself also support this conclusion. CPS-I induced by Se, therefore, is clearly an acquired proten contributing to the differertiated expression of the mature hepatocyte.

Thus in our studies, we have demonstrated that various tumor cells can be induced to differentiate by Se both *in vitro and in vivo* into cells with normal characteristics (Yu et al. 1988). The effects mainly included: induction of differentiation of transplantable hepatoma ascites cells in mice, as indicated by increases in cAMP, protein kinase A isozyme type II, as well as CPS-I, and suppressions of cGMP, protein kinase A isozyme type I and aspartate carbamyl transferase which are associated with cell proliferation (Lu et al. 1989); the differentiating effects of Se on cultured human hepatoma cell lines, QGY-7701 and SMMC-7721, and human pulmonary adenocarcinoma cell lines, LTEP-a-2 and SPC-A-1 were also shown *in vitro*, as indicated by an increase in adhesiveness of cells and decrease in the extent of saturation density. Furthermore a down-regulation on *c-myc* gene expression and stimulation of the *c-fos* gene expression by Se in hepatoma cells were demonstrated (Yu 1990). On improvement on the differentiation, 98% of the cells were still viable, but the cell proliferation was reduced; their tumorigenicity in animals was suppressed; prolongation of survival times of animals inoculated with Se-treated tumor cells were observed. (Ao et al.,1987; Lu et al.1987). This observation is similar to that reported by Nano et al. (1989) who demonstrated the growth of human colon cancer cells Caco 2,incubated in the presence of 10 µM of Se, was inhibited by 50%, whereas 90～100% of the cells were still viable. These findings suggest that Se, an essential nutrient for humans and animals, may play an important role in regulation of cell differentiation and proliferation. The studies have also shown that stopping cell multiplication by Se-inducing differentiation to mature cells can correct the genetic abnormalities that give rise to malignancy. These observations merit further exploration on the possible usefulness of Se in cancer prevention and treatment.

REFERENCES

Ao, P., Zhao, M. and Yu, S.Y.(1987): In vitro differential effects of sodium selenite on the growth of human hepatoma cells and human embryonic liver cells. *Biol. Trace Elem. Res.* 14, 1-18.

Ao, P., Zhao, M. and Yu, S.Y.(1987): Some differentiating effects of selenium on the cultured human hepatoma cells and human pulmonary adenocarcinoma cells in vitro. *Biol. Trace Elem. Res.* 14, 19-26.

Ao, P., Zhao, M. and Yu, S.Y.(1987): Differential effects of selenium on the proliferation of human pulmonary adenocarcinoma cells and human embryonic lung diploid cells in vitro. *Biol. Trace Elem. Res.* 14, 29-42.

Broghamer, W.L. et al.(1976): Relationship between serum selenium levels and patients with carcinoma. *Cancer* 37, 1384-1388.

Clayton, C.C. and Baumann, C.A.(1949): Diet and azo dye tumors: Effect of diet during a period when the dye is not fed. *Cancer Res.* 9, 575-582.

Huang, S. et al.(1982): Studies on the mechanism of carcinogenesis VI. The immunochemistry of carbamyl phosphate synthetase in rat liver and hepatoma induced by diethylnitrosamine. *Acta Biochim. et Biophys. Sinica.* 14, 407-415.

Hu, X. and Zhang, Y.(1990): Effects of selenium deficiency and supplementation on tumor immune response in mice. *Chinese J. of Oncology* 12, 328-331.

Jacobs, N.M.(1983): Selenium inhibition of 1,2-dimethylhydrazine-induced colon carcinogenesis. *Cancer Res.* 43, 1646-1649.

Lewko, W.M. and McConnell, K.P.(1982): Biphasic influence of selenium on cell growth and the synthesis of collagens in cultured mammary tumor cells. *Federation Proc.* 41, 623.

Li, S., Fan, M. et al.(1977): Studies on the mechanism of carcinogenesis. I. Interrelationship between the changes in proliferation and tissue-specific enzyme activities of rat liver during development and carcinogenesis by diethylnitrosamine. *Acta Biochim. et Biophys. Sinica* 9, 113-130.

Lowry, O.H., Rosebrough, N.J. et al(1951): Protein measurement with the Folin phenol reagent. *J. Biol. Chem.* 193, 205-275.

Lu, X. and Yu. S.Y.(1987): The influence of sodium selenite on the membrane fluidity and carcinogenicity of the hepatoma cells. *Chinese Bioch. J.* 3, 449-454.

Lu, X. et al.(1989): The effects of sodium selenite on the induction of tissue-specific enzyme CPSase I and inhibition of cell proliferation-related enzyme ACTase in AH_{22} mouse hepatoma ascites cells. *Chinese Biochem. J.* 5, 235-239(in Chinese)

Medina, D. and Oborn, C.J.(1981): Differential effects of Se on the growth of mouse mammary cells in vitro. *Cancer Lett.* 13, 333-344.

Milner, J.A. and Hsu, C.Y.(1981): Inhibitory effects of selenium on the growth of L1210 leukemic cells. *Cancer Res.* 41,1652-1656.
Murakami, A. et al.(1983): In vivo study of developmental changes in carbamyl phosphate synthetase-I in rat of liver: repression of the enzyme synthesis immediately after birth. *Biochim. Biophys. Acta* 739:66-72.
Nano, J.L., Czerucka, D. et al.(1989): Effect of selenium on the growth of three humen colon cancer cell lives. *Biol Trace Elem. Res.* 20,31-43.
Nyunoya, H. et al.(1985): Characterization and derivation of the gene coding for mitochondrial carbamyl phosphate synthetase I of rat. *J. Biol. Chem.* 260:9346-9356.
Schillaci, M., Martin, S.E. et al.(1982): The effects of dietary selenium on the biotransformation of 7,12-dimethyl-benz[anthracene. *Mutat. Res.* 101, 31-37.
Schrauzer, G.N. White, D.A., et al.(1977): Cancer mortality correlation studies. III statistical association with dietary selenium intakes *Bioinorg. Chem.* 7, 23-34.
Shamberger, R.J. and Willis, C.E.(1971): Selenium distribution and human cancer mortality. *CRC Crit Rev. Clin. Lab. Sci.* 2, 211-221.
Spallholz, J.E.(1981): Selenium: What role in immunity and immune cytotoxicity? In *Selenium in Biology and Medicin.* ed. J.E. Spallholz, J.L. Martin, and H.E. Ganther, p103-107. AVI Publishing Co., Westport, CT.
Thomas, P.S.(1980): Hybridization of denatured RNA and small DNA fregments transferred to nitrocellulose. *Proc. Nat. Acad. Sci. USA.*, 77, 5201-5205.
Thompson, H.J. and Becci, P.J.(1980): Selenium inhibition of N-methyl-N-nitrosoures-induced mammary carcinogenesis in rat. *J. Natl. Cancer Inst.* 65, 1299-1301.
White, B.A. et al.(1982): Cytoplasmic dot hybridization. *J. Biol. Chem.* 257:8569-8572.
Wu, S. et al.(1987): Cloning of CPS-I cDNA and the changes in CPS-I mRNA contents during hepatocarcinogenesis in rat. *Scientia Sinica(B)* 5:518-522.
Yu, S.Y., Ao, P. et al.(1988): Biochemical and celluler aspects of the anticancer activity of selenium. *Biol. Trace Elem. Res.* 15, complete 243-256.
Yu, S.Y., Lu, X.P. et al.(1990): The regulatory effects of selenium on the expression of oncogenes associated with proliferation and differentiation on tumor cells. In *Metal ions in Biology and Medicine.* ed. Ph. Collery, L.A. Poirier, M. Manfait, J.C. Etienne pp. 487-489. Paris, John Libbey Eurotext.
Yu, S.Y. and Zhu, Y.J. et al.(1985): Regional variation of cancer mortality incidence and its relation to selenium levels in China. *Biol. Trace Elem. Res.* 7, 21-29.
Yu, S.Y. and Zhu, Y.J. et al.(1988): Selenium chemoprevention of liver cancer in animals and possible human applications. *Biol. Trace Elem. Res.* 15, 231-241.

Metal Ions in Biology and Medicine, vol. 2. Eds. J. Anastassopoulou, Ph. Collery, J.C. Etienne, Th. Theophanides. John Libbey Eurotext, Paris © 1992, pp. 157-162

Carcinogenicity interactions between nickel and magnesium

Neil A. Littlefield, Lionel A. Poirier

Division of Comparative Toxicology, National Center for Toxicological Research, United States Food and Drug Administration, Department of Health and Human Services, Jefferson, Arkansas, USA

Mg is essential for several different and varied metabolic and physiological functions and participates in almost all anabolic and catabolic functions. Deficiencies are not common since the metal is abundant in the food supply; however, the symptoms for deficiency include muscle wasting, apathy, numbness, convulsions, deliria, ventricular fibrillation, tachycardia, and CNS depression.

Both epidemiological and experimental evidence show an association between Mg deficiency and the development of leukemia and other cancer. One of the first indications of this occurred when Bois (1964) showed that rats fed a Mg-deficient diet for 95 days developed tumors of the thymus. There were no tumors of the thymus found in rats that had adequate Mg in the diet. Jasmin (1968) showed that up to 40% of the rats which survived 40 days of dietary Mg depletion developed thymomas. Another early study that was intended to characterize the clinical signs of a Mg-deficient diet demonstrated that Mg deficiency was more effective in producing leukemia than was the carcinogen N-2-fluorenylacetamide (Battifora et al., 1968). Table 1 is reproduced from some of his data.

Table 1. Summary of Experiments (Battifora et al., 1968)

Group No.	Dietary Regimen (mg/100 gm) Magnesium	Carcinogen	Percent of Rats Developing Leukemia
1	65	0	0
2	5	0	25.0
3	5	0	9.5
4	5	60	33.3
5	65	60	1.5

When Mg was present in the diet at 65 mg/100 gm, the incidence of leukemia was nonexistent or very low, whereas at 5 mg/100 gm then the incidence of leukemia was high. As shown in group 5, the incidence of leukemia was also low when Mg was present at the same time as the carcinogen. Hass et al. (1989) demonstrated that Mg deprivation favors an increased incidence of reticuloendothelial tumors, presumably attributable to suppression of development of immunity to this class of neoplasms, or interference in maturation of immunocytes. Solid epithelial cancers were slightly reduced in incidence and malignancy by Mg deprivation.

The epidemiological evidence is supplemented and supported by other experimental studies. It was demonstrated by Rubin et al. (1981) and Rubin (1982) that Mg was a second messenger in the action of mitogens, as shown by the fact that Mg-deprived transformed cells became serum dependent for DNA synthesis and resembled non-transformed cells in appearance, serum requirements, and response to cell populations density. This effect was transient.

Mills et al. (1984) used male Fischer 344 rats with implanted and established tumors to demonstrate that a Mg-deficient diet for 32 days would retard the tumor growth solely by dietary Mg depletion (Table 2).

Also, as shown in the work of Mills et al. (1984) and of Cameron and Smith (1989), tumor cells contained less Mg and potassium but more sodium and chloride than the rapidly dividing normal cells.

Table 2. Effect of Magnesium Depletion on Tumor Weight

Diet Group	# Rats	Tumor Wt.(g)	Tumor Magnesium (μ/g)
Control	7	18.4 ± 4.09	194 ± 7.56
Deficient	9	9.8 ± 1.90	118 ± 13.5

Kasprzak and Waalkes (1986) reviewed the roles of several essential metals and their effects of carcinogenesis. They indicated that Mg and zinc tends to inhibit carcinogenesis and that the deficiency of Mg increased the incidence of neoplasia in both humans and animals. There is a simple correlation between the inhibitions of carcinogenesis by the Mg and zinc supplementation and the reduction of carcinogen binding to cells and DNA. Although there are various studies showing correlations between Mg deficiencies in the diets to disorders such as lung tumors, thymomas, leukemias, chromosomal aberrations, mammary adenomas, and inhibitions of injections site tumors, they concluded that no definite conclusions regarding the role of Mg in carcinogenesis could be formulated. They did conclude that inhibiting effects seem to prevail in Mg-supplemented states, while Mg deficiency appears to enhance carcinogenesis. Durlach et al. (1986) postulated that Mg acts as an anticancer agent in some instances and in others it induces a carcinogenic effect. They also indicated that Mg appears to be a non-competitive antagonist of Ni. They showed that carcinogenesis induces Mg distribution disturbances with Mg depletion in non-neoplastic tissue. Theophanides (1984) stated that the Mg ion binds directly to the guanine N7 atom and to 06 and to the negative oxygens of the phosphate through the water molecules of hydration. The Mg atom is found to be near the N7 site of the purine base interacting with the M7 site in a reversible manner. This could prevent this site from being attacked, which could explain why Mg could be preventive for cancer.

Carcinogenic divalent metals, such as Ni, and physiologically essential divalent metals such as Mg, are often antagonistic. Mg has the capacity to inhibit Ni uptake by target tissues <u>in vivo</u> and to inhibit Ni-induced disturbances in DNA synthesis, also <u>in vivo</u>. A popular hypothesis is that Ni causes damage on genetic material by oxidative reactions. Kurokawa et al. (1989), demonstrated that $NiCl_2$ acted as a promoter in renal carcinogenesis. Costa (1989) showed that water-soluble (<u>in vitro</u>) Ni ions display cell transforming activity. Ni ions bind poorly to DNA in comparison to their relatively high affinity for certain amino acids in cellular protein.

The respective capacity of physiologically essential metals to antagonize DNA binding (Zn > Mg > Ca) parallels their <u>in vivo</u> capacity to antagonize Cd-induced carcinogenesis (Waalkes and Poirier, 1984). Preventive effects of physiologically essential metals against metal-induced carcinogenesis may result from reduced binding at target sites. This appears to be especially true for Mg (Poirier et al., 1983). In a study designed to examine the antagonism between Mg and calcium and the tumorigenic metals Ni and lead, Ni and lead salts administered alone produced a significant increase in lung adenomas in mice. However, when administered with doses of calcium acetate or Mg acetate neither carcinogenic metal showed any significant tumorigenic activity (Poirier et al., 1984). The results indicate the existence of an antagonism between Mg and calcium and the tumorigenic metals.

The respective extracellular concentrations of Mg appears to be important. Conway et al., 1987) showed that raising the extracellular level of Mg ions inhibited Ni-induced DNA strand breaks, DNA-protein crosslinks, sister chromatid exchanges, chromosomal aberrations and cell transformation. $NiCl_2$ was added at concentrations of 250 to 1000 μM and Mg at 0.8 to 20 mM. Rodriguez and Kasprzak (1989) gave strain A mice multiple i.p. injections of Ni acetate and Mg acetate and demonstrated that the Ni-induced pulmonary adenoma incidence was prevented by the Mg acetate. Mg decreased Ni accumulation in pulmonary cell nuclei and cytosol, but not in mitochondria or microsomes, and prevented Ni-induced unscheduled pulmonary DNA synthesis. Kasprzak et al. (1986) determined that the ability of selected physiologically essential divalent cations to reduce the binding of Ni to DNA as Mg > Mn > Ca > Zn = Cu.

The general approach of our studies consists of conducting a series of <u>in vitro</u>

studies under conditions in which the Mg content of media have been altered. Ni will be added as the carcinogenic agent to study possible interactions between Mg and a carcinogenic metal. Lymphocytes, isolated from the spleen, will be used since Mg has been shown to influence the incidence/development of leukemia and also because of its role in immune surveillance. This triad of Mg-Ni-lymphocytes was chosen because of demonstrated metabolic/interactive relationships as outlined in the background discussion.

Using a factorial approach of two Ni concentrations (50 + 10 μM), along with Mg sufficient and deficient RPMI 1640 media, a transformed human-derived lymphocyte B cell line (TK-6) showed that Mg and Ni both influenced the growth (Fig. 1). Ni was present at concentrations of 10 and 50 μM and Mg was either present at normal concentrations or absent. Mg and Ni had opposite responses and the positive effect from the Mg at these concentrations were not sufficient to overcome the effect of Ni.

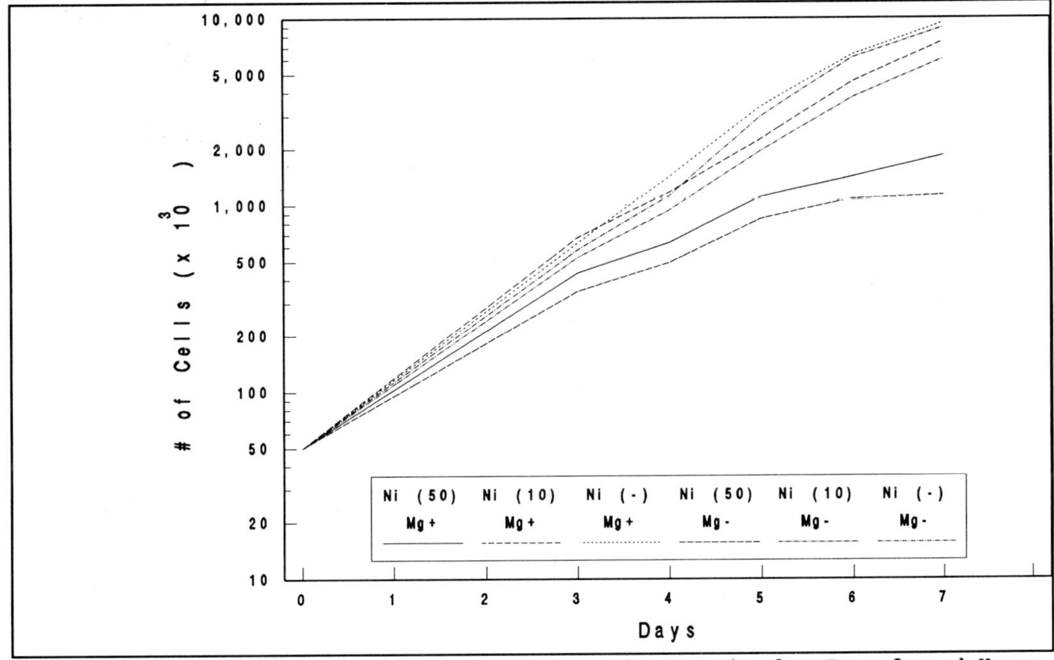

Figure 1. The Effect of Ni/Mg Interactions on the Growth of a Transformed Human-Derived Lymphocyte B Cell Line (TK-6)

This same general design will be used to examine the effects and interactions between Ni and Mg. The initial investigation will include, but not be limited to DNA synthesis and damage, effects on the cell cycle, viability, growth, and transformation events. Transit through the cell cycle will be analyzed using flow cytometry techniques with a FACScan Cell Cycle Analyzer. RPMI 1640 media that is initially Mg-free will be used as the growth media. Mg and Ni will be added as dictated in the respective treatment groups. The analysis of the data will principally use factorial analysis statistics.

In other studies, we incubated various mixtures of Ni, Mg, H_2O_2, and ascorbate in the presence of 2'-deoxyguanosine (dG) as shown in Table 3. Incubation of dG resulted in formation of 8-OH-dG in easily detectable amounts when H_2O_2 and Ascb were both present in the incubation mixture. Trace amounts appeared in three other instances after 24 hours when H_2O_2 was absent and Ascb was present (samples 3, 7 and 15). Aside from these seven incubation mixtures, there was no evidence of formation of 8-OH-dG. In instances in which 8-OH-dG was formed, neither the presence of Ni nor Mg had any effect on incubations at 37°C for as long as 24 hours. When the 8-OH-dG was formed in the mixtures with both H_2O_2 and Ascb present, it was detectable within one hour of incubation time.

Table 3. Formation of Guanine and 8-OH-dG from 2-deoxyguanosine (percent of dG deglycosylated to Gu or hydroxylated to 8-OH-dG as calculated by HPLC peak area ratio)

Sample #	Incubation Mixture	Guanine 1 Hr.	Guanine 3 Hr.	Guanine 24 Hr.	8-OH-dG 1 Hr.	8-OH-dG 3 Hr.	8-OH-dG 24 Hr.
1	Ni, Mg, H2O2, Ascb	1.03	1.52	76.46	0.85	1.09	2.23
2	Ni, Mg, H2O2,		--	--	0.16	--	--
3	Ni, Mg, Ascb	--	0.02	1.26	--	--	0.17
4	Ni, Mg	--	--	0.08	--	--	--
5	Ni, H2O2, Ascb	1.00	1.71	68.65	1.00	1.09	2.06
6	Ni, H2O2	--	--	0.43	--	--	--
7	Ni, Ascb	--	--	1.23	--	--	0.01
8	Ni	--	--	0.07	--	--	--
9	Mg, H2O2, Ascb	1.20	1.60	46.19	1.02	1.15	1.77
10	Mg, H2O2	0.01	0.03	0.10	--	--	--
11	Mg, Ascb	--	0.02	1.59	--	--	--
12	Mg	--	0.07	0.01	--	--	--
13	H2O2, Ascb	1.66	2.04	27.46	1.26	1.50	2.08
14	H2O2	0.01	0.05	0.04	--	--	--
15	Ascb	--	--	1.52	--	--	0.11
16		0.01	0.02	0.03	--	--	--

Ascb had a greater influence in the production of the 8-OH-dG than did the H_2O_2 as shown by traces of 8-OH-dG that occurred after 24 hours in instances where only Ascb was in the reaction mixture. The only indication that the Mg may have influenced the formation of 8-OH-dG was in the mixture in which Mg was incubated along with H_2O_2, dG, and Ascb (sample 9), where the amount of 8-OH-dG at 24 hours was less than that of the other mixture in which Ni was also present (samples 1 and 5), or was not included (sample 13). The sampling of the incubation mixtures did not continue past 24 hours since prior studies by Kasprzak and Hernandez (1989) showed little reaction after 24 hours.

The deglycosylation of dG was also measured. As in the 8-OH-dG analysis, the greatest amounts of guanine (Gu) occurred when both H_2O_2 and Ascb were present, especially after incubation of dG for 24 hours. All mixtures containing Ascb produced Gu after 24 hours. Unlike the 8-OH-dG analysis, the presence (or absence) of the metals appeared to influence the formation of Gu. The greatest amounts of Gu occurred when Ni was present in the ion mixture. A combination of Ni and Mg produced the highest concentration of Gu. Ni alone produced more Gu than when Mg alone was present in a similar incubation mixture with both H_2O_2 and Ascb present. When neither Ni nor Mg was present along with H_2O_2 and Ascb, the Gu, although still substantially high, was lower than when H_2O_2 and Ascb were present with Ni and/or Mg. If H_2O_2 was missing from the mixture, but Ascb present, the influence from the respective metals, both Ni and Mg, was not evident. (Samples 3, 7, 11, and 15). The analysis at 3 hours presents evidence of an effect by the metals. When Ni is present, there is little or no formation of Gu except when both H_2O_2 and Ascb are present, whereas in all of the incubation mixtures where Ni is absent (except where Ascb is the only additive), the Gu appears in small amounts in the 3 hour analysis.

When these studies were repeated several times, it was evident that the reaction mixtures were very sensitive to even slight variations. The effects of pH were quite marked. Originally, the reaction mixtures were prepared from 50 mM Tris/HCl buffer that was adjusted to pH 7.4. To determine the influence of pH, incubation mixture 1 (Ni, Mg, H_2O_2, Ascb, and 2-dG) was duplicated and adjusted to a respective pH as shown in Table 4, ranging from 6.2 to 7.8 with 0.2 step increments. Tris buffer has a pKa of 8.1 and a buffering range of 7.0 to 9.1. Several samples were intentionally included that were outside of this range.

The pH change after 24 hours of incubation, as well as the formation of Gu and 8-OH-dG, (Table 4) shows that the formed products are far greater at the lower pH and decrease with increasing pH. The pH change over the 24 hours correlates with the activity of the mixture; i.e., the greater the pH change, the more activity in the mixture. Between pH 7.0 and 7.2, which is at the lower range of the buffer, there was a precipitous change in both activity and pH change. From these data, it is obvious that production of Gu and 8-OH-dG is directly influenced by pH.

Table 4. Effect of pH on Formation of Gu and 8-OH-dG

pH at Start	pH at 24 Hours	Δ pH	Gu % Ratio	8-OH-dG % Ratio
6.2	2.74	3.46	85.82	12.79
6.4	2.90	3.50	52.61	8.18
6.6	3.06	3.54	38.43	7.12
6.8	3.34	3.46	19.68	5.40
7.0	3.61	3.39	15.95	4.68
7.2	5.90	1.30	3.31	3.66
7.4	6.54	0.86	2.68	2.28
7.6	6.87	0.73	2.18	0.55
7.8	7.25	0.55	1.99	0.00

In view of the evidence cited above, there is ample evidence that Mg is important in the maintenance of the general integrity and sound physiology of the biological system, and as such can be used to study mechanisms and actions of various aspects of toxicology and carcinogenicity. The most prominent effects of Mg in cancer prevention may be its role in the control of immunity and growth. The approach to study the Mg-Ni interaction will concentrate on the lymphocyte for these specific reasons: (1) they are a very active differentiation cell system; (2) the tendency for promotion of neoplastic transformation by Mg deprivation is restricted to cells concerned principally with the immune system, particularly lymphocytes; and (3) immune dysfunctions associated with Mg deficiency may be a direct effect on T-cell function or indirect by influencing T-cell maturation. Lymphocytes will be exposed to factorial combinations and doses of Ni and Mg using both _in vitro_ and _in vivo_ techniques. Cytokines, such as interleukin-2 (Il-2) and granulocyte-macrophage cell stimulating factor (GM-CSF), will provide another variable factor. Both primary and immortalized cells will be used in the _in vitro_ studies.

REFERENCES

Battifora, H.A., McCreary, P.A., Hahneman, B.M., Laing, G.H., and Hass, G.M. 1968): Chronic magnesium deficiency in the rat. Arch. Path. 86, 610-620.

Bois, P. (1964): Tumour of the thymus in magnesium-deficient rats. Nature 204, 1316.

Cameron, I.L. and Smith, N.K.R. (1989): Cellular concentration of magnesium and other ions in relation to protein synthesis, cell proliferation, and cancer. Magnesium 8, 31-44

Conway, K., Wang, X. Xu, L., and Costa, M. (1987): Effect of magnesium on nickel-induced genotoxicity and cell transformation. Carcinogenesis 8, 1-1121.

Costa, M. (1989): Perspectives of the mechanism of nickel carcinogenesis gained from models of _in vitro_ carcinogenesis. Environ. Health Per. 81, 73-76.

Durlach, J., Bara, M., Guiet-Bara, A., and Collery, P. (1986): Relationship between magnesium, cancer, and carcinogenic or anticancer metals. Anticancer Research 6, 1353-1362.

Hass, G.M., Galt, R.M., Laing, G.H., Coogan,, P.S., Maganini, R.O., and Friese, J.A. (1989): Inductions of a rat T cell lymphoma-leukemia by magnesium deficiency - A study of fetal defense against maternal neoplasia. Magnesium 8, 45-55.

Jasmin, G. (1968): Action of hormones on the progression of magnesium deficiency in rats. Dans endocrine aspects of disease processes. Edie par G.Jasmin, p356. St. Louis, Warren H. Green Publishers, Inc.

Kasprzak, K.S., Hernandez, L. (1989): Enhancement of hydroxylation and deglycosylation of 2'-deoxyguanosine by carcinogenic nickel compounds. Cancer Res., 119:5965-5968.

Kasprzak, K., Waalkes, M., and Poirier, L. (1986): Antagonism by essential divalent metals and amino acids of nickel(II)-DNA binding _in vitro_. Tox. Appl. Pharm. 82, 336-343.

Kasprzak, K.S., and Waalkes, M.P., (1986): The role of calcium, magnesium, and zinc, in carcinogenesis. Adv. Exp. Med. Biol. (Essent. Nutr. Carcinog.) 206, 497-515.

Kurokawa, Y., Takahashi, M. Maekewa, A., and Hayashi, Y. (1989): Promoting effect of metal compounds on liver, stomach, kidney, pancreas, and skin carcinogenesis. J. Amer. Col. Toxicol. 8, 1235-1239.

Mills, B.J., Broghamer, W.L., Higgens, P.J., and Lindeman, R.D. (1984): Inhibition of tumor growth by magnesium depletion of rats. J. Nutr. 114, 739-745.

Poirier, L.A., Kasprzak, K.S., Hoover, K.L., and Wenk, M.L. (1983): Effects of calcium and magnesium acetates on the carcinogenicity of cadmium chloride in Wistar rats. Cancer Res. 43, 4575-4581.

Poirier, L.A., Theiss, J.C., Arnold, L.J., and Shimkin, M.B. (1984): Inhibition by magnesium and calcium acetates of lead subacetate- and nickel acetate-induced lung tumors in strain A mice. Cancer Res. 44, 1520-1522.

Rodriguez, R.E., and Kasprzak, K.S. (1989): Antagonists to metal carcinogens. J. Amer. Coll. Toxicol. 1265-1269.

Rubin, H., Vudair, C. and Sanui, H. (1981): Restoration of normal appearance, growth behavior, and calcium content to transformed 3T3 cells by magnesium deprivation. Proc. Natl. Acad. Sci. USA. 78, 2350-2354.

Rubin, H. (1982): Effect of magnesium content on density-dependent regulation of the onset of DNA synthesis in transformed 3T3 cells. Cancer Res. 42, 1761-1766.

Theophanides, T. (1984): Metal ions in biological systems. Internat. J. Quantum Chem. 26, 933-941.

Waalkes, M.P. and Poirier, L.A. (1984): In vitro cadmium-DNA interactions: Cooperativity of calcium binding and competitive antagonism by calcium, magnesium, and zinc. Toxicol. Appl. Pharm. 75, 539-546.

Metal Ions in Biology and Medicine, vol. 2. Eds. J. Anastassopoulou, Ph. Collery, J.C. Etienne, Th. Theophanides. John Libbey Eurotext, Paris © 1992, pp. 163-166

Budotitane : preclinical and clinical development of a new tumor-inhibiting titanium complex

B.K. Keppler*, C. Friesen*, E. Vogel*, M.E. Heim**

*Anorganisch-Chemisches Institüt der Universität Heidelberg, Im Neuenheimer Feld 270, W-6900 Heidelberg, Germany. ** Sonnenberg-Klinik, Hardtstr. 13, W-3437 Bad Sooden-Allendorf, Germany*

In the development of tumor-inhibiting non-platinum complexes, budotitane (INN), *cis*-diethoxybis(1-phenylbutane-1,3-dionato)titanium(IV) (Fig. 1), is among the most advanced. It is undergoing clinical trials today. Phase I studies with chronic application will have been finished by the end of this year.

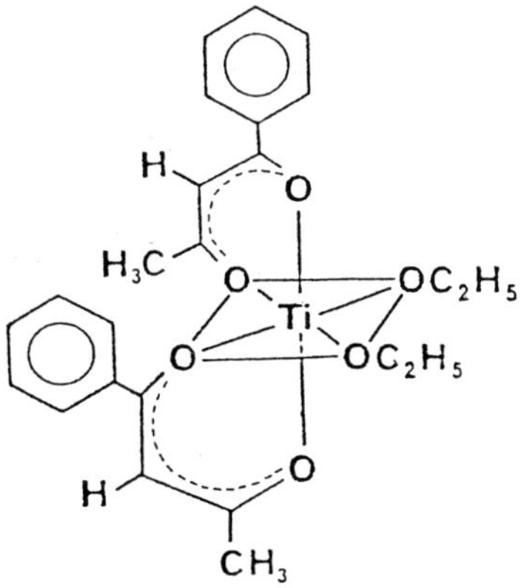

H
O
H_3C
O
OC_2H_5
Ti
O
OC_2H_5
O
H
CH_3

Fig. 1: Budotitane (INN), *cis*-diethoxybis(1-phenylbutane-1,3-dionato)titanium(IV), $Ti(bzac)_2(OEt)_2$, KP 102.

We have carried out extensive investigations into structure-activity relations, which have shown a clear dependence of antitumor activity on the central metal and the diketonato ligand. When exchanging the central metal of the compound, which belongs to the class of bis(β-diketonato) metal complexes, antitumor activity decreases in the order titanium > zirconium > hafnium > molybdenum > tin > germanium. The tumor-inhibiting effect is also highly dependent on the nature of the diketonato ligand. This ligand should be substituted with planar aromatic ring systems such as the phenyl rings in budotitane, because they provide the steric requirements of a good antitumor activity. Most of the tumor-inhibiting bis(β-diketonato) complexes are *cis*-configurated. Compounds that are *trans*-configurated show medium activity, which may be due to the formation of the *cis*-configuration taking place after the replacement with water of the space-filling group X, which is responsible for the formation of the *trans*-configuration. The *cis*-configurated compounds with an unsymmetrically substituted β-diketonate as ligand are in an equilibrium between three possible isomers in solution at room temperature, due to the fact that the diketonate can rotate via a twist mechanism. In low-temperature NMR experiments it became clear that the isomer shown by the structure of budotitane above is responsible for about 60 % of all isomers, whereas the other two isomers, taken together, account for about 40 % (Fig. 2).

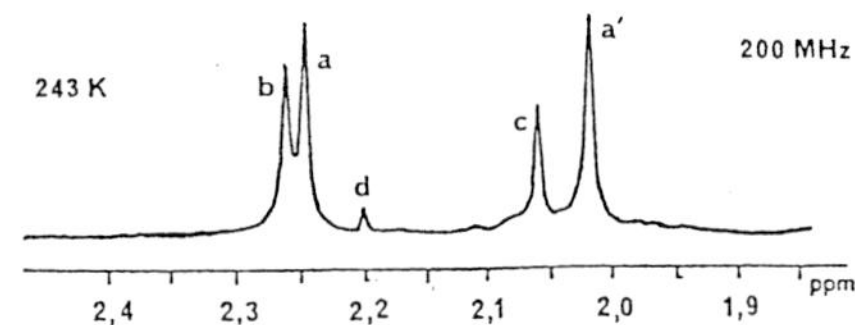

Fig. 2: a, a' = signals of the two C<u>H</u>$_3$ groups of the isomer shown above;
b, c = signals of the possible other two *cis*-isomers;
d = signal of the CH_3 protons of the free ligand (in traces).

The phenyl groups in budotitane should be in coplanar conjugation to the metal enolate ring. This could not be found out directly, by X-ray analyses of budotitane, as the quality of crystals was not good enough, but it was evidenced by X-ray analyses of a direct derivative of budotitane, *cis*-$Ti(bzbz)_2(OEt)_2$ (Fig. 3), which show that three of the four phenyl rings are coplanar to the metal enolate ring while only one of the phenyl rings is drawn out of the plane for steric reasons. Due to the fact that budotitane has only two phenyl rings in the molecule, rather than four, it may be concluded that these are coplanar to the metal enolate ring.

The easily hydrolizable group in the bis(β-diketonato) complexes does not play a major role in antitumor activity, but it is important for the galenic formulation in the clinic. The ethoxy group as leaving group in budotitane hydrolizes at a slower rate than the corresponding halides.

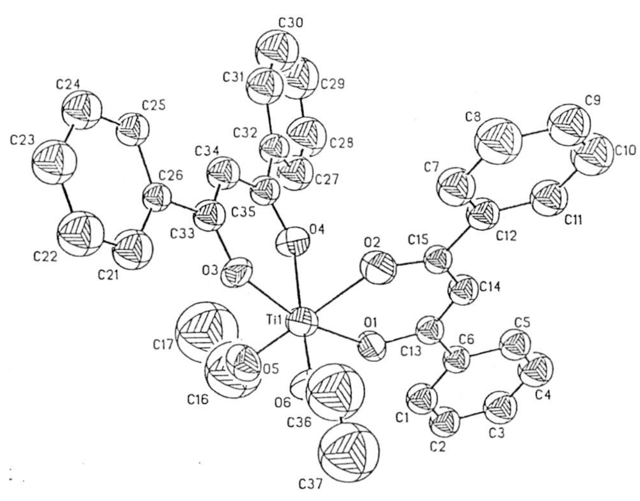

Selected bond distances (Å) and angles (°):

Ti(1)-O(1)	1.999 (9)	O(1)-Ti(1)-O(2)	82.6 (4)
Ti(1)-O(2)	2.057 (10)	O(2)-Ti(1)-O(4)	82.3 (4)
Ti(1)-O(4)	2.074 (11)	O(4)-Ti(1)-O(3)	81.9 (4)
Ti(1)-O(3)	1.996 (9)	O(3)-Ti(1)-O(5)	98.2 (4)
Ti(1)-O(5)	1.792 (11)	O(5)-Ti(1)-O(6)	98.4 (5)
Ti(1)-O(6)	1.793 (12)	O(6)-Ti(1)-O(1)	100.1 (5)

Fig. 3: X-Ray Structure of *cis*-Diethoxybis(1,3-diphenylpropane-1,3-dionato)titanium(IV), *cis*-Ti(bzbz)$_2$(OEt)$_2$, KP 117.

Budotitane is active in several transplantable tumors and shows promising activity in an autochthonous colorectal tumor model, which is highly predictive for the clinical situation. Side-effects include mild hepatotoxicity and nephrotoxicity. These preclinical findings have been confirmed in clinical phase I studies. The clinical starting dose was chosen according to animal toxicity studies as 1/10 acute LD_{10} in rats. In the single-dose application, 7 dose levels of 1, 2, 4, 6, 9, 14, and 21 mg/kg B.W. were evaluated. All patients were treated over 2 or 3 dose levels with at least a 6-week interval between applications. The first drug-related toxicity was observed at a dose of 9 mg/kg B.W., when a patient complained about a reversible impairment of the sense of taste shortly after the infusion. A moderate increase in liver enzymes and LDH was observed at a dose of 14 mg/kg B.W. Nephrotoxicity with an increase in urea and creatinine of WHO grade 2 was dose-limiting at the 21 mg/kg B.W. dose level in 2 patients. In both patients, pretreatment creatinine clearance had been normal. Urea and creatinine returned to normal values over a period of 10 weeks.

Nephrotoxicity was accompanied by nausea, weakness and malaise. Myelosuppression was not observed at any of the tested dose levels. The maximum tolerated single-dose of budotitane thus was between 14 and 21 mg/kg B.W. The recommendation for the repeated dose application is 21 mg/kg B.W. (800 mg/m^2 B.S.A.) total dose divided into 8 applications of 100 mg/m^2 B.S.A. twice a week over a 4-week period. So far 3 patients at each dose level have been treated with 100, 120, and 150 mg/m^2 B.S.A. 8 times in 4 weeks. No hepatotoxicity or nephrotoxicity were observed at these dose levels, while all patients experienced the described gustatory changes. At a dose of 14 mg/kg B.W. of budotitane, the titanium concentration in the serum reached values between 2 and 5 μg/g, and at a dose of 21 mg/kg B.W. values between 5 and 12 μg/g. Titanium could be detected in the serum 7 days and, in one case, even 4 weeks after a single-dose application. In red blood cells titanium was detected at concentrations of 1-2 μg/g.
After the chronic application studies with budotitane, clinical phase II studies will show the ultimate value of this new drug in cancer therapy.

References

(1) Keppler, B.K., Berger, M.R., Klenner, T., Heim, M.E. (1990) Metal Complexes as Antitumour Agents. Advances in Drug Research 19, 243-310.

(2) Keppler, B.K. (1990) Metal Complexes as Anticancer Agents. The Future Role of Inorganic Chemistry in Cancer Therapy. New J. Chem. 14, 389-403.

(3) Keppler, B.K., Friesen, C., Moritz, H.G., Vongerichten, H., Vogel, E. (1991) Tumor-inhibiting bis(β-diketonato) metal complexes. Budotitane, *cis*-Diethoxybis(1-phenylbutane-1,3-dionato)titanium(IV), the first transition metal complex after platinum complexes to have qualified for clinical trials. Structure & Bonding 78, 97-127.

Acknowledgements

This work was supported by the *Deutsche Krebshilfe,* Bonn, FRG, and the *Fonds der Chemischen Industrie,* Frankfurt, FRG.

Metal Ions in Biology and Medicine, vol. 2. Eds. J. Anastassopoulou, Ph. Collery, J.C. Etienne, Th. Theophanides. John Libbey Eurotext, Paris © 1992, pp. 167-172

Therapeutic index of gallium, orally administered, as chloride, in combination with cisplatinum and etoposide in lung cancer patients

Philippe Collery, Hervé Vallerand, Alain Prevost, Dragisa Milosevic, Michel Morel, Jean-Pierre Dubois, Bernard Desoize, Claude Pechery, Jean-Marie Dubois de Montreynaud, Hervé Millart, Henri Choisy

Centre Hospitalier Universitaire Régional, 51092 Reims Cedex, France

1-Introduction

The in vitro cytotoxic activity of Gallium (Ga) depends on its extracellular concentration, and moreover on the duration of the contact with the cancer cells (1). In cancer therapy, the daily oral administration of gallium chloride ($GaCl_3$) could allow a permanent contact between Ga and the tumor cells, during a long time, up to several months or years, with a more selective uptake than after parenteral use (2). Ga is also a biological response modifier, through its antagonism with divalent ions (Mg, Fe, Zn and Ca), reducing their concentrations in tissues (3), particularly in tumors (4). The modulation on ionic transfer of monovalent ions (Na, K) observed in experimental conditions (5) may be a consequence of the action on ATPase (6). The effect of Ga on the ionic cellular concentrations and transfers, as well as its action on DNA polymerase (7) and its ability to block the cells in phase G1 (8), could induce an inhibition of the tumor growth or a reduction of the tumor growth according to the Ga cellular concentrations. This cellular Ga concentration depends on the plasma Ga concentration reached after daily oral administration of $GaCl_3$ and is also influenced by serum transferrin levels, tumor volume, the histology of the primary tumor and the site of metastases (9,10). An individual adaptation of the doses could then be useful if the therapeutic index could be defined, in order to avoid toxicity and to optimize efficacy. This therapeutic index will not be the same when $GaCl_3$ would be administered alone or in combination therapy with other cytotoxic agents. The plasma Ga concentration required to obtain an inhibition of the tumor growth with $GaCl_3$ alone has already been determined (11). We are now investigating the therapeutic index of $GaCl_3$ administered in conjunction with a chemotherapy by cisplatinum (CDDP) and etoposide.

2-Before determining the therapeutic index of $GaCl_3$ in combination with CDDP and etoposide, an adaptation of CDDP and etoposide doses has been first defined, with 400 mg/24h $GaCl_3$.

2-1- The first step has been to maintain the same area under the curve (AUC) in serum total platinum and etoposide concentrations during the 5 days of each infusion .

CDDP and etoposide were administered as continuous intravenous infusions for 120 hours. The AUC was calculated for time 0 to 64 hours (AUC_{0-64}) and time 0 to 120 hours (AUC_{0-120}) of each infusion by determining serum total Pt and etoposide concentrations at the following hours after the beginning of the infusion: 0, 16, 24, 40, 48, 64, 72, 88, 96, 112 and 120 hours.

Total Pt concentrations were determined by AAS and serum etoposide concentrations by HPLC. AUC results were expressed in $\mu g.l^{-1}.h$ for total serum Pt concentrations and in $\mu mol.l^{-1}.h$ for etoposide. Dosages were 15 $mg/m^2/24h$ for CDDP and 25 $mg/m^2/24h$ for etoposide during the first course and during the first 64 hours of the second course.

The drug dosages were adapted at time 64h of the second course in order to obtain the same AUC during the 120 hours of the second course ($AUC_{(0-120)\,2}$ than during the first course $AUC_{(0-120)1}$, according to a mathematical formula. This one has been based on the hypothesis that AUC is a function of the drug dosage (D) according to the equation : **AUC = K . D** with K (coefficient of proportionality) constant during the 5 days of infusion (K_1 for the first cycle, K_2 for the second cycle,...). The total dose of CDDP or etoposide given from 0 to 64 h has been expressed by $D_{(0-64)1}$ for the first course and by $D_{(0-64)2}$ for the second course; the total dose of CDDP or etoposide given from 0 to 120 h by $D_{(0-120)1}$ for the first course and by $D_{(0-120)2}$ for the second course. The AUC observed during the first 64 h of the infusion has been noted $AUC_{(0-64)1}$ for the first course and $AUC_{(0-64)\,2}$ for the second course. We know $D_{(0-64)1}$ and $D_{(0-64)2}$ as well as $D_{(0-120)\,1}$

We wish to calculate $D_{(64-120)2}$ in order to obtain $AUC_{(0-120)2} = AUC_{(0-120)1}$

When replacing $AUC_{(0-120)}$ by $K.\,D_{(0-120)}$ for the corresponding cycles, the last equation becomes : $K_2 \cdot D_{(0-120)\,2} = K_1 \cdot D_{(0-120)\,1}$

As $K_2 = AUC_{(0-64)2} / D_{(0-64)2}$ and $K_1 = AUC_{(0-64)1} / D_{(0-64)1}$

then $\{AUC_{(0-64)2} / D_{(0-64)2}\} \cdot D_{(0-120)2} = \{AUC_{(0-64)1} / D_{(0-64)1}\} \cdot D_{(0-120)\,1}$

and as $D_{(0-120)\,2} = D_{(0-64)2} + D_{(64-120)\,2}$

we can change this term in the equation , and then isolate what we are looking for, that is $D_{(64-120)\,2}$

The solution is :

$$\mathbf{D_{(64-120)2} = D_{(0-64)2} \cdot \{[D_{(0-120)1} / D_{(0-64)1}].[AUC_{(0-64)1} / AUC_{(0-64)2}]-1\}}$$

The same calculation can be repeated for the next courses.

In fact, the dosage is only modified once at time 72h of each course, according to the drug concentrations measured on the first 6 blood samples, including those at time 64h.

This method was applied in 9 patients with inoperable lung cancer. The results were given during the first international symposium on metal ions in biology and medicine (12).

If the differences between $AUC_{(0-120)2}$ and $AUC_{(0-120)\,1}$ were about 20 % , they were only near 5% between the third and the second cycles. This method seems then suitable to obtain nearly constant $AUC_{(0-120)}$. This can avoid the cumulative toxicity of CDDP but moreover allows to use the average of several courses of chemotherapy and compared it with the toxicity and the efficacy:

- no toxicity superior to grade 2 was noted in this study.

- among 8 evaluable patients, the $AUC_{(0-120)}$ for serum total platinum were significantly higher ($p \leq 005$, Wilcoxon test) for the 4 responders (82292 ± 8222 $\mu g.l^{-1}.h$) than for the 4 non responders concerning (48540 ± 6748 $\mu g.l^{-1}.h$). The $AUC_{(0-120)}$ for serum etoposide were also higher, but not significantly, in responders (165 ± 38 $\mu mol.l^{-1}.h$) than in non-responders (108 ± 51 $\mu mol.l^{-1}.h$) . These results were observed in patients receiving 400 mg $GaCl_3$, daily, without adaptation of $GaCl_3$ dosage.

2-2- The second step has been the CDDP and etoposide dosage adjustement in order to obtain, as soon as the first cycle, the AUC observed in the responders of the preceeding trial.

The aim was then to obtain an $AUC_{(0-120)}$ of 80000 µg.l^{-1}.h for serum total Pt and of 200 µmol.l^{-1}.h for etoposide.

The regression curve AUC $_{(0-120)}$ / AUC $_{(0-64)}$ plotted with the results of the first course of the preceeding trial, in which the doses were constant (15 mg/m^2/24h for CDDP and 25 mg/m^2/24h for etoposide) has been used to determine the adaptation formula (Fig.1).

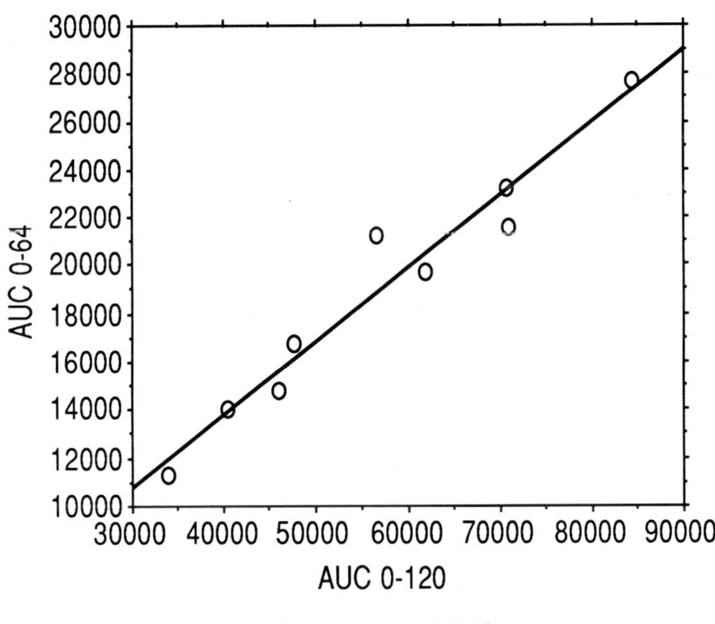

$$AUC_{(0-120)} = 3.2 \times AUC_{(0-64)} - 6000$$

Fig.1: regression curve for AUC in serum total platinum, in the absence of dose adjustement

The formula to obtain an AUC of 80000 µg.l^{-1}.h for serum total platinum during the first course of chemotherapy has been calculated according this coefficient of regression:

$$D_{(72-120)}/2 = [\{ (2.5 * 80000) / (3.2 * AUC_{0-64}) - 6000 \} - 1,5] * \{D_{(0-72)}/3\}$$

According to the regression curve for etoposide (not plotted), the adaptation to obtain during the first course of chemotherapy an AUC of 200 µmol.l-1.h for etoposide has been :

$$D_{(72-120)}/2 = [\{(2.5 * 200) / (2.3 * AUC_{0-64}) - 26 \} - 1,5] * \{D_{(0-72)}/3\}$$

This method was applied to 12 cancer patients without prior treatment : 9 non small cell lung cancer (NSCLC) and 3 small cell lung carcinomas (SCLC).The courses of chemotherapy were repeated every 3 weeks . $GaCl_3$ was daily administered at the dosage of 400 mg/24h during each course of chemotherapy, but also between these courses, without neither interruption nor adaptation. Plasma Ga assays were performed in the same time than serum total Pt and etoposide.

The results have already been reported (13):

- no clinical toxicity was observed except some nausea and vomiting; no biological toxicity was superior to grade 2.

- 4 partial responses and 1 complete response were observed among the 9 NSCLC, without any significant difference neither for AUC total platinum between responders (89598 ± 20843 $\mu g.l^{-1}.h$) and non responders (83820 ± 13455 $\mu g.l^{-1}.h$), nor for AUC etoposide (227 ± 41 $\mu mol.l^{-1}.h$ in responders and 211 ± 30 $\mu mol.l^{-1}.h$ in non responders). The results obtained in the 3 SCLC, who were responders, were also similar : 88081 ± 15431 $\mu g.l^{-1}.h$ for AUC Pt and 217 ± 29 for AUC etoposide. By contrast, significant differences were observed in NSCLC, according to Wilcoxon's test, between responders and non-responders, for plasma Ga at the 3rd course of chemotherapy: the average of the maximal plasma Ga concentrations observed for each patient were respectively 244 ± 34 µg/l and 113 ± 57 µg/l ($p< 0.01$). In SCLC, the results were similar to those obtained in NSCLC with a regression of the tumor volume (243 ± 132 µg/l).

For potentiating CDDP and etoposide by $GaCl_3$, it seems necessary to obtain plasma Ga concentrations as high as 200 µg/l. On the other hand, when the plasma Ga concentrations do not reach this value, no partial reponse has to be expected, even though the adaptation of CDDP and etoposide dosages could achieved the same AUC as in responders of the preceeding trial. The standard deviation was less than 20% for total Pt and in etoposide AUC and this method of adaptation is suitable. We could use it in the next trial, in which an escalation of GaCl3 dosages will be performed, in order to increase the plasma Ga concentrations in non-responders.

3- Modulation of $GaCl_3$ dosages with the same adaptation of CDDP and etoposide dosages:

A dose-escalation of GaCl3 has been performed in 17 patients with lung cancer, from 400 to 1200 mg/24h, all of them treated by CDDP and etoposide according to the defined schedule of treatment. 400 mg/24h of $GaCl_3$ was administered the first day of the first course of chemotherapy by CDDP and etoposide and maintened until the second course. At that time, the $GaCl_3$ dose was increased to 800 mg/24h when there was a lack of significant reduction in the tumor volume, according to the chest X ray radiography. Once again, the GaCl3 was increased to 1200 mg/24h at the beginning of the third course in absence of regression. In 3 patients in whom the tumor of the volume could not be evaluate by the chest X ray radiography, the dose-increase only occurred after the third course after a more complete evaluation with endoscopy, computed tomography, liver ultrasonography and bone scintigraphy. Among the 17 patients, there were 9 squamous cell carcinomas, 4 adenocarcinomas, 4 large cell carcinomas. The mean age was 58 (range:44-75). Staging : 6 patients with a stage III and 8 with a stage IV; 3 patients in post-surgery.

During 103 courses, evaluable for the toxicity, 1 septicemia, 1 vascular purpura and 1 confusion (reversible) occurred.

3-1- A renal toxicity (creatinemia > 140 µmol/l , but less than 200 µmol/l) has been observed in 9/103 courses of chemotherapy. For these 9 courses, there was a significant increase ($p<0.001$, Wilcoxon's test) in plasma Ga concentrations (521 ± 121 µg/l) by comparison to the other courses, in which plasma Ga concentrations were found to be 248 ± 152 µg/l. On the other hand, no significant difference has been observed for AUC in total Pt or etoposide (Table I).

Table I: relationship between renal insufficiency and pharmacokinetic parameters

	creatinemia > 140 µmol/l	creatinemia < 140 µmol/l	p
AUC total Pt	93014 ± 31683	88388 ± 17225	N.S
AUC etoposide	227 ± 35	217 ± 47	N.S
plasma Ga concentration	521 ± 121	248 ± 152	< 0.001

According to these results, with an AUC in serum total Pt of near 90000 µg.l-1.h, plasma Ga concentrations lower than 400 µg/l could avoid a renal insufficiency.

3-2- <u>The hematological toxicity</u> is shown in table II.

Table II: hematological toxicity (103 evaluable courses of chemotherapy)

	grade 0	grade 1	grade 2	grade 3	grade 4	Total
hemoglobinemia	27	38	25	11	2	103
neutrophils	80	11	10	2	0	103
platelets	97	2	2	1	1	103

This hematological toxicity has not been related to the pharmacokinetic parameters (Table III), but to serum transferrin levels, serum iron and ferritinemia (Table IV).

Table III: relationship between the hematological toxicity and the pharmacokinetic parameters

	grade 0,1,2	grade 3,4	p
AUC total Pt	89007 ± 19032	87225 ± 17182	N.S
AUC etoposide	270 ± 167	291 ± 173	N.S
plasma Ga concentration	220 ± 40	222 ± 57	N.S

Table IV: relationship between hematological toxicity and serum transferrin, iron and ferritin

	grade 0	grade 1	grade 2	grade 3 and 4
serum transferrin (mg/l)	2.6 ± 0.3	2.3 ± 0.6	2.5 ± 0.5	1.8 ± 0.3 *
p	< 0.0001	< 0.02	< 0.05	
ferritin (mg/l)	605 ± 225	705 ± 679	427 ± 260	1205 ± 780 *
p	N.S	N.S	< 0.02	
serum iron (µmol/l)	16 ± 10	12 ± 9	16 ± 15	7 ± 5 *
p	< 0.005	< 0.05	< 0.05	

4-In conclusion :

It is possible to determine a therapeutic index of GaCl3 , administered in combination with CDDP and etoposide. With an AUC in serum total Pt between 80000 and 100000 $\mu g.l^{-1}.h$ and an AUC in etoposide between 200 and 400 $\mu mol.l^{-1}.h$, this therapeutic index is defined by the plasma Ga concentration. With plasma Ga concentrations lower than 200 µg/l, no efficacy has to be expected . With plasma Ga concentrations higher than 400 µg/l, renal insufficiency may occur.

The optimum dosage of $GaCl_3$ must allow plasma Ga concentrations between 200 and 400 µg/l, as soon as the first course of this combined treatment. To avoid the hematological toxicity, patients must have serum transferrin values higher than 2.1 mg/l. We shall define the efficacy of this schedule of treatment in the further clinical trial.

5- References:

(1) RASEY J.S., NELSON N.J., LARSON S.M. (1981): Relationship of iron metabolism to tumor cell toxicity of stable gallium salts. Intern. J. Nucl. Med. Biol. 8: 303-313.

(2) COLLERY Ph., MILLART H., SIMONEAU J.P.et al. (1983): Selective uptake of Gallium administered orally, as chloride, by tumor cells.13th International Congress of Chemotherapy, Vienna. New Concepts in Cancer Chemotherapy, K.H.Spitzy, K. Karrer eds., part. 284, PS 12 -11, p. 35-43.

(3) VISTELLE R., COLLERY Ph, MILLART H (1989): In vivo distribution of gallium in healthy rats after oral administration and interactions with iron, magnesium and calcium.Trace Elem. Med. 6: 27-32

(4) COLLERY Ph ., MILLART H ., PLUOT M. , ANGHILERI L.J (1986): Effects of gallium chloride oral administration on transplanted C3HBA mammary adenocarcinoma: Ga, Mg, Ca and Fe concentration and anatomopathological characteristics. Anticancer Res. 6: 1085 - 1088.

(5) BARA M. , GUIET-BARA A., COLLERY P. , DURLACH J. (1985): Gallium action on the ionic transfer through the isolated human amnion. I. Effect on the amnion as a whole and interaction between Gallium and Magnesium. Trace Elements in Med. 2 : 99 - 102.

(6) ANGHILERI L.J. (1982) : Isomorphous ionic replacement : experimental evidence hypothesis proposed to explain gallium-67 accumulation . J. Nucl. Med. Allied Sci. 26 : 113-115.

(7) ADAMSON R.H., CANELLOS G.P., SIEBER S.M. (1975): Studies on the antitumor activity of gallium nitrate and other group III A metal salts. Cancer Chemother . Rep. 59: 599-610.

(8) CARPENTIER Y., LIAUTAUD-ROGER F., COLLERY Ph., LOIRETTE M., DESOIZE B., CONINX P. (1990) : Effect of gallium on the cell cycle of tumor cells in vitro. in: Metal Ions in Biology and Medicine.Eds.Ph.Collery et al. John Libbey Eurotext, Paris : pp.406-408.

(9) COLLERY Ph., MILLART H., LAMIABLE D.et al. (1989): Clinical pharmacology of gallium chloride after oral administration in lung cancer patients. Anticancer Res. 9: 353- 356.

(10) COLLERY P ., MILLART H ., CHOISY H .et al. (1989): Magnesium alterations and pharmacokinetic data in gallium treated lung cancer patients. Magnesium 8 : 56 -64 .

(11) COLLERY Ph., MILLART H., FERRAND O. et al. (1985): Gallium chloride treatment of cancer patients after oral administration ; a pilot study. Chemiotherapia 4 : 1165-166.

(12) COLLERY Ph., MOREL M., MILLART H. et al (1990): Oral administration of gallium in conjunction with platinum in lung cancer treatment.in: Metal Ions in Biology and Medicine. eds. Ph.Collery, L.A.Poirier, M.Manfait, J.C.Etienne. John Libbey Eurotext, Paris : pp.437-442.

(13)COLLERYPh., MOREL M., DESOIZE B. et al. (1991): Combination chemotherapy with cisplatinum, etoposide and gallium chloride: individual adaptation of doses. Anticancer Res.11:1529-1532.

Metal Ions in Biology and Medicine, vol. 2. Eds. J. Anastassopoulou, Ph. Collery, J.C. Etienne, Th. Theophanides. John Libbey Eurotext, Paris © 1992, pp. 173-175

New gallium complexes for a cisplatin combination therapy

Ph. Collery*, H. Millart*, C. Pechery**, F. Kratz***, B.K. Keppler***

** Médecine Interne, Cancérologie, Clinique des Maladies Respiratoires, Hôpital Maison Blanche, 45, rue Cognacq-Jay, 51092 Reims Cedex, France. ** Les Laboratoires Méram, avenue de la Libération, 77020 Melun Cedex, France. *** Anorganisch-Chemisches Institut der Universität Heidelberg, Im Neuenheimer Feld 270, W-6900 Heidelberg, Germany*

In clinical studies Collery could show that a combination therapy of cisplatin, VP 16 and gallium chloride in patients with inoperable non-small cell lung tumors has distinct advantages over a therapy with cisplatin and VP 16 alone (1). Gallium chloride potentiates the effect of chemotherapy. Simple gallium salts proper have a certain tumor-inhibiting activity, which, however, was not very promising in monotherapy.

For a combination therapy with cisplatin, the daily oral administration of gallium has been proposed to allow permanent contact with the malignant cells and a more selective uptake than after parenteral infusion. To be effective, the plasma gallium concentrations have to reach values as high as 750 μg/l (2). When using the chloride salt of gallium, the plasma concentrations may be too low to be efficient (3). In order to improve the bioavailability of gallium, we have synthesized new gallium complexes and investigated their intratissular concentrations in comparison with $GaCl_3$.

The following three gallium compounds of differing lipophilia show marked differences in their bioavailability in comparison to gallium chloride.

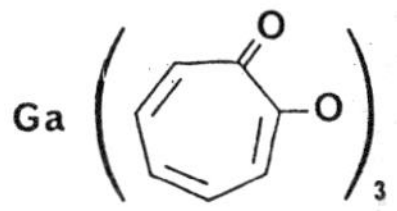

Tris(tropolonato)gallium(III), KP 41

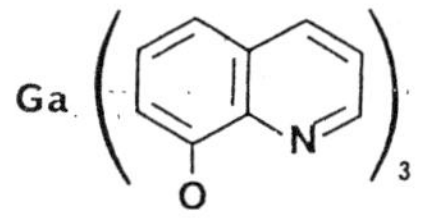

Tris(8-chinolinolato)gallium(III), KP 46

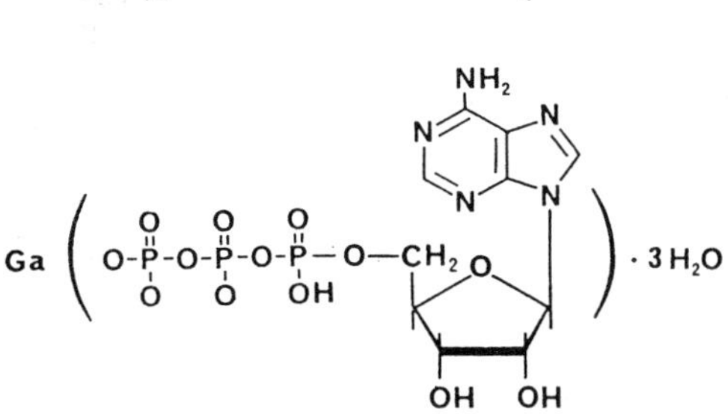

Adenosine-5-triphosphate-gallium(III)-trihydrate, KP 951

All compounds as well as gallium chloride were administered orally at a daily equimolar dose of 1.35 mmol/kg. Organ and serum levels were investigated by means of atom absorption spectroscopy (see diagrams below; the numbers above the columns indicate the standard deviations). The hydroxychinoline complex, KP 46, shows a bioavailability so high that in this case the experiment had to be disrupted after only three applications as a result of increasing substance toxicity. The diagrams below show that high plasma levels were reached after only three days. These levels could not be reached with the other compounds, which were all administered daily over nine days, not even after this nine day application. In the case of the adenosine triphosphate compound of gallium this is probably due to its higher hydrophilia and lower stability against hydrolysis, and in the case of the tropolonato complex, which should be similarly lipophil as the hydroxychinoline complex, it may be attributed to a lower complex stability.

The highest levels of KP 46 were found in the serum, with about 1400 μg/l. The next highest levels were found in the liver (ca. 20 μg/l) and in the bone (ca. 35 μg/l). Spleen (ca. 9 μg/l) and heart (ca. 6 μg/l) follow, whereas the ovaries show levels of only about 2 μg/l and the brain only 0.2 μg/l. Thus the necessity of reaching a gallium plasma concentration of 750 μg/l is met by the treatment with KP 46, which reaches gallium levels of about 1400 μg/l.

After it became clear in these first experiments that it is possible to obtain far higher gallium levels in the tissue with the tris(8-hydroxychinolinolato)gallium(III) complex, KP 46, than with gallium chloride or other gallium compounds, further investigations into the combination therapy with cisplatin are now to follow.

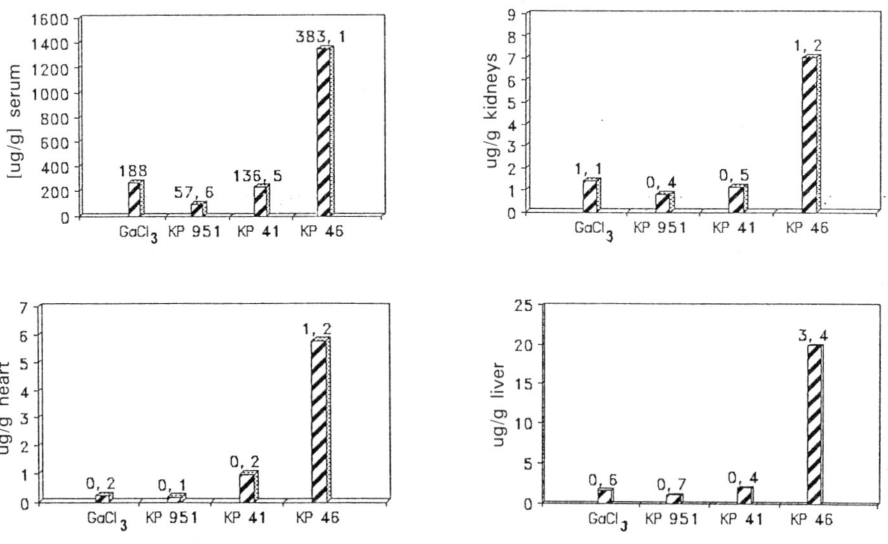

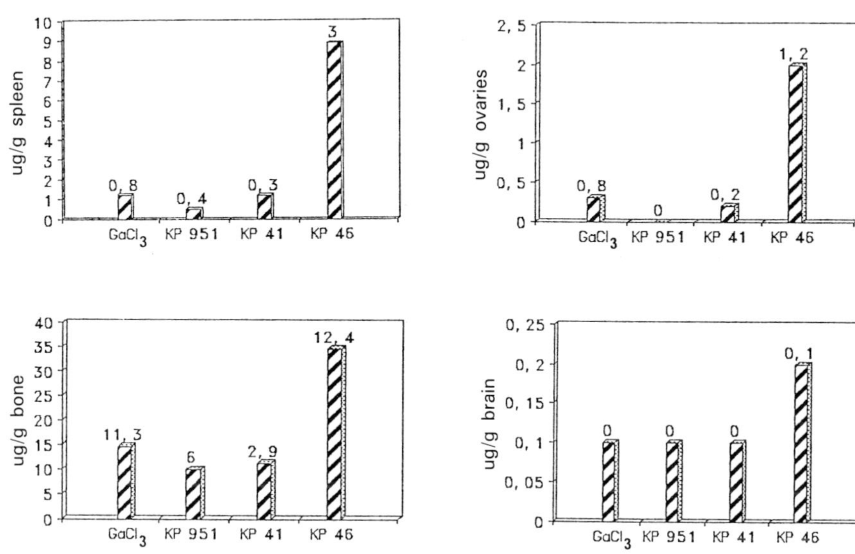

References

(1) Collery, Ph., Morel, M. (1990) Oral administration of gallium in conjunction with platinum in lung cancer treatment. In: Metal Ions in Biology and Medicine. Ph. Collery, L.A. Poirier et al. eds. John Libbey Eurotext, Paris, pp. 437-442.

(2) Collery, Ph., Millart, H. et al. (1985) Gallium chloride treatment of cancer patients after oral administration. A pilot study. Chemotherapia 4, 1165-1166.

(3) Collery, Ph., Millart, H. et al. (1989) Clinical pharmacology of gallium chloride after oral administration in lung cancer patients. Anticancer Res. 9, 353-356.

Acknowledgements

This work was supported by the *Deutsche Krebshilfe,* Bonn, FRG, and the *Fonds der Chemischen Industrie,* Frankfurt, FRG.

Metal Ions in Biology and Medicine, vol. 2. Eds. J. Anastassopoulou, Ph. Collery, J.C. Etienne, Th. Theophanides. John Libbey Eurotext, Paris © 1992, pp. 176-177

Tumor growth inhibition by gallium chloride after oral administration in tumor-bearing mice

Philippe Collery*, Léopold J. Anghileri**, Michel Morel*, Gilles Tran****, Pierre Rinjard***, Jean-Claude Étienne*

** Centre Hospitalier Universitaire, 51092 Reims, Cedex France. ** Laboratoire de Biophysique, Hôpital Central, 54000 Nancy, France. *** Centre de Recherche, Coopération Pharmaceutique Française, 77000 La Rochette, France. **** Laboratoire Meram, 4, rue Amelot, 75011 Paris, France*

Parenterally administered gallium nitrate has demonstrated antitumor activity for a variety of murine tumor models (1).Preclinical studies performed in various type of experimental animals showed the dose-limiting toxicity to be renal, but hepatic, pulmonary, gastrointestinal, hematologic, and integumentary systems are also involved (2,3).In order to reduce the toxicity effects of galium, we have studied the action of gallium chloride wich was orally administered on both, growth evolution of the murine mammary adenocarcinoma C3HBA, and the toxic effects on the host.

Material and methods :

Right after subcutaneous inoculation of C3HBA adenocarcinoma, groups of 30 female C3HHeJ mice (18-20 g body weight) were treated by a daily ingestion of 400 mg/kg of Gacl3 dissolved in the drinking water. The tumor growth evolution was controlled by measuring its diameters with a caliper, and the tumor volume was calculated by means of the formule $(D \times d^2)/2$ where D is the longer diameter and d is the shorter one. Using the Wilcoxon's test, the tumor volume values of the treated groups were compared to the values corresponding to a control group without gallium chloride. The systemic toxicity was evaluated on groups of tumor-bearing and control (non inoculated) aminals, which were treated or not with the same dose of gallium chloride used to study the effects on tumor growth evolution.

Results :

Concerning the tumor growth evolution, a significant reduction of the tumor volume was observed between 27 and 49 days after tumor inoculation, during the exponential phase of the tumor growth ($p<0.05$). After this period , the tumor reached a plateau and no significant differences were noted between the 2 groups (figure 1). The same difference of the efficacy between the exponential growth and the plateau phase was already observed after intraperitoneal inoculation of $GaCl3$ in tumor-bearing mice (4). On the other hand, the systemic toxicity, assessed as body weight modification for tumor-bearing and control animals, was absent for either of them (figure 2).

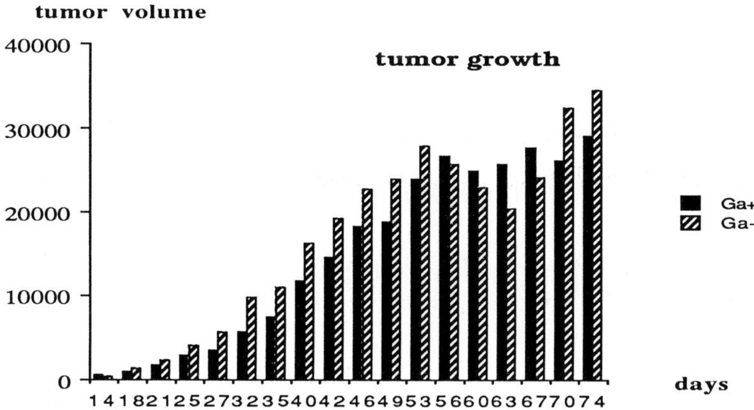

figure 1: tumor volume values corresponding to gallium-treated (Ga+) and control animals (Ga-)

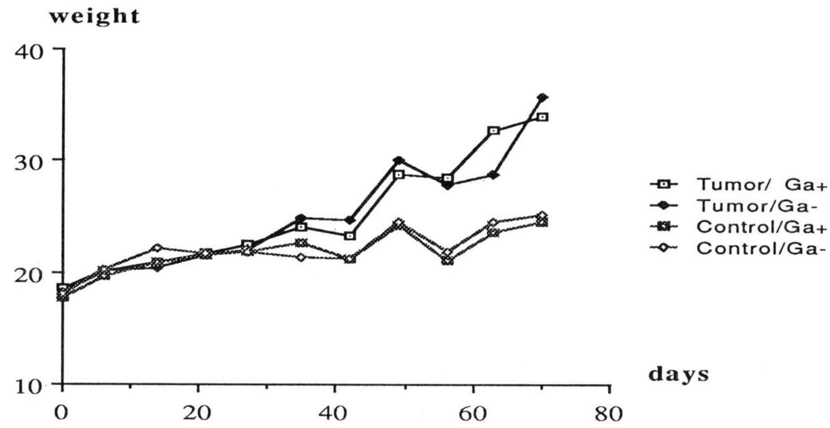

figure 2: body-weight of gallium-treated (Ga+) and control animals (Ga-)

Conclusion : According to these experimental results we can state that oral administration of gallium chloride allows a reduction of the tumor growth during the exponential phase of the tumor growth. Thanks to this effect and the lack of toxicity, $GaCl_3$ has been used as a potentiator of a conventional chemotherapy.

References:

(1) Adamson, R.H., Canellos, G.P., Sieber, S.M. (1975) : studies on the antitumor activity of gallium nitrate and other group IIIa metal salts. Cancer Chemother. Rep. 59: 599-610.

(2) Dudley, H.C., Levine, M.D. (1949) : studies of the toxic action of gallium. J. Pharmacol. Exp. Ther. 95 : 487 - 493.

(3) Newman, R.A., Brody, A.R., Krakoff, I.H. (1979) : gallium nitrate induced toxicity in the rat: a pharmacologic, histopathologic and microanalytical investigation. Cancer 44: 1728-1740.

(4) Carpentier, Y., Liautaud-Roger, F., Labbe, F., Loirette, M., Collery, P., Coninx, P. (1987): effect of gallium at two phases of the CA 755 tumour growth . Anticancer Res. 7: 745-748

Metal Ions in Biology and Medicine, vol. 2. Eds. J. Anastassopoulou, Ph. Collery, J.C. Etienne, Th. Theophanides. John Libbey Eurotext, Paris © 1992, pp. 178-179

Effect of gallium on anthracycline uptake in sensitive and resistant K562 cancer cells

J.-M. Millot*, H. Morjani*, Ph. Collery**, M. Polissiou***, M. Manfait*

** Laboratoire de Spectroscopie Biomoléculaire, Faculté de Pharmacie, 51096 Reims, France. ** Centre Hospitalier Universitaire, Hôpital Maison Blanche, 51092 Reims, France. *** Laboratory of General Chemistry, Agricultural University of Athens, 11855 Athens, Greece*

Recent studies have shown that Gallium is an antagonist of iron (1), particularly at the level of the carrier protein transferrin (2). Moreover, iron chelators induce a modulation of anthracycline cytotoxicity in cancer cells (3). Thus, it is possible to expect an influence of Gallium on the cellular uptake of anthracyclines in K562 cells. For this purpose, microspectrofluorometry was used to measure intranuclear concentrations of doxorubicin (DOX).

MATERIAL AND METHODS

Cells

K562 is a human leukemia cell line, established from a patient with chronic myelogenous leukemia in blast transformation. The K562-DOX cell line, resistant to doxorubicin, was obtained by continuous exposure to increasing DOX concentrations, and was maintained in RPMI containing DOX (100 nM). This subline exhibited the multidrug resistance.
Cells in exponential growth phase at $5x10^5$/ml density in RPMI were treated by $GaCl_3$ (1 µM and 10 µM) during 48h in a moist air/CO_2 incubator at 37°C. Cells were washed twice and incubated in doxorubicin at the concentration of 2 µM. After 4 hours, cells were washed free of drug and were seeded on a petri dish containing PBS for the drug uptake measurements by confocal laser microspectrofluorometry.

Microspectrofluorometric analysis (4)

Fluorescence emission spectra from a microvolume within a living cell were recorded with a microspectrofluorometer (modified Raman spectrometer OMARS 89, Dilor, Lille, France) (4). Using an optical microscope (Olympus BH2) equipped with a 100X water phase contrast immersion objective (Leitz fluotar), a laser beam (457.9 nm) (Spectra Physics Ar^+ 2020/03) was focused to a spot of less than 1 µm in diameter.
The fluorescence emission spectrum arising from the nucleus of a DOX-treated cell, can be expressed as a sum of spectral contributions of free drug, DNA-bound drug and intranuclear autofluorescence. Each of these contributions has a characteristic spectral shape and the fluorescence yield of the free form is 48 times higher than that of the bound-DNA form. Thus, the DOX concentration in a cell nucleus was determined from these spectral contributions and by means of the corresponding fluorescence yields.

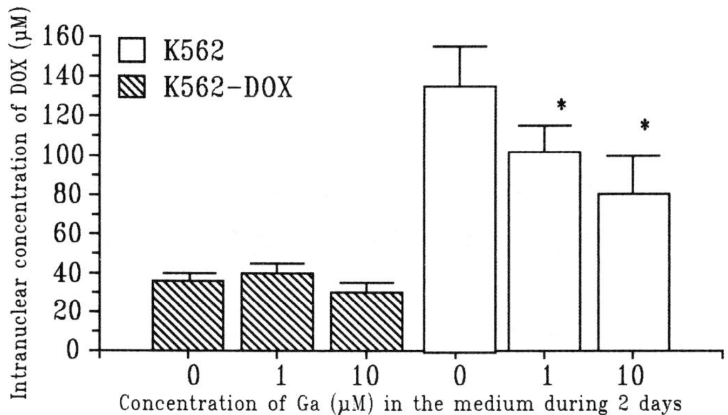

Figure 1 : Intranuclear concentrations of DOX in K562 and K562-DOX cells, in function of Gallium concentration in the medium (* : $p<0.01$)

RESULTS

For K562 sensitive cells, the means (± SD) of the intranuclear concentrations of doxorubicin, expressed in µM, are 137 ± 30 in untreated cells, 100 ± 22 in 1 µM Ga-treated cells, 82 ± 33 in 10 µM Ga-treated cells. These results indicate a significant decrease of intranuclear concentrations of doxorubicin in both Ga-treated cells, as compared to control ($p<0.01$) (Fig. 1).
For K562-DOX resistant cells, the means (± SD) of the intranuclear concentrations of doxorubicin are 35.7 ± 9 in untreated cells, 36.6 ± 8 in 1 µM Ga-treated cells, 29.9 ± 9 in 10 µM Ga-treated cells. In the same incubation conditions, doxorubicin intranuclear concentrations were lower in K562-DOX cells than in K562 cells, but they were not modulated by Gallium (Fig. 1).

CONCLUSION

From our data, the Ga-treated cells showed decreased intranuclear concentrations of doxorubicin as compared to the untreated cells. This inhibition of anthracycline uptake by Ga has been described on K562 sensitive cells but not on K562-DOX cells. Previous results on ionic transfer through the isolated human amnion have described that Ga induced a decrease of ionic fluxes through the amnion and modified the membrane potential (5). Thus, our present result is in accordance with the hypothesis that Ga is a modulator of cell permeability by altering the membrane potential in cancer cells.

REFERENCES

1- Collery Ph., Vistelle R., Arsac F., Habets F., Millart H., Choisy H. (1990) : Effects of $GaCl_3$-CDDP combination on the intratissular concentrations of Ga, Pt, Mg, Fe and Ca in heathly mice. In : Metal ions in biology and medicine. Eds Ph. Collery, L.A. Poirier, M. Manfait, J.C. Etienne. John Libbey Eurotext, Paris, 412-414.
2- Sephton R., De Abrew S. (1990) : Mechanism of Gallium uptake in tumours. In : Metal ions in biology and medicine. Eds Ph. Collery, L.A. Poirier, M. Manfait, J.C. Etienne. John Libbey Eurotext, Paris, 393-397.
3- Bergeron R.J., Ingeno M.J. (1987) : Microbial iron chelator-induced cell cycle synchronization in L1210 cells. Cancer Res., 47: 6010-6016.
4- Gigli M., Doglia S., Millot J-M., Valentini L., Manfait M. (1988) : Quantitative study of doxorubicin in living cell nuclei by microspectrofluorometry, Biochim. Biophys. Acta., 950, 13-20.
5- Bara M., Guiet-Bara A., Collery P., Durlach J. (1985) : Gallium action on ionic transfer through the isolated human amnion. I.Effect on the amnion as a whole and interaction between gallium and magnesium. Trace elements in Med. 2: 99-102.

Metal Ions in Biology and Medicine, vol. 2. Eds. J. Anastassopoulou, Ph. Collery, J.C. Etienne, Th. Theophanides. John Libbey Eurotext, Paris © 1992, pp. 180-181

Bone reconstruction of a lytic rib metastase after chemotherapy with cisplatinum, etoposide and gallium in a lung cancer patient

Philippe Collery, Dominique Perdu

Departement des Maladies Respiratoires, Centre Hospitalier Universitaire, 51092 Reims Cedex, France

Introduction: Bone metastases are frequent in lung cancer patients and ribs are one of the most common sites with lytic aspects on X ray radiograph. Their pronostic is poor and reconstruction of a lytic rib metastase is unusual. We report such a case after chemotherapy including gallium (Ga) which has been demonstrated to have biological effects on bone.

Case report: A 49 year old man was hospitalized in august 1990 for evaluation of a lung adenocarcinoma few weeks after a left pneumonectomy (T2 N2 M0). Biopsies on the bronchic scar of pneumonectomy revealed the presence of malignant cells and bone asymptomatic metastases were evocated by Technetium scintigraphy on the first right rib, two controlateral ribs, the upper part of the right hip and the lower zone of the right femoral diaphyse. The first right rib was destroyed in X-ray radiography. Computed tomography did not show any residual tumor in the thorax and there was neither hepatic, nor cerebral metastase. Calcemia was normal but phosphatases alcalines were moderatly increased (140 U.I/l) as well as phosphatemia (1.58 mmol/l).

A chemotherapy with cisplatinum (CDDP) and etoposide as 5 days continuous infusions every 3 weeks was then started in combination with a daily oral gallium chloride ($GaCl_3$) administration. Individual adaptation of the doses of the three drugs was performed to improve the efficacy and tolerance of this treatment.

Doses were 15 mg/m^2/24h for CDDP and 25 mg/m^2/24h for etoposide at the beginning of the first cycle with an adaptation at hour 72 of the infusion, according to total platinum and etoposide concentrations, in order to obtain an AUC between 80000 and 90000 μg.l^{-1}.h for total plasma platinum and between 200 and 230 μmol.l^{-1}.h for etoposide, as already described (3). For the next courses the initial dosage was the fith of the total dose of the preceeding cycle during the first three days and an adaptation was then again realized at hour 72 with the same goal. $GaCl_3$ was initialy given with the daily oral dosage of 400 mg/24h. During the next courses, dosages were modified between 400 and 1200 mg/24h, in order to maintain a plasma Ga concentration between 200 and 400 μg/l.

After 3 courses of chemotherapy no significant differences were observed concerning the tumor evaluation except for the first right rib which could be seen again in part in chest radiograph. Malignant cells were still present on the bronchic scar of pneumonectomy. By contrast, differences were marked after 6 additional courses with lack of neoplastic cells on endoscopic biopsies, a complete reconstruction of the first right rib on X ray radiography and a significant regression of the number of scintigraphic hyperfixations. A total of 12 courses of chemotherapy could be administered, permitting a nearly complete regression of the bone scintigraphic abnormalities, except on the cotyle. Blood phosphatemia and phosphatases alcalines were normalized (respectively 1.30 mmol/l and 95 U.I./l). Thanks to the adaptation of the drug dosages, no clinical toxicity was noted and the biological toxicity was moderate. A radiotherapy could be given on the last metastatic site, that means on the lytic area of the cotyle. No recurrence has been noted in february 1992.

Comments: About this case report, we would like to emphasize the role of Ga on bone. The great affinity of Ga for bone has been demonstrated, and particularly after oral administration (5). Several biological effects of Ga on bone have also been demonstrated (4): an increase of calcium and phosphate content, a decrease of osteoclastic activity, a dose-dependant inhibition of seeded hydroxyapatite crystal formation and growth, due to adsorption of gallium onto hydroxyapatite crystal surface, a concentration-dependant increase in collagen synthesis and finally an increase of bone formation in vitro. That could explain the unusual reconstruction of the lytic metastase in our observation, which could not have been observed neither according to the natural evolution of bone metastases in lung cancer nor by the 2 other drugs or an associated disease. Moreover, this observation illustrates the need for a long time of treatment in order to obtain the best efficacy with Ga as modifyer of the biological response (1,5). The plasma Ga concentration remaining at a steady-state, an accumulation of Ga will occur in tissues , particularly in bone (5). Ga can also potentiate a chemotherapy with CDDP and etoposide (2) and this combination chemotherapy allows a progressive reduction of the bone metastases as noted by the different scintigraphies .

References :

1) Collery, Ph., Millart, H., Pluot, M., Anghileri, L.J. (1986): effects of gallium chloride oral administration on transplanted C3HBA mammary adenocarcinoma: Ga, Mg, Ca and Fe concentration and anatomopathological characteristics. Anticancer Res. 6 : 1085-1088.

2) Collery, Ph.,Morel M., Millart, H., Desoize, B., Cossart, C.,Perdu, D.,Vallerand, H., Bouana,J.C., Pechery, C.,Etienne, J.C., Choisy, H., Dubois de Montreynaud, J.M. (1990): oral aministration of gallium in conjunction with platinum in lung cancer treatment. in: Metal lons in Biology and Medicine. Collery Ph, Poirier L.A., Manfait M.,Etienne J.C . Eds .John Libbey Eurotext, Paris : pp 437-442.

3) Collery, Ph.,Morel M., Desoize, B.,Millart, H., Perdu, D., Prevost, A., Vallerand, H., Pechery, C., Choisy, H., Etienne, J.C., Dubois de Montreynaud, J.M. (1991): combination chemotherapy with cisplatin, etoposide and gallium chloride for lung cancer: individual adaptation of doses. Anticancer Res. 11: 1529-1532.

4)Todd, P.A., Fitton, A. (1991): gallium nitrate. A review of its pharmacological properties and therapeutic potential in cancer-related hypercalcemia. Drugs 1991, 42, 261-273.

5)Vistelle, R., Collery, Ph., Millart, H. (1989): in vivo distribution of gallium in healthy rats after oral administration and its interaction with Fe, Mg and Ca. Trace El. Med. 6: 27-32.

Metal Ions in Biology and Medicine, vol. 2. Eds. J. Anastassopoulou, Ph. Collery, J.C. Etienne, Th. Theophanides. John Libbey Eurotext, Paris © 1992, pp. 182-183

Bayesian estimation of cisplatin pharmacokinetics during five-day continuous infusions

B. Desoize*, R. Dufour*, Ph. Collery**, S. Urien***

** GIBSA, Institut J. Godinot, BP171, 51056 Reims Cedex, France. **Hôpital Maison Blanche, 45, rue Cognacq-Jay, 51092 Reims Cedex, France. *** Faculté de Médecine, 8, rue du Général-Sarrail, 94010 Créteil, France*

We previously reported that the toxicity and the efficacy of cisplatin, when administered as 5-day continuous infusion, was related to the plasma concentration or the AUC of total platinum [Pt,] (1,2). We then decided to adjust the dose of cisplatin for each patient to reach the therapeutic window. We established a mathematical model for an adjustment to the cisplatin AUC during the 3rd day of the cycle (2). But, the Bayesian pharmacokinetics based on population pharmacokinetics, proposed by Sheiner et al and Iliadis et al (4,6), allow the dose to inject before the treatment cycle to be calculated. Favre et al (3) used such a model, but for technical reason we could not use it in our laboratory. In this work, we evaluated the efficacy of the Bayesian model and compared the results to those obtained by the ordinary least-square nonlinear regression.

PATIENTS and METHODS

For the Bayesian pharmacokinetics we have sampled a population of reference, including 14 patients from l'Institut J. Godinot, with a cancer lung, breast or of the mediastinum. Each patient received cisplatin as a 5-day continuous infusion. For each patient, the Pt concentration of 7 blood samples per course during 3 cycles, i.e. 21 assays per patient, was determined. The blood samples were withdrawn just before and at the end of the infusion, and every morning (8:30 am) during the infusion. The pharmacokinetic parameters of these patients were determined with the "MicroPharm" program (for IBM compatible computers), created by one of us (Copyright 1990 INSERM).

To evaluate the Bayesian method to predict individual pharmacokinetic parameters, we used the Pt concentrations of 7 patients from the same Institute during 3 following cycles, the number of blood samples was from 14 to 20 per patient. For some patients the cycles were the number 1, 2 and 3 (2), the number 2, 3 and 4 (2), 3, 4 and 5 (1) or 4, 5 and 6 (2). Parameters were estimated with the same computer program, using each time either the Bayesian method or the least-square nonlinear regression. The results obtained by the least-square nonlinear regression of all the data from the patients were used as references.

RESULTS and DISCUSSION

The clearance of cisplatin (Cl) in the reference population was 0.166 ± 0.045 l/h (mean ± SD), the volume of distribution (Vd) was 66.6 ± 15.5 l, and the half life (t½) was 12.3 ± 4.0 days. No correlation was found between the weight nor the body surface and any of the pharmacokinetic parameters, but the serum protein content was significantly correlated to the Pt clearance ($p<0.017$, $r=0.645$). All the data of the patients were also computed with the Bayesian method. For 6 patients the results were similar to the reference population : the mean Cl was 112 % ± 9 of the references, 98 % ± 10 for the Vd and 94 % ± 22 for the t½. But, for one patient the values were obviously differents : 34, 237 and 709 % respectively, according to the graph (not shown here) the Bayesian estimation gave clearely the best fit, so it was used as reference for the 7th patient.

The average of the three parameters (Cl, Vd and t½) yielded by the Bayesian estimation of all the data of the first cycle alone, was 104 % of the reference, and the average of the SD was 24, when the non–Bayesian estimation yielded respectively 141 % and 27. This indicates that after the first cycle of cisplatin one needs the help of the Bayesian pharmacokinetic approach to calculate patient parameters.

The parameters were also estimated with only three points of the first cycle : the Pt concentration before, in the middle and at the end of the cycle. The average of the three parameters were comparable and close to reference (108 % and 110 % respectively), but the dispersion of the results was much lower with the Bayesian approximation (19 and 62 respectively). These results indicate that for this chemotherapy, one can estimate the pharmacokinetic parameters with only 3 blood samples

Usually one needs data during the decrease of the plasma drug concentration, for this reason the same computations were run with a fourth data point : the concentration measured just before the following cycle. This value improved the non–Bayesian computation, mainly the t½, the average of the three parameters was 116 % and the SD 23. The parameters obtained with the Bayesian estimation were only slightly better : 110 % and 19 respectively. The last evaluation was run with [2 cycles x 3 points], i.e. 6 data points. The Bayesian estimation yielded again better results than non–Bayesian : 103 % and 16 versus 113 % and 47. The differences between the reference, Bayesian and non–Bayesian simulations are depicted for one patient in the figure 1.

To evaluate the accuracy of results one needs references, as the true values are not available we used the estimation obtained with 14 to 20 data points. In all these calculations made with the same number of data, the Bayesian estimation yielded always more accurate parameters. These results indicated that this method is suitable to cisplatin injected in 5–day continuous infusion. It allows to know in advance the patients kinetic parameters with better accuracy than the least–square nonlinear regression. Furthermore, this prediction can be obtained with a limited blood sampling, we obtained with 3 to 4 samples equivalent results to those obtained with 14 to 20 samples. The use of limited sampling models is important since it will allow enough data to be collected for population pharmacodynamic studies (5,6). Ratain and Vogelzang wrote that Bayesian models are not simple (5), but we must state that in our case the Bayesian estimation is as simple to compute than the least–square nonlinear regression. It is reasonable to think that such a model will enable the blood concentration to be predicted during the following cycle. Then, it seems possible to anticipate a high blood concentration which will induce toxicity, or a low blood level which will prevent efficacy. The extreme blood concentrations will be then avoided by the drug dosage adjustment.

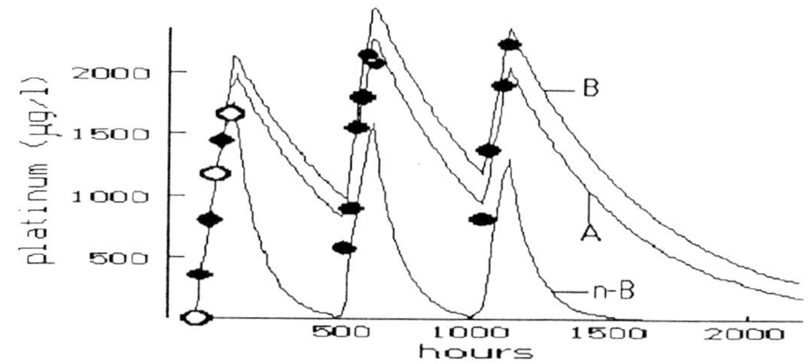

Fig.1– Simulation of the plasma concentration of Pt versus time by the least–square nonlinear regression with all the samples (16, A), Bayesian simulation with 3 points (open circles, B) and least–square non linear regression simulation with the same 3 points (n–B).

REFERENCES

1– Desoize B, Maréchal F, Millart H, Cattan A. Biomed Pharmacother, 1991, **45**, 203–207

2– Collery P, Morel M, Millart H, Desoize B et al. In "Metal Ions in Biology and Medicine", P. Collery et al ed., J. Libbey, London, 1990, 437–442

3– Favre R, Charbit M, Rinaldi Y A et al. Bull cancer, 1988, **75**, 541–550

4– Sheiner LB, Beal S, Rosenberg B et al. Clin Pharmacol Ther, 1979, **26**, 294–205

5– Ratin MJ, Vogelzang NJ. Cancer Treat Rep, 1987, **71**, 935–939

6– Iliadis A, Bachir–Rako M, Bruno R et al. J Pharmacokinet Biopharm, 1985, **13**, 101–115

Metal Ions in Biology and Medicine, vol. 2. Eds. J. Anastassopoulou, Ph. Collery, J.C. Etienne, Th. Theophanides. John Libbey Eurotext, Paris © 1992, pp. 184-185

Biologically active complexes of Zn (II) and Cd (II) with 5-bromouracil

V.K. Rastogi, Babu Lal, Y.C. Sharma*, C.L. Jain**

*Department of Physics, LR College (Meerut University), Sahibabad-201 005, India. * Department of Physics, NAS College, Meerut, India and ** Department of Chemistry, MMH College, Ghaziabad-201 002, India*

INTRODUCTION

Metal complexes play an important role in the biological activity of drugs, as the complex formation has been suggested one of the important mechanism for the drug interaction. Recent spectroscopic studies of uracil derivatives and its metal complexes have been motivated by their biological importance (Rastogi et al, 1990, 1991; Singh et al, 1987). DNA normally contains uncommon nucleotides usually in very small amount. 5-bromouracil (5-BU) is one of the well known uncommon nucleotide bases and have the ability to bind metals or to bind to tissues via metals. Hence, in order to understand the mechanism by which the metal ions intervene in the function of nucleic acid bases, and to find the coordinating sites in 5-BU, we have undertaken the present study. Here we report the isolation of the complexes of Zn(II) and Cd(II) with 5-BU. Chemical analyses are used to determine stoichiometries and vibrational spectroscopy is used to illucidate the vibrational modes and sites of coordination.

EXPERIMENTAL

The metal complexes were isolated by mixing the hot appropriate hydrated metal nitrate solution (1 m mole) prepared in ethanol (14 ml)-water (100 ml) mixture and hot alcoholic soluton of 5-bromouracil (1 m mole). The resulting mixture was heated to about 65°C and the NaOH was added to adjust the pH to about 4-6. The white precipitate thus obtained was filtered, washed several times with ethyl alcohol and recrystallised from the same solvent. The residue was dried in an oven at about 90°C.

RESULTS AND DISCUSSION

The complexes formed possess 1:1 stoichiometry and are insoluble in common organic solvents. The chemical composition (Table 1)

Table 1 Physicochemical data of the Complexes

Complex	Colour	m.p.	Found/(Calc.) %			
			M	C	H	N
$Zn(L)(OH)_2.3H_2O$	White	315°C	18.94	13.86	3.18	8.18
			18.98	13.92	3.19	8.13
$Cd(L)(OH)_2.3H_2O$	White	310°C	28.70	13.00	2.89	8.00
			28.72	12.26	2.81	7.15

corresponds to the molecular formula $[M(L)(OH)_2.3H_2O]$; M = Zn(II), Cd(II) and L = $C_4H_3N_2O_2Br$.

The vibrational spectra of the complexes show some band shifts which confirm the coordination modes of the ligand well. The $\nu(C_2 = O)$ and $\nu(C_4 = 0)$ modes in the spectra of free ligand appears as strong bands at 1700/1720 cm^{-1} and 1655/1670 cm^{-1} (IR/Raman) respectively. In the spectra of the complexes $\nu(C_4 = 0)$ band is shifted to lower frequencies by 30 cm^{-1}, while $\nu(C_2 = O)$ band remains unaffected, suggesting that the ligand coordinates to the metal ion through $C_4 = O$ group and not with $C_2 = O$ group. The further evidence of bonding of oxygen with metal is provided by the appearance of a band $\sim$ 250 cm-1 in the far IR spectra of the complexes. The medium broad band appearing in the region 950-940 cm^{-1} in the spectra of the complexes has been assigned as OH bridging. The weak bands appearing in 3325-3350 cm^{-1} region have been attributed to $\nu(OH)$ of water. The appearance of bands at 360 cm^{-1} in Zn(II) complex and at 340 cm^{-1} in Cd(II) complex due to ν(M-O) (aquo) confirm the presence of coordinated water molecules in these complexes. The bands due to ν(N-H) and ν(C-Br) modes remain unaltered, indicating the non-involvement of these groups in complexation. Thus a octahedral polymeric structure has been suggested for these complexes as shown in Fig. The ligand 5-BU and Zn(II) complex have been found to possess antitumour activity. Thus it is concluded that this nucleic acid base act as donor towards transition metal ions and interact with metals during the transcription and/or translation processes.

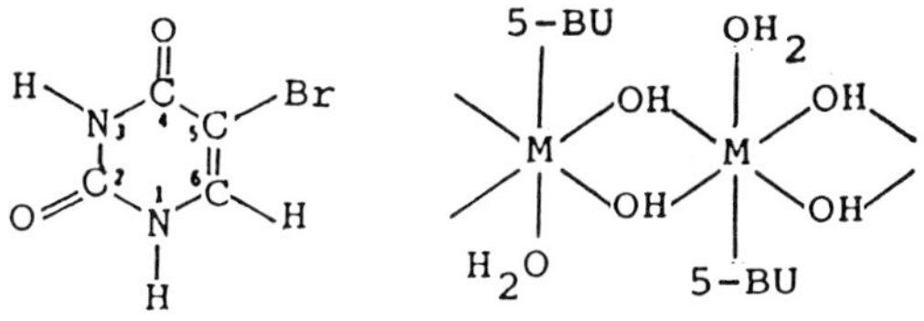

REFERENCES

Rastogi V K, Mital H P and Sharma S N (1990) : Indian J Phys. : 64B pp.312-316.

Rastogi V K, Arora Sushma, Gupta S L and Sharma D K (1991): Spectroscopy of biological molecules, eds R E Hester and R B Girling. Lodon : Royal Society of Chemistry.

Singh B, Khan S A and Uday Bhanu (1987) : Indian J Chem : 26A pp.1066-1068.

Metal Ions in Biology and Medicine, vol. 2. Eds. J. Anastassopoulou, Ph. Collery, J.C. Etienne, Th. Theophanides. John Libbey Eurotext, Paris © 1992, pp. 186-187

NCI anticancer *in vitro* pre-screening of diorganotin (IV) compounds against a panel of sixty human tumor cell lines

Marcel Gielen*, Rudolph Willem**

*Free University of Brussels VUB, * Department of General and Organic Chemistry of the Faculty of Engineering and ** High Resolution NMR Centre, Room 8G512, Pleinlaan 2, B-1050 Brussels, Belgium*

Substituted bis[di-n-butyl(salicylato)tin] oxides were recently tested *in vitro* against the human A 204 rhabdomyosarcoma tumour, MCF-7 mammary carcinoma, T24 bladder carcinoma, WiDr colon carcinoma and IgR-37 melanoma cell lines and were found more active than cis-platin (Bouâlam **et al.**, 1990, Ross **et al.**). Among these, bis[di-n-butyl(4-aminosalicylato)tin] oxide, compound **1** (see figure 1) was found (Ross **et al.**) to be 8 times more active than cis-platin in A 204 cultures, 20 times more against MCF-7, 4 times more against T24, 3 times more against WiDr and only slightly more against IgR-37.

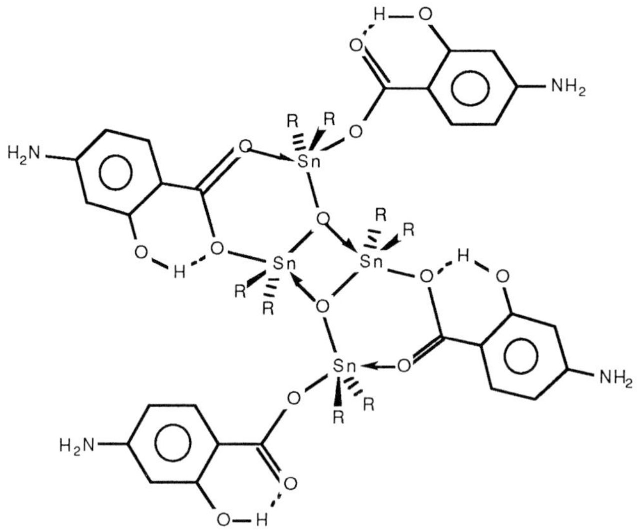

Fig. 1: Structure of compounds **1** (R = n-Bu) and **2** (R = Ph) in the crystalline state and in $CDCl_3$ solution [Bouâlam **et al.** (1991)]

Because of the strong cytotoxic activity of compound **1**, its diphenyltin analog, bis[diphenyl(4-aminosalicylato)tin] oxide, compound **2**, and several other analogous compounds of the type

$[n\text{-}Bu_2(X(2\text{-}HO)\text{-}C_6H_3COO)Sn]_2O$, compounds **3** (X = 3-Me), **4** (X = 4-Me), **5** (X = 5-Me) and **6** (X = 3-MeO), bis[di-n-butyl(3,5-diiodosalicylato)tin] oxide, compound **7** and bis[di-n-butyl(2-aminobenzoato)tin] oxide, compound **8**, were synthesized. All were tested *in vitro* at the National Cancer Institute, Bethesda, Maryland. Our purpose was to confirm the trend to high activities on a wider panel of cancer cells.

Compound **1** scores globally satisfactorily since four of the five relevant selectivity or sensitivity parameters (Gielen & Willem) calculated by the NCI display statistically significantactivity values [D_{GI50} (67 > 50), D_{TGI} (69 > 50), D_H (81 > 75) and MGD_H (77 > 75)]. The same conclusion holds for compounds **6** and **8**. Compounds **2**, **3** and **7** are less satisfactory because only three of these five parameters are statistically significant. Compounds **4** and **5** provide poor results. The National Cancer Institute decided to refer only compounds **1** and **2** to the Biological Evaluation Committee.

The fact that compound **1**, a di-n-butyltin compound, displays a higher *in vitro* activity than its diphenyltin analog, compound **2**, is in contrast to the results of previous screenings on murine P388 and L1210 *in vivo*, where diphenyltin compounds generally scored much better than their corresponding di-n-butyltin analogs (Ross **et al.**, Crowe, Meinema **et al.**).

Whereas compound **3** gives test results that are not very different from those obtained for compound **1**, its isomers, compounds **4** and **5**, are much less selective and exhibit no subpanel sensitivity.

These preliminary results show that more research should be performed in the field of novel organotin compounds with potential antitumour activity, especially in the area of structure-activity correlations (Atassi).

REFERENCES

Atassi, G. (1985): Antitumor and Toxic Effects of Silicon, Germanium, Tin and Lead Compounds, *Rev. Si, Ge, Sn & Pb Cpds.* **8**: 219-235

Bouâlam, M., Gielen, M., Meriem, A., de Vos, D. & Willem, R. (Pharmachemie B.V.) (1990): *Eur. Pat.* 90202316.7-, 21/09/90, Anti-tumor compositions and compounds

Bouâlam, M., Willem, R., Biesemans, M., Mahieu, B., Meunier-Piret, J. & Gielen, M. (1991): Synthesis, characterization and *in vitro* antitumour activity of diorganotin derivatives of substituted salicylic acids and analogs. Crystal structure of bis(5-methoxysalicylato-di-n-butyltin) oxide, *Main Group Met. Chem.* **14**: 41-56

Crowe, A.J. (1988): The Antitumour Activity of Tin Compounds. In: Metal-Based Antitumour Drugs (Gielen, M.F., ed.), Freund Publ. House, London, pp. 103-149

Gielen, M. & Willem, R. (1992), Cytotoxic activity of bis-[di-n-butyl(4-aminosalicylato)tin] oxide, NSC: 628561, bis-[diphenyl(4-aminosalicylato)tin] oxide, NSC: 628562, and some related compounds, against a series of human tumour cell lines. *Anticancer Res.*: in press

Meinema, H.A., Liebregts, A.M., Budding, H.A. & Bulten, E.J. (1985): Synthesis and Evaluation of Organometal-Based Anti-tumor Agents of Germanium and Tin, *Rev Si, Ge, Sn & Pb Cpds.* **8**:157-168

Ross, M., Gielen, M., Lelieveld, P. & de Vos, D. (1992): Cytotoxic Activity of Di-n-butyltin(IV)(X-A-B-X) Compounds Related to Salicylic Acid against Human Tumour Cells. *Anticancer Res.* **11**: 1089-1091

Metal Ions in Biology and Medicine, vol. 2. Eds. J. Anastassopoulou, Ph. Collery, J.C. Etienne, Th. Theophanides. John Libbey Eurotext, Paris © 1992, pp. 188-189

In vitro cytotoxic activity against a panel of sixty human tumor cell lines of some diorganotin (IV) 1,2-ethylenediamine N,N'-diacetates, N-(2-hydroxyethyl)- and N-(carbamoylmethyl)-iminodiacetates, and ortho-aminobenzoates

Marcel Gielen*, Rudolph Willem**

*Free University of Brussels VUB, * Department of General and Organic Chemistry of the Faculty of Engineering and ** High Resolution NMR Centre, Room 8G512, Pleinlaan 2, B-1050 Brussels, Belgium*

Several organotin compounds synthesized in our laboratory provided satisfactory *in vitro* screening results against two human tumour cell lines, MCF-7, a mammary tumour, and WiDr, a colon carcinoma (Mancilla **et al**.; Meriem **et al**., 1990).

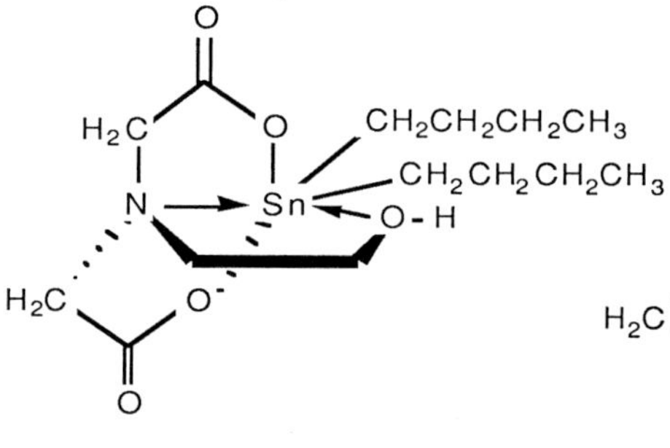

Compound **1**, NSC 628566

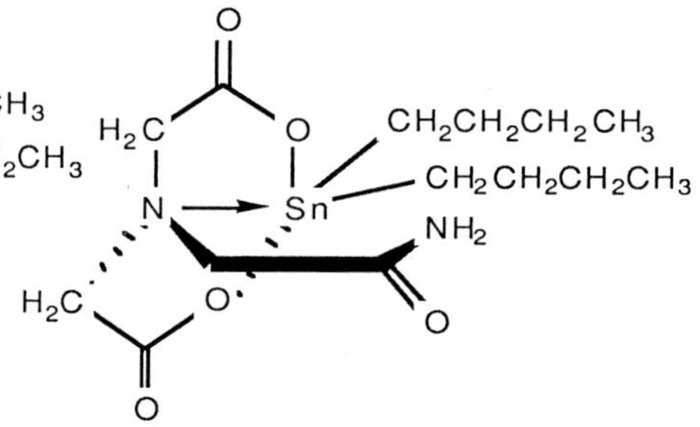

Compound **2**, NSC 628568

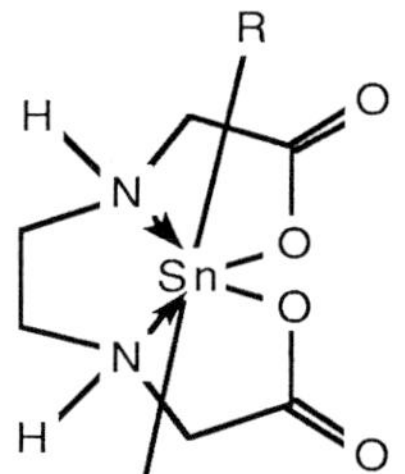

R = n-Bu, compound **3**, NSC 628574

R = n-Oct, compound **4**, NSC 628575

R = Me, compound **5**, NSC 628576

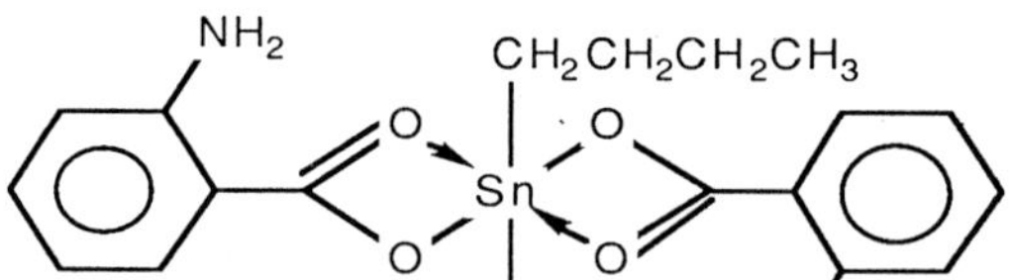

Compound **6**, NSC 628572

Fig. 1: Structures and NSC numbers of compounds **1** to **6**

Especially di-n-butyltin(IV) N-(2-hydroxyethyl)- and N-(carbamoylmethyl)-iminodiacetates, compounds **1** and **2** (Meriem **et al**., 1989), di-n-butyl-, di-n-octyl- and dimethyltin(IV) ethylene diamine N,N'-diacetates, compounds **3**, **4** and **5** (Mancilla) and di-n-butytin bis-o-aminobenzoate, compound **6** (Meriem, 1990) (see fig. 1) are worth outlining. Therefore, the NCI tested these compounds against the extensive panel of human tumour cell lines available there.

Compounds **1** and **2** gave NCI *in vitro* screening results (Gielen & Willem) quite comparable to those obtained for bis[di-n-butyl(4-aminosalicylato)tin] oxide [NSC: 628561]: they score globally satisfactorily since four of the five relevant selectivity or sensitivity parameters meet the criteria of statistically significant activity [D_{GI50}, D_{TGI} or $D_{LC50} > 50$, D_H and $MGD_H > 75$)]. Compounds **4** and **6** score satisfactorily for only three. Compound **3** provided satisfactory D_H and MGD_H parameters but showed no subpanel sensitivity.

Compound **5**, the dimethyltin derivative, is inactive, as expected (Mancilla **et al**.; Meriem **et al**., 1990).

These data are quite encouraging and show that organotin compounds are reasonable candidates as active antitumour drugs except dimethyltin compounds. More research in this promising field is however needed to develop an organotin compound suitable for clinical trials.

REFERENCES

Gielen, M. & Willem, R. (1992), Cytotoxic activity against a series of human tumour cell lines of some diorganotin(IV) 1,2-ethylenediamine N,N' diacetates, N-(2-hydroxyethyl)- and N-(xcarbamoylmethyl)-iminodiacetates, and ortho-aminobenzoates, *Anticancer Res.*, in press

Mancilla, M., Farfán, N., Castillo, D., Molinero, L., Meriem, A., Willem, R., Mahieu, B.& Gielen, M. (1989): Synthesis and characterization of a series of diorganotin compounds of the type $R_2Sn(O\text{-}C_6H_4\text{-}o\text{-}NH\text{-}CH_2CH_2\text{-}NH\text{-}C_6H_4\text{-}o\text{-}O)$, *Main Group Met. Chem.* **12**: 213-223

Meriem, A., Willem, R., Meunier-Piret, J. & Gielen, M. (1989): Diorganotin(IV) derivatives of N-(2-hydroxyethyl)- and N-(carbamoylmethyl)-iminodiacetic acid: Synthesis, spectroscopic characterization, X-ray structure analysis and *in vitro* antitumour activity, *Main Group Met. Chem.* **12**: 187-198

Meriem, A., Willem, R., Meunier-Piret, J., Biesemans, M., Mahieu, M. & Gielen, M. (1990): Synthesis, spectroscopic characterization and antitumor activity of diorganotinbis(ortho-aminobenzoates) and some N-substituted derivatives thereof. X-Ray structure determination of di-n-butyltinbis(ortho-aminobenzoate), *Main Group Met. Chem.* **13**: 167-180

Metal Ions in Biology and Medicine, vol. 2. Eds. J. Anastassopoulou, Ph. Collery, J.C. Etienne, Th. Theophanides. John Libbey Eurotext, Paris © 1992, pp. 190-191

In vitro anticancer activities of triphenyltin carboxylates against human tumor cell lines

M. Gielen*, R. Willem***, M. Bouâlam***, A. El Khloufi*, D. de Vos****

*Free University of Brussels VUB, * Department of General and Organic Chemistry of the Faculty of Engineering and ** High Resolution NMR Centre, Room 8G512, Pleinlaan 2, B-1050 Brussels, Belgium. *** Université de Tétouan, Faculté des Sciences, Département de Chimie, Tétouan, Morocco. **** Medical Department, Pharmachemie BV, NL-2003 RN Haarlem, The Netherlands*

Organotin compounds exhibit antitumor activity like platinum compounds such as cisplatin, cis-$(NH_3)_2Cl_2Pt$,(Bouâlam **et al.**, 1990, 1991a; Gielen & Willem).

	X	Y	Z	MCF-7	WiDr
1	H	H	2-OCH_3	16	15
2	H	H	4-F	15	14
3	H	3-F	5-F	18	17
4	H	H	2-$OCOCH_3$	13	9
5	H	2-OH	5-Cl	11	18
6	H	2-OH	5-NH_2	14	17
7	H	2-OH	5-OCH_3	6	15
8	H	2-OH	5-SO_3H	100	131
9	2-OH	3-$CH(CH_3)_2$	5-$CH(CH_3)_2$	8	13
Cis-platin				850	624
Etoposide				187	624
Doxorubicin				63	31
Mitomycin C				3	17

Table 1: Inhibition doses ID_{50} in ng/mL of substituted triphenyltin benzoates, $(C_6H_5)_3Sn$-O-CO-C_6H_2XYZ, against two human tumor cell lines, MCF-7, a mammary tumor, and WiDr, a colon carcinoma

The present work describes substituted triphenyltin benzoates Ph_3Sn-O-CO-C_6H_2XYZ possessing considerable antitumor activity (see table 1) (Bouâlam **et al.**, 1991b).

Among organotin compounds, many possessing antitumor activity were **di**organotin compounds (R_2SnXY): Narayanan (1983) reported that, of 129 diorganotin compounds tested by the National Cancer Institute, 48% were found active *in vivo* against P388 leukemiaon murine mice, whereas, of 132 triorganotin compounds tested, only 9% were active. Several di-n-butyltin compounds studied previously (Gielen **et al.**, 1992) exhibit inhibition doses of about 50 ng/mL against MCF-7. Compounds **1** to **7** and compound **9** are about four to ten times more active than these di-n-butyltin compounds *in vitro* against MCF-7 and much more active than cis-platin. They were found almost as active as mitomycin C. Against WiDr, the same di-n-butyltin derivatives were much less active, giving ID_{50} values of 70 or more (Gielen **et al.**, 1992). Compounds **1** to **7** and compound **9** are five to ten times more active as the most active di-n-butyltin compounds and score again comparably to mitomycin C.

REFERENCES

Bouâlam, M., Willem, R., Gelan, J., Sebald, A., Lelieveld, P., de Vos, D. & Gielen, M. (1990): Synthesis, characterization and *in vitro* antitumor activity of a series of substituted 2,2-di-n-butyl-4-oxo-benzo-1,3,2-dioxastannins, *Appl. Organomet. Chem.* **4** : 335-343

Bouâlam, M., Gielen, M., Meriem, A., de Vos, D. & Willem, R. (Pharmachemie B.V.) (1990): Anti-tumor compositions and compounds, *Eur. Pat.* 90202316.7-, 21/09/90

Bouâlam, M., Willem, R., Biesemans, M., Mahieu, B., Meunier-Piret, J. & Gielen, M. (1991): Synthesis, characterization and *in vitro* antitumor activity of diorganotin derivatives of substituted salicylic acids and analogs. Crystal structure of bis(5-methoxysalicylato-di-n-butyltin) oxide, *Main Group Met. Chem.* **14** : 41-56

Bouâlam, M., Gielen, M., El Khloufi, A., de Vos, D. & Willem, R. (Pharmachemie B.V.) (1991): Novel organotin compounds having anti-tumour activity and anti-tumour compositions, Eur. Pat. 91202746.3-, 22/10/91

Gielen, M. & Willem, R. (1992): Cytotoxic Activity of Bis-[di-n-butyl(4-aminosalicylato)tin] oxide, NSC: 628561, Bis-[diphenyl(4-aminosalicylato)tin] oxide, NSC: 628562, and some related compounds, against a series of human tumor cell lines, *Anticancer Res.*, in press

Gielen, M., Lelieveld, P., de Vos, D. & Willem, R. (1992): *In vitro* antitumor activity of organotin compounds, in "Metal-Based Antitumor Drugs", M. Gielen, Ed., Freund Publ. House, Tel Aviv, Israel, in press

Narayanan, V.L. (1983): Strategy for the discovery and development of novel anticancer agents, in "Structure-activity relationships of antitumor agents", ed. Reinhoudt, D.T., Connors, T.A., Pinedo, H.M. & van de Poll, K.W., Martinus Nijhoff, pp.16-33

Metal Ions in Biology and Medicine, vol. 2. Eds. J. Anastassopoulou, Ph. Collery, J.C. Etienne, Th. Theophanides. John Libbey Eurotext, Paris © 1992, pp. 192-193

In vitro cytotoxic activity of some di- and triorganotin oxinates and thio-oxinates against a panel of sixty human tumor cell lines

M. Gielen*, R. Willem**, J. Holecek***, A. Lycka****

*Free University of Brussels VUB, * Department of General and Organic Chemistry of the Faculty of Engineering and ** High Resolution NMR Centre, Room 8G512, Pleinlaan 2, B-1050 Brussels, Belgium. ***Institute of Chemical Technology, 53210 Pardubice, Czechoslovakia. ****Research Institute of Organic Syntheses, 53218 Pardubice-Rybitví, Czechoslovakia*

Organotin(IV) compounds generally display a lower antitumour activity than the platinum-based antitumour drugs when tested against murine P388 or L1210 leukemiae (Crowe; Meinema **et al**.). However, several series of organotin(IV) compounds were recently found to be more active *in vitro* than cis-platin (Bouâlam **et al**.; Ross **et al**.)against the human cell lines of the A 204 rhabdomyosarcoma, MCF-7 mammary carcinoma, T24 bladder carcinoma, WiDr colon carcinoma and IgR-37 melanoma. Accordingly a series of di- and triorganotin oxinates and thio-oxinates were tested by the National Cancer Institute against the human tumour cell lines of the extensive panel (Gielen & Willem) recognized nowadays to be relevant in an anti-cancer prescreening strategy.

The compounds examined have the following general structures (Ross **et al**.):

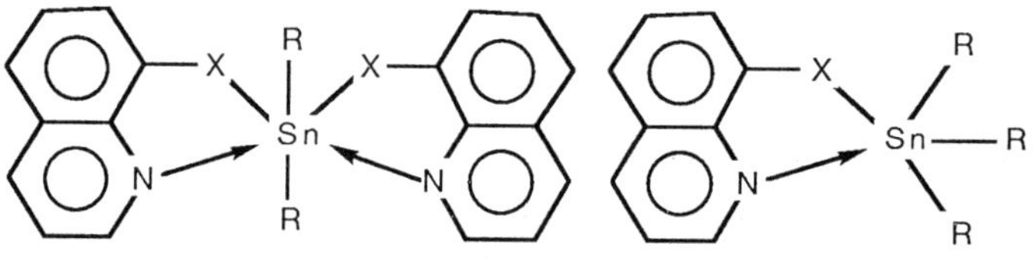

R = CH=CH$_2$, X = O, NSC 628593, **1**

R = CH=CH$_2$, X = S, NSC 628594, **2**

R = (CH$_2$)$_3$CH$_3$, X = O, NSC 628587, **3**

R = (CH$_2$)$_3$CH$_3$, X = S, NSC 628588, **4**

R = C$_6$H$_5$, X = O, NSC 628591, **5**

R = C$_6$H$_5$, X = S, NSC 628592, **6**

R = C$_6$H$_5$CH$_2$, X = O, NSC 628589, **7**

R = C$_6$H$_5$CH$_2$, X = S, NSC 628590, **8**

R = C$_6$H$_5$, X = O, NSC 628585, **9**

R = C$_6$H$_5$, X = S, NSC 628586, **10**

The National Cancer Institute decided to refer compound **1** to the Biological Evaluation Committee because two of its D_{GI50}, D_{TGI} and D_{L50} values were larger than 50, and the D_H and MGD_H values were greater than 90. Compound **3** scores comparably but no pending action was decided by NCI.

Compounds **2**, **5**, **6** and **8** exhibit no subpanel sensitivity because they are characterized by D_{GI50}, D_{TGI} and D_{LC50} values generally lower than 50. Compound **9** also scores very poorly, and compounds **4**, **7** and **10** are hardly better.

Clearly, only the divinyltin and, to a smaller extent, the di-n-butyltin oxinates, are active. The tin-sulfur bond might have too strong a covalent character to allow the thiooxinates to exhibit sufficient activity but this is obviously not the only determinant factor.

The triphenyltin compounds are not that promising, in agreement with earlier *in vivo* and *in vitro* observations (Crowe; Meinema **et al**.).

These data suggest that diorganotin compounds might be reasonable candidates as active antitumour drugs. More research in this promising field is however needed to get a better insight into structure-activity relationships.

REFERENCES

Atassi, G. (1985): Antitumor and Toxic Effects of Silicon, Germanium, Tin and Lead Compounds, *Rev. Si, Ge, Sn & Pb Cpds.* **8**: 219-235

Bouâlam, M., Gielen, M., Meriem, A., de Vos, D. & Willem, R. (Pharmachemie B.V.) (1990): Anti-tumor compositions and compounds, *Eur. Pat.* 90202316.7-, 21/09/90

Crowe, A.J. (1988): The Antitumor Activity of Tin Compounds. In: Metal-Based Antitumor Drugs (Gielen, M.F., ed.), Freund Publ. House, London, pp. 103-149

Gielen, M., Willem, R. (1992), Cytotoxic activity of bis-[di-n-butyl(4-aminosalicylato)tin] oxide, NSC: 628561, bis-[diphenyl(4-aminosalicylato)tin] oxide, NSC: 628562, and some related compounds, against a series of human tumor cell lines, *Appl. Organomet. Chem.*, in press

Meinema, H.A., Liebregts, A.M., Budding, H.A. & Bulten, E.J. (1985): Synthesis and Evaluation of Organometal-Based Anti-tumor Agents of Germanium and Tin, *Rev Si, Ge, Sn & Pb Cpds.* **8**: 157-168

Ross, M., Gielen, M., Lelieveld, P. & de Vos, D. (1992): Cytotoxic Activity of Di-n-butyltin(IV)(X-A-B-X) Compounds Related to Salicylic Acid against Human Tumour Cells. *Anticancer Res.* **11**: 1089-1091

Metal Ions in Biology and Medicine, vol. 2. Eds. J. Anastassopoulou, Ph. Collery, J.C. Etienne, Th. Theophanides. John Libbey Eurotext, Paris © 1992, p. 194

Inorganic Tin (IV) dithiocarbamates as cytostatic agents

C. Preti*, M. Tagliazucchi*, A. Furlani**, A. Papaioannou**, V. Scarcia**, V. Cherchi***[(1)], L. Sindellari***

** Departement of Chemistry, University of Modena, Italy. ** Institute of Pharmacology and Pharmacognosy, University of Trieste, Italy. *** Departement of Inorganic, Metallorganic and Analytical Chemisty, University of Padova, Italy. [(1)]Boehringer-Mannheim SpAgrant*

Recently we reported on Tin(II) and Tin(IV) dithiocarbamate complexes that have been studied for their cytostatic activity against two tumoral cell lines, an epidermoid human carcinoma (KB) and murine leukemia(L 1210)[1,2].
The very high *in vitro* cytostatic effect displayed by some Tin(IV) inorganic derivatives prompted us to explore the *in vitro* antiproliferative effect of new series of inorganic Tin(IV) compounds with alkyl, cycloalkyl and heterocyclic dithiocarbamates.
The present note deals with synthesis, characterization and cytostatic activity tests of new Tin(IV) dithiocarbamate complexes (L), of formula SnL_4, SnL_2Cl_2 ed SnL_3Cl. The compounds were studied in comparison with alkyl, cycloalkyldithiocarbamate analogs and heterocyclic, in an attempt to correlate chemical structure and biological activity.
Almost all compounds showed very pronounced antiproliferative activity against both cell lines,although the leukemic cells appeared to be in general more responsive than the KB cell line. For many Tin derivatives the IC_{50}[(a)] values were similar or often lower than those displayed by cisplatin, determined by us under the same experimental conditions (0.37 μM and 0.56 μM against KB and L1210 cells respectively).
The substituents at the nitrogen seem to influence the cytostatic effect. Moreover the properties of the complexes depend strongly on the stoichiometry of the compounds.
Further *in vivo* assays against some tumour systems will be carried out on the most *in vitro* active complexes.

(a) Concentration inducing 50% cell growth inhibition

1. V.Scarcia, A.Furlani, A.Papaioannou, C.Preti, G.Fracasso, D.Marton and L. Sindellari, in: "Metal ions in Biology and Medicine; P.Collery, L.A. Poirer, M.Mainfait, J.C. Etienne edts. John Libbey Eurotext, Paris 1990.

Metal Ions in Biology and Medicine, vol. 2. Eds. J. Anastassopoulou, Ph. Collery, J.C. Etienne, Th. Theophanides. John Libbey Eurotext, Paris © 1992, pp. 195-196

Novel structural features of tetrakis (μ-carboxylato) dirhodium (II), an antitumor agent, bound to azathioprine, a biologically active mercaptopurine derivative

H.T. Chifotides*, K.R. Dunbar*, J.H. Matonic*, N. Katsaros**

* *Department of Chemistry, Michigan State University, E. Lansing, MI 48824, USA.*
** *NRCS « Demokritos », 15310 Ag. Paraskevi Attikis, Greece*

There is considerable interest in interactions of tetrakis (μ-carboxylato) dirhodium (II) complexes with nucleic acid bases because they function as antitumor agents against many types of tumors by inhibiting DNA and protein synthesis. These complexes react with adenosine and polyadenosine nucleotides, single stranded DNA, sulphur containing amino acids and proteins, but they do not react with polyguanylic or polycytidylic acid. Azathioprine (6-[1-methyl-4-nitroimidazol-5-yl) thio] purine, AZA) is an immunosuppressively and cytostatically active, yet masked, prodrug of 6-mercaptopurine (6-MP), which is used as an established clinical agent for the therapy of human leukemias (Van Scoik *et al.*, 1985). In AZA, the sulphydryl group of 6-MP is substituted with the nitroimidazolyl group in order to avoid in vivo methylation of the -SH group, alter the metabolism of the drug and improve the targeting of 6-MP toward tumor cells by preferentially liberating the thiopurine in the tumor. The cytostatic activity of these antimetabolites is attributed to: (a) feedback inhibition of the first enzyme in de novo ribonucleotide synthesis, (b) inhibition of purine ribonucleotide interconversion, (c) incorporation into DNA after intracellular conversion to 6-thioguanine (Van Scoik *et al.*, 1985). Besides, it has been found that certain metal complexes of 6-MP show enhanced antitumor activity with respect to the free ligand (Kirschner *et al.*,1966).

Crystal structures of biologically active ligands with metals are important for the understanding of factors affecting metal transport, issues that are related to the design of new metal-mediated repository, slow release or long acting drugs. The considerable biological activity of AZA combined with the electronically and stereochemically versatile binding sites of AZA led us to investigate the chemistry of AZA with dirhodium tetraacetate. The X-ray crystallographic study of the bis-adduct $[Rh_2(OAc)_4(AZA)_2] \cdot 4$ DMAA (**1**) was undertaken (Fig. 1) in order to elucidate the stereochemistry of the different interactions and understand the factors affecting metal transport and potentiation of DNA-binding drugs by metals. Unlike the few known purines which bind to the dirhodium tetraacetate through the imidazole ring N(7) or N(9) sites (Rubin *et al.*, 1991), AZA coordinates to the axial positions of the dirhodium tetraacetate cage through the purine N(3), while (**1**) resides on a crystallographic center of inversion at the midpoint of the Rh-Rh bond. The structure is further stabilized by hydrogen bonding between the N(9)-H atom of the imidazole ring with the acetate O(2), as is evidenced by the N(9)-O(2) distance of 3.00 Å. This hydrogen bonding resembles that formed between rhodium carboxylate oxygens and the exocyclic N(6) group of N(7) bound 1-methyladenosine (Rubin *et al.*, 1991) and polyadenylic acid bases. Presumably, steric constraint imposed by the octahedral environment about the rhodium atom together with the bulk of the imidazole ring on S(1) of the mercaptopurine inhibits N(7) binding. For the same steric reasons rhodium carboxylates do not react with polycytidylic acid in which N(3), the preferable binding site for other metals, is flanked by the bulky carbonyl

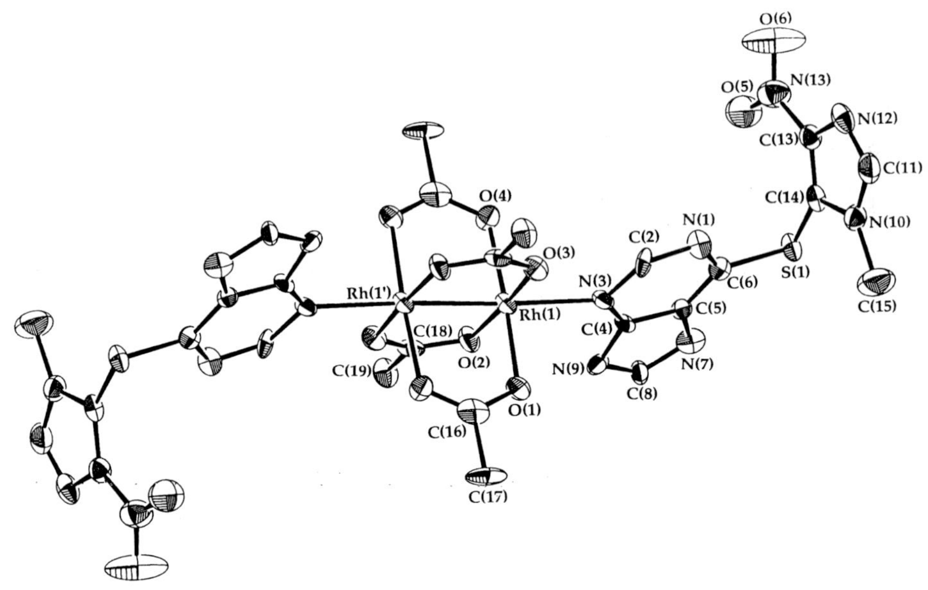

Fig. 1. ORTEP representation of the bis-adduct $[Rh_2(OAc)_4(AZA)_2] \cdot 4DMAA$ (**1**) with 50 % probability elipsoids.

O(2) group which itself cannot hydrogen bond to the acetates (Aoki &Yamazaki, 1984). From a biological point of view, preliminary tests of (**1**) on different tumor cell lines (L1210 and Sarcoma 180) show positive antitumor activity and need to be further investigated.

To sum up, the similarities of our unusual structure with the known rhodium tetraacetate complexes of nucleotides, imply the fact that for an octahedral complex to have antitumor activity not only the electronegativity of the various binding sites of the ligand play a major role, but stereospecific interligand interactions as well. These selective binding properties of the rhodium complexes are promising as a useful tool in understanding the mechanism of action of various chemotherapeutic agents.

REFERENCES

Aoki, K. and Yamazaki, H. (1984): Stereospecific interactions between tetrakis (μ-carboxylato) dirhodium (II) antitumor agents and nucleic acid bases. Crystal structure of $[Rh_2(acetato)_4.(AAMP)]_n$ (AAMP = 4-amino-5-aminomethyl)-2-methylpyrimidine). *J. Am. Chem. Soc.*, 106, 3691.

Kirschner, S.; Wei, Y. K.; Francis, D. and Bergman, J. G. (1966): Anticancer and potential antiviral activity of complex inorganic compounds. *J. Med. Chem.* 9, 369.

Rubin, J. R.; Haromy, T. P. and Sundaralingam M. (1991): Structure of the anticancer drug complex tetrakis (μ-acetato)-bis (1-methyladenosine) dirhodium (II) monohydrate. *Acta Cryst.*, C47, 1712.

Van Scoik, K.; Johnson, C. A. and Porter, W. R. (1985): The pharmacology and metabolism of the thiopurine drugs 6-mercaptopurine and azathioprine. *Drug Metabolism Reviews*, 16, 157.

Metal Ions in Biology and Medicine, vol. 2. Eds. J. Anastassopoulou, Ph. Collery, J.C. Etienne, Th. Theophanides. John Libbey Eurotext, Paris © 1992, pp. 197-198

Alpha-methyl glucose uptake : a sensitive and specific markor of platine induced damage on LLC-PK$_1$ cells

Isabelle Dupin, Joël Poupon, Laurent Benel, Philippe Chappuis, François Rousselet

Laboratoire de Biochimie Métabolique et Clinique-Faculté des Sciences Pharmaceutiques et Biologiques - Paris V, 4, avenue de l'Observatoire, 75270 Paris Cedex 06, France

The lack of sensitive markors of cellular impairment constitutes a serious drawback for in vitro studies, which often use cell viabilities as assessed by the neutral red uptake method.

We adapted to LLC-PK$_1$ cells treated with a nephrotoxic compound, cisplatin (CDDP), a technique developped by BOOGARD et al (1989), the α Methyl-Glucose (αMG) uptake and used, for comparison, the neutral red uptake technique. Another comparison between these 2 techniques was also assessed using a cotreatment including CDDP and a compound suspected to act as a chemoprotector of CDDP toxicity, selenomethionine (SeMet).

MATERIAL AND METHODS

LLC-PK$_1$ cells were grown in MEM supplemented with 10 % (v/v) fetal calf serum, until they reached optical confluence (3 days). One day after, a subsequent treatment with CDDP alone or CDDP + SeMet was achieved during 24 hours. The αMG transport was determined by the rate of incorporation of α [^{14}C]MG. The final medium displayed an activity of 0,05 μCi/ml and was not supplemented with glucose, fetal calf serum nor antibiotics. After 2 hours incubation, the radioactivity was determined by liquid scintillation counting. Results were calculated per mg protein and expressed as percentage of control dishes (non treated cells).The cell viabilities were assessed by the neutral red uptake method adapted from BORENFREUND and PUERNER (1984).

RESULTS

- The αMG uptake progressively increased until day 7, together with the renal brush border membrane enzymes such as γ glutamyl transpeptidase (GGT) and alkaline phosphatase (PAL) (Fig. 1).

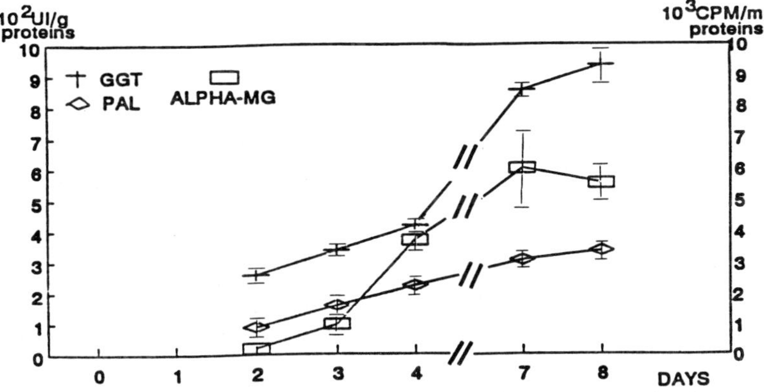

Fig. 1 : GGT and PAL activities and αMG uptake according to the days of culture.

- CDDP toxicity : unlike the viabilities, the decrease of αMG was regular and already noticeable for low CDDP levels (ie, at 8 μM CDDP, no alteration of the viability against a 30 % decrease of αMG uptake, see Fig. 2).

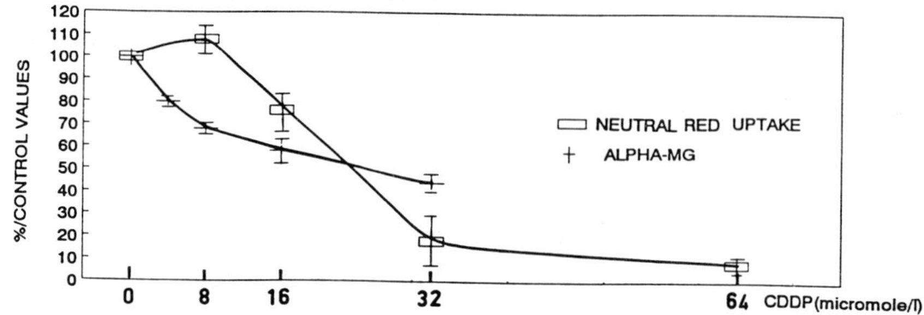

Fig. 2 : αMG uptake and viabilities assessed by the Neutral Red uptake technique as a function of CDDP concentrations.

The results obtained with the combination CDDP + SeMet (Fig. 3) kept well with those mentionned above : the αMG uptake decrease was clearly related to CDDP concentrations whereas viabilities, at first, remained unchanged then dropped for CDDP values above 16 μM (lag-phase phenomenon).

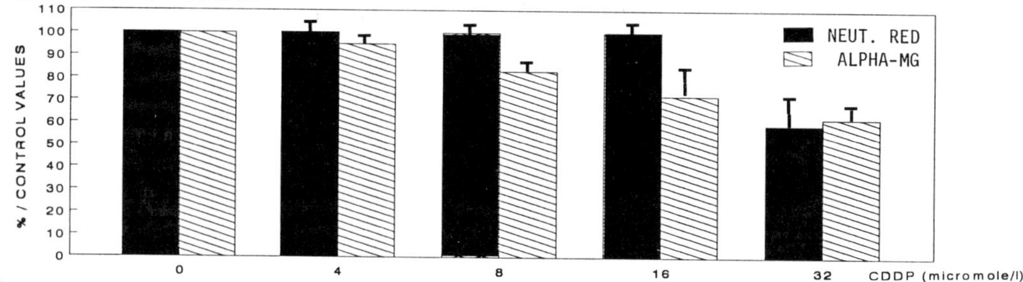

Fig. 3 : Comparison of viabilities and αMG uptake according to CDDP in presence of 10^{-4}M SeMet.

DISCUSSION

The concomittant increase of αMG transport together with the renal brush border enzymes (Fig. 1) reflects an important function of the tubular cell that is its capacity for transport of an analog of glucose, αMG. Moreover, a sensible and specific inhibitor of the brush border glucose carrier, the phloridzine, impedes almost completely this transport (data not shown).

Both Fig. 2 and 3 are the reflect of a similar evolution : concentration dependant effect for αMG uptake against an unchanged effect followed by a marked drop for viabilities. The consequence of this, is that using the viability criteria alone could lead to partially incomplete data. Indeed, the protective effect of SeMet on CDDP toxicity, which is clear using the viability criteria is somewhat lessened using the αMG uptake criteria.

CONCLUSION

The difference of these 2 techniques may be explained by the fact that a slight modification of glucose uptake by the cell does not disturb the cell viability, thus reflecting an early impairment of cell functions. Therefore, αMG uptake constitutes for LLC-PK_1 cells a sensible and specific markor which could be applied to study the cytotoxicity of low levels of heavy metals, such as platinum compounds.

BIBLIOGRAPHY

- Boogard, P.J., Mulder, G.J., Nagelkerke, J.F. (1989) : Isolated proximal tubular cells from rat kidney as an in vitro model for studies on nephrotoxicity. Toxicol. Appl. Pharmacol. 101 : I, 135-143.
- Borenfreund, E., Puerner, J.A. (1984) : Toxicity determined in vitro by morphological alterations and neutral red absorption. J. of Tissue Cult. Meth. 9 : 7-9.

Metal Ions in Biology and Medicine, vol. 2. Eds. J. Anastassopoulou, Ph. Collery, J.C. Etienne, Th. Theophanides. John Libbey Eurotext, Paris © 1992, pp. 199-200

Development of In-111 labeled activated carbon microspheres and analysis of mammary lymph flow by double isotope method

Takakazu Kawanishi, Yoshiaki Karaki, Masatoshi Maeda*, Toshio Saeki, Masao Fujimaki, Hikaru Seto**, Takashi Honda*

*Second Department of Surgery, * Radioisotope Laboratory, ** Department of Radiological Science, Toyama Medical and Pharmaceutical University, 2630 Sugitani, Toyama, Japan*

The establishment of an empirical method of the mammary lymph nodes in which mammary lymph flow analysis is considered may simplify future breast cancer surgery. As volume and direction of flow in the mammary lymph tract cannot be presumed only on the basis of anatomical manifestations, and as no radiopharmaceutical which was macroscopically visible as well as usefull in analysis of both lymph flow and lymphoscintigraphy was available, we previously developed Tc-99m labeled activated carbon microspheres(^{99m}Tc-CH44), which have affinity for lymph and can be macroscopically identified, and have been confirmed to be useful in quantitative analysis of mammary lymph flow in patients with breast tumors(Maeda et al., 1988; Saeki et al., 1990).

We have developed In-111 labeled activated carbon microspheres(^{111}In-CH44)for use in analysis of mammary lymph flow by double isotope method (Katayama et al., 1985; Nishimura et al., 1990). ^{111}In-CH44 was made by the NaI complex method(Fig. 1). The labeling rate immediately after preparation was more than 99% at pH11 and 37℃, and stability was maintained for 24hr under continuous shaking. The rate of release In-111 from ^{111}In-CH44 was found to be 23% at 6hr in a simulation model. The result of analysis of lymph flow in 19 rats and of popliteal lymphoscintigraphy in rabbits suggested that ^{111}In-CH44 is useful in mammary lymphoscintigraphy and the detail analysis of mammary lymph flow. When 1mℓ(0.3mCi, 11.1MBq) of ^{111}In-CH44 was injected into the mammary glands of 2 patients with breast tumors, the axillary and parasternal lymph nodes were visualized clearly(Fig. 2). In 8 patients with breast cancer studied by the double isotope method, 1mℓ(0.3mCi, 11.1 MBq)of ^{111}In-CH44 was injected before operation into the outer side of the mammary gland, and 1mℓ(2.0mCi, 74MBq)of ^{99m}Tc-CH44 into the inner side, and radioactivity of each isotope in surgically dissdissected lymph nodes was counted. In 3 patients with parasternal lymph nodes dissection, percent uptake by total dissected nodes of ^{111}In-CH44 was about 0.42% and that of ^{99m}Tc-CH44 was 0.06%. Mean distribution of radioactivity of, respectively, ^{111}In-CH44 and ^{99m}Tc-CH44 in each regionallymph node group was as follows: brachial and subscapular, 2.3% and 0.5%; central, pectoral and subpectoral 81.4% and 74.1%; interpectoral 0% and 1.8%; infraclavicular 1.9% and 5.7%; highest infraclavicular 0.4% and 0%; and parasternal 16.3%and 19.1%(Fig. 3). Thus mammary lymph flow in the same

$^{111}InCl_3$ 2mCi ┐
(74MBq) │ stir + 5% activated carbon microspheres(CH44)
NaI 5mg ┘ ↓

pH adjustment by 1/10N NaOH

Fig. 1. Preparation of ^{111}In-CH44 by NaI complex method

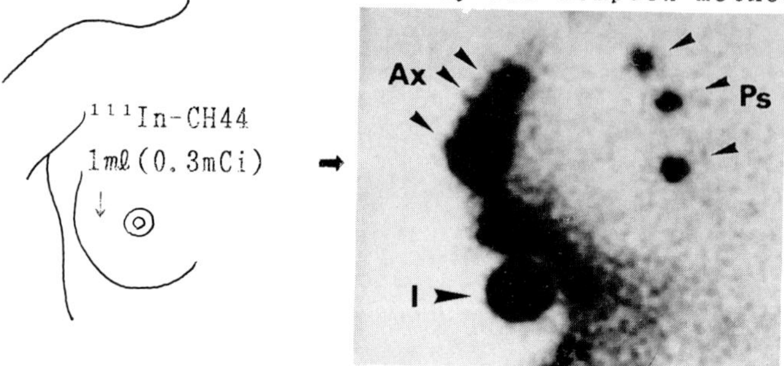

I :injected site
Ps:parasternal LN
Ax:axillar LN

Fig. 2. Lymphoscintigraphy using ^{111}In-CH44

	uptake by total dissected nodes (%)	mean distribution of radioactivity(%)						
		regional lymph nodes						
		1a	1b	1c	2	2h	3	total
^{111}In(outer)	0.42	2.3	81.4	0.0	1.9	0.4	16.3	100
^{99m}Tc(inner)	0.06	0.5	74.1	1.8	5.7	0.0	19.1	100

Fig. 3. Analysis of mammary lymph flow by double isotope method in 3 patients breast cancer undergone extended radical mastectomy (regional lymph nodes:1a brachial 1b central,pectoral and subpectoral 1c interpectoral 2 infraclavicular 2h highest infraclavicular 3 parasternal)

patient can be evaluated using two isotopes at the same time.

These results suggest that double isotope method using ^{111}In-CH44 and ^{99m}Tc-CH44 is useful in the detailed analysis of mammary lymph flow.

REFERENCES

Maeda,M.,Saeki,T.,Karaki,Y.,et al.(1988):Study of mammary lymph node scintigraphy by Tc-99m labeled activated carbon microspheres.The Japanese Jounal of Nuclear Medicine 25:809-810.

Saeki,T.,Karaki,Y.,Fujimaki,M.,et al.(1990):Dvelopment of Tc-99m labeled activated carbon microspheres and clinical application.Jounal of Japan Surgical Society 91:729-740.

Katayama,K.,Yonemura,Y.,Hashimoto,T.,et al.(1985):Studies of Gastoric lymphatics using double isotope method.The Japanese Jounal of Gastroenterological Surgery 18:1750.

Nishimura,G.,Yamaguchi,A.,Ishida,T.,et al.(1990):Lymphatic drainage from the rectum as demonstrated by double isotope method.The Jounal of the Japan Society of the colo-proctology 43:153-158.

4 NEPHROLOGY CARDIOLOGY HYPERTENSION

Metal Ions in Biology and Medicine, vol. 2. Eds. J. Anastassopoulou, Ph. Collery, J.C. Etienne, Th. Theophanides. John Libbey Eurotext, Paris © 1992, pp. 203-208

Intracellular magnesium in cardiovascular disease

Abraham S. Abraham

Department of Medicine B, Shaare Zedek Medical Center, Jerusalem, Israel

ACUTE MYOCARDIAL INFARCTION

Each year, 1,500,000 persons have an acute myocardial infarction (AMI) in the United States, and some 550,000 die of ischemic heart disease (Levy, 1984). Some 60-65 per cent of all deaths from coronary artery disease are sudden and occur outside hospital (Braunwald, 1980). Of those patients who survive to be admitted to hospital, some 15-20 per cent will succumb there (Abraham **et al.**, 1980). The major cause of these early deaths is ventricular fibrillation (VF).

Physiology

Magnesium (Mg) is second only to potassium (K) as the most plentiful intracellular cation. The constant activity of Na+K+ ATPase, an enzyme located in the myocardial cell membrane and dependent on Mg as a co-factor for its function (Skou **et al.**, 1971) is responsible for keeping the inside of the cell electrically negative with respect to the outside. A fall in intracellular Mg will result in a fall in the activity of the enzyme with a consequent decrease in the intracellular K concentration. (Solomon, 1986).

Hirche **et al.** (1980) monitored the rate of increase of extracellular K in ventricular muscle made ischemic by coronary artery ligation and found that extracellular K started to increase about 10 seconds after occlusion. Kraft **et al.** (1980) have shown that ventricular muscle cells exposed to a high K medium show a reduction of negative resting potential and of action potential amplitude. The addition of Mg to the medium produced an attenuation of these effects.

Thus, within minutes after coronary occlusion, there is a marked alteration in electrophysiological properties of ventricular myocardial cells with shortening of action potential and decrease in amplitude, upstroke velocity and resting potential (Downar **et al.**,1977). The reduction in the K gradient across the cell must result in membrane depolarization, an increase in automaticity and an increased arrhythmogenicity. The stage is set for ventricular tachycardia (VT) or VF.

Watanabe and Dreifus (1972) demonstrated that an increase in extracellular Mg increased the negative resting membrane potential, action potential amplitude, maximal rate of depolarization and action potential duration of ventricular fibres. These effects of a high Mg concentration were prominent even at K concentrations that were sufficiently high to decrease these parameters. We have shown (Abraham **et al.**, 1986), in a study of 215 patients with acute myocardial infarction, that mononuclear cell K increased nearly twice as much in patients with ventricular tachyarrythmias when compared to patients without such arrhythmias. Mononuclear cell Mg also increased, and those patients in whom high levels were found had a significant decrease in the rate of ventricular tachyarrhythmias. We suggested that mononuclear cell K and Mg levels mirror myocardial interstitial (or extracellular) levels of these cations and that a high interstitial Mg level has a protective effect on the increased excitability of the ischemic nyyocardial cell due to, and in spite of, a high interstitial K level. One possible explanation is that the accumulation of Mg ions in the extracellular space may, by virtue of their ability to restrict K efflux, neutralize the electrochemical changes which such efflux would produce (Shine and Douglas, 1974). This would therefore either delay or completely prevent the fatal arrhythmias that often follow the acute coronary occlusion.

Woods and Chapman (1984) have shown that raising the extracellular Mg concentration from 0.85 to 3.4 mmol/l reduced the rate of spontaneous depolarisation of hypoxic canine tissue and returned the resting muscle potential to normal. The threshold for electrically induced VT or VF increased when normal and digitalized dogs were treated with Mg (Ghani and Rafah, 1977).

Studies on the use of intravenous magnesium in patients with AMI.

Malkiel-Shapiro (1958) was the first to use parenteral MgSO4 in AMI in an open trial claiming a mortality of 1.6 per cent in 64 patients up to 4-6 weeks following the infarct. However it is only in the last decade that a number of controlled trials have been published on the use of parenteral Mg in patients with AMI. Summarising the 7 placebo-controlled trials that have so far been published (Morton **et al.**, 1985; Smith **et al.**, 1986; Rasmussen **et al.**, 1986; Abraham **et al.**, 1987; Feldstedt **et al.**, 1988; Ceremuzynski, 1989; Shechter **et al.**, 1990), 657 patients with AMI received IV Mg and 648 placebo. The placebo group had more arrhythmias (34 per cent versus 18 per cent and a higher mortality - 3.8 per cent versus 8.0 per cent, $p < 0.005$) (Teo **et al.**, 1990; Editorial, 1991).

In a series of 276 consecutive patients with AMI, 250 (mean age 67 years) were treated with a continuous infusion of MgSO4 over 24 hours - 10 mmol (elemental Mg) in the first 30 minutes, then 12 mmol every 8 hours, with a mean increase in serum Mg from 0.82 to 1.15 mmol/l. Nine patients were excluded because of advanced AV block, 11 because of a systolic blood pressure on admission of 100 mm Hg or less, and in 6 the Mg infusion had to be discontinued because of the development of transient hypotension. No patient had sustained VT with hemodynamic instability requiring electrical defibrillation. The total in-hospital mortality (mean of 12 days) was 3.6 per cent amongst these 250 patients and 5.4 per cent for all the 276 patients (Abraham **et al.**, 1990a).

How does magnesium prevent arrhythmias after AMI.

Most studeis have shown no correlation between the level of serum Mg and the frequency of arrhythmias in patients with AMI (Rasmussen, 1988). A fall in serum Mg levels has been demonstrated not only in patients with AMI, but also in normal labor and in patients with acute medical and surgical disease (Abraham **et al.**, 1980). Also, although there is a fall in serum Mg levels immediately following an AMI, the levels nevertheless remain within the normal range (Abraham **et al.**, 1977). It is probable that the antiarrhythmogenic effect of IV Mg is due to a direct pharmacological effect and not due to a correction of the fall in serum Mg.

How does Mg reduce early mortality following AMI?

We have shown that, in the presence of an increased mononuclear cell K, the presence of a high mononuclear cell Mg is associated with a statistically significant lower mortality than when intracellular Mg levels were not increased, and the ratio of the maximum rise in intr1acellular K to the maximum rise in intracellular Mg is a good predictor of in-hospital mortality following AMI ($p<0.007$) (Abraham **et al.**, 1988a).

The most likely mechanism by which the administration of intravenous Mg reduces early mortality after AMI is by a reduction in infarct size. Experimentally, Chang **et al.** (1985) have shown that dogs fed a Mg deficient diet developed larger infarcts than did control animals. There is a loss of Mg from the myocardium following experimentally induced myocardial acute necrosis (Abraham **et al.**, 1981). A reduction in infarct size in patients with AMI has also been shown (Morton **et al.**, 1985). We have recently presented preliminary results from an as yet ongoing study in which patients with acute myocardial infarction have been randomized into two primary treatment groups to receive either IV Mg or IV Propranolol on admission (Abraham **et al.**, 1990). So far 59 patients have been studied, half in each group. The maximum enzyme (CPK, GOT, LDH) rise was significantly lower in the group receiving Mg. Secondly, using a QRS scoring system (Wagner **et al.**, 1982), we found that patients in the Mg group had a lower electrocardiographic score at one month than those that received Propranolol. Both these preliminary findings tend to confirm that there is indeed a reduction in infarct size in patients who receive IV Mg. The reduction in infarct size will result in a reduction in the incidence of congestive heart failure and cardiogenic shock with less likelihood of intractable arrhythmias, all important causes of early death after AMI.

Yet another mechanism by which infarct size may be reduced is by vasodilation of spastic coronary arteries surrounding the infarct site (Turlapaty and Altuna, 1980) and the administration of Mg to patients with acute coronary spasm has been shown to lead to a resolution of the resultant electrocardiographic changes (Chadda 1986). These mechanisms have recently been reviewed by Altura (1988).

Finally, it has been shown that Mg inhibits platelet aggregation in vitro (Hughes and Tonks, 1965), severely reduces the extent of platelet attachment to exposed subendothelial tissue (Kurgan **et al.**, 1980) and prevents thrombosis during microvascular surgery (Ackland, 1972).

Side effects

The main side effect of intravenous Mg infusion is a feeling of flushing when patients are given an initial bolus dose (Abraham **et al.**, 1987). In most of these, reduction of the rate of infusion results in a return of the blood pressure to normal. The use of this treatment has proven to be safe (Rasmussen **et al.**, 1986; Abraham **et al.**, 1987; Shechter **et al.**, 1990) and no special monitoring is needed.

Conclusion

Intravenous Mg is a safe and inexpensive drug whose use has been shown to reduce the incidence of serious arrhythmias, infarct size and early mortality following acute myocardial infarction.

CONGESTIVE CARDIAC FAILURE

The corner stone of treatment for congestive heart failure or for mild to moderate hypertension has, for many years, been thiazide or loop diuretics with a Potassium supplement. The effect of these drugs in causing hypokalemia (in spite of supplementation with Potassium) is well known with its concomitant effects, the most serious of which is the development of ventricular arrhythmias (Harrington **et al.**, 1982).

The effect of these drugs on Magnesium are less widely known nor is the fact that the resultant hypomagnesemia is an important contributor to refactory Potassium depletion and to ventricular ectopic arrhythmias (Hollifield, 1984; Whang **at al.**, 1985).

In a study of 38 patients with mild to moderate hypertension, it has been shown that there is a good correlation between theazide therapy, hypokalemia and increased incidence of ventricular ectopic beats- (Hollifield, 1989).

Dyckner and Wester (1987) have also shown that there is a good correlation between duration of thiazide therapy and serum and skeletal muscle Potassium and Magnesium levels. In addition these workers have shown that intracellular potassium deficiency could not be corrected by an infusion of magnesium (Dyckner and Wester,1969).

The status of mononuclear cell Potassium and Magnesium levels in these patients has been less well studied.

A prospective, randomized study was carried out on 155 patients who were followed up for 6 months after acute myocardial infarction (Abraham **et al.**, 1986b). Of the 85 patients who were in congestive heart failure, 48 received Furoxemide with Potassium supplements amd 37 received a combination of Hydrochlorothiazide with Amiloride (Moduretic). The remaining 70 patients did not require diuretics and served as controls. At 6 months, serum levels were unchanged in all groups. Mononuclear cell K levels were 37.0 $\pm$ 0.8, 40.0 $\pm$ 1.6 fmol/cell in patients who did not receive diuretics or who received Moduretic, respectively, and 25.4 $\pm$ 1.4 fmol/cell ($p < 0.001$) in those who received Furosemide with Potassium. Mononuclear Mg levels were 5.0 $\pm$ 0.1, 4.7 $\pm$ 0.2 and 1.5 $\pm$ 0.2 fmol/cell, respectively ($p < 0.001$).

In a retrospective study (Abraham **et al.**, 1988c), 45 patients receiving diuretics for from 6-60 months were examined. Thirty one patients were being treated for congestive heart failure and 14 for hypertension without congestive failure. Of the 31 patients with congestive failure 9 received Furosemide alone, 12 Furosemide with Potassium supplementation and 10 received Moduretic. Of the 14 patients with hypertension, 6 received Chlorothiazide alone and 8 received Moduretic. Serum Potassium was significantly lower than controls (4.25$\pm$0.05 and 3.2$\pm$0.33 mmol/l respectively; $p<0.01$) in the patients receiving Chlorothiazide with no difference in the other groups. On the other hand, mononuclear cell Potassium was significantly lower in patients receiving either loop or thiazide diuretics than in either controls or patients receiving Moduretic.

In addition, the longer patients had received loop or thiazide diuretics the lower the potassium levels in their mononuclear cells ($r=0.558$; $p<0.001$). Mononuclear cell Magnesium levels also tended to be lower in these groups although the difference from controls or patients receiving Moduretic did not reach statistical significance.

The effects of an ACE inhibitor, Enalapril, were studied in 15 elderly patients (mean age 74, range 67-86 years) in severe refractory congestive heart failure (8 in New York Heart Association class IV, 6 in class III and 1 in class II)(Abraham **et al.**, 1988b). All were receiving optimal therapy with digitalis, diuretics and vasodilators and were either in a steady state for at least 1 week before entry into the trial or deteriorating. 10 patients received 5 mg and out 10 mg of Enalapril daily. During the 12 week follow-up period 1 patient died of intracerebral hemorrhage and 2 were lost to follow-up. There was a significant improvement in the functional capacity of the remaining patients with no significant change in serum creatinine or blood urea nitrogen or in the Potassium or Magnesium levels of mononuclear cells.

HYPERTENSION

Sixteen patients with a mean age of 68 years with mild to moderate hypertension were treated with either Diltiazem or Hydrochlorothiazide for 6 weeks followed by Enalapril for a further 6 weeks (Abraham **et al.**, 1991). A second group of 40 patients (mean age 71 years) were treated with either Hydrochlorothiazide or Enalapril for 12 weeks, the non-responders receiving both drugs for 8 weeks.

Treatment with Hydrochlorothiazide or Enalapril resulted in a lowering of both systolic and diastolic blood pressure, but diastolic pressure was lower in patients treated with Enalapril (89$\pm$2 and 82$\pm$2 mmHg respectively; $p<0.05$). Treatment with Diltiazem resulted in a fall in diastolic pressure only. Treatment with Hydrochlorothiazide resulted in a fall of 17 per cent in serum potassiun ($p<0.05$) which returned to normal when Enalapril was substituted. Hydrochlorothiazide also produced a 23 per cent fall in mononuclear cell sodium content ($p<0.01$) at 4 weeks with a further 15 per cent fall at 12 weeks ($p<0.05$). Mononuclear cell potassium and magnesium also fell at 12 weeks by 18 per cent and 16 per cent, respectively ($p<0.05$). All these effects were reversed when Enalapril was substituted. A similar pattern of events was seen with Diltiazem, again reversed with Enalapril. Finally, there was no relationship between changes in mononuclear cell sodium or other cation content and changes in blood pressure.

REFERENCES

Abraham, A.S., Eylath, U., Weinstein, M. & Czackes, E. (1977): Serum magnesium levels in patients with acute my ca di l in ar ti n. New Eng l. J. Med . 29 , 862-863.

Abraham A.S., Shaoul R., Shimonovitz S., Eylath U. & Weinstein M. (1980): Serum magnesium levels in acute medical and surgical conditions. Biochem. Med. 24, 21-26.

Abraham, A.S., Bar-On, E. & Eylath, U. (1981): Changes in the magnesium content of tissues following myocardial damage in rats. Med. Biol., 59, 99-102.

Abraham, A.S., Rosenmann, D., Meshulam, Z., Zion, M.M. & Eylath, U. (1986a): Serum, lymphocyte and erythrocyte potassium, magnesium and calcium concentrations and their relation to tachyarrhythmias in patients with acute myocardial infarction. Am. J. Med. 81, 983-988.

Abraham, A.S., Rosenmann, D., Meshulam, Z., Balkin, J., Zion, M.M. & Eylath, U. (1986b): Intracellular cations and diuretic therapy following acute myocardial infarction. Arch. Int. Med. 146, 1301-1303.

Abraham, A.S., Rosenmann, D., Kramer, M., Balkin, J., Zion M.M., Farbstein, H. & Eylath, U. (1987): Magnesium in the prevention of lethal arrhythmias in acute myocardial infarction. Arch. Int. Med. 147, 753-755.

Abraham, A.S., Rosenmann, D. & Zion, M.M. (1988a): Lymphocyte potassium and magnesium concentrations as prognostic factors after acute myocardial infarction. Cardiology 75, 194-199

Abraham, A.S., Balkin, J., Rosenmann, D., Brooks, B.A., Eylath, U. & Zion, M.M. (1988b): Effects of Enalapril on lymphocyte sodium, potassium, magnesium and calcium levels in patients with severe congestive heart failure. Cardiology 75, 338-343.

Abraham, A.S., Meshulam, Z., Rosenmann, D. & Eylath, U. (1988c): Influence of chronic diuretic therapy on serum, lymphocyte and erythrocyte Potassium, Magnesium and Calcium concentrations. Cardiology 75, 17-23.

Abraham, A.S., Balkin, J., Rosenmann, D., Eylath, U., & Zion, M.M. (1990a): Continuous intravenous infusion of magnesium sulfate after acute myocardial infarction. Mag. Trace Elements 9, 137-142.

Abraham, A.S., Rosenmann, D., Balkin, J., Ilan, M., Shaheen, J. & Zion, M.M. (1990b): IV magnesium or propranolol in acute myocardial infarction. Preliminary report of a randomized trial. Mag. Res. 3,71.
Abraham, A.S., Brooks, B.A., Grafstein, Y., Barchilon, E., Nubani, N., Eylath, U. & Shemesh, D. (1991): Effects of Hydrochlorothiazide Diltiazem and Enalapril on mononuclear cell Sodium and Magnesium levels in systemic hypertension. Am. J. Cardiol. 68, 1357-1361.
Acland, R. (1972): Prevention of thrombosis in microvascular surgery by use of magnesium sulphate. Br. J. Plast. Surg. 25, 292-299.
Altura, B.M. (1988): Ischemic heart disease and magnesium. Magnesium 7,57-67.
Braunwald, E. (1980): Heart disease. A textbook of cardiovascular medicine, p. 778 (Saunders, Philadelphia).
Ceremuzynski, L., Jurgiel, R., Kulakowski, P. & Gebalska, J. (1989): Threatening arrythmias in acute myocardial infarction are prevented by intravenous magnesium sulfate. Am. Heart J. 118, 1333-1334.
Chadda, K.D. (1986): Clinical hypomagnesemia, coronary spasm and cardiac arrhythmias. Magnesium 5, 47-52.
Chang, C., Varghese, P.J., Downey, J. & Bloom, S. (1985): Magnesium deficiency and myocardial infarct size in the dog. J. Am. Coll. Cardiol. 5, 280-289.
Downar, E., Janse, M.J. & Durrer, D. (1977): The effect of acute coronary occlusion on subepicardial transmembrane potential in the intact porcine heart. Circulation 56, 217-224.
Dyckner, T. & Wester, P.O. (1969): Ventricular extrasystoles and intracellular electrolytes before and after Potassium and Magnesium imfusion in patients on diuretic treatment. Am. Heart. J. 97, 12-18.
Dyckner, T. & Wester, P.O. (1987): Plasma and skeletal muscle electrolytes in patients on long term diuretic therapy for arterial hypertension and/or congestive heart failure. Acta. Med. Scand. 222, 231-236.
Editorial (1991): Magnesium for acute myocardial infarction. Lancet 338, 667-668.
Feldstedt, M., Bochelouche, P. & Svenningsen, A. (1988): Failing effect of magnesium substitution in acute myocardial infarction. Eur. Heart J. 9, 226.
Ghani, M.B. & Rafah, M. (1977): Effects of magnesium chloride on electrical stability of the heart. Am. Heart J. 94, 600-602.
Harrington, J. T., Isner, J.M. & Kassirer, J.P. (1982): Our national obsession with Potassium. Am. J. Med. 73, 155-159.
Hirche, H.J., Franz, L., Bus, R., Bissing, R.L. & Schramm, M. (1980): Myocardial extracellular K+ and H+ increase and noradrenaline release as a possible cause of early arrhythmias following acute coronary occlusion in pigs. J. mol. cell. Cardiol. 12, 579-593.
Hollifield, J.W. (1984): Potassium and Magnesium abnormalities: diuretics and arrhythmias in hypertension. Am. J. Med. 77 (suppl.5A), 28-32.
Hollifield, J.W. (1989): Thiazide treatment of systemic hypertension. Effects on serum Magnesium and ventricular ectopic activity. Am. J. Cardiol. 63, 22G-25G.
Hughes, A. & Tonks, R.S. (1965): Platelets, magnesium and myocardial infarction. Lancet 1, 1044-1046.
Kurgan, A., Gertz, S.D., Wajnberg, R.S., Eldor, A., Jersky, J. & Nelson, E. (1980): Effect of magnesium sulfate on platelet deposition in rabbits following temporal artery occlusion with surgical clips. Surgery 87, 390-396.
Kraft, L.F., Katholi, R.E., Woods, W.T. & James, T.N. (1980): Attenuation by magnesiun of the electrophysiological effects of hyperkalemia on human and canine heart cells. Am. J. Cardiol. 45, 1189-1195.
Levy, R.L. (1984): The decline in coronary heart disease mortality. Status and perspectives on the role of cholesterol. Introduction. Am. J. Cardiol. 54,1c.
Malkiel-Shapiro, B. (1958): Further observations on parenteral magnesium sulphate therapy in coronary heart disease: a clinical appraisal. S. A. Med. J. 32, 1211-1215.
Morton, B.C., Nair, R.C., Smith, F.M., McKibbon, T.G. & Poznanski W.J. (1985): Magnesium therapy in acute myocardial infarction - a double blind study. Magnesium 3, 346-352.
Rasmussen, H.S., McNair, P., Norregard, P., Backer, S., Lindeneg, O. & Balslov, S. (1986): Magnesium infusion in acute myocardial infarction. Lancet 1, 234-236.
Rasmussen, H.S. (1988): Justification for intravenous magnesium therapy in acute myocardial infarction. Mag. Res. 1, 59-73.
Shechter, M., Hod, H., Marks, N. & Rabinowitz, B. (1990): Magnesium therapy and mortality in acute myocardial infarction. Am. J. Cardiol. 66, 271-274.
Shine, K.I. & Douglas, A.M. (1974): Magnesium effects on ionic exchange and mechanical function in rat ventricles. Am. J. Physiol. 222, 317-322.
Skou, J.C., Butler, K.W. & Hanson, O. (1971): Effect of nagnesium, ATP P1 and sodium on the inhibition of (Na+K)-activated enzyme system by g-strophanthidin. Biochimica et Biophysica Acta. 241, 443-461.
Smith, L.F., Heagerty, A.M., Bing, R.F. & Barnett, D.B. (1986): Intravenous infusion of magnesium sulphate after acute myocardial infarction: effects on arrhythmias and mortality. Int. J. Cardiol. 12, 175-180.
Solomon, R.G. (1986): Ventricular arrhythmias in patients with myocardial infarction and ischemia: the role

of serum potassium. Drugs 31 (suppl.4), 112-120.
Teo, K., Held, P., Collins, R. & Yusuf, S. (1990): Effect of intravenous magnesium on mortality in myocardial infarction. Circ. 82, III-393.
Turlapaty, P.D.M.V. & Altura, B.M. (1980): Magnesium deficiency produces spasms of coronary arteries: relation to etiology of sudden death ischemic heart disease. Science 208, 198-200.
Wagner, G.S., Freye, C.J., Palmeri, S.T., Roark, S.F.,Stack, N.C., Ideker, R.E., Harrel, F.E., & Selvester, R.H. (1982): Evaluation of a QRS scoring system for estimating myocardial infarct size. Circ. 65, 342-347.
Watanabe, Y. & Dreifus, L.S. (1972): Electrophysiological effects of potassium and its interactions with magnesium. Cardiovasc. Res. 6, 79-88.
Whang, R., Flink, E.B., Dyckner, T., Wester, P.O., Aikawa, J.K., & Ryan, M.P. (1985): Magnesium depletion as a cause of refractory Potassium repletion. Arch. Int. Med. 145, 1686-1689.
Woods, W.T.Jr. & Chapman, G.D. (1984): Preservation of resting potential by magnesium in hypoxic canine cardiac cells. Am. J. Cardiol. 53, 528-530.

Metal Ions in Biology and Medicine, vol. 2. Eds. J. Anastassopoulou, Ph. Collery, J.C. Etienne, Th. Theophanides. John Libbey Eurotext, Paris © 1992, pp. 209-214

Zinc deficiency : an ignored side effect of antihypertensive treatment

Theodore D. Mountokalakis

Third Department of Medicine, Medical School, Athens University, Sotiria General Hospital, CP 15696, 152 Mesogion avenue, Athens, Greece

In the last 20 years, the adverse side effects of drugs have assumed increasing importance in the management of hypertension. It is now apparent that metabolic side effects, such as hyperlipidemia, glucose intolerance, hypokalemia or hypomagnesemia, can upset the balance between the benefit and risks of treatment, in cases of mild elevations of the blood pressure. Recent observations suggest that zinc deficiency may represent a potential hazard additional to the known side effects of chronic antihypertensive treatment. Two groups of commonly used antihypertensive agents have been studied in this respect: diuretics and angiotensin converting enzyme inhibitors.

DIURETICS

Renal clearance studies in man have indicated that the renal handling of zinc may depend on urine flow (or a flow-related parameter) rather than on tubular transport mechanisms (Prasad and Oberleas, 1970; Steele, 1973; Theodoulou *et al*, 1987).
That thiazide diuretics increase urinary zinc excretion was first noted in the early '70s (Pak *et al*, 1972; Wester, 1973). In a subsequent randomized trial in untreated hypertensive patients, Wester (1980) found that urinary zinc excretion increased by 60 percent during long-term treatment with bendroflumethiazide, chlorthalidone and hydrochlorothiazide and much less during treatment with loop diuretics (furosemide, bumetanide) or triamterene. Serum zinc remained unchanged during treatment. The author remarked that "it is unclear if the increased urinary losses of zinc will lead to a zinc deficiency of clinical significance" and that "since diuretic treatment is very common and zinc has been recognized as an essential element for human health, the diuretic-zinc problem calls for further attention".

To assess whether diuretic-induced zinc losses can result in zinc deficiency we measured hair zinc in 20 patients with mild hypertension who had been treated with thiazides, alone or in combination with beta-blockers or methyldopa for 6 to 36 months before study; and in 19 patients with mild hypertension who had not been given any diuretic treatment for at least six months before study. Mean (±SEM) hair zinc was found to be significantly ($p<0.01$) lower in the patients treated with diuretics (2.18±0.10 μmol/g) than in the control group (3.46±0.19 μmol/g).

Serum zinc did not differ significantly between the two groups (Mountokalakis *et al*, 1984).

Although not appropriate for the assessment of rapid changes in zinc metabolism because of its slow turnover, the concentration of zinc in hair is nevertheless used as an estimate of body zinc stores (Prasad & Cossack, 1983). The finding of low hair zinc levels in patients treated with diuretics may, therefore, be regarded as indicative of tissue zinc depletion.

ANGIOTENSIN CONVERTING ENZYME INHIBITORS

The search for an association between angiotensin converting enzyme inhibitors (ACEI) and zinc has been triggered by the fact that a number of side effects of the ACEI captopril, such as skin changes and disorders of taste and smell, are also observed in zinc deficiency (McNeil *et al*, 1979). To test the hypothesis that these side effects might be due to alterations of zinc metabolism, Zumkley *et al* (1985) measured zinc concentrations in the plasma and red blood cells of 14 hypertensive patients treated with captopril in combination with other antihypertensive drugs; and of 13 untreated hypertensives who served as a control group. Plasma zinc was found to be slightly decreased and erythrocyte zinc to be slightly increased in the patients treated with captopril as compared to the control group.
As stated by the authors, decreased plasma zinc concentrations were mainly found in 5 patients who developed disorders of taste and smell or pruritus or ekzematous skin changes during captopril therapy.

In a more elaborated study, Abu-Hamdan *et al* (1988) assessed taste acuity and measured plasma zinc and urinary zinc excretion in 11 hypertensive patients treated with captopril for more than 6 months; 17 hypertensive patients treated with captopril for less than 6 months; and 17 hypertensive patients not receiving captopril, who served as controls. Compared to controls, patients on long-term captopril treatment had significantly higher taste-detection and taste-recognition thresholds, lower plasma zinc levels and higher urinary zinc excretion. The short-term captopril group did not differ significantly from the control group except for higher taste-recognition threshold for salty and sweet. It must be noted, however, that as it is also true for the study published by Zumkley *et al* (1985), many of the captopril-treated patients were also receiving diuretic treatment and thus the increased urinary zinc losses in these patients could be attributed to the effect of the diuretic.

Yet data from a subsequent study came to add to the confusion. Golik *et al* (1990) measured urinary zinc to urinary creatinine ratio in five groups of hypertensive patients and in a control group of healthy subjects. Hypertensive patients were either untreated or treated for at least three months with captopril alone, hydrochlorothiazide alone, captopril combined with hydrochlorothiazide, or captopril combined with furosemide.
Treated patients exhibited significantly increased urinary zinc to urinary creatinine ratios in comparison to control subjects and untreated hypertensives. However, patients receiving combination therapy had lower urinary zinc to urinary creatinine ratios than patients treated with either captopril alone or hydrochlorothiazide alone. According to the authors, thiazide diuretics and furosemide "might inactivate the zincuric effect of captopril by binding to its suplhydryl group within the tubular lumen".

In view of these controversial findings we measured serum zinc, fractional zinc clearance and hair zinc in four groups of patients with essential hypertension; 22 patients who had been treated with thiazide diuretics, alone or in combination with beta-blockers, calcium antagonists or methyldopa, for at least six months before study; 17 patients who had not received any diuretic or ACEI treatment for at least six months before study; 18 patients who had been treated with ACEI (captopril 11, enalapril 5, perindopril 1, lisinopril 1) in combination with thiazide diuretics for at least 6 months before study; and 22 patients who had been treated with ACEI inhibitors alone (captopril 12, enalapril 10) for at least 6 months before study. The results are shown in table 1.

Table 1. Serum zinc (SZn), fractional zinc clearance (FCZn) ad hair zinc (HZn) in the four groups of hypertensive patients. Mean±SD.

Patient group	SZn (μmol/l)	FCZn (x100)	HZn (μmol/g)
Patients on thiazides	14.8±2.8 (n=22)	0.55±0.25 (n=22)	2.39±0.26 (n=18)
Patients not receiving diuretics or ACEI	14.2±1.7 (n=17)	0.45±0.24 (n=17)	2.73±0.48 (n=10)
Patients on ACEI and thiazides	13.8±1.8 (n=18)	0.70±0.46 (n=18)	2.35±0.69 (n=10
Patients on ACEI alone	14.7±2.0 (n=22)	0.44±0.20 (n=22)	2.21±0.66 (n=18)

Serum zinc did not differ significanlty among the three groups. Fractional zinc clearance was significantly ($p<0.05$) higher in patients treated with ACE in combination with thiazides than in patients not receiving diuretics or ACEI or in patients treated with ACEI alone. On the other hand, hair zinc was significantly ($p<0.05$) lower in each of the groups of patients treated with either thiazides or ACEI, alone or in combination, than in the group of patients who had not been given diuretics or ACEI for at least 6 months before study. The above findings suggest that although ACEI do not cause considerable renal zinc loss, long-term treatment with these drugs may be associated with tissue zinc depletion. This effect seems to be shared by all agents tested in this study. As to the possible mechanism by which ACEI exert their effect on zinc metabolism, it is noteworthy that the angiotensin converting enzyme is a zinc containing enzyme on which ACEI act as zinc ligands. As postulated by Zumkley *et al* (1985) ACEI may interact with other zinc binding sites in the body and cause tissue zinc depletion.

IMMUNE DYSFUNCTION

Among several other trace metals zinc seems to regulate immune response, particularly cell-mediated immunity (Chandra, 1983). Lymphoid atrophy, depletion of lymphocytes, and a significant reduction in the proportion of helper T cells and in the activity of natural killer cells have been observed in patients with acrodematitis enteropathica or acquired zinc deficiency (Barnes & Moynahan, 1973; Allen *et al*, 1983). In several occasions, these changes have been corrected by zinc supplementation (Barnes & Moynahan, 1973; Tarazoglou *et al*, 1985). Since chronic diuretic treatment is associated with increased urinary zinc losses and a decreased concentration of zinc in hair, indicative of zinc depletion, we have examined whether T cell subpopulations are affected by prolonged administration of diuretics in hypertension. Serum zinc, hair zinc, and peripheral T lymphocyte sub-populations were measured in 10 hypertensive patients who have been treated with thiazide diuretics, alone or in combination with beta-blockers or reserpine for 6 to 36 months before study; and in 9 hypertensive patients who had not been given any diuretic or ACEI treatment for at least 6 months before study. Two of them were taking beta-blockers, 4 methyldopa, and one nifedipine. The results are shown is table 2.

Table 2. Serum zinc (SZn), hair zinc (HZn), and lymphocyte subpopulations in the two groups of hypertensive patients. (Mean±SD).

Patient group	SZn (μmol/l)	HZn (μmol/g)	Lymphocyte subpopulations T3(%)	T4(%)	T8(%)	T4/T8
Patients receiving diuretics	16.1 ±2.12	2.04* ±0.41	79.0 ±6.2	30.9** ±11.1	57.3** ±12.0	0.61* ±0.38
Patients not receiving diuretics	15.3 ±1.53	3.13 ±1.04	76.0 ±13.4	51.1 ±15.0	34.0 ±17.4	2.12 ±1.52

*p<0.01, **p<0.005; significance of difference between the two groups by ANOVA

As can be seen, low hair zinc concentrations in patients treated with diuretics were associated with a decrease in circulating T helper (T4) cells, an increase in circulating T suppressor (T8) cells, and a decrease in the T4/T8 ratio.

Two of the diuretic-treated patients were studied for a second time, before and after the oral administration of zinc aspartate, 150 mg daily, for one month. As can be seen from table 3, zinc supplementation resulted in reversal of the existing abnormalities in T lymphocyte subpopulations.

Table 3. Effect of zinc supplementation for one month on serum zinc (SZn), hair zinc (HZn), and lymphocyte subpopulations in two hypertensive patients receiving diuretics.

	SZn (μmol/l)	HZn (μmol/g)	Lymphocyte subpopulations T3(%)	T4(%)	T8(%)	T4/T8
Before	13.8	2.05	85	40	55	0.74
After	15.1	2.31	95	78	16	4.87
Before	13.6	2.00	83	30	65	0.46
After	14.1	2.16	80	61	20	3.05

The above findings suggest that long-term treatment of hypertension with thiazide diuretics results in changes in T cell subpopulations indicative of depressed cellular immune function, and that these changes can be reversed by zinc supplementation.

CONCLUSIONS

Chronic treatment of hypertension with diuretics is associated with continuous urinary zinc losses which may result in tissue zinc depletion. Tissue zinc depletion may also occur in prolonged treatment of hypertension with ACEI, but the underlying mechanism remains uncertain.
Impaired immune response, disturbed sense of taste and smell, and possibly other clinical manifestations related to zinc deficiency may be regarded as additional side effects of antihypertensive treatment. However, further information is needed before one can safely advise zinc supplementation in every patient treated with diuretics. Not only the evaluation of zinc status is difficult, but also the upper limits of the amounts of zinc considered safe are not well defined (Bogden *et al*,. 1990).

REFERENCES

Abu-Hamdan, D.K., Desai, H., Sondheimer, J., Felicetta, J., Mahajan, S., Mc Donald, F. (1988): Taste acuity and zinc metabolism in captopril-treated hypertensive male patients *Am.J.Hypert.* 1, 3035-3085.

Allen, J,.I., Perri, R.I., McClain, C.J., Kay, N.E. (1983): Alterations in human natural killer cell activity in patients with zinc deficiency with sickle cell disease. *J. Lab. Clin. Med.* 105, 19-22.

Barnes, P.M. & Moynahan, E.J. (1973): Zinc deficiency in acrodermatitis enteropathica: Multiple dietary intolerance treated with synthetic diet. *Proc. Roy. Soc. Med.* 66, 327-329.

Bogden, J.D., Oleske, J.M., Lavenhar, M.A., Munves, E.M., Kemp, F.W., Bruening, K.S., Holding, K.J., Denny, T.N., Guarino, M.A., Holland, B.K. (1990): Effects of one year of supplementation with zinc and other micronutrients on cellular immunity in the elderly. *J. Am. Coll. Nutr.* 9, 214-225.

Chandra, R.K. (1983): Nutrition, immunity and infection: Present knowledge and future directions. *Lancet* 1:688-691.

Golik, A., Averbuhh, Z., Cohn, M, Maor, J., Berman, S., Shahed, U., Modai, D. (1990): Effect of diuretics on captopril - induced urinary zinc excretion. *Eur. J. Clin. Pharmacol.* 38, 359-361.

Mc Neil, J.J., Anderson, A., Christophidis, N., Jarrot, B., Louis, W.J. (1980): Taste loss associated with oral captopril treatment. *Br. Med. J.* 2, 1555-1556.

Mountokalakis, T., Dourakis, S., Karatzas, N., Maravelias, C., Koutselinis, A. (1984): Zinc deficiency in mild hypertensive patients treated with diuretics. *J. Hypertens.* 2 (suppl 3): 571-572.

Pak, c.Y.c., Ruskin, B., Diller, E. (1972): Enhancement of renal excretion of zinc by hydrochlorothiazide. *Clin. Clim. Acta* 39:511-517.

Prasad, A.S. & Cossack, Z.T. (1983): Zinc in sickle cell disease. *Trans. Assoc. Am. Physicians* 96, 246-249.

Prasad, A.S. & Oberleas, D. (1970): Binding of zinc to amino acids and serum proteins in vitro. *J. Lab. Clin. Med.* 7, 416-425.

Steele, T.H. (1973): Dissociation of zinc excretion from other cations in man. *J. Lab. Clin. Med.* 81: 205-213.

Tarazoglou, E., Prasad, A.S., Hill, G., Brewer, G., Kaplan, J. (1985): Decreased natural killer cell activity in patients with zinc deficiency with sickle cell disease. *J. Lab. Clin. Med.* 105, 19-22.

Theodoulou, G., Dourakis, S., Mayopoulou-Symvoulidou, D., Mountokalakis, T. (1987): Relationship between zinc excretion and urine flow in healthy volunteers. *Kidney int.* 31, 866.

Wester, P.O. (1973): Trace elements in serum and urine from hypertensive patients

before and during treatment with chlorthalidone. *Acta Med. Scand.* 194, 505-512.
Wester, P.O. (1980): Urinary zinc excretion during treatment with different diuretics. *Acta Med. Scand.* 208, 209-212.
Zumkley, H., Bertram, H.P., Yetter, H., Zidek, W., Losse, H. (1985): Zinc metabolism during captopril treatment. *Horm. Metabol. Res.* 17, 256-258.

Metal Ions in Biology and Medicine, vol. 2. Eds. J. Anastassopoulou, Ph. Collery, J.C. Etienne, Th. Theophanides. John Libbey Eurotext, Paris © 1992, pp. 215-219

Serum aluminium : its relation with anemia and iron metabolism in uraemic patients on intermittent haemodialysis program

M. Gonzalez Enguita, A. Garcia de Jalon Comet, M.L. Calvo Ruata*, D. Zapatero Gonzalez, J. Escanero Marcen*

Unidad de Nutrición y Metales, Servicio de Bioquímica Clínica, Hospital Miguel Servet y Hospital Clínico Universitario, INSALUD. Zaragoza, España*

INTRODUCTION

The risk of aluminium (Al) absorption from Al-containing phosphate binders is almost worldwide accepted. Although some Al-free phosphate binders have been synthetised, they require further evaluation; meanwhile, Al-containing phosphate binders remain the standard drug for reducing serum phosphorous in chronic renal failure (CRF).

In recent years great interest has centred on studying the likely factors modulating gastrointestinal Al absorption; this has been well documented, but its mechanism is still unknown or poorly understood.

Aluminum loading has been recently implicated as a contributing factor in the normochromic normocytic anemia, non-iron deficient, found in a great proportion of patients with chronic renal failure. The precise mechanisms by which an excess of aluminum induces anemia are still to be elucidated. Several hypothesis have been postulated: a disturbance in heme synthesis, decreased globin synthesis, an increased hemolysis (suggested by a decreased osmotic fragility and by a mild reticulocytosis), or an interference with the normal metabolism of iron (Fe) (aluminum could act alone influencing anemia, or perhaps, may interact with other metals such as iron, lead, or zinc).

Some similarities seem to exist between iron and aluminum. Plasma Al has recently been shown to be bound to transferrin and could thereby enter the pathways of iron distribution and metabolism in aluminum overloaded patients. Recent reports suggest that might exist an interaction into the gastro-intestinal tract between them, and like other metals, both might share a common pathway of gut absorption, thus emphasizing the potential risk of the trace element toxicity in iron deficiency.

METHODS AND MATERIALS.

We have measured and evaluated serum aluminum and ferritin concentrations in 71 patients with CRF undergoing maintenance hemodialysis (47 males and 24 females).

Dialysis was perfomed for four hours three times a week. All patients were prescribed oral antacids containing aluminum hidroxide as a phosphate binder for the duration of their long-term dialysis. They all were treated with a dialysate containing negligible amounts of aluminum (less than 10 μg/l).

Serum aluminum levels were measured by flameless atomic absorption spectrophotometry with graphite furnace (HGA-700, autosampler AS-70), using a single beam spectrophotometer (Perkin-Elmer®, model 1100-B), with L´vov platform and deuterium background correction. Care was taken to avoid contamination in handling the samples. The accuracy of this procedure has been validated by participation in an international quality control survey (Worldwide Interlaboratory Quality Control Aluminum, Poitiers, France). Reproducibility of the procedure was ± 5%; detection limit (2 SD of determinations of the zero standard) has been 0.8 μg/l; characteristic mass obtained (amount of Al yielding an absorbance signal of 0.0044 A): 11 pgs. The normal range for serum aluminum obtained in our laboratory has been 2-14 μg/l.

Serum ferritin was quantitated by enzyme-immunoanalysis (ELISA). Hematological parameters have been determinated using a Technicon H6000 counter.

Serum ferritin is clearly the most useful diagnostic aid for assesing iron stores in patients on chronic hemodialysis. This study investigates whether hemodialysis patients with different iron stores (low-normal, normal or high ferritin values), have different patterns of Al absorption.

The patients were separated into three groups according to their serum ferritin values:

Group I: Serum ferritin below 100 ng/ml (low-normal ferritin group).
Group II: Serum ferritin 100-250 ng/ml (normal ferritin group).
Group III: Serum ferritin above 250 ng/ml (high ferritin group).

Statistical analysis of data was perfomed by using the nonparametric Kruskall-Wallis test with separate estimates of variance for calculations of statistical significance, based on the mean value in each group. Relationships between hematological parameters and degree of aluminum overload were examined by a linear regression analysis. Values in tables and text are expressed as mean ± 1 standard deviation (SD). A p value of < 0.05 was regarded as significant.

RESULTS

As shown in Table 1 Group III had a mean serum ferritin almost 9 times higher than Group I and significantly higher ($p < 0.05$) hemoglobin concentration.

Table 1: Details of patients divided into three groups based on the same serum ferritin.

	Group I	Group II	Group III
Serum ferritin (ng/ml)	**< 100**	**100-250**	**> 250**
Mean serum ferritin	45.04 ± 21	148.4 ± 47	378.3 ± 108.6
Number of patients	48	9	14
(mean age)	50.3 ± 15.1	57.7 ± 15.3	46.3 ± 17
Hemoglobin (g/dl)	9.38 ± 1.4*	9.39 ± 1.3	10.45 ± 1.2*
Serum Al level (μg/l)	50.3 ± 46.7	36.2 ± 26.6	29.4 ± 23.2

*** p< 0.05.**

We haven´t found statistically significant correlation between serum ferritin and aluminum levels, ($p = 0.335$), although it can be seen that serum Al is higher as iron stores get lower; this is also confirmed by lineal regression analysis, as no statiscally correlation can be found once again (Fig. 2: $r = -0.16$; $p = 0.1821$).

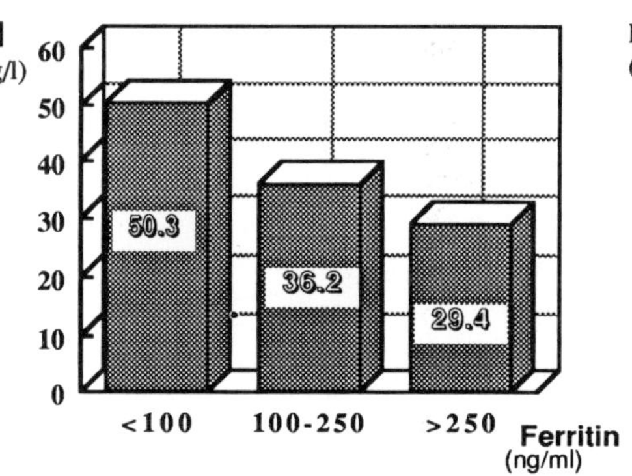

Fig. 1.- Al levels according ferritin groups

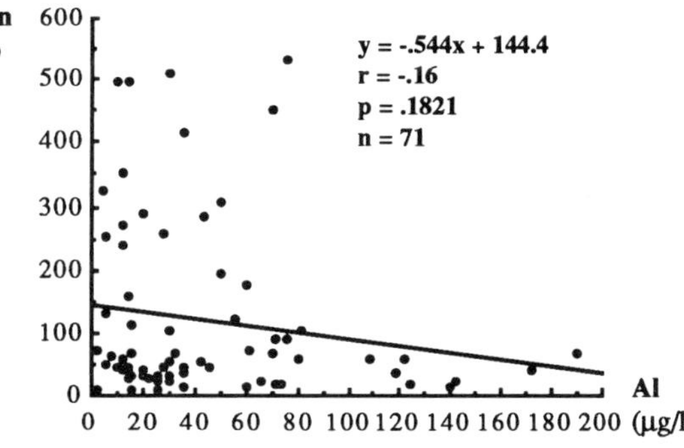

Fig. 2.- Relation between serum Al and ferritin.

We have howewer found, and **only** in Group I (serum ferritin < 100 ng/ml) (Fig. 3), a statiscally significant relation between serum Al levels and total mean amount of $Al(OH)_3$ ingested as phosphate binder ($r = 0.34$; $p = 0.0169$).

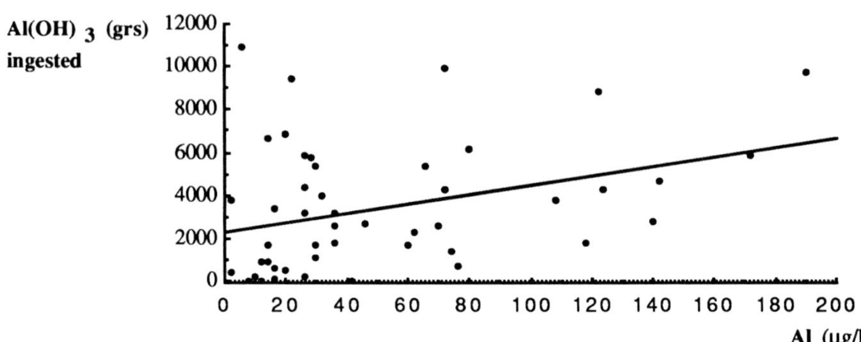

Fig. 3.- Relationship between serum Al and amount of Al $(OH)_3$ ingested in patients (n = 48) with ferritin < 100 ng/ml.

By lineal regression (figs. 4 and 5), we have found that serum Al levels well correlate (negatively and significantly) with hematological parameters of anemia (Hb: $r = -0.51$, $p = 0.0001$; Hto: $r = -0.48$, $p = 0.0001$; MCV: $r = -0.28$, $p = 0.0186$; MCHb: $r = -0.27$, $p = 0.0214$).

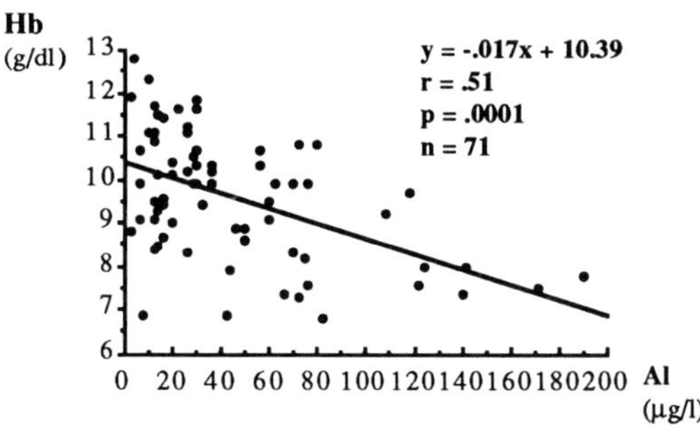

Fig. 4.- Hemoglobin and serum Al levels.

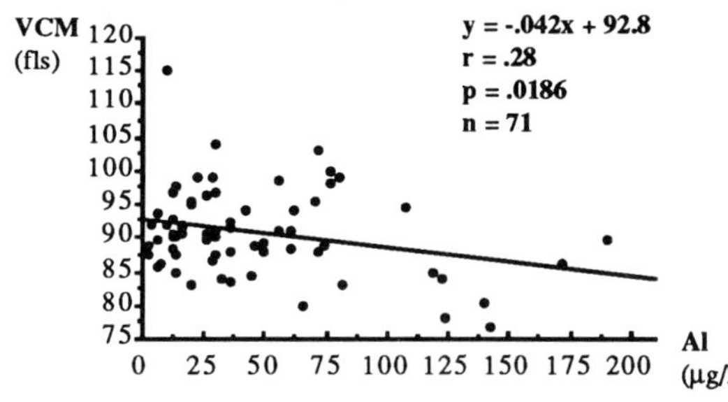

Fig.5.- VCM and serum Al levels.

As above, we have found that correlation between serum Al levels with hemoglobin (Hb), mean corpuscular volume (MCV) (Fig.6) and mean corpuscular hemoglobin (MCHb) is **only** statiscally significant in patients with low-normal iron stores (ferritin values < 100 ng/ml): Hb: $r = -0.49$; $p = 0.0004$; VCM: $r = -0.321$; $p = 0.0262$; MCHb: $r = -0.37$; $p = 0.0104$.

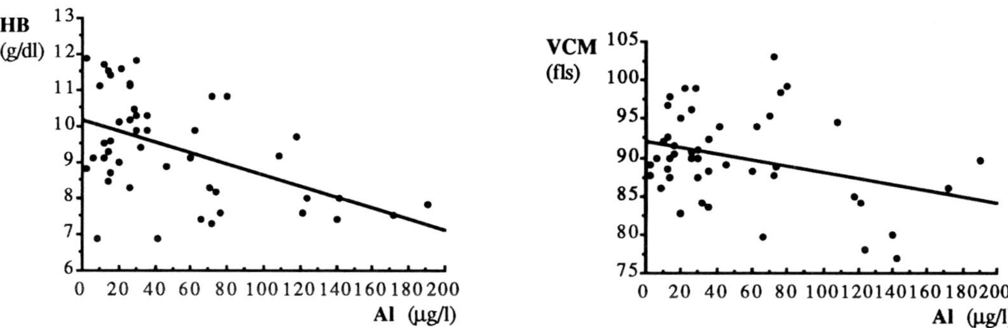

Fig.6.- Relationships of serum Al with Hb and VCM in patients with low-normal iron stores (ferritin < 100 ng/ml).

CONCLUSIONS.

1.- From our findings we could think that levels of serum ferritin might be a useful index to predict Al gastrointestinal absorption, and to select patients at risk of Al hyperabsorption; patients with low-normal iron stores have higher risk to increase their serum Al levels ("Al hyperabsorber patients").

2.- Serum Al levels well and negatively correlate with the hematological parameters of the anemia from uraemic patients on intermittent HD.

3.- Correlation between serum Al values with Hb, MCV and MCHb is **only** statiscally significant in patients with ferritin levels lower than 100 ng/ml.

BIBLIOGRAPHY.

1.- Cannata J, Suárez C, Cuesta V, Rodriguez R, Allende M, Herrera J, Pérez J. (1984): Gastrointestinal aluminum absorption: is it modulated by the iron-absortive mechanism?. Proc Eur Dial Transpl Assoc. 21, 354-359.

2.- D´Haese PC, Van de Vyver FL, De Wolff FA, De Broe ME. (1985): Measurement of aluminum in serum, blood, urine and tissue of chronic hemodialysed patients by use of electrothermal atomic absorption spectrometry. Clin. Chem. 31, 24-29.

3.- Drüeke T, Lacour B, Touam M, Jucquel JP, Plachot JJ, Cournot-Witmer G, Galle P. (1986): Effect of aluminum on hematopoiesis. Kidney Int. 29 (Suppl. 18), S45 - S48.

4.- Fernández I, Fernández JL, Rodriguez R, Sanz A, Cannata JB. (1989): Influencia del grado de saturación de los depósitos de hierro en la absorción gastrointestinal de aluminio. Rev Esp Fisiol. 45, 33 - 40.

5.- Moreb J, Popovtzer M, Friedlaender M, Konijn A, Hershko C. (1983): Evaluation of iron status in patients on chronic hemodialysis: relative usefulness of bone marrow hemosiderin, serum ferritin, transferrin saturation, mean corpuscular volume and red cell protoporphyrin. Nephron 35, 196-200.

Metal Ions in Biology and Medicine, vol. 2. Eds. J. Anastassopoulou, Ph. Collery, J.C. Etienne, Th. Theophanides. John Libbey Eurotext, Paris © 1992, pp. 220-223

Relathionship between metal ions Ca^{++} Mg^{++} K^{+} and Na^{+} during the sudden changes of arterial pressure (AP) in man

Th. Galeas*, D. Mylonas*, A. Kritikos**, N. Tsianas***, M. Lemoni****

B′ Internal Medicine Clinic Cardiology Dept** Artificial Kidney Unit*** Microbiology Dept**** Trikala General Hospital, Greece*

INTRODUCTION

Results of epidemiologic studies show the existence of a relationship between Ca^{++} Mg^{++} K^{+} Na^{+} and AP (Reed et al.,1985). Renal patients with end-stage renal failure, treated with hemodialysis, have all the "advantages" to be under intensive surveillance of their vital,biochemical and hematologic parameters during hemodialysis treatment. Arterial hypotension and hypertension are the most common complications of hemodialysis (Agrapfiotis Th.,1984; Sombolos K.,1984).This work aimed to study the Behaviour of Ca^{++} Mg^{++} K^{+} and Na^{+} ionsduring the sudden changes of AP,in hemodialysed patients, confirming epidemiologic studies.

MATERIAL-METHODS

Material of the study were 27 renal patients of the artificial kidney unit in Trikala General Hospital, 17 male and 10 female, average age 54,74 $\pm$ 11,73 who had been under hemodialysis for 12-120 months. Of them 6 patients were under mild anti-hypertensive medication (b-blockers, calcium antagonists or angiotensin converting enzyme inhibitors) without having any problem. Also, with 3 patients who did not care about the proper liquid intake in their nutrition we had to proceed to ultrafiltration because they manifested congestive cardiac insufficiency-heart failure-pulmonary edema owing to liquid overload. All the patients included in the study, read and accepted the protocol which is internationally admitted and according to the prototype of the study of Athens (Moulopoulos S.,1963; Adamopoulos P., 1983). It was divided in three stages. During the first stage (before connection to the unit) AP of every patient, in a state of relaxation,was measured. Blood taking followed to define serum Ca^{++} Mg^{++} K^{+} and Na^{+}.
In the second and third stages that followed, AP was measured in every patient who complained of subjective symptoms of elevation or fall of AP. At the same time blood samples were taken to define serum Ca^{++} Mg^{++} K^{+} and Na^{+}. All measurements were conducted in the hospital biochemical laboratory with the use of an electrolyte electrode-analyser for $Ca^{++}K^{+}$and Na^{+} and the chromometric method for the measurement of Mg^{++}.

For the measurement of AP a sphygmomanometer was used by a trained nurse who had been appointed before and was unaware of the research protocol. The whole procedure took 6 months. For the statistical analysis of the results pair-t-test method with 11 degrees of liberty was used.

RESULTS

Table 1 is indicative of the results:

Total number of examined (27)	serum(mmol/l) $Ca^{++} \pm SD$	serum(mmol/l) $Mg^{++} \pm SD$	serum(meq/l) $K^{+} \pm SD$	serum(meq/l) $Na^{+} \pm SD$
Relaxation	$1,14 \pm 0,15$	$1,02 \pm 0,1$	$5,46 \pm 0,71$	$141,7 \pm 4,03$
(normal rates)	1,14 – 1,30	0,65 – 1,05	3,5 – 5	135 – 145
Sudden elev of AP	$1,30 \pm 0,15$	$1,0 \pm 0,88$	$5,5 \pm 1,00$	$145,33 \pm 3,31$
	t=4,92	t=2,81	t=6,82	t=2,07
	P<0,01	P<0,05	P<0,0001	NON SS
Sudden fall of AP	$1,27 \pm 0,24$	$0,82 \pm 0,13$	$3,5 \pm 0,29$	$134,4 \pm 1,51$
	t=2,22	t=3,82	t=6,15	t=2,01
	NON SS	P<0,05	P<0,01	NON SS

a)when AP is in normal rates a relatively "fragile equilibrium" appears in the relationship between Ca^{++} Mg^{++} K^{+} and Na^{+}.
b)During sudden elevation of AP an increase of Ca^{++}statistically extremely significant, is observed, as well as significant Mg^{++}level decrease, and significant K^{+} level increase without any changes in Na^{+} levels.
c)During the sudden fall of AP a trend is observed to confirm the "hypomagnisemia, hypokalemia, hypocalcemia" triad.

DISCUSSION

The outbreak of knowledge that came from the basic biological research and the efforts to control a critical problem of public health led to the immense development of hypertension bibliography the last years. From a first point of view, we can say that hypertension morbidity is a result of work overload that is imposed on heart and the damage of blood vessels at the points of minimum resistance. There have also been written and published studies on special subjects related to hypertension such as angiotensin, catecholamines, adrenal glands hormones, central nervous system, hemodynamics, vessel reactivity, vasodilative substances and kidneys. Besides,opinions suggest mechanisms related to prostaglandins, kallikrein, quinine and hypertensive lipids as aetiological factors of hypertension (Hurst 1978). forty years ago Page also expressed the theory of mosaic of hypertension to support that it is logical to consider hypertension as a disease where numerous regulator-mechanisms remain in a state of interaction to keep arterial pressure elevated (Page 1949). After some years Kobayashi referred to the existence of a relationship between cardiovascular abnormalities and hardness of the river water in Japan, emphasizing the existence of ions as an aetiology of hypertension and apoplexy (KObayashi 1960). The same year Schroeder from USA found a negative relationship between hardness of potable water and deaths from ischemic hypertensive cardiopathy giving an emphasis on the relationship between $Ca^{++}$and Mg^{++}(Schroeder.,1960). In Texas the Ca-Mg relationship was directly correlated to hypertension (Dawson 1978). Other studies showed that administration of Mg^{++}increased the low $Mg^{++}$and K^{++}in muscles, increasing hypertension at the same time (Dyckner 1983).

That is supplemantation of Mg^{++} together with K^{+} could have an antihypertensive effect (Zawada,1987; Hollifield, 1984). Galeas (1989) in epidemiologic studies, examined the relationship of $Ca^{++}$and Mg^{++} and the incidence on cardiovascular diseases. In a clinical study by the same team, a positive effect of Ca^{++} on the therapy of mild hypertension was found (Galeas,1990; 1991). In the present clinical study further knowledge comes to light which together with epidemiologic studies show that the above mentioned electrolytes are closely correlated to the changes of AP. Some researchers support that excess of $Ca^{++}$is a cause of high AP (Resncik 1983; McCarron,1989) and some others that hypertensives have Ca^{++} deficiency (McCarron,1982;1985). K^{+} was found to have a protective effect on vessels and to be the cause of a possible decrease of AP (Langford, 1983). It was supported that Mg^{++} has a vasodilative effect and that its deficiency caused increase of AP (Seeling, 1974; Sharrett, 1975). When Ca^{++} Mg^{++} K^{+} and Na^{+} are in a state of electrolyte-electric equilibrium then we have the relationship of LOEB (Gunther, 1981; Enciclopedia Medica Italiana 1982):

$$K= \frac{Na^{++}}{Ca^{++}} + \frac{K^{+}}{Mg^{++}} + \frac{OH^{-}}{H^{+}}$$

We could support that sudden elevation or fall of AP activate mechanisms which disturb the ion balance relationship of LOEB, thus causing rapid transportation of ions from the extracellular to the intracellular area and inversely. This transportation could interfere into the mechanism of AP balance in man and disturb it. However, we are not in the position to know which mechanism could initially interfere. Our clinical findings give us the priority to support the interrelationship of the above mentioned ions as a uniform factor of the AP balance. Every disturbance of this factor could give a start to mechanisms that contribute simultaneously to the disturbance of the relationship between AP and these ions.

In conclusion sudden elevation or fall of AP during hemodialysis has a relation with the changes of Ca^{++} Mg^{++} and K^{+} concentrations and seems to be independent of Na^{+} concentrations. We could say that AP should also be examined as a disease regulated by Ca^{++} Mg^{++} K^{+} and Na^{+}electrolytes.

REFERENCES

Agrafiotis Th.(1984): Artificial kidney.Parisianos Gr.eds.p.154,158,159. Athens

Adamopoulos P.(1983).Coronary heart disease and its risk factor. Treatment of risk factors in community."The study of Athens" Academic disertation. Athens.

Dawson E.B, Frey M.J,Moore T.D and McGanity W.J (1978). Relationship of metal metabolism to vascular disease mortality rate in Texas.Am.J.Clin. Nutr. 31:1188-1197

Dyckner T and Wester P.O.(1983). Effect of magnesium on blood pressure. Br.Med.J. 286:1847-1849

Enciclopedia Medica Italiana.(1982) Ed USES, 9,35

Galeas Th, Klotsotyras G, Mylonas D,Sideris D.(1989) Geographical distribution of acute infarction in Trikala,Greece.Hellenic Cardiological review. 212-217.

Galeas Th,Papadopoulos A,Bardas Hr,Agoritsa D, Papanikolaou E, Apostolakis K.(1989) Geochemical environment of alluvial soil and its relationship to essential hypertension in Trikala.Proceedings of the 4th Northhellenic Conference. Thessaloniki.
Galeas Th,Lappas Chr,Papadopoulos A and Founta P.(1990).Strategies in the treatment of hypertension in unknown etiology end-stage nephropathy.Renal Failure.53 (abstract)
Galeas Th,Papdopoulos A.(1991).Strategies in the treatment of unknown etiology end-stage renal failure.Medical Annals 14:90-96
Gunther T.(1981).Magnesium Bulletin.3:91
Hollifield J.(1984).Potassium and magnesium abnormalities;diuretics and arrhythmias in hypertension.Am.J.Med.77:28-32
Hurst W.(1978).The heart.Michalopoulos eds.3:1789-1803.Athens.Mc Graw-Hill Book Company
Kobayashi J.(1960).A chemical study of the average quality and characteristics of river waters in Japan.Ber.Ohara Inst.Landw Forsch 11:313-357
Langford HG.(1983).Dietary potassium and hypertension.Epidemiologic data. Ann.Int.Med.98(suppl):770-772
McCarron DA,Young EW,Bukoski RD,Morris CD.(1989)Calcium metabolism and arterial pressure.In Retting R,Ganten D,Luft F eds.Salt and Hypertension. Springer-Verlag.176
McCarron D,Morris C, Cole C.(1982.Dietary calcium in human hypertension. Science 217:267-269
McCarron D,Morris C.(1985) Blood pressure response to oral calcium in persons with mild to moderate hypertension.Am.Int.Med.103:825-831
Moulopoulos S.(1963).Techniques of blood pressure measurement In:Cardiomechanics.Thomas,Springfield,III pp 5-20
Page I.H.(1949).Pathogenesis of arterial hypertension.J.A.M.A. 14:451
Reed D,McGec D,Yamo K,Haukin J.(1985)Diet,blood pressure and multicollinearity.Hypertension 7:405-411
Resncik LM,Laragh JH.(1983). The hypotensive effect of short term oral calcium loading in essential hypertension.Clin Res.31:334 (abstract)
Schroeder H.A.(1960).Relations between mortality from cardiovascular diseases and treated water supplies.J.A.M.A. 172:1902-1908
Seeling MS,Heggtveit HA.(1974).Magnesium interelationships in ischemic heart disease. A review.Am . J. Clin. Nutr. 27:59-63
Sharrett AR,Feinleib M.(1975).Water constitutions and trace demands in relation to cardiovascular diseases. Prev. Med 4:20-25
Sombolos K.(1984). Hemodialysis.pp 212-214,220,225.University Studio Press Thessaloniki
Zawada E, Zerwee J, McClung Dan.(1989) Magnesium prevents acute hypercalcemic hypertension.Nephron.47:109-114

Metal Ions in Biology and Medicine, vol. 2. Eds. J. Anastassopoulou, Ph. Collery, J.C. Etienne, Th. Theophanides. John Libbey Eurotext, Paris © 1992, pp. 224-225

Intracellular Mg^{++} concentrations under diuretic treatment in mild essential hypertensive patients

K. Kisters, K.H. Rahn, W. Zidek

Medizinische Poliklinik der Universität W-4400 Münster, Albert-Schweitzer-Str. 33, Germany

Summary

Whereas diuretic-induced changes of plasma Mg^{++} concentrations have often been described, comparatively few data on intracellular Mg^{++} concentrations under diuretic treatment are known. Therefore we studied the effect on intracellular Mg^{++} concentrations of a thiazide diuretic (trichlormethiazide 4 mg/d) in red blood cells of 14 patients with mild essential hypertension, and of a combination of a thiazide diuretic and a potassium-sparing diuretic (trichlormethiazide and amiloride 2 mg/d each) in red blood cells of 11 patients with mild essential hypertension. Measurements were performed by atomic absorption spectroscopy before starting treatment and after 4-6 and 8-12 weeks' diuretic treatment. Intracellular Mg^{++} concentrations decreased significantly under thiazide therapy, whereas there was a significant increase in intracellular Mg^{++} concentrations under thiazide and potassium-sparing combined diuretic therapy ($p< 0,05$). The results show that the combination of a thiazide diuretic and a potassium-sparing diuretic is a useful means to avoid intracellular Mg^{++} loss.

Key words: Mg^{++} - diuretic treatment - mild essential hypertension

Introduction

It is well known that diuretic treatment can result in Mg^{++} depletion, since many diuretics inhibit the reabsorption of filtered magnesium in the proximal and distal tubule (Dyckner & Wester, 1984; Kisters et al., 1990). Changes in plasma Mg^{++} concentrations have often been described (Brednan & Milligran, 1987; Hollifield, 1986; Ryan, 1987), but comparatively few data on cellular Mg^{++} concentration under diuretic treatment are known.
Therefore we studied the effect on intracellular Mg^{++} concentrations of a thiazide diuretic and a combination of a thiazide and a potssium-sparing diuretic in red blood cells of mild essential hypertensive patients.

Patients and methods

Red blood cells of 11 patients with mild essential hypertension, who got a combination of a thiazide and a potassium-sparing diuretic and of 14 patients with mild essential hypertension, who were thiazide treated, were investigated.

Methods: 10 ml heparinized blood were drawn and centrifuged with 2500 g. Then plasma was removed. The red blood cells were washed twice with an isotonic lithium acetate solution. Measurements were performed in the hemolysate after freezing and rethawing the red blood cell pellet. Intracellular total Mg^{++} concentrations in red blood cells were measured with atomic absorption spectroscopy, using the Thermo Jarrell Ash Video 12 apparatus. Calibration curves were established using solutions with known Mg^{++} concentrations, in the lower, upper and intermediate range (Seronorm charge No 176, Merck, Pathonorm H charge No 21, Nyegaard, Pathonorm L charge No 20, Nycomed). For each sample a mean value was calculated from 3 measurements. All measurements were done in one series at room temperature. Intraassay variability was 5,7% in 10 subsequent measurements.

Results

Table 1 shows mean values and standard deviations of intracellular Mg^{++} content (Mg_i^{++}) before and after diuretic treatment (mmol/l, *=p< 0,05).

	before	after 4-6 weeks	after 8-12 weeks
trichlormethiazide	1,86±0,14	1,90±0,24	1,62±0,30 *
trichlormethiazide/ amiloride combination	1,83±0,15	1,83±0,17	1,98±0,11 *

The results show that intracellular Mg^{++} concentrations decreased significantly under thiazide therapy, whereas there was a significant increase in intracellular Mg^{++} concentrations under thiazide and potassium-sparing combined diuretic therapy (p< 0,05).

Discussion

In contrast to plasma Mg^{++} concentration under diuretic treatment, intracellular Mg^{++} concentration has not been studied in detail yet. Extracellular Mg^{++} constitutes only about 3% of total body Mg^{++}. Therefore plasma Mg^{++} concentration may not be adequate for assessing the Mg^{++} status of the body. For this reason intracellular Mg^{++} concentrations under diuretic treatment were determined. Our results show that the combination of a thiazide diuretic and a potassium-sparing diuretic is a useful means to avoid intracellular Mg^{++} loss.

References

Brednan, J.M., Milligran,K. (1987): Diuretic-associated hypomagnesemia in the elderly. In Arch. Intern. Med. 147: 1768-1771.

Dyckner, T., Wester, P.O. (1984): Intracellular magnesium loss after diuretic administration. In Drugs 28 (Suppl.1): 161-166.

Hollifield, J.W. (1986): Thiazide treatment of hypertension. In Am. J. Med. 80 (Suppl.4A): 8-12.

Kisters, K., Zidek, W., Fehske, K., Kwapisz, A., Rahn, K.H. (1990): Mg^{++} metabolism under diuretic treatment with the loop diuretic piretanide. In Metal Ions in Biology and Medicine. John Libbey Eurotext, Paris: 172-176.

Ryan, M.P. (1987): Diuretics and potassium/magnesium depletion. In Am. J. Med. 82 (Suppl.3A): 38-47.

Metal Ions in Biology and Medicine, vol. 2 Eds. J. Anastassopoulou, Ph. Collery, J.C. Etienne, Th. Theophanides. John Libbey Eurotext, Paris © 1992, pp. 226-227

Intracellular aluminium concentrations in renal insufficiency and after renal transplantation

Klaus Kisters, Claus Spieker, Hans-Peter Bertram*, Michael Barenbrock, Karl-Heinz Rahn, Walter Zidek

*Medizinische Poliklinik der Universität, *Institut für Pharmakologie und Toxikologie W-4400 Münster, Albert-Schweitzer-Str. 33, Germany*

Summary

Intracellular aluminum concentrations were determined in lymphocytes of 15 patients on regular hemodialysis treatment as compared to 15 controls and 14 patients, studied 14,6±2,8 months after renal transplantation. Lymphocytic aluminum content was referred to lymphocytic protein, which was determined by the Bradford method. Lymphocytic aluminum content was measured by atomic absorption spectroscopy. Aluminum concentrations in lymphocytes of patients on regular hemodialysis treatment for 3,5±1,6 years were 23,8±5,2 compared to 18,4±5,4 in controls and 14,9±8,6 µg Al/g lymphocytic protein in patients after renal transplantation (means±SD). The results indicate that besides the well known alterations in aluminum blood plasma concentrations in patients on regular hemodialysis treatment, intracellular aluminum concentrations are significantly increased as compared to controls ($p< 0,05$). After renal transplantation intracellular aluminum content is significantly lowered as compared to hemodialysis patients ($p< 0,05$).

Key words: aluminum - lymphocytes - renal insufficiency - renal transplantation

Introduction

In patients with renal insufficiency or in patients undergoing chronic intermittent hemodialysis treatment blood plasma aluminum concentrations are frequently found increased (Zumkley & Kisters, 1990; Kisters et al., 1992). In different kinds of tissues, e. g. in brain (Alfrey et al., 1976; Ledermann & Henry, 1978), bone (Cournot-Witmer et al., 1981; Hodsman et al., 1982) or gastric mucous membrane (Kisters et al., 1990), elevated aluminum concentrations have also been described. Only few data exist on intracellular aluminum content. Furthermore it is still unknown, whether intracellular aluminum concentrations are lowered after renal transplantation. Therefore intracellular aluminum concentrations were determined in lymphocytes of patients on regular hemodialysis treatment as compared to controls and patients after renal transplantation.

Patients and methods

15 patients with normal renal function, who had never been aluminum exposed before

served as controls. 15 patients on regular hemodialysis treatment for 3,5±1,6 years and 14 patients 14,6±2,8 months after renal transplantation were studied. Intracellular aluminum concentrations were measured in lymphocytes of each patient from which 10 ml of heparinized blood was removed. Intralymphocytic aluminum concentration was referred to lymphocytic protein content. Lymphocytic protein content was determined by Bradford's method using Coomassie Blue. Lymphocytes were isolated by the density gradient method using Lymphoprep. The suspension of lymphocytes was then washed twice in bidistilled water. For lysis of the cells, the suspension was frozen to -18°C and then rethawed. The measurements of aluminum concentrations in lymphocytes were performed by atomic absorption spectroscopy using a Perkin-Elmer 500 HGA-apparatus. Lymphocytic aluminum content was expressed as µg Al/g lymphocytic protein content.

Results

In controls 18,4±5,4 µg Al/g lymphocytic protein (mean±SD) was measured versus 23,8±5,2 µg Al/g lymphocytic protein in hemodialysis patients. The findings indicate significantly elevated aluminum concentrations in lymphocytes of hemodialysis patients as compared to controls ($p< 0,05$). Intralymphocytic aluminum content was measured 14,9±8,6 µg Al/g lymphocytic protein in patients after renal transplantation (serum creatinine 1,0±0,1 mg/dl). After renal transplantation intracellular aluminum content is significantly lowered as compared to hemodialysis patients ($p < 0,05$).

Discussion

The results indicate that in patients on regular hemodialysis treatment intracellular aluminum concentrations are significantly increased as compared to controls ($p< 0,05$), whereas after renal transplantation intracellular aluminum content of lymphocytes normalizes. In earlier studies it has already been shown that aluminum incorporation depends on the degree of renal insufficiency. It is well known that variations in plasma aluminum concentrations insufficiently reflect changes in the whole body stores. For this reason intracellular aluminum concentrations, for example in lymphocytes, may be more suitable to assess the whole aluminum body content. Whether elevated intracellular aluminum concentrations in lymphocytes over prolonged periods of time may impair lymphocytic function and hence exhibit immunosuppressive effects has still to be discussed.

References

Alfrey, A.C., Le Gendre, G.R., Kaehny, W.D. (1976): Dialysis encephalopathy syndrome. In New Engl. J. Med. 294: 184-188.

Cournot-Witmer, G., Zingraff, J., Piachot, J.J., Escaig, F., Lefevre, R., Boumati, P., Bourdeau, A., Garaledian, M., Galle, P., Bourdon, R., Drueeke, T., Balsan, S. (1981): Aluminum Localization in Bone from Hemodialysed Patients: Relationship to Matrix Mineralisation. In Kidney Int 20: 375-378.

Hodsman, A.B., Sherrard, D.J., Alfrey, A.C., Ott, S., Brickmann, A.S., Miller, N.L., Malony, N.A., Coburn, D.W. (1982): Bone Aluminum and Histomorphometric Features of Renal Osteodystrophy. In J Clin Endocrinol Metab 54: 539-544.

Kisters, K., Spieker, C., Zidek, W., Fetsch, T., Bertram, H.P., Fromme, H.G., Zumkley, H., Rahn, K.H. (1990): Aluminum concentrations and localisation in gastric mucous membrane before and after therapy with aluminum-containing antacids. In Trace Elements in Medicine 4: 199-202.

Kisters, K., Spieker, C., Bertram, H.P., Rahn, K.H., Zidek, W. (1992): Aluminum concentrations in lymphocytes of patients on regular hemodialysis treatment. In Trace Elements in Medicine 1: 25-27.

Ledermann, R.J., Henry, C.E. (1978): Progressive dialysis encephalopathy. In Ann Neurol 4: 199-202.

Zumkley, H., Kisters, K. (1990): Spurenelemente. Wissenschaftliche Buchgesellschaft, Darmstadt, pp.3-9.

Metal Ions in Biology and Medicine, vol. 2. Eds. J. Anastassopoulou, Ph. Collery, J.C. Etienne, Th. Theophanides. John Libbey Eurotext, Paris © 1992, pp. 228-229

Plasma and intracellular electrolytes in preeclampsia

K. Kisters, C. Spieker, W. Niedner*, I. Fafera*, K.H. Rahn, W. Zidek

*Medizinische Poliklinik der Universität, *Frauenklinik der Universität W-4400 Münster, Albert-Schweitzer-Str. 33, Germany*

Summary

In 27 patients with preeclampsia and in 22 healthy pregnant women plasma and intraerythrocytic Mg^{++} concentrations were determined. In preeclamptic women Mg^{++} concentrations were measured before and after institution of treatment with Mg^{++} salts and after delivery. Plasma Mg^{++} concentration in preeclamptic and healthy pregnant women was not significantly different. Intraerythrocytic Mg^{++} concentration before treatment with Mg^{++} was significantly lower in preeclamptic patients as compared to healthy pregnant women ($1,33 \pm 0,29$ mmol/l versus $1,12 \pm 0,16$ mmol/l, $p < 0,05$) and increased after treatment with magnesium to $1,19 \pm 0,24$ mmol/l. Mg^{++} measurements were performed by atomic absorption spectroscopy. Intraerythrocytic sodium and potassium concentrations, determined by flame photometry, were not significantly different in preeclamptic and healthy pregnant women. Lowered cellular Mg^{++} concentrations in preeclampsia may contribute to the development of hypertension in this disorder.

Key words: intracellular electrolytes - preeclampsia - hypertension

Introduction

Preeclampsia was treated with magnesium salts since the turn of the century (Volhard, 1918). From the therapeutic effects of Mg^{++} salts and from the known vasodilating properties of Mg^{++}, Mg^{++} deficiency was suggested to play a role in the development of vasoconstriction in preeclampsia (Seelig, 1980; Altura et al., 1983). Body Mg^{++} stores cannot be assessed adequately by measurements of plasma Mg^{++} concentration, since plasma contains less than 3% of body Mg^{++} stores. Therefore intracellular Mg^{++} concentration in preeclampsia was of interest.

Patients and methods

27 patients with preeclampsia and 22 healthy pregnant women were studied. The diagnosis of preeclampsia was made, when blood pressure was $\geq 140/\geq 90$ mm Hg or when an increase of systolic pressure by > 30 mm Hg or of diastolic pressure by > 15 mm Hg was observed at least at two independent measurements, and when urinary protein excretion exceeded 0,3 g/l.
For statistical analysis paired and unpaired Student's t test was used.
Intraerythrocytic Na^+ and K^+ concentrations were determined by flame photometry.

Mg^{++} concentration in plasma and in erythrocytes were measured with an atomic absorption spectroscope (Thermo Jarrell Ash Video 12, Thermo Jarrell, Dortmund, Germany). 10 ml heparinized blood was drawn and centrifuged with 2500 g. Then plasma for Mg^{++} determinations was removed. The erythrocytes were washed twice with an isotonic lithium acetate solution adjusted to pH 7,4. Mg^{++} was measured in the hemolysate at room temperature after freezing and rethawing the erythrocyte pellet in Mg^{++} free tubes. Calibration curves were established using solutions with known Mg^{++} concentrations.

Results

The results are given in figure 1.

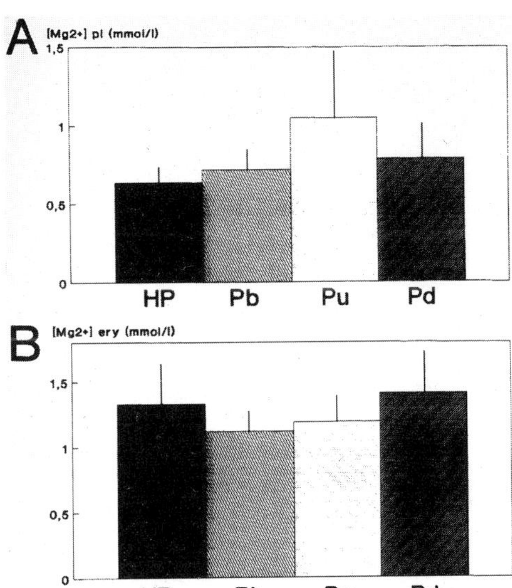

Fig. 1. A: Plasma Mg^{++} concentrations in healthy pregnant women (HP), patients with preeclampsia before (Pb) and under (Pu) institution of treatment with Mg^{++} salts and after delivery (Pd).

Fig. 1. B: Intraerythrocytic Mg^{++} concentrations in healthy pregnant women (HP), patients with preeclampsia before (Pb) and under (Pu) institution of treatment with Mg^{++} salts and after delivery (Pd). Mean values and standard deviations are noted.

Intraerythrocytic Na^{+} and K^{+} concentrations were not significantly different in preeclamptic and healthy pregnant women.

Discussion

In contrast to plasma Mg^{++} concentrations, intracellular Mg^{++} concentrations in preeclampsia have not yet been studied in detail (Hall, 1957). Mg^{++} measurements in erythrocytes were preferred in the present study, because the Mg^{++} concentration can be assessed directly. After supplementation of Mg^{++}, an increase in the plasma Mg^{++} concentration compared with untreated patients was noted. However, the intracellular Mg^{++} concentration remained decreased despite the normal plasma Mg^{++} concentration. This suggests a disturbance in transmembrane Mg^{++} distribution in preeclampsia, which cannot be completely corrected by an increase in the extracellular Mg^{++} concentration. The results show that a Mg^{++} deficiency, e.g. due to a decreased Mg^{++} intake, is not sufficient to explain the decrease in intracellular Mg^{++} concentration. The demonstration of an intracellular Mg^{++} deficiency in the present study may explain the successful use of Mg^{++} in the treatment of preeclampsia.

References

Altura, B.M., Altura, B.T., Carella, A. (1983): Magnesium deficiency-induced spasms of umbilical vessels: relation to preeclampsia, hypertension, growth retardation. In Science 221: 376-378.

Hall, D.G. (1957): Serum magnesium in pregnancy. In Obstet Gynecol 9: 158-162.

Seelig, M.S. (1980): Magnesium deficiency in the pathogenesis of disease. In New York: Plenum.

Volhard, F. (1918): Bilateral haematogenic renal disease (in German). In Berlin:Springer.

Metal Ions in Biology and Medicine, vol. 2. Eds. J. Anastassopoulou, Ph. Collery, J.C. Etienne, Th. Theophanides. John Libbey Eurotext, Paris © 1992, pp. 230-231

Intracellular Mg^{++} content in essential and renal hypertension

K. Kisters, C. Spieker, M. Tepel, K.H. Rahn, W. Zidek

Medizinische Poliklinik der Universität W-4400 Münster, Albert-Schweitzer-Str. 33, Germany

Summary

Using fluorescence indicators numerous measurements of intracellular free electrolyte content in lymphocytes and platelets have already been performed in patients with essential hypertension. Therefore it was of interest to develop a method to determine total Mg^{++} content in lymphocytes offering advantages for routine measurements as compared to fluorescence methods. Intracellular Mg^{++} measurements were performed in lymphocytes of 12 normotensive (NT), 18 essential hypertensive (EH) and 10 renal hypertensive (RH, patients with a chronic glomerulonephritis). Mg^{++} content was referred to lymphocytic protein, which was determined according to Bradford's method, using Coomassie Blue. Mg^{++} measurements were performed by atomic absorption spectroscopy (Video 12 apparatus, Thermo Electron, Dortmund, D). The results show that in patients with essential hypertension intralymphocytic Mg^{++} content is significantly lowered as compared to controls (0,07±0,05 versus 0,11±0,04 mmol Mg/g lymphocytic protein content, $p < 0,01$). In renal hypertensive patients intracellular Mg^{++} content was measured 0,35±0,12 mmol Mg/g lymphocytic protein content (means±SD), which was significantly increased as compared to normotensive or essential hypertensive patients ($p < 0,01$).

Key words: intracellular Mg^{++} - lymphocytes - essential and renal hypertension

Introduction

Mg^{++} has been implicated in the pathogenesis of essential hypertension. Whereas plasma Mg^{++} concentrations have often been investigated, comparatively few data on intracellular Mg^{++} concentrations are available. Furthermore the role of intracellular Mg^{++} content in essential hypertension is also controversely discussed. Decreased intracellular free Mg^{++} concentrations in erythrocytes have been described in essential hypertension (Resnick et al., 1984), whereas other authors were unable to confirm this finding (Woods et al., 1988). Therefore it was of interest to develop a method to determine total Mg^{++} content in lymphocytes offering advantages for routine measurements as compared to other methods.

Patients and methods

Patients: In 18 patients (10 males, 8 females, aged 52,1±9,8 years, blood pressure 177,1±14,3/104±13,7 mm Hg, means±SD) with essential hypertension, 10 renal hypertensives with chronic glomerulonephritis (5 males, 5 females, aged 49,5±8,5 years, blood pressure 182±11,7/111,4±7,9 mm Hg) and 12 normotensives (6 male, 6 female, aged 47,4±13,6 years, blood pressure 115,2±10,8/85,3±7,4 mm Hg) were studied. Methods: 20 ml heparinized blood was drawn of each patient. Lymphocytes were isolated by the density gradient method using Lymphoprep[R]. The suspension of lymphocytes was then washed twice in bidistilled water. For lysis of the cells, the suspension was frozen to -18°c and then rethawed. Thereafter, in the sample Mg^{++} concentration was determined by atomic absorption spectroscopy (Video 12 apparatus of Thermo Electron, Dortmund, D). Protein concentration was measured using the Coomassie Blue method. Lymphocytic Mg^{++} content was then expressed as mmol Mg/g lymphocytic protein content.

Results

Table 1. Intralymphocytic Mg^{++} concentrations in normotensive (NT), essential hypertensive (EH) and renal hypertensive patients (RH) (means±SD, mmol Mg^{++}/g lymphocytic protein content, *=p< 0,01).

		Mg^{++}	
NT	(n=12)	0,11±0,04	*
EH	(n=18)	0,07±0,05	*
RH	(n=10)	0,35±0,12	

The results show that in patients with essential hypertension intralymphocytic Mg^{++} content is significantly lowered as compared to controls (p< 0,01). In renal hypertensives intracellular Mg^{++} content is significantly increased as compared to normotensive or essential hypertensive patients (p< 0,01).

Discussion

Our data support Mg^{++} deficiency or a depletion of intracellular Mg^{++} in essential hypertension. Intralymphocytic Mg^{++} content is significantly lowered in essential hypertensives as compared to controls (p< 0,01). Determination of free intracellular Mg^{++} or intraerythrocytic Mg^{++} content is still controversely discussed (Resnick et al., 1984; Woods et al., 1988; Kjeldsen et al., 1989).
For this reason we developed a new method to determine total intracellular Mg^{++} content in lymphocytes, which may offer advantages for routine measurements. Furthermore an increased intracellular Mg^{++} content was found in renal hypertensive patients, due to renal insufficiency. The results obtained in renal hypertensives show that the decrease of lymphocytic Mg^{++} content is not an unspecific effect associated with arterial hypertension per se, but may be the consequence of a specific defect in transmembrane Mg^{++} transport.

References

Kjeldsen, S.E., Sejersted, O.M., Leren, F.P., Eide, I.K. (1989): Increased erythrocyte Mg^{++} in untreated essential hypertension. In Journal of Hypertension 7: 156-7.

Resnick, L.M., Gupta, R.K., Laragh, J.H. (1984): Intracellular free magnesium in erythrocytes of essential hypertension: relation to blood pressure and serum divalent cations. In Proc Natl Acad Sci USA 81: 6511-6515.

Woods, K.L., Walmsley, D., Heagerty, A.M., Turner, D.L., Lian, L.Y. (1988): ^{31}p nuclear magnetic resonance measurement of free erythrocyte magnesium concentration in man and its relation to blood pressure. In Clin Sci 74: 513-517.

Metal Ions in Biology and Medicine, vol. 2. Eds. J. Anastassopoulou, Ph. Collery, J.C. Etienne, Th. Theophanides. John Libbey Eurotext, Paris © 1992, pp. 232-233

Intracellular calcium concentrations in platelets of spontaneously hypertensive rats are increased by erythropoietin. Pathogenetic aspects of primary hypertension

M. Tepel, H. Wischniowski, K. Kisters, K.H. Rahn, W. Zidek

Med. Univ.-Poliklinik, University of Muenster, Albert-Schweitzer-Str. 33, W-4400 Muenster, Germany

Introduction:

Hypertension is a common side effect of erythropoietin (EPO) treatment of renal anemia (Raine, 1988). However, the mechanisms by which EPO increases blood pressure are still not completely understood. Recently it was reported that EPO-induced vasoconstriction of vascular resistance vessels was dependend on the presence of calcium (Heidenreich et al., 1991). On the other hand, there is considerable evidence of abnormal cellular calcium handling in hypertension. Several investigators have focused on impaired calcium metabolism as a pathogenic factor in the development of hypertension (Erne et al., 1984). The present investigation was undertaken to examine the different effects of EPO on cytosolic free calcium concentrations in intact blood platelets from spontaneously hypertensive and normotensive rats using the new fluorescent dye technique.

Methods:

Blood was collected from 9 spontaneously hypertensive rats (SHR) from Muenster strain, weighting 300-400 g, and 9 age-matched normotensive Wistar-Kyoto rats (WKY). Heparinized rat blood was centrifuged at 240 g for 15 minutes to obtain platelet rich plasma, which was centrifuged at 240 g for 20 minutes, and the platelet pellet resuspended in Hanks balanced salt solution containing 136 mM NaCl, 5.40 mM KCl, 0.44 mM KH_2PO_4, 0.34 mM Na_2HPO_4, 5.60 mM D-glucose and 1 mM $CaCl_2$. The platelet suspension was incubated with 1 μM fura-2-acetoxymethylester (Sigma, Deisenhofen, Germany) for 60 minutes at 37°C. After centrifugation at 240 g for 10 minutes to remove extraneous dye the platelet pellet was again resuspended in Hanks balanced salt solution. The fluorescence intensity of 1000 μl suspension of fura2 loaded platelets (100,000/μl) in a thermostatized quarz cuvette with constant stirring was measured in a Fluorescence Spectrophotometer Model F-2000 (Hitachi Ltd. Tokyo, Japan) with excitation wavelengths of 340 and 380 nm and an emission wavelength of 510 nm. Calcium concentrations in intact cells were obtained according to the established method described by Grynkiewicz et al. (1985). Prior to fluorescence measurements platelets were incubated with 250 U/ml EPO (Behringwerke, Marburg, Germany) for 30 minutes at 37°C. For statistical evaluation of the data Wilcoxon's test was used and two-tailed p values of less than 0.05 were considered to be significant.

Results:

In resting platelets cytosolic free calcium concentration was significantly higher in SHR compared to WKY (171.9 ± 21.5 nM vs 93.1 ± 19.7 nM, mean ± SEM, $p<0.05$, Fig. 1). Incubation with 250 U/ml EPO significantly increased cytosolic free calcium concentration in platelets of SHR to 197.5 ± 27.8 nM ($p<0.05$ compared to resting value). After preincubation with EPO cytosolic free calcium concentration was significantly higher in platelets of SHR compared to WKY (197.5 ± 21.5 nM vs 93.0 ± 20.0 nM, $p<0.01$, Fig. 1).

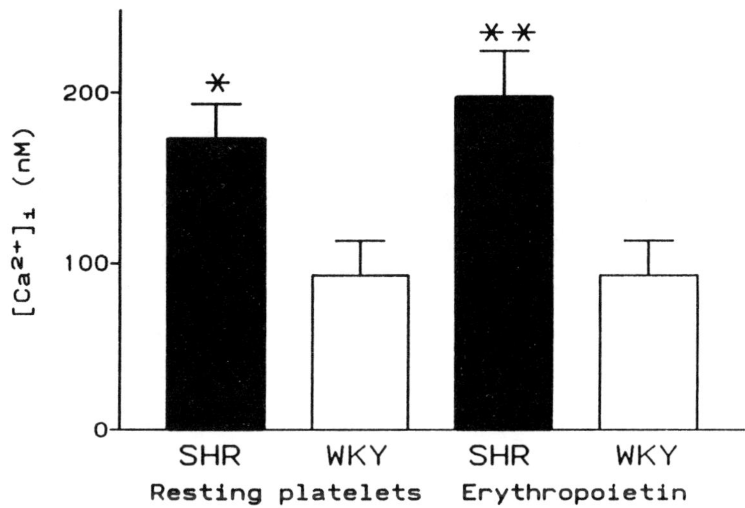

Fig. 1: Cytosolic free calcium concentration $[Ca^{2+}]_i$ in intact platelets from spontaneously hypertensive rats (SHR) and from normotensive Wistar-Kyoto rats (WKY) loaded with fura2. $[Ca^{2+}]_i$ (mean ± SEM) in resting platelets and after preincubation with 250 U/ml erythropoietin are shown. Significance levels (SHR vs WKY) are indicated: *$p<0.05$; **$p<0.01$.

Addition of 0.15 U/ml thrombin rapidly rised cytosolic free calcium concentration in platelets. Further, incubation with 250 U/ml EPO significantly increased thrombin induced changes of cytosolic free calcium concentration in platelets of SHR (306.6 ± 74.3 nM vs 193.6 ± 36.2 nM, $p<0.01$). In contrast, preincubation with 250 U/ml EPO had no effect on thrombin induced changes of cytosolic free calcium in platelets of WKY (135.3 ± 37.4 nM vs 111.9 ± 27.1 nM).

Discussion:

An increased cytosolic free calcium concentration was observed in intact platelets of SHR compared to WKY. This observation was confirmed by several investigators (Bruschi et al. 1984). Therefore it may be concluded that increased cytosolic free calcium concentration is a prerequisite in primary hypertension and may play an important role in the pathogenesis of hypertension.

In this study it was clearly demonstrated that EPO had different effects on cytosolic free calcium concentration in platelets from SHR and WKY. EPO increased cytosolic free calcium concentration and thrombin induced changes of cytosolic free calcium in platelets from SHR but not in platelets from WKY. Therefore it may be concluded that hypertensive cells are more sensitive to external stimuli causing increased cytosolic free calcium concentration.

References:

Bruschi, G., Bruschi, M.A., Caroppo, M., Orlandini, G., Spaggiari, M., and Cavatorta, A. (1985): Cytoplasmic free $[Ca^{2+}]$ is increased in the platelets of spontaneously hypertensive rats and essential hypertensive patients. Clin. Sci. 68, 179-184.

Erne, P., Bolli, P., Bürgisser, E., and Bühler, F.R. (1984): Correlation of platelet calcium with blood pressure. Effect of antihypertensive therapy. N. Engl. J. Med. 310, 1084-1088.

Grynkiewicz, G., Poenie, M., and Tsien, R.Y. (1985): A new generation of Ca^{2+} indicators with greatly improved fluorescence properties. J. Biol. Chem. 260, 3440-3450.

Heidenreich, S., Rahn, K.H., and Zidek, W (1991): Direct vasopressor effect of recombinant human erythropoietin on renal resistance vessels. Kidney Int. 39, 259-265.

Raine, A.E.G. (1988): Hypertension, blood viscosity, and cardiovascular morbidity in renal failure: implications of erythropoietin therapy. Lancet i, 97-100.

Metal Ions in Biology and Medicine, vol. 2. Eds. J. Anastassopoulou, Ph. Collery, J.C. Etienne, Th. Theophanides. John Libbey Eurotext, Paris © 1992, pp. 234-235

Importance of cytosolic free sodium and related sodium-transport-systems in the pathogenesis of primary hypertension

M. Tepel, S. Husseini, H. Wischniowski, K. Kisters, K.H. Rahn, W. Zidek

Med. Univ.-Poliklinik, University of Muenster, Albert-Schweitzer-Str. 33, W-4400 Muenster, Germany

Introduction:

Several abnormalities in sodium content and in sodium transport systems, e.g., Na-K-ATPase or Na-H-exchange, have been attributed to primary hypertension (Blaustein, 1984; Hilton, 1986). Further, changes of sodium-calcium-exchange may play an important role in the pathogenesis of primary hypertension. However, most of the experimental data on intracellular sodium content were based on measurements using destructed cells. In the present study the novel sodium-sensitive fluorescent dye sodium-binding-benzofuran-isophthalate (SBFI) was used for measurements of cytosolic free sodium concentrations in intact platelets from spontaneously hypertensive rats (SHR) and normotensive Wistar-Kyoto rats (WKY).

Methods:

Blood was collected from 13 SHR from Muenster strain, weighting 300-400 g, and 13 age-matched normotensive WKY. Heparinized rat blood was centrifuged at 240 g for 15 minutes to obtain platelet rich plasma, which was centrifuged at 240 g for 20 minutes, and the platelet pellet resuspended in Hanks balanced salt solution containing 136 mM NaCl, 5.40 mM KCl, 0.44 mM KH_2PO_4, 0.34 mM Na_2HPO_4, 5.60 mM D-glucose, 1 mM $CaCl_2$ and 10 mM N-2-hydroxyethyl-piperazine-N'-2-ethanesulfonic acid, pH 7.4. Measurements of cytosolic free sodium concentrations using the fluorescent dye technique were performed according to recently described methods (Harootunian et al., 1989; Borin and Siffert, 1990). Briefly, the platelet suspension was incubated with 3 μM SBFI-acetoxymethylester (Calbiochem, Frankfurt, Germany) and 0.1% (w/v) non-ionic detergent Pluronic F-127 (Molecular Probes, Eugene, USA) for 60 minutes at 37°C. After centrifugation at 240 g for 10 minutes to remove extraneous dye the platelet pellet was again resuspended in Hanks balanced salt solution. The fluorescence intensity of 1000 μl suspension of SBFI loaded platelets (100,000/μl) in a thermostatized quarz cuvette with constant stirring was measured in a Fluorescence Spectrophotometer Model F-2000 (Hitachi Ltd. Tokyo, Japan) with excitation wavelengths of 340 and 385 nm and an emission wavelength of 500 nm. The fluorescence excitation ratio at 340/385 nm was calculated. The excitation ratio was calibrated in terms of cytosolic free sodium concentration in situ on each platelet preparation by equilibration of intracellular sodium content with known extracellular sodium concentrations in the presence of ionophors. For statistical evaluation of the data Wilcoxon's test was used and two-tailed p values of less than 0.05 were considered to be significant.

Results:

Resting cytosolic free sodium concentrations were not significantly different in intact platelets of SHR and WKY (21.9 ± 4.6 mM vs 13.8 ± 2.3 mM, mean ± SEM, Fig. 1). Inhibition of Na-K-ATPase by 1 mM ouabain for 30 minutes significantly rised cytosolic free sodium concentration in platelets of SHR (38.3 ± 5.3 mM, $p<0.01$ compared to resting value) and in platelets of WKY (24.1 ± 3.7 mM, $p<0.01$). However, no differences could be observed between SHR and WKY in regard to inhibition of Na-K-ATPase (Fig. 1).
Activation of Na-H-exchange by 0.15 U/ml thrombin increased cytosolic free sodium concentration in SHR by 23.9 ± 4.4 mM and in WKY by 37.0 ± 5.5 mM, showing no significant differences.

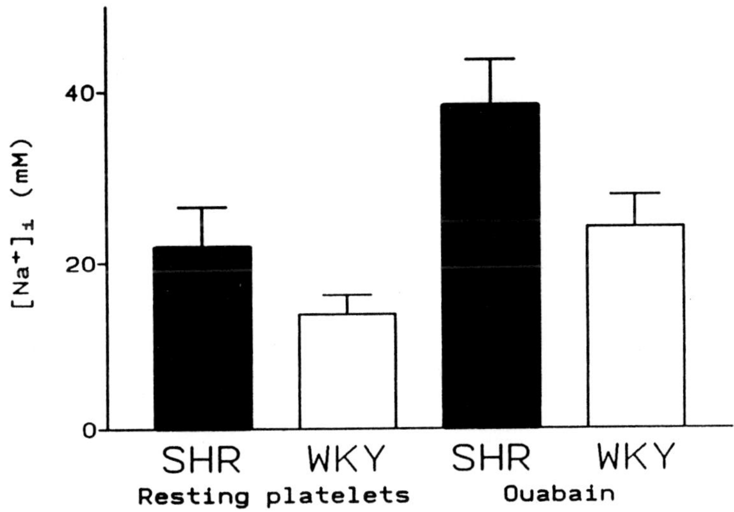

Fig. 1: Cytosolic free sodium concentration $[Na^+]_i$ in intact platelets of spontaneously hypertensive rats (SHR) and normotensive Wistar-Kyoto rats (WKY). $[Na^+]_i$ (mean ± SEM) in platelets loaded with sodium-binding-benzofuran-isophthalate at resting state and 30 minutes after incubation with 1 mM ouabain are shown.

Discussion:

In the present study the novel fluorescent dye technique was used to obtain cytosolic free sodium concentrations in intact cells of SHR and WKY. In contrast to previous measurements in destructed cells there was no significant difference of resting cytosolic free sodium concentrations between SHR and WKY. In addition, it was shown that neither Na-K-ATPase nor Na-H-exchange were altered in primary hypertension. These new data indicate that the role of sodium in the pathogenesis of hypertension need to be reinvestigated in intact cells.

References:

Blaustein, M.P. (1984): Sodium transport and hypertension. Where are we going? Hypertension 6, 445-453.

Borin, M. and Siffert, W. (1990): Stimulation by thrombin increases the cytosolic free Na^+ concentration in human platelets. J. Biol. Chem. 265, 19543-19559.

Harootunian, A.T., Kao, J.P.Y., Eckert, B.K., and Tsien, R.Y. (1989): Fluorescence ratio imaging of cytosolic free Na in individual fibroblasts and lymphocytes. J. Biol. Chem. 264, 19449-19457.

Hilton, P.J. (1986): Cellular sodium transport in essential hypertension. N. Engl. J. Med. 314, 222-229.

Metal Ions in Biology and Medicine, vol. 2. Eds. J. Anastassopoulou, Ph. Collery, J.C. Etienne, Th. Theophanides. John Libbey Eurotext, Paris © 1992, pp. 236-237

Effects of different sodium salts on blood pressure in spontaneously hypertensive rats (SHR)

P. Laurant, * P. Lambropoulos, E. Gaillard, A. Berthelot

*Laboratoire Physiologie Pharmacie, UFR Médecine et Pharmacie, 25030 Besançon Cedex, France. * Hydroxydase Société des Eaux Minérales Naturelles, 63340 Le Breuil-sur-Couze, France*

Sodium (Na) intake has been found to be implicated in the increase of blood pressure and in the development of arterial hypertension (HTA). However, some workers have shown that only Na as the chloride salt (NaCl) increased blood pressure while Na given with other anions did not (Kurtz and Morris, 1983 ; Kurz and al, 1987 ; Luft and al, 1988 ; 1990). These findings have some interest in public health because some european mineral waters contains high levels of Na in different salt forms as the bicarbonate salt ($NaHCO_3$) (Wollbeck, 1986). So, it is of interest to study the effect of one such mineral water on the development of HTA in SHR.

Methods : Male SHR (4 weeks old) were randomized in 4 groups. One control group was given demineralized water (C). One group was given mineral water Hydroxydase containing high Na level (1945 mg/l) (group H). Two groups were given equimolar amounts of Na as NaCl (group A) and as $NaHCO_3$ (group B) in demineralized water. Blood pressure was determined by tail cuff method in unanesthetized and prewarmed rats during 10 weeks. Na and K levels were determined in plasma and urine by flame photometry at 3 and 9 weeks of treatment.

Results : After 4 weeks of treatment, systolic blood pressure was significantly higher in group A and was lower in groups B and H as compared to blood pressure in group C (Fig. 1). These changes in blood pressure levels were not associated with changes in natremia at any stage of experimentation while kalemia was significantly higher ($p < 0.05$) in group A (5.24 ± 0.06 mM) as compared to group C (4.83 ± 0.12 mM) and kaliemia was significantly lower ($p < 0.001$) in group B (4.65 ± 0.11 mM) and in group H (4.50 ± 0.10 mM) as compared to group A. The administration of Na as NaCl, $NaHCO_3$ or mineral water Hydroxydase resulted in higher urinary excretion of Na at 3 weeks (1.70 ± 0.13 mM in group A ; 1.65 ± 0.09 mM in group B ; 1.52 ± 0.02 mM in group H) as compared to group C (0.56 ± 0.02 mM). Since urinary excretion of Na remained elevated at 9 weeks in SHR receiving Na-containing drinking waters, natriuresis was found to be more higher ($p < 0.001$) in group A (1.48 ± 0.08 mM) as compared to group B (0.96 ± 0.07 mM) and group H (1.02 ± 0.05 mM). At 3 weeks, kaliuresis was significantly decreased in group A (0.63 ± 0.07 mM, $p > 0.001$) and significantly increased in group B (1.26 ± 0.10 mM, $p < 0.05$) and in group H (1.25 ± 0.05, $p < 0.05$) as compared to group C (1.03 ± 0.06 mM). However, after 9 weeks, the urinary excretion of K was significantly increased in group A (0.87 ± 0.03 mM, $p < 0.01$) and in group H (0.88 ± 0.04 mM, $p < 0.01$) but was not change in group B (0.68 ± 0.05 mM) as compared to control group C (0.72 ± 0.03 mM).

Discussion : Drinking water containing NaCl increased blood pressure while drinking water containing $NaHCO_3$ attenuated the development of HTA in SHR. In addition, we found that mineral water Hydroxydase attenuated the development of HTA in the same manner that $NaHCO_3$ dit it. Since mineral water Hydroxydase contains high levels of Na as $NaHCO_3$ salt, it is suggested that the decrease in blood pressure levels in Hydroxydase-treated rats could be mediated by $NaHCO_3$. The decrease in blood pressure induced by $NaHCO_3$-containing drinking waters is not accompanied by an enhanced natriuresis. On the contrary, after 9 weeks, natriuresis was found to be lower in these 2 groups as compared to the group receiving NaCl. Since kaliuresis was increased and kaliemia was decreased in groups B and H, it is suggested a leak of K in rats receiving $NaHCO_3$ and Hydroxydase. Na retention and urinary K leak seem to be incompatible with the decrease in blood pressure of Hydroxydase -and $NaHCO_3$- treated rats. So, the mechanisms by which $NaHCO_3$ and mineral water Hydroxydase operate to decrease blood pressure in SHR remain unknown.

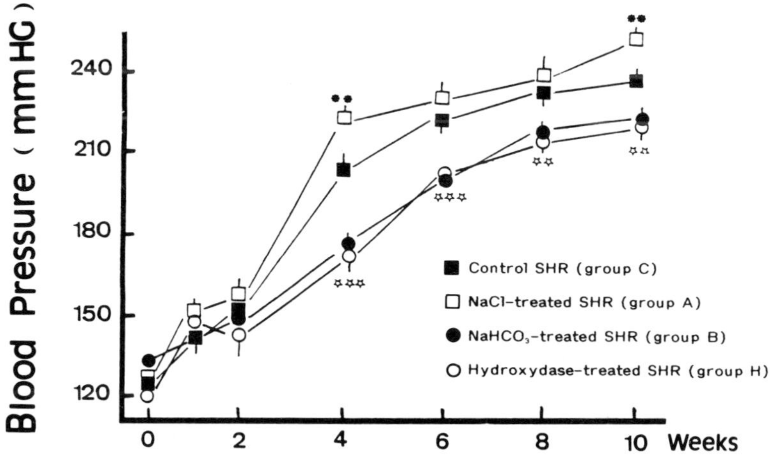

Fig. 1 : Blood pressure levels during 10 weeks of experiment in SHR.
**$p < 0,01$ group A vs group C
☆☆$p < 0,01$, ☆☆☆$p < 0,001$ groups B and H vs group C

References :

Kurtz, T.W., and Morris, R.C. (1983) : Dietary chloride as a determinant of "sodium-dependent" hypertension. Science 222 : 1139-1141.

Kurtz, T.W., Al-Bander, H.A., and Morris, R.C. (1987) : "Salt-sensitive" essential hypertension in men : is the sodium ion alone important ? N. Engl. J. Med. 317 : 1043-1048.

Luft, F.C., Steinberg, H., Ganten, U., Meuer, D., Gless, K.H., Lang, R.E., Fineberg, N.S., Rascher, W., Unger, T., and Ganten, D. (1988) : Effect of sodium chloride and sodium bicarbonate on blood pressure in stroke prone spontaneously hypertensive rats. Clin. Sci. 74 : 577-585.

Luft, F.C., Zemel, M.B., Sowers, J.A., Fineberg, N.S., and Weinberger, M.H. (1990) : Sodium bicarbonate and sodium chloride: effect on blood pressure and electrolyte homeostasis in normal and hypertensive man. J. Hypertens. 8 : 663-670.

Wollbeck, D. (1986) : Mineral und Heilwaesser in der natriunmarmen Ernaeherung. Ernaeherung-Umschau 33 : 389-392.

Metal Ions in Biology and Medicine, vol. 2. Eds. J. Anastassopoulou, Ph. Collery, J.C. Etienne, Th. Theophanides. John Libbey Eurotext, Paris © 1992, pp. 238-239

Serum aluminium : epidemiological features of its toxicity on hemodialysis patients

A. Garcia de Jalon Comet, M. Gonzalez Enguita, D. Zapatero Gonzalez, M.L. Calvo Ruata, J. Perez Perez*

Unidad de Nutrición y Metales, Servicios de Bioquímica Clínica y Nefrología, Hospital Miguel Servet, INSALUD, Zaragoza, España*

The syndrome of aluminum (Al) toxicity is now well recognized in patients with chronic renal failure (CRF), particularly those treated by hemodialysis (HD). In this population group, sources of aluminum intoxication are more important and effective. In adittion, excess aluminum, ordinarily eliminated by the kidneys (main excretion pathway), cannot occur in the dialysis patients. So, striking elevations of serum aluminum concentrations occur, with an important toxicity risk.

METHODS AND MATERIALS.

In our hospital, we measured and evaluated serum aluminum concentrations in 71 patients with CRF undergoing maintenance hemodialysis (47 males and 24 females). They were 50 ± 15.6 (mean ± SD) years of age, ranging from 18 to 73 years. They had been on maintenance hemodialysis for 4 to 168 months (53 ± 39.2).

Dialysis was perfomed for four hours three times a week. All patients were prescribed oral antacids containing aluminum hidroxide as a phosphate binder for the duration of their long-term dialysis. They all were treated with a dialysate containing negligible amounts of aluminum (less than 10 μg/l).

Serum aluminum levels and dialysis fluid aluminum content were measured by flameless atomic absorption spectrophotometry (graphite furnace HGA-700, autosampler AS-70), using a single beam spectrophotometer (Perkin-Elmer®, model 1100-B), with deuterium background corrector.

RESULTS.

Control group (n= 74):
Serum Al levels were 8.36 ± 2.74 μg/l (range: 2-14 μg/l). There were no significant differences according to sex (Table 1). We have found, however, a positive correlation between serum Al levels and age ($r = 0.283$; $p = 0.015$) (there was a significant serum Al increase proportional to the increase of age).

HD patients (n= 71):
Serum Al levels in the 71 chronic HD patients were 44.33±41.61 μg/l (range: 2-190 μg/l), much higher than in controls ($p < 0.001$) (Table 1). There was no relation, neither with sex (males: 43.91 ± 35.58; females: 45.33 ± 52.20) nor different groups of age ($p = 0.649$).

Table 1.- Serum Al values ($\mu g/l$)

	Patients on HD	Controls
Mean serum Al:	44.39 ± 41.57* (range: 2-190)	8.01 ± 3.56* (range: 2-14)
• Males	(n = 47): 43.91 ± 35.6	(n = 40): 7.8 ± 3.49
• Females	(n = 24): 45.33 ± 52.2	(n = 34): 8.26 ± 3.69

* p= 0.0001

We have found (figs.1 and 2) however, a positive correlation between serum aluminum levels and length of dialysis (r = 0.34; p = 0.0039).

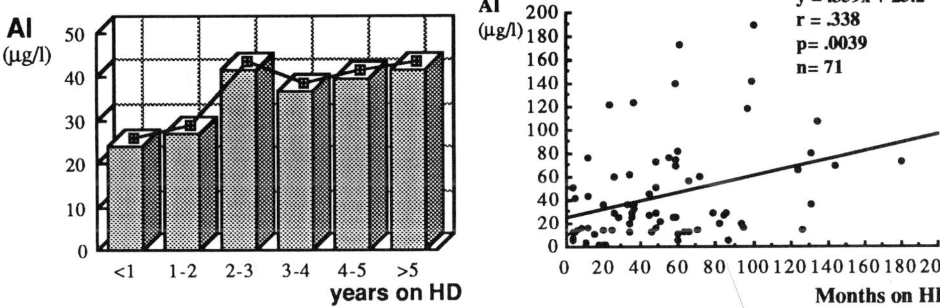

Fig.1.- Serum aluminum and length of dialysis.

Fig.2.- Relationship of serum Al level to months of dialysis therapy.

In adittion, a statistically significant relationship between serum Al levels and the amount of daily ingested aluminum hydroxide ($Al(OH_3)$) (Fig.3), was found (r = 0.26; p = 0.0287).

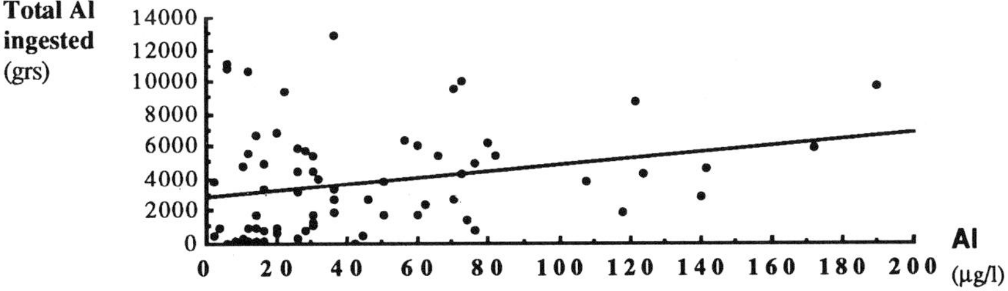

Fig.3.- Serum Al levels and total aluminum hydroxide ingested in HD patients.

BIBLIOGRAPHY:

1.- **Cannata JB, Serrano M, Fernández I, Fernández JL, Olaizola I.** (1989): Minimizing the risk of oral aluminum exposure in chronic renal failure. In: Traeger J, Cantarovich F, Olmer M. (eds.) : Present-day concepts in the treatment of chronic renal failure. Contrib. Nephrol. Basel, Karger, vol 71, pp 81-89.

2.- **D'Haese PC, Van de Vyver FL, De Wolff FA, De Broe ME.** (1985): Measurement of aluminum in serum, blood, urine and tissue of chronic hemodialysed patients by use of electrothermal atomic absorption spectrometry. Clin. Chem. 31, 24-29.

3.- **McCarthy J, Milliner D, Kurtz S, Johnson W, Moyer Th.** (1986): Interpretation of serum aluminum values in dialysis patients. Am. J. Clin. Pathol. 86, 629-636.

4.- **Van de Vyver FL, Silva FJ, D'Haese PC, Verbueken AH, De Broe ME.** (1987): Aluminum toxicity in dialysis patients. Contrib. Nephrol. 55, 198-220.

Metal Ions in Biology and Medicine, vol. 2. Eds. J. Anastassopoulou, Ph. Collery, J.C. Etienne, Th. Theophanides. John Libbey Eurotext, Paris © 1992, pp. 240-241

Comparison of a hemoperfusion charcoal filter versus a hemofiltration dialyzer for reducing blood levels of cis-platinum

Peter S. Turk, James F. Belliveau*, James W. Darnowski, Harold J. Wanebo

*Brown University/Roger Williams Medical Center, Providence, RI 02908, USA and *Providence College, Providence, RI, 02918, USA*

The removal of drugs and poisons by extracorporeal hemofiltration and hemoperfusion spans the last four decades and is used in the treatment of overdoses/poisonings (Culter et al., 1987) and regional arterial infusion chemotherapy (Dedrick et al., 1984). The technology of extracorporeal devices has advanced to where one primarily chooses between commercially available hollow tube dialysis membrane hemofiltration units (Muchmore et al., 1991) or coated charcoal hemoperfusion cartridges (Cohan et al., 1982). Comparison studies indicate that hemoperfusion is more effective than hemofiltration with many organic compounds and also, with limited data, suggest the same result for chelated metal ions (Cutler et al., 1987; Winchester, 1984). The specific aim of this research is to evaluate these two extracorporeal techniques using regional (pelvic) intra-arterial chemotherapy for the inorganic cancer chemotherapeutic agent, cis-platinum, and compare the results to a representative organic drug, 5-fluorouracil.

MATERIALS AND METHODS

Commercially available hemoperfusion charcoal cartridges (Alukart, 01-6003-6) and hemofiltration cellulose acetate hollow fiber dialyzers (Travenol, CL*M151L) were used to evaluate the in vivo reduction of drug blood levels. Three experimental protocols were compared in a canine model using 30 minute infusions of both cis-platinum (40 mg/m^2) and 5-fluorouracil (400 & 1600 mg/m^2): 1) regional (pelvic) intra-arterial chemotherapy via the infrarenal aorta without extracorporeal removal (RIA); 2) regional (pelvic) intra-arterial chemotherapy with concomitant hemoperfusion via an infrarenal aorta-IVC circuit for 60 minutes (RIAC-HP); and 3) regional (pelvic) intra-arterial chemotherapy with concomitant hemofiltration via an infrarenal aorta-IVC circuit for 60 minutes (RIAC-HF).

Blood and dialysis filtrate samples were collected at various times after the start of drug infusion in dogs (22-32 kg) at the large animal operating facilities at Brown University. Samples were stored at -20°C until analyzed. Samples were assayed for platinum content using conventional 3-electrode d-c argon plasma emission spectroscopy (Forastiere, et al., 1988) and for 5-fluorouracil by HPLC (Darnowski et al., 1985). Efficiencies of the hemoperfusion charcoal cartridge and hemofiltration dialysis membrane were evaluated as the % decrease of drug plasma blood levels immediately before entering and after exiting the filter or membrane.

RESULTS AND DISCUSSION

Table 1. presents data which show that the hemoperfusion charcoal filter is more efficient at removing both cis-platinum and 5-fluorouracil than the hemofiltration dialysis membrane. The removal efficiency data for the dialysis membrane correlated with the percentage of total drug recovered in the filtrate. Sixteen percent of the cis-platinum (range 12-18%, n=2) and ten per cent of the 5-fluorouracil (range 8.4-12%, n=2) were recovered in the dialysis filtrate over a one hour period from the beginning of drug infusion. These relative drug removal efficiencies resulted in remote systemic platinum levels for RIAC-HP being 1/3 those of RIA, versus those for RIAC-HF being 2/3 those of RIA during the 60-minute period after the start of drug infusion. The efficiency of the hemoperfusion charcoal cartridge decreases with time for cis-platinum compared to the organic drug, 5-fluorouracil, probably due to the combined effects of protein binding and conversion to ionic forms of the platinum complex, both platinum species having decreased binding capabilities on the coated charcoal surface. Thirty minutes after the completion of cis-platinum infusion with the hemoperfusion cartridge, a negative efficiency of -13% was obtained which may mean that the charcoal surface was acting as a source of drug as blood levels decreased after drug administration. The binding of cis-platinum to the charcoal surface appears to be controlled by kinetic rather than thermodynamic factors, in that, a 1st order half-life of adsorption of 16 minutes was obtained in a static, in vitro system with 100 ml of 54 ppm cis-platinum in saline being put in contact with 6.0 gms of coated charcoal (comparable values to the canine system for aqueous plasma volume, cis-platinum concentration and charcoal mass).

Given the above results with cis-platinum, the hemoperfusion system is more efficient in rapidly removing metal ion complexes than the hemofiltration system. The hemoperfusion system is also simpler to use, in that, it does not need a filtrate removal mechanism or a substitution fluid mechanism. Also, drug removal efficiencies can be easily decreased by decreasing the flow through the charcoal cartridge relative the systemic flow or increased by putting charcoal cartridges in parallel or tandem. Thus the commercial hemoperfusion system seems preferred over the hemofiltration system for regulating levels of metal ion complexes.

Table 1. In vivo removal efficiencies of cis-platinum and 5-fluorouracil by hemoperfusion charcoal filters and hemodialysis dialysis membranes.

	Dose (mg/m^2)	Removal Efficiency after 5 minutes into infusion	Removal Efficiency at end of infusion (30 min)
Charcoal Filter			
cis-platinum	40	84 % (n=8)	31 % (n=8)
5-fluorouracil	400	80 % (n=5)	75 % (n=5)
5-fluorouracil	1600	83 % (n=3)	86 % (n=3)
Dialysis Membrane			
cis-platinum	40	13 % (n=3)	11 % (n=3)
5-fluorouracil	1600	5 % (n=2)	10 % (n=2)

ACKNOWLEDGEMENTS

The following students at Providence College assisted in this research: Sheila Fitzpatrick and Leslie Kelly. Thanks are extended to Elizabeth Kill and the personnel at the Chemistry and Materials Laboratories of Texas Instruments, Inc., Attleboro, MA 02703 for permission to use their plasma emission spectrometers and for their invaluable technical assistance.

REFERENCES

Cohen, S.L., Winchester, J.F. and Gelfand, M.C. (1982): Treatment of intoxication with charcoal hemoperfusion. *Drug Metabolism Reviews* 13, 681-693.

Cutler, R.E., Forland, S.C., St. John Hammond, P.G. and Evans, J.R. (1987): Extracorporeal removal of drugs and poisons by hemodialysis and hemoperfusion. *Ann. Rev. Pharmacol. Toxicol.* 27, 161-191.

Darnowski, J.W., Sawyer, R.C., Stolfi, R.L., Martin, D.S. and Lau-Cam, C.A. (1985): Decreased host toxicity in vivo during chronic treatment with 5-fluorouracil. *Cancer Chemother. Pharmacol.* 14, 63-69.

Dedrick, R.L., Oldfield, E.H. and Collins, J.M. (1984): Arterial drug infusion with extracorporeal removal. I. Theoretical basis with particular reference to the brain. *Cancer Treat. Rep.* 68, 373-380.

Forastiere, A.A., Belliveau, J.F., Goren, M., Vogel, W.C., Posner, M.C. and O'Leary, G.P. (1988): Pharmacokinetic and toxicity evaluation of five-day continuous infusion versus intermittent bolus cis-diamminedichloropaltinum (II) in head and neck cancer patients. *Cancer Res.* 48, 3869-3874.

Muchmore, J.H., Krementz, E.T. Carter, R.D., Preslan, J.E. and George, W.J. (1991): Treatment of abdominal malignant neoplasms using regional chemotherapy with hemofiltration. *Arch. Surg.* 126, 1390-1396.

Winchester, J.F. (1984): Poisoning-active treatment methods. *Dialysis & Transplantation* 13, 21-24.

Metal Ions in Biology and Medicine, vol. 2. Eds. J. Anastassopoulou, Ph. Collery, J.C. Etienne, Th. Theophanides. John Libbey Eurotext, Paris © 1992, pp. 242-243

Influence of furosemide and ramipril on the cisplatinum-induced nephrotoxicity

Erik Klaus, Horst Grötsch, Max Hropot

Hoechst AG, POB 800320, W-6230 Frankfurt am Main 80, Germany

Cisplatinum (Cp) is widely used for cancer chemotherapy, but like other heavy metals, it has an associated dose-limiting nephrotoxic effect. It has been shown in rats that after 3 to 5 days Cp treatment histopathological changes are the most profound, predominantly in the straight portion of the renal proximal tubule (Safirstein et al., 1981). It was suggested that urinary glutathione-S-transferase is a marker for proximal renal tubular injury from Cp (Feinfeld et al., 1981). Moreover, increased urinary alanine-aminopeptidase (AAP) and gamma glutamyl-transpeptidase (GGT) have been also found in rats treated with Cp and simultaneous administration of Cp and furosemide even worsen the enzymuria (Scholz et al., 1984). The aim of this study was to examine the interaction between Cp, furosemide and the ACE inhibitor ramipril with regard to enzymuria during multiple treatment and recovery periods. It has been well established that ACE inhibitors not only decrease elevated systemic blood pressure, but also reduce overt proteinuria and may retard the progression of renal disease (Keane et al., 1989).

METHODS

Experiments were performed in 36 male Wistar rats with an initial body weight of about 170 g and were placed in single metabolism cages with free access to food and tap water. The rats were randomized in 6 groups and urine was collected daily (24-hour urine samples). During a run-in period of 3 days initial values of each group were evaluated on the day before treatment. Thereafter the rats were treated with vehicle (control), Cp (1.5 mg/kg intravenously), furosemide (128 mg/kg orally), ramipril (0.5 mg/kg orally) and with combinations of all three drugs on 4 consecutive days. After the treatment period a recovery period of 4 days followed and four 24 hour samples were collected again. The following parameters were determined in the urine: volume, AAP, GGT, N-acetylglucosaminidase (NAG), lactate dehydrogenase (LDH), electrolytes, protein, creatinine and osmolality. For statistical evaluation the median and the standard error of the median of each group were calculated.

RESULTS AND DISCUSSION

As shown in Fig. 1 furosemide, as a loop diuretic, caused pronounced excretion of urine (A) and AAP (C) as compared to control and ramipril group, whereas the urinary excretion of protein (B) and GGT (D) was not changed in these groups. The groups treated with furosemide and Cp showed an additional increase in all urinary parameters. The nephrotoxic effect of Cp was still present in the recovery period as indicated by diuresis (A) and GGT deficiency (D). However, in Cp groups the addition of ramipril exerted slight protective effects concerning urinary protein (B) and AAP output (C). In this acute study, all other parameters mentioned in methods were not influenced in groups where ramipril was present.

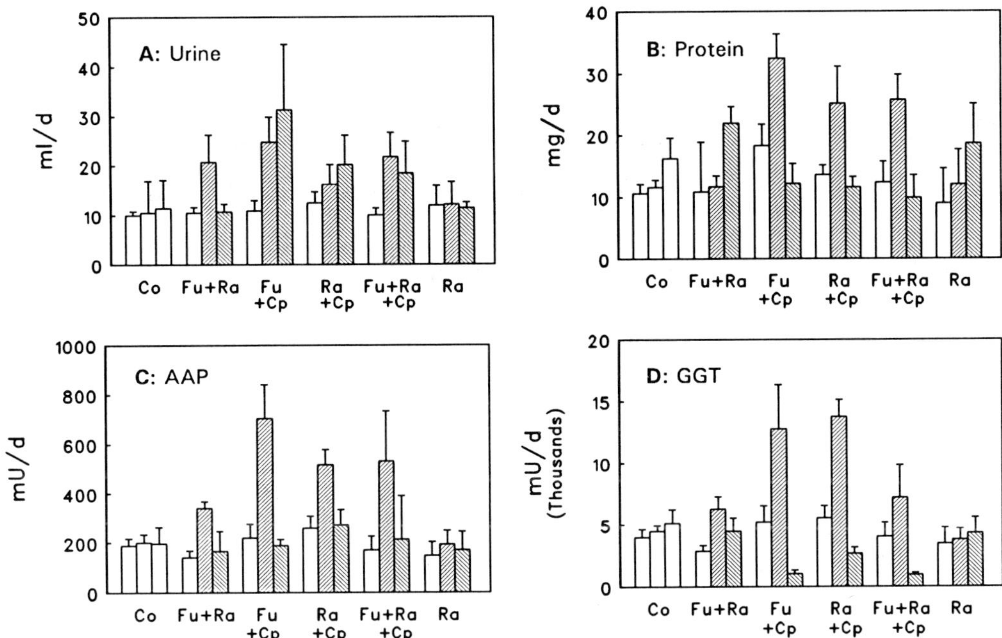

Fig. 1. Excretion of urine (**A**) and urinary protein (**B**), AAP (**C**), and GGT (**D**) in rats treated with vehicle (Co), furosemide (Fu), ramipril (Ra), and cisplatinum (Cp). The bars of each group from left to right display the means of initial values, of the treatment and of the recovery periods. For the calculation of treatment and recovery periods the values from the third and fourth day were included, respectively. [Medians ± standard errors of the medians, n = 6].

The results demonstrate enhanced effects of the combined treatment with Cp and furosemide on the urinary excretion of the enzymes AAP, GGT, NAG and LDH (data of NAG and LDH not shown in Fig. 1). Persistent high-level diuresis in the recovery period in groups where Cp was present indicates a disturbance of renal concentrating mechanism (Safirstein et al., 1981). Furosemide was shown to reinforce the injurious effect of Cp on the proximal tubule, probably because of the interaction of both compounds at the secretion site, indicating prolonged retention of Cp in the kidney (Choie et al., 1980). Several studies suggest, that ACE inhibitors may retard the progression of diabetic nephropathy. Moreover, in the present study there was a moderate reduction of Cp-induced nephrotoxicity by the addition of ramipril. It is very likely that a prolongation of the experiment would deliver more conclusive results.

REFERENCES

Choie, D.D., Delcampo, A.A., Guarino, A.M. (1980): Subcellular localisation of cis-dichlorodiamine-platinum(II) in rat kidney and liver. *Toxicol. Appl. Pharmacol.* **55**, 245-252.

Feinfeld, D.A., Fleischner, G.M., and Arias, I.M. (1981): Urinary ligandin and glutathione-S-transferase in gentamicin-induced nephrotoxicity in the rat. *Clin. Sci.* **61**, 123-125.

Keane, W.F., Anderson, S., Aurell, M., de Zeeuw, D., Narins, R.G., and Povar, G. (1989): Angiotensin converting enzyme inhibitors and progressive renal insufficiency. *Ann. Intern. Med.* **111**, 503-516.

Safirstein, R., Miller, P., Dikman, S., Leyman, N., and Chapiro, C. (1981): Cisplatinum nephrotoxicity in rats - defect in papillary hypertonicity. *Amer. J. Physiol.* **241**, F175-F185.

Scholz, W., Grötsch, H., Hropot, M. Kief, H., and Klaus, E. (1984): Enhancement of cis-platinum-induced emzymuria by furosemide in rats. *Human Toxicology* **3**, 447.

5 PHARMACOLOGY TOXICOLOGY

Metal Ions in Biology and Medicine, vol. 2. Eds. J. Anastassopoulou, Ph. Collery, J.C. Etienne, Th. Theophanides. John Libbey Eurotext, Paris © 1992, pp. 247-252

Metal ions from the environment to the function in living organisms

I. Bertini, L. Messori

Laboratorio di Chimica Inorganica e Bioinorganica, Universita' degli Studi di Firenze, via G. Capponi 7, 50121 Firenze, Italia

ABSTRACT
The roles of metal ions in living systems are discussed, particular focus being given to the structure and function of metalloproteins. Examples of metalloproteins with either electron transfer or catalytic functions are illustrated. The processes through which transition metal ions are incorporated in living organisms and the strategies for metal uptake are described.

METAL IONS: ROLES IN BIOLOGICAL SYSTEMS

Metal ions are essential for living processes (Bertini et al., 1992b). Intra and intercellular communications rest largely on the concentration gradients of potassium, sodium and calcium; blood clotting and muscle contraction depend on calcium concentrations; the capture of light depends on the magnesium containing pigment chlorophyll; electron transfer processes are mainly based on iron proteins; oxidative metabolism is almost always dependent on iron and copper catalysts; transport of oxygen requires iron and copper proteins; the capture of nitrogen is obtained through the intervention of complex metal clusters containing iron, molibdenum, and, sometimes, vanadium; the zinc fingers play an important role in the regulation of DNA transcription. Metal ions have been integrated in biomolecules and biological processes at such an extent that we cannot even think of life in the absence of metals. Here we will give some insights into the structural complexity of metalloproteins and its relationship to function, and will survey the processes through which transition metal ions are extracted from the environment and integrated in the biological macromolecules.

EVOLUTION AND METALLOPROTEINS

The actual structure of metalloproteins, the one that we find today in higher organisms, is the result of an evolutionary process which took billion years. The ultimate goal of the process has been that of constructing more and more efficient and specialized biomolecular machines which could take advantage of the favourable and unique chemical properties of metal ions. As their efficiency increased, these biochemical machines have become increasingly complex from a structural point of view. The present structures have been achieved thanks to the extraordinary versatility of the organic matter, i.e. to the possibility of obtaining a virtually infinite number of primary sequences starting from a limited number of building blocks. Biological efficiency has been the driving force of this evolution.

Proteins have evolved in such a way to generate architecturally composite structures consisting of the assembly of β–sheets, α–helices, turns and loops, capable of accomodating individual metals, or even cluster of metals, in functionally appropriate environments. The chemical properties of the region surrounding the metal center(s) play a key role in modulating the overall reactivity. Indeed, at variance with metal ions and coordination compounds in solution, metal ions in metalloproteins are located well inside a polypeptide chain which provides the ligands and tunes the hydrophobic or hydrophylic character of the region around them, the local electric fields and the acid base properties. It follows that the reactivity of metal ions in the active site of proteins may be completely changed with respect to the conventional solution chemistry. The iron sulfur proteins containing the Fe_4S_4 cluster, and the zinc enzyme carboxypeptidase are good examples to demonstrate the peculiarity of metal ion chemistry inside the active site of proteins.

IRON SULFUR PROTEINS WITH A Fe_4S_4 CLUSTER.

Let us consider the general organization of the iron sulfur proteins containing the Fe_4S_4 cluster, namely ferredoxins and high potential iron sulfur proteins (HIPIPs). The structure of the Fe_4S_4 cluster and its linkage to the protein backbone is shown in Figure 1. Probably, in both types of proteins, the cluster serves as an electron transfer center.

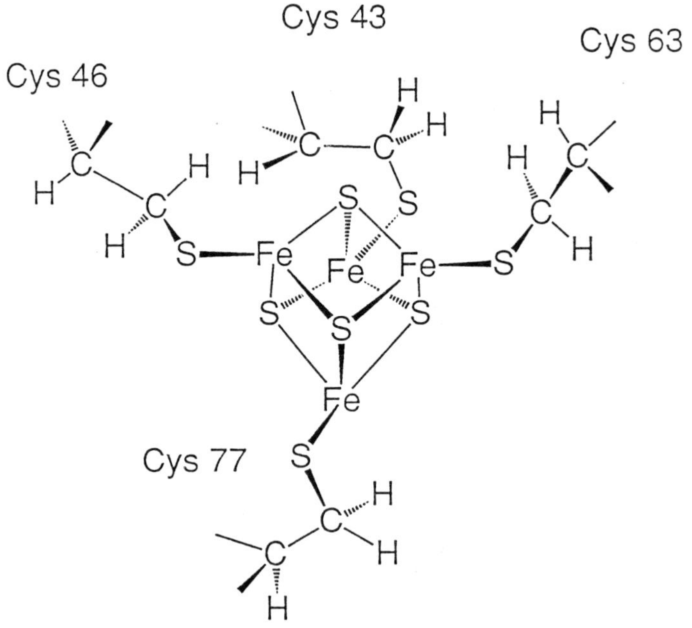

Figure 1. Schematic drawing of the Fe_4S_4 cluster.

The formal oxidation states of the iron ions in the Fe_4S_4 cluster of HIPIP correspond to three Fe(III) and one Fe(II) in the oxidized state and two Fe(III) and two Fe(II) in the reduced state. The reduction potentials range from 450 to 250 mV. On the contrary, in ferredoxins, formally we find two Fe(III) and two Fe(II) in the oxidized state and three Fe(II) and one Fe(III) in the reduced state. The reduction potential is around –400 mV.

The redox properties of Fe_4S_4 iron sulfur proteins have been rationalized in terms of three accessible oxidation states, the upper two of which would correspond to the redox couple of HIPIP and the lower two to the redox couple of ferredoxin.

^1H NMR studies, together with Mossbauer results, have provided a deeper insight into the electronic structure of these fascinating clusters permitting the accurate determination of the magnetic coupling interactions (Bertini et al., 1991; Bertini et al., 1992a). In oxidized HIPIP there is a mixed valence pair with oxidation state +2.5; the other two iron ions are in the oxidation state +3. From inspection of the X–ray structure it appears that the cluster is at the surface of an hydrophobic region. The mixed valence iron pair and one iron(III) ion are partially exposed to the solvent; the other iron(III) ion is completely buried. Upon reduction, a cluster corresponding to that of oxidized ferredoxin is obtained: all the iron ions are in the 2.5 oxidation state with apparent electronic delocalization, at least pairwise. The ground state is S=0.

The electronic situation of oxidized ferredoxin is virtually equivalent to that of reduced HIPIP. At variance, reduced ferredoxins have been studied at a lesser extent; it appears, however, that in the latter species there is a pair with a 2.5 oxidation state plus two isolated iron(II) ions.

The most striking aspect in the chemistry of Fe_4S_4 iron sulfur proteins is that, in spite of the strong structural similarity of the iron clusters, the actual redox potentials of the two proteins are different at such an extent that in HIPIP the active redox couple is not the same as in ferredoxin. This means that the nature of the local environment and the overall backbone folding around the cluster has a large influence in modulating the redox properties.

CARBOXYPEPTIDASE AS AN EXAMPLE

Carboxypeptidase, a zinc protease, provides a clear example of how the coupling of protein and metal properties permits to reach high degrees of catalytic efficiency. Carboxypeptidase A is a zinc enzyme which catalyzes the hydrolysis of the carboxy terminal aminoacid in a peptidic chain (Vallee and Auld, 1990). The enzyme shows preference for aromatic aminoacids. Extensive crystal data on bovine carboxypeptidase A allow deep insight into the structural features of the enzyme (Christianson and Lipscomb, 1989). Figure 2 shows a schematic drawing of the active site of Carboxypeptidase A. Near the metal center there is a hydrophobic pocket which is able to accomodate the aromatic ring of the substrate.

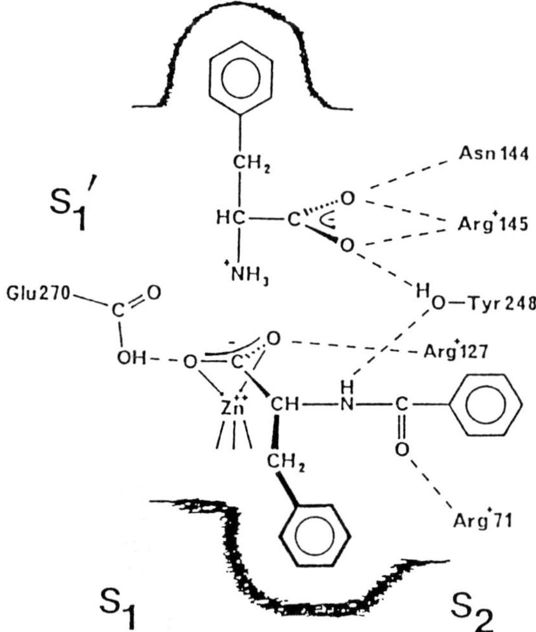

Figure 2. Active site of carboxypeptidase

Two nearby residues are important for the stabilization of the enzyme–substrate adduct: an arginine (Arg 145), at the bottom of the cavity, forms a hydrogen bond with the carboxylate group of the incoming peptide; a tyrosine (Tyr 248) forms a hydrogen bond with the peptidic amide group. Today, it is current opinion that the peptidic carbonyl interacts with Arg 127 and is activated for the nucleophilic attack (Christianson and Lipscomb, 1989). The zinc(II) ion is coordinated by two histidines (His 69, His 196) and one glutamate (Glu 72). Moreover, zinc is coordinated to a water molecule which, on its turn, is hydrogen bonded with Glu 270. The latter interaction plays a strategic role in the whole catalytic process, by modulating the nucleophilic properties of the zinc coordinated water. As a proof of its importance we can remind that, in the absence of Glu 270, the genetically engineered enzyme results to be inactive. The proposed zinc–hydroxo species is perfectly oriented to perform the nucleophilic attack on the carbonyl carbon of an aminoacid residue arranged in the cavity as previously described. Once the attack is performed one proton is provided by Tyr 248 which takes it back from the indissociated form of Glu 270. Then, the products leave and the hydrogen bond between the zinc coordinated water and Glu 270 forms again.

Overall, the above reaction scheme pinpoints how the concerted action of the metal and of a few uncoordinated residues is crucial to function. Anyway, a dynamic concept of the protein structure would be needed to better understand all the steps of the catalytic mechanism in relation to active site flexibility. Under this respect Molecular Dynamics simulation techniques are going to occupy a central role in the near future.

SELECTIVE UPTAKE OF METAL IONS FROM THE ENVIRONMENT

Now we move to describe briefly the way through which essential metal ions are extracted from the environment and integrated in metalloproteins. The overall process of metal uptake, transport, storage and delivery to the sites of utilization in higher organisms is a very complex one being the result of a long evolutionary history. However, even the mechanisms that we find in microorganisms appear to be very sophisticated and specialized. Neilands has described the strategies used by microorganisms to extract iron(III) from the environment in spite of its scarce availability; these mechanisms comprise the synthesis of specialized ligands, the siderophores, and a series of genetic processes that ensure iron homeostasis (Neilands, 1983).

In synthesis, the main problems in the process of metal assumption from the environment are represented by the natural abundance and availability of the metal in question, the competition of hydrolysis processes, the selectivity problem, the need of ligands sufficiently strong to bind the metal but also capable to release it, the ability to cross biological membranes, the competition of poisonous metals, the intrinsic toxicity of many metals and the requirement of an accurate regulation of metal concentration in biological fluids.

TRANSFERRINS

Transferrins, the iron transport proteins in mammalians, are a paradigmatic example for the illustration of the above concepts. Transferrins are proteins designed to bind trivalent metal ions. They are all monomeric proteins, of molecular mass 80,000, with the capacity of binding tightly but reversibly, two iron(III) ions together with two carbonate anions. The relationship between the metal and the anion is strongly synergistic in the sense that neither is bound tightly in the absence of the other; this is a key aspect to understand metal reactivity. Crystallographic analyses of diferric human lactoferrin and rabbit serum transferrin have defined the location and the nature of the iron sites in transferrins (Anderson et al., 1989). All transferrins have essentially the same bilobal structure, with one iron site in each lobe, located in a cleft between two domains (Figure 3). The iron ligands (two tyrosines, one histidine, one aspartate and the bidentate carbonate) are the same in every case, giving rise to a distorted octahedral geometry.

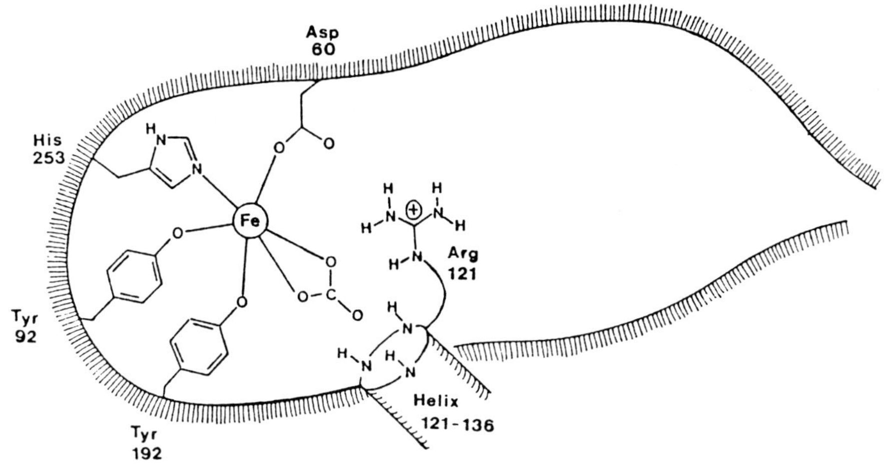

Figure 3. Active site of transferrins.

Yet, the molecular mechanism of metal uptake and release from transferrins has not been elucidated in detail. Physiologically metal release occurs when iron transferrin binds a membrane receptor and the resulting complex is internalized in the cytoplasm. Then metal release occurs either by acidification or by a reductive mechanism or by a conformational change. Presently, the first hypothesis seems to be the favored one.

Interestingly, it is possible to set up in vitro systems to simulate physiological metal release from transferrins. Analysis of the rate of release under different solution conditions provides hints concerning the actual molecular mechanism (Chasteen, 1989). A reaction scheme of the following type has been proposed on the basis of kinetic experiments:

1) $\mathrm{Fe(III)Tf{-}CO_3{}^{2-} = Fe(III){-}Tf{-}CO_3{}^{2-\,\#}}$

2) $\mathrm{Fe(III){-}Tf{-}CO_3{}^{2-\,\#} + Chel = Chel{-}Fe(III){-}Tf{-}CO_3{}^{2-}}$

3) $\mathrm{Chel{-}Fe(III){-}Tf{-}CO_3{}^{2-} = Fe(III){-}Chel + Tf{-}CO_3{}^{2-}}$

4) $\mathrm{Tf{-}CO_3{}^{2-} + H^+ = Tf + HCO_3{}^-}$

In this scheme the first step, corresponding to a conformational change of the protein from a "close" to an "open" state, is the rate limiting step. Then, the "open" protein easily delivers the metal to the incoming ligand (Chel). This proposal has been supported by recent crystallographic data on apolactoferrin as compared to iron lactoferrin. Local unfolding of the protein structure occurs preferentially at low pH values upon weakening of the protein–synergistic anion interaction.

So, transferrin represents a very specialized system capable of binding iron(III) very tightly when it is needed, but also capable of delivering it easily at the utilization sites when particular conditions are met, like a more acidic and/or a reducing environment. In conclusion, transferrin is the expression of the need of providing the living organisms with the essential iron(III) species in spite of the high insolubility of the latter at physiological pH values.

METALLOTHIONEIN

We like to conclude this short report on metalloproteins with some remarks on a very particular protein: metallothionein. Metallothioneins are small proteins with a high content of cysteines; they can bind up to seven zinc(II) or cadmium(II) ions per molecule, in two thiolate clusters of four and three metals. The overall structure has been solved both in the crystal state and in solution through X–ray and 2D NMR studies (Kaegi et al., 1988). A schematic drawing of cluster arrangement is shown in Figure 4.

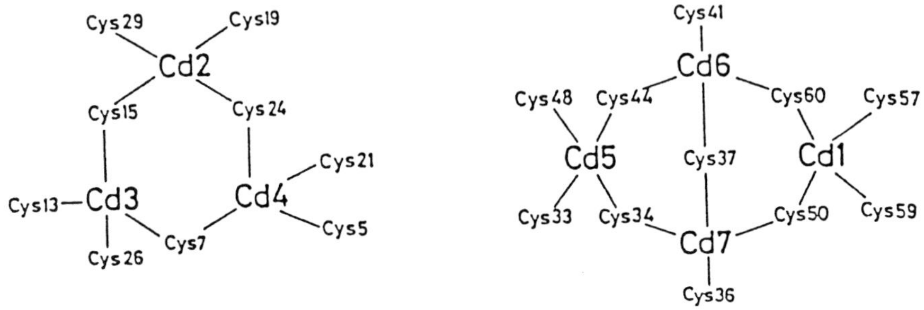

Figure 4. Metal clusters in metallothionein.

The mechanism of cluster formation has been analyzed by replacing the native zinc(II) ion with paramagnetic cobalt(II) (Bertini et al., 1989). Given the high metal content, metallothioneins probably serve as storage proteins for the essential zinc(II). But there is another, even more important function for metallothioneins. Metallothioneins can bind strongly the toxic heavy metal ions like cadmium and mercurium. So they can sequester these metals and perform a general detoxification function. A clear indication in favor of the latter hypothesis is provided by the observation that these proteins are highly inducible in response to cadmium(II) injection.

REFERENCES.

Anderson, B.F., Baker, H.M., Norris, G.E., Rice, D.W., Baker, E.N. (1989): Structure of Human Lactoferrin, J. Mol. Biol. 209, 711–734.

Bertini, I., Luchinat, C., Messori, L., Vasak, M. (1989): Proton NMR Studies of the Cobalt(II) Metallothionein System, J. Am. Chem. Soc. 111, 7296–7300.

Bertini, I., Briganti, F., Luchinat, C., Scozzafava, A., Sola, M. (1991): 1H NMR spectroscopy and the electronic structure of the high potential iron sufur protein from Chromatium vinosum. J. Am. Chem. Soc. 113, 1237–1245.

Bertini, I., Capozzi, F., Ciurli, S., Luchinat, C., Messori, L., Piccioli, M. (1992): Identification of the iron ions of HIPIP from Chromatium vinosum within the protein frame through 2D NMR experiments, J. Am. Chem. Soc. in press.

Bertini, I. et al., (1992): "Bioinorganic Chemistry", University Science Books, Mill Valley, California.

Chasteen, N.D. (1983): Transferrin: a perspective, Adv. Inorg. Biochem. 5, 201–233.

Christianson, D.W., Lipscomb, W.N. (1989): Carboxypeptidase A, 22, 62–69.

Kaegi, J.H.R., Schaeffer, A. (1988): Biochemistry of metallothionein, Biochemistry, 23, 8509–8515.

Neilands, J.B. (1983): Siderophores, Adv. Inorg. Biochem. 5, 137–166.

Vallee, B.L., Auld, D.S. (1990): Zinc enzymes and proteins, Biochemistry, 29, 5647–5659.

Metal Ions in Biology and Medicine, vol. 2. Eds. J. Anastassopoulou, Ph. Collery, J.C. Etienne, Th. Theophanides. John Libbey Eurotext, Paris © 1992, pp. 253-258

Relevance of aluminium-acid complex equilibria to aluminium bioavailability

Guy Berthon

INSERM U305, Equipe « Bioréactifs : Spéciation et Biodisponibilité », 38, rue des Trente-six Ponts, 31400 Toulouse, France

INTRODUCTION

Aluminium is the third most prevalent element and the most abundant metal in the earth's crust. There is, however, no evidence that it has any essential function in animals, particularly in humans (Bertholf *et al.*, 1988). The first reason for this is certainly the natural lack of availability of aluminium to living species. Life originally developed in the presence of large amounts of chemically available metal ions; living species ultimately used small fractions of these as essential constituents whilst protecting themselves against excesses through specific homeostatic processes. In contrast with this, the "hard" Al^{3+} ions remained sequestered in soils in the form of insoluble salts during successive steps of evolution. Therefore, neither were these used as essential components of living species, nor had they to be protected against. This rationale presumably accounts for the fact that aluminium toxicity went unnoticed until recently (Sorenson *et al.*, 1974).

Given the above rationale, it does not seem surprising that aluminium toxicity was first discovered in patients receiving long term hemodialysis (Alfrey *et al.*, 1976), i.e. as the result of a direct contamination of the blood. It was only later that oral aluminium toxicity was noticed, after the removal of aluminium from the water used in dialysis baths proved insufficient to eradicate the so-called dialysis encephalopathy and its associated symptoms (Kaehny *et al.*, 1977a). Aluminium-containing phosphate binders administered orally were then recognized as the main agents of aluminium toxicity (Andreoli *et al.*, 1984). Aluminium-containing antacids were also proven to induce aluminium gastrointestinal absorption, but to different extents depending on the nature of the aluminium salt administered (Kaehny *et al.*, 1977b). Aluminium intrusion in everyday life is also now increasing because of the direct use of aluminium cookware, and also because of industrial pollution. The huge amounts of acids injected into the atmosphere of the northern hemisphere are turned into acid rains which dissolve the aluminium normally sequestered in soils, hence introducing it into the food chain (Williams, 1987).

Since the discovery of oral aluminium toxicity, many investigations relative to the different factors likely to influence aluminium bioavailability have been conducted by toxicologists. Given the chemical properties of the Al^{3+} ion, anions containing oxygen as a donor atom are especially prone to associate with it. It is thus no surprise that acids commonly present in food have been found to play a leading role with respect to aluminium absorption (Partridge *et al.*, 1989) as well as excretion (Domingo *et al.* 1986).

Physiological observations made with respect to the presence of different chemical associations including an aluminium salt and different alternate ligands provide macroscopic information on the effect of metabolic changes, but do not allow any insight into these changes at the molecular level. Likewise, although direct analysis of the main biofluids of treated animals permit the distinction between protein-bound and non protein-bound aluminium pools, they cannot give access to the distribution of low-molar-mass (l.m.m.) species which are the only active ones in terms of metal translocation. The speciation of aluminium within its ultrafiltrable fractions in given biofluids can fortunately be investigated through computer simulation, provided formation and solubility product constants applicable to physiological conditions are known beforehand. A few characteristic examples of applications based on constants determined in our group (Berthon & Daydé, 1992) are given below.

ALUMINIUM-ACID INTERACTIONS IN GASTROINTESTINAL FLUID AND BLOOD PLASMA

The bioavailability of aluminium depends to a determining extent on the nature of the l.m.m. species into which it is distributed in the two main biofluids for metal balance, i.e. gastrointestinal fluid and blood plasma.

In the gastrointestinal fluid, two types of effects can be expected from the numerous acids commonly found in food: (i) the first condition for a metal to be absorbed from the gastrointestinal tract is solubility, and conjugate anions of dietary acids can be present in sufficient concentrations to dissolve otherwise insoluble aluminium salts; (ii) metal ion transport across membranes is generally facilitated by its coordination into electrically neutral species, and, among their different complexes with Al^{3+} ions, anionic forms of dietary acids can give rise to appreciable amounts of such species. It may also be that the acid ingested does not form any neutral complex with aluminium, but once the aluminium salt is dissolved by this acid, the free ions released can be coordinated into neutral forms by other nutrients present in the gastrointestinal tract.

Thus, aluminium complex equilibria determine the respective fractions of metal which can be absorbed by the gastrointestinal membrane or will be directly eliminated into the faeces. Similarly, aluminium complex equilibria occurring in the blood plasma condition the fate of the metal in this biofluid. Schematically, electrically charged l.m.m. species tend to be directly eliminated via the urine, whereas neutral species will be capable of diffusing into tissues, part of these being directed to hepatic cells from where aluminium can be excreted through the bile. The absorption of dietary acids is followed by an increase in the concentration of corresponding conjugate anions in plasma. Therefore, aluminium metabolism may be influenced towards excretion or tissue diffusion, depending on the nature and on the physico-chemical properties of the complexes predominantly formed. Synergistic or antagonistic effects can thus be registered for dietary acids with respect to their gastrointestinal influence.

Aluminium-acid complex equilibria in the gastrointestinal fluid

Citric acid was the first dietary constituent to be recognized as a major factor in the toxicity of oral aluminium-containing therapeutic compounds (Slanina *et al.*, 1986). All complex equilibrium calculations run using formation constants either far from physiological conditions (Slanina *et al.*, 1986) or estimated (Martin, 1986), and then determined under appropriate conditions (Venturini & Berthon, 1989), concurred to substantiate this clinical observation: an appreciable fraction of aluminium hydroxide dissolved in the presence of citric acid occurs as a neutral complex which may induce aluminium absorption.

Following these first results, further studies were undertaken as to the influence of dietary constituents on aluminium intestinal absorption. In particular, the aggravating role of citrate towards aluminium absorption was confirmed by investigations on perfused intestines of anesthetized rats (Partridge *et al.*, 1989). In the same study, a number of organic acids commonly present in the diet were found to delay the precipitation of aluminium hydroxide normally observed near pH 4.5 (Partridge *et al.*, 1989) up to values above 8. Concurrently, the influence of dietary acids on the solubility of aluminium hydroxide was investigated by computer-aided speciation through ECCLES (May *et al.*, 1978) and SOLGASWATER (Eriksson, 1979) programs, corresponding results being in line with the above observations made on rats (Daydé & Berthon, 1990a; 1990b).

Furthermore, the distributions of various concentrations of aluminium, simulated with revised versions of SPE and SPEPLOT programs (Martell & Motekaitis, 1988) in the presence of different levels of dietary acids, showed that several of these compounds could neutralise significant fractions of Al^{3+} ions, rendering them potentially absorbable (Berthon & Daydé, 1992).

Among the dietary constituents investigated, namely citric, oxalic, malic, tartaric, succinic, aspartic and glutamic acids, tartaric acid was found to induce the largest percentage of neutral aluminium complex, malate or citrate ranking second depending on the metal concentration. Given as examples, Fig. 1 and Fig. 2 show simulated distributions of aluminium as a function of pH at two different concentrations. The first of these (0.0005 M) corresponds to 2.7 mg of metal, i.e. about half the average 5 mg normally ingested per day (Bertholf *et al.*, 1988), in 200 cm^3. The second (0.05 M) corresponds to 270 mg of metal, i.e. the aluminium contained in 2 tablets of Maalox, in the same volume of water. The concentration of tartrate in these two examples is 0.02 M, which corresponds to 200 cm^3 of white wine (Ribereau-Gayon *et al.*, 1977). The distribution profile of the neutral complex $Al_2Tra_2H_{-2}°$ (written here with a negative number of protons to signify that the complex may be due to the deprotonation of the tartrate hydroxy groups as well as to the dissociation of two molecules of coordinating water) can be compared with that of the AlCta° neutral species formed by citrate at the same 0.02 M concentration (this corresponding to 25 cm^3 of lemon juice diluted in 200 cm^3 of water (Slanina *et al.*, 1986).

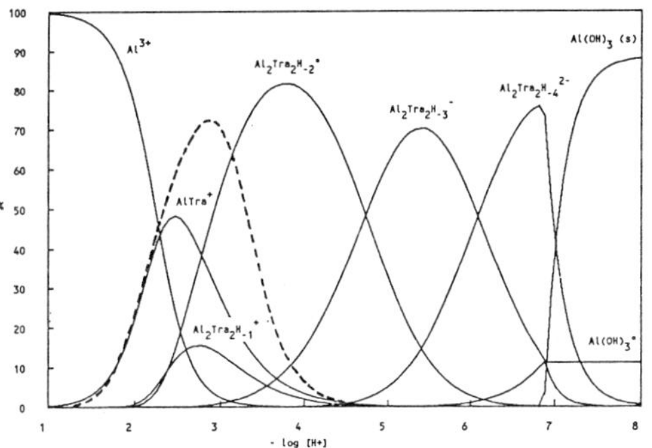

Fig. 1. Aluminium distribution (C_{Al} = 0.0005 M) in the presence of tartrate (C_{Tra} = 0.02 M). The dashed profile stands for AlCta° under identical conditions (i.e. C_{Cta} = 0.02 M).

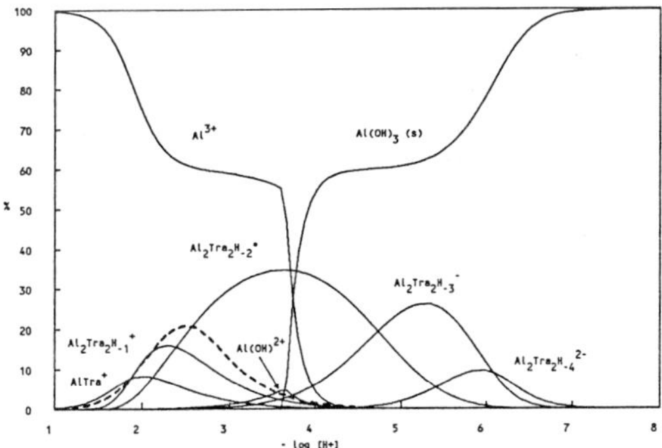

Fig. 2. Aluminium distribution (C_{Al} = 0.05 M) in the presence of tartrate (C_{Tra} = 0.02 M). The dashed profile stands for AlCta° under identical conditions (i.e. C_{Cta} = 0.02 M).

Clearly, the neutral complex of tartrate spans over a larger pH interval than that of citrate, and reaches a larger maximum percentage for both aluminium concentrations. Tartrate should thus be still a more aggravating factor of aluminium absorption than citrate. In fact, the exactness of this prediction will largely depend on the concentration of phosphate in the intestinal lumen.

Phosphate has been shown to co-precipitate with aluminium hydroxide in the intestine (Partridge *et al.*, 1989). This is also corroborated by speciation studies. Simulations run for varying levels of phosphate do indeed show that tartrate complexes progressively regress as the concentration of phosphate is raised. With aluminium and tartrate concentrations of 0.05 M and 0.02 M for example, the maximum percentage of $Al_2Tra_2H_{-2}°$ (34.7% at pH 3.59) remains unchanged for phosphate concentrations up to 0.01 M, but declines to 18.1% at pH 3.45 for C_{PO4} = 0.02 M (Fig. 3). For C_{PO4} = 0.025 M, it is reduced to 6.8% at pH 3.24, and is no longer significant (0.6% at pH 3.1) when C_{PO4} reaches 0.05 M (Fig. 4). The effect of phosphate on the extent of the AlCta° neutral complex formed with a citrate concentration equivalent to that of tartrate (i.e. C_{Cta} = 0.02 M) is similar, although not to the same extent: unchanged up to C_{PO4} = 0.01 M (about 20% near pH 2.5), the maximum percentage of AlCta° is brought down to 13.7 at pH 2.54 for C_{PO4} = 0.02 M, then to 9.7% at pH 2.68 for C_{PO4} = 0.025 M, but still amounts to 4.5% at pH 2.96 for C_{PO4} = 0.05 M, and is not yet negligible for C_{PO4} = 0.075 M (1.9% at pH 3.1).

The role of phosphate illustrated above with respect to aluminium bioavailability, due to the combined effect of the two species $AlPO_4(s)$ and $Al_2PO_4(OH)_2^+$ formed in parallel, has recently been demonstrated to be the reason for the safer therapeutic use of aluminium phosphate with respect to the hydroxide (Berthon & Daydé, 1992). Another remark can also be deduced from the above calculations: although inferior to that of tartrate per se, the aggravating effect of citrate towards aluminium absorption is comparatively less sensitive to the influence of phosphate. Furthermore, the lower the aluminium concentration, the larger this difference in sensitivity to phosphate. Consequences of this are worth taking into account in normal dietary circumstances as well as under aluminium-based therapeutic conditions. To conclude with this, it has been noted by Partridge *et al.* (1989) that all the compounds elevating the pH of precipitation of aluminium hydroxide possessed aluminium-binding groups on two adjacent atoms in the carbon chain backbone. It can now be added that tricarboxylic acids like citric acid should a priori be more hazardous than dicarboxylic ones in respect of aluminium absorption, since their main neutral aluminium complex forms outside the pH range within which both $AlPO_4(s)$ and $Al_2PO_4(OH)_2^+$ species coexist.

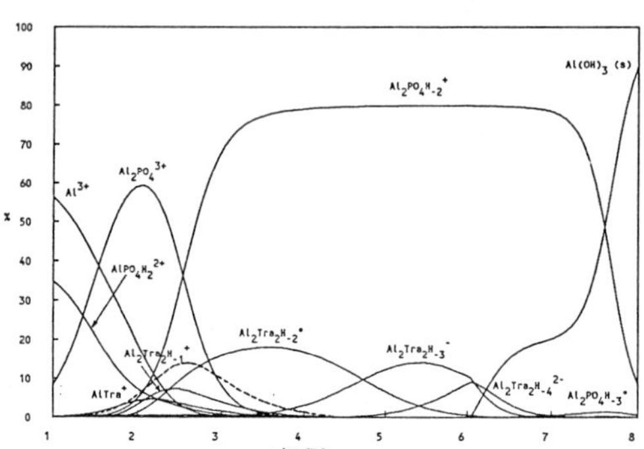

Fig. 3. Aluminium distribution (C_{Al} = 0.05 M) in the presence of tartrate (C_{Tra} = 0.02 M) and phosphate (C_{PO4} = 0.02 M). The dashed profile stands for AlCta° under identical conditions (i.e. C_{Cta} = 0.02 M).

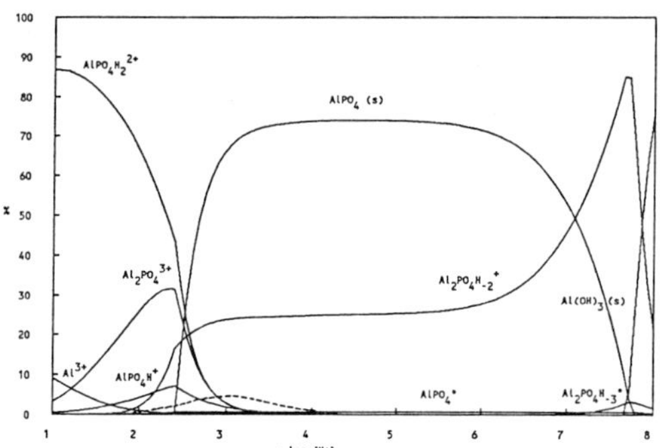

Fig. 4. Aluminium distribution (C_{Al} = 0.05 M) in the presence of tartrate (C_{Tra} = 0.02 M) and phosphate (C_{PO4} = 0.05 M). The dashed profile stands for AlCta° under identical conditions (i.e. C_{Cta} = 0.02 M).

Aluminium-acid complex equilibria in blood plasma

Aluminium complex equilibria occurring in the gastrointestinal fluid are determining for aluminium absorption. The effect of this absorption in respect of final aluminium body loading can, however, be modulated by the new complex equilibria ensuing in blood plasma. Transferrin has definitely been characterised as the ultimate carrier of aluminium in plasma (Martin, 1986). However, aluminium tissue penetration as well as excretion mainly rests on the physico-chemical properties of the predominant complexes of its l.m.m. fraction. Recent simulations run with the ECCLES program (May *et al.*, 1978) have shown (Daydé *et al.*, 1990) that $Al(OH)_3°$ and $AlPO_4°$ accounted for a large percentage of this fraction, the next species,

$Al_2PO_4(OH)_2^+$, representing only 7%. This is significantly at variance with former conclusions which did not take account of the soluble neutral species above (Martin, 1986).

Once a reference simulation model for the distribution of a given metal in plasma has been established, it becomes possible to analyse the relative effects of increasing plasma concentrations of a ligand on the fate of this metal. Normal equilibria to which in vivo stationary states are roughly assimilated may indeed be shifted so that the l.m.m. fraction of the metal is raised at the expense of its protein-bound pool. Simulations run with the ECCLES program (May *et al.*, 1978) in this respect have shown that the ligands investigated could mobilise transferrin-bound aluminium in the order phosphate > citrate >> malate ≈ oxalate (Daydé, 1990). As to the derived effect on aluminium balance, phosphate is expected to exert a changing influence: forming mainly neutral complexes at "normal" free concentrations of aluminium (which tends to facilitate aluminium tissue penetration), it progressively gives rise to predominantly charged species as the free concentration of aluminium rises (Daydé *et al.*, 1990). Increasing citrate levels are shown to be in favour of aluminium urinary excretion, which corroborates physiological observations made on mice (Domingo *et al.* 1986). In contrast, tartrate cannot exert any mobilising influence even for high concentrations up to 0.1 M. Therefore, contrary to citrate, tartrate cannot counteract in plasma the influence it exerts on aluminium gastrointestinal absorption. Again, this tends to confirm in vivo observations made on the neurotoxic effects of aluminium tartrate (Boegman & Bates, 1984).

CONCLUSION

These results show that the influence of dietary constituents on aluminium tissue penetration is by no means simple. In the gastrointestinal stage, this influence depends, not only on the concentrations of aluminium and of the constituent directly involved, but also on that of other constituents present in the gastrointestinal tract. In this respect, phosphate is shown to be a limiting factor of aluminium absorption. In blood plasma, the situation is not more straightforward since the same ligand can favour or inhibit aluminium urinary excretion depending on the aluminium level. In addition, some dietary constituents, such as citrate (Daydé & Berthon, 1990b), can attenuate in plasma the result of their unfavourable gastrointestinal influence while others, such as tartrate, cannot. Many studies of this nature are still necessary before effective prevention can be established against the side-effects of hitherto irreplaceable aluminium-containing drugs, although the present results have already induced a better awareness of the problems involved.

REFERENCES

Alfrey, A.C., Legendre, G.R., and Kaehny, W.D. (1976): The dialysis encephalopathy syndrome. Possible aluminium intoxication. *N. Engl. J. Med.* 294, 184-188.

Andreoli, S.P., Bergstein, J.M., and Sherrard, D.J. (1984): Aluminium intoxication from aluminium-containing phosphate binders in children with azotemia. *N. Engl. J. Med.* 310, 1079-1084.

Bertholf, R.L., Wills, M.R., and Savory, J. (1988): Aluminum. In *Handbook on Toxicity of Inorganic Compounds*, eds H.G. Seiler, H. Sigel and A. Sigel, pp. 55-64. New York: Marcel Dekker.

Berthon, G., and Daydé, S. (1992): Why aluminum phosphate is less toxic than aluminum hydroxide. *J. Amer. Coll. Nutr.* in press.

Boegman, R.J., and Bates, L.A. (1984): Neurotoxicity of aluminum. *Can. J. Physiol. Pharmacol.*, 62, 1010-1014.

Daydé, S. (1990): Etude des équilibres de complexation et spéciation simulée de la fraction ultrafiltrable de l'aluminium dans le plasma sanguin et le fluide gastro-intestinal. Implications pour la toxicité de l'aluminium. *Thèse de Doctorat de l'Université Paul Sabatier*, Toulouse.

Daydé, S., and Berthon, G. (1990a): Potential toxicity of presumably insoluble aluminium salts in presence of common dietary acids. *Food Add. Contam.* 7, S155-S157.

Daydé, S., and Berthon, G. (1990b): Origin of the double role of citrate towards aluminium intoxication. *J. Inorg. Biochem.* 36, 348.

Daydé, S., Filella, M., and Berthon, G. (1990): Aluminum speciation studies in biological fluids. Part 3. Quantitative investigation of aluminum-phosphate complexes and assessment of their potential significance in vivo. *J. Inorg. Biochem.* 38, 241-259.

Domingo, J.L., Llobet, J.M., Gomez, M., and Corbella, J. (1986): Acute aluminium intoxication: a study of the efficacy of several antidotal treatments in mice. *Res. Comm. Chem. Pathol. Pharmacol.* 53, 93-103.

Eriksson, G. (1979): An algorithm for the computation of aqueous multi-component, multiphase equilibria. *Anal. Chim. Acta* 112, 375-383.

Kaehny, W.D., Alfrey, A.C., Holman, R.E., and Shorr, W.J. (1977a): Aluminum transfer during hemodialysis. *Kidney Int.* 12, 361-365.

Kaehny, W.D., Hegg, A.P., and Alfrey, A.C. (1977b): Gastrointestinal absorption of aluminum from aluminum-containing antacids. *N. Engl. J. Med.* 296, 1389-1390.

Martell, A.E., and Motekaitis, R. (1988): Determination and use of stability constants. Weinheim: VCH.

Martin, R.B. (1986): The chemistry of aluminium as related to biology and medicine. *Clin. Chem.* 32, 1797-1806.

May, P.M., Linder, P.W., and Williams, D.R. (1978): Computer simulation of metal ion equilibria in biofluids: models for the low-molecular-weight complex distribution of calcium(II), magnesium(II), manganese(II), iron(III), copper(II), zinc(II), and lead(II) ions in human blood plasma. *J. Chem. Soc. Dalton* 588-595.

Partridge, N.A., Regnier, F.E., White, J.L., and Hem S.L. (1989): Influence of dietary constituents on intestinal absorption of aluminum. *Kidney Int.* 35, 1413-1417.

Ribereau-Gayon, J., Peynaud, E., Ribereau-Gayon, P., and Sudraud, R. (1977): Sciences et Techniques du Vin, Paris: Dunod.

Slanina, P., Frech, W., Ekström, L.-G., Lööf, L., Slorach, S., and Cedergren, A. (1986): Dietary citric acid enhances absorption of aluminium in antacids. *Clin. Chem.* 32, 539-541.

Sorenson, J.R.J., Campbell, I.R., Tepper, L.B., and Lingg, R.D. (1974): Aluminum in the environment and human health. *Environ. Health Persp.* 8, 3-95.

Venturini, M., and Berthon, G. (1989): Aluminium speciation studies in biological fluids. Part 2: quantitative investigation of aluminium citrate complexes and appraisal of their potential significance in vivo. *J. Inorg. Biochem.* 37, 69-90.

Williams, R.J.P. (1987): Comparative biochemistry of aluminium. *Rec. Trav. Chim. Pays-Bas* 106, 401.

Metal Ions in Biology and Medicine, vol. 2. Eds. J. Anastassopoulou, Ph. Collery, J.C. Etienne, Th. Theophanides. John Libbey Eurotext, Paris © 1992, pp. 259-264

Role of zinc in the endocrine and neuroendocrine function

Sam J. Bhathena, Moshe J. Werman

Carbohydrate Nutrition Laboratory, Beltsville Human Nutrition Research Center, USDA, Beltsville, Maryland 20705, USA

Zinc has been recognized as an essential trace element in animal and human nutrition. Though overt zinc deficiency in humans is rare, it has been demonstrated in humans, especially after prolonged total parental nutrition. Zinc has been shown to be either a component of an enzyme or is required as a cofactor for the enzyme activity in at least 200 different enzymes. Some of these enzymes are involved in hormone and neuropeptide processing. Thus, like copper, it can affect hormonal, neuropeptide and opiate function. Conversely hormones and opiates also affect zinc metabolism.

ZINC AND BRAIN FUNCTION

The essentiality of zinc in animal nutrition has been known since 1930 and in humans primarily through the work of Prasad and Sandstead since 1960s. The role of zinc in brain development is relatively recent. In the 1970s, Hurley and colleagues demonstrated teratogenic effects on brain development in fetus of dams fed low zinc diet. The possible involvement of zinc deficiency in CNS deformation in humans was suggested by Sever and Emanuel in 1973. Studies on the role of zinc in brain development and function have been extensively reviewed (Frederickson et al., 1984; Rogers et al., 1985; Prohaska, 1987; Dreosti, 1989). Among the trace elements, the concentrations of zinc in the brain is second only to iron. Zinc is more concentrated in some areas of the brain where it has been suggested to play a significant biological function. Among the various brain areas examined, the highest concentration of zinc is found in the hippocampus especially in mossy fiber axons, where zinc ions have been postulated to modulate the functions of opiate, GABA receptors and the mediation of synaptic transmission. The level of zinc in hippocampus increases with age. In animals fed zinc deficient diet, there is a decrease in brain size, underdevelopment of cerebellar cortex, decreased dendritic growth in the cortex and an abnormal development of Purkinje cells (Dvergsten et al., 1984). Both the excess as well as the deficiency of zinc have been implicated in several neurological disorders (Ebadi & Hama, 1986) notably schizophrenia, Pick's disease, alcoholism, Wilson's disease, Alzheimer and epilepsy (Pfeiffer & Braverman, 1982; Wallwork, 1987). The involvement of zinc in fifth day fits in newborn (Xie & Smart 1991) has been questioned (Ben-Ari & Cherubini 1991). Among the subcellular fractions of several brain areas, synaptosomes contain higher concentration of zinc than myelin and mitochondria (Rajan et al., 1976) though in a recent study zinc distribution was shown to be equally distributed between myelin, synaptosomes and mitochondria (Saito et al., 1988).Though in adults, brain zinc levels are stable, zinc is actively taken up by mossy fibers of hippocampus in culture and stored in synaptic vesicles in nerve terminals (Howell et al., 1984; Assaf & Chung 1984). Electrical stimulation of nerve fiber tracts also induces the release of stored zinc (Howell et al., 1984). In several areas of brain, such as the hippocampus and cerebellum, zinc is bound to proteins that resemble liver metallothionein (Ebadi and Hama, 1986) and this protein may be involved in zinc homeostasis and possibly in synaptic functions.

INTERACTIONS OF ZINC

Zinc has been shown to interact with several metals especially divalent ions such as copper, aluminum, cadmium, lead, selenium, iron and calcium. In some biological process, zinc and copper are interchangeable while in others they antagonize each other's action. Superoxide dismutase contains both copper and zinc. Interactions of zinc with essential fatty acids, vitamins A and C and phytate have also been reported. Zinc and copper have been shown to interfere with each other's absorption and zinc toxicity can be reversed by copper. Similarly, excess zinc ingestion reversibly causes copper deficiency and sideroblastic anemia. Zinc absorption is also affected by protein in the diet. In brain, however, zinc has been reported to interact with copper, aluminum, cadmium and lead. Thus, high zinc can decrease the level of these metals and vice versa. The therapeutic uses of zinc have been suggested in copper, aluminum, lead and cadmium neurotoxicity.

Zinc also interacts and forms complexes with hormones and opiates. Like copper, zinc forms coordination compounds with enkephalins. Zinc-met-enkephalin is more analgesic than morphine or met-enkephalin alone (Gromov and Serdiuk, 1990). The interaction between zinc and insulin is well established. Luteinizing hormone releasing hormone (LHRH) may be active in inducing ovulation only when combined with zinc, copper or nickel (Kozlowski et al., 1990). Zinc also binds to growth hormone (GH) and forms a GH dimer with two zinc ions per dimer. The dimer appears to be more resistant to denaturation in guanidine-HCl than the monomeric form of GH. The dimer associated with zinc may be a preferred form of storage of GH in secretory granules (Cunningham et al., 1991). Zinc is also required for structural stability of nerve growth factor (Pfeiffer & Braverman, 1982). Zinc finger motifs are part of DNA-binding domain of nuclear hormone receptors and dimerization may be responsible for the biological effects (Forman and Samuels, 1990).

CONTROL OF ZINC BY HORMONES AND OPIATES

Several hormones have been reported to control plasma zinc levels. A detailed discussion is beyond the scope of this review. Increase growth hormone and corticosterone decreases plasma zinc while the decrease of these hormones increases plasma zinc levels. Progesterone, but not estrogen, decreases plasma zinc levels (Henkin, 1976). Glucagon infusion in dogs has been shown to increase zinc excretion. This is also true for metabolic conditions such as diabetes, trauma, starvation or glucagonoma in which either plasma glucagon is increased or insulin is decreased. In mixed lymphocyte cultures, insulin and calcitonin together with mitogen increase zinc influx (Chausmer et al., 1991). Monokines such as interleukin-1 and 6 and tumor necrosis factor cause redistribution of zinc (Klasing & Johnstone, 1991). Whether any of these hormones or monokines have any effect on brain zinc level is not clear and needs to be investigated. One recent report by Gulya et al. (1991) indicates that in addition to hormones, opiates also play a role in controlling brain zinc levels. They injected δ opioid agonist enkephalin analogs (D-Pen 2, D-Pen 5)enkephalin intracerebroventrally and observed a significant time and dose dependent decrease in zinc in three different regions of the brain.

Since pretreatment with naloxone abolished this effect it appeared that the effect of enkephalinamide was through opiate receptors.

ZINC ENZYMES IN BRAIN

More than 200 zinc dependent enzymes are known, but only a few have been reported in the brain. These enzymes are primarily involved in myelination, protein synthesis, catecholamine and other neurotransmitters synthesis and metabolism and in opiate and neuropeptide processing and function. Compared to copper deficiency, zinc deficiency has less effect on cerebellar myelination. Hypomyelination observed in zinc deficiency could be due to the lower activities of 2',3'-cyclic nucleotide 3'-phosphohydrolase and alkaline phosphatase (Dreosti, 1989) or may be due to reduced level of T_3 (Prohaska 1987). The enzymes involved in neurotransmitter functions namely glutamic acid dehydrogenase, dopamine-β-hydroxylase and phenylethanolamine N-methyl transferase are increased in zinc deficiency which may explain the increase in catecholamines in severe (Wallwork et al., 1982) but not mild (Halas et al., 1982) zinc deficiency. Superoxide dismutase present in synaptosomes may be involved in protecting catecholamines from superoxide mediated oxidation (Dreosti 1989). Zinc is also involved in the γ-aminobutyric acid (GABA) metabolism in brain. At physiological doses zinc stimulates glutamic acid decarboxylase (GAD) possibly via stimulating pyridoxal kinase to form pyridoxal phosphate. However, in pharmacological doses zinc inhibits GAD. Thus zinc has both stimulatory and inhibitory effect on synaptic transmitters in the hippocampus (Ebadi et al. 1984). Zinc also regulates GABA receptors in hippocampus and is a potent non-competitive antagonist of N-methyl-D-aspartate (NMDA) responses in hippocampus (Peters et al., 1987; Westbrook & Mayer, 1987). Zinc also attenuates the NMDA stimulated cholecystokinin octapeptide from cerebral cortex (Bandopadhyay & Belleroche, 1991).

Recently several zinc dependent peptidases have been demonstrated in brain. Many of these are involved in neuropeptide and opiate processing in brain, pituitary and hypothalamus. Pekary et al., (1991) recently reported that in zinc deficiency, the conversion of prepro TRH to TRH in hypothalamus, brain and pituitary is decreased, possibly due to a decrease in posttranslational processing enzyme such as carboxypeptidase H. Zinc is also a cofactor for TRH biosynthesis (Garfinkel, 1986). The decreased TRH synthesis may be due to a reduction in one or more zinc dependent enzymes. It is important to note that many peptides in pituitary and hypothalamus are active only in amidated or acetylated form. Zinc (along with copper and ascorbate) is required for α-amidation of peptides. Endopeptidase 24.15, a zinc-metalloenzyme is also present in brain (Acker et al., 1987). Zinc is involved in the degradation of biologically active peptides and hormones such as neurotensin, bradikinin, substance P, LHRH. Zinc is also involved in opiate processing and converts dynorphin, α- and β-neoendorphin to enkephalins. Another zinc-metallopeptidase involved in hormone and opiate processing is dipeptidyl aminopeptidase present in brain and pituitary (Lee & Snyder, 1982). It is involved in the degradation of enkephalins and angiotensin II, by removing dipeptides from N-terminus. The enzyme is not active if the N-terminus is blocked or modified by amidation or acetylation. This may explain why some short chain peptides are biologically active only in the amidated or acetylated form. An enzyme which hydrolyses amidated peptides at both terminals has also been reported (Yokosawa et al., 1983; Skidgel & Erdos, 1985). Whether this is also a zinc dependent enzyme is not clear. Angiotensin converting enzyme (peptidyl dipeptidase A) also hydrolyses amidated peptides such as substance P (Turner, 1986). Zinc is also implicated in the regulation of activity of cerebral adenylate cyclase (Baba et al., 1981). The enzyme is inhibited by zinc (and copper) in the absence of dithiothreitol.

ZINC AND OPIATE RECEPTORS

Marzullo and Friedhoff (1977) first demonstrated that zinc inhibited opiate binding in vitro and this action was more potent than copper. The inhibition depends on the potencies with which zinc (and copper) bind to protein sulphydryl groups. It is important to note that unlike copper, zinc has only one valency and hence does not undergo oxidation-reduction. Its modification of opiate receptor is possibly through the oxidation-reduction of thiols (Marzullo & Hine, 1980). This is also supported by the data of Stengaard-Pedersen et al. (1981) who showed that inhibition of enkephalinamide (2-D-Ala-5-L-methionine) to opiate receptors in the hippocampus by zinc is reversed by thiol reductants. They also reported decreased binding by zinc to other areas of brain - cerebral cortex, the basal ganglia and the rest of the forebrain. The decrease binding was due to decreased affinity of the receptor without significant change in the number of receptor (Stengaard-Pederson et al., 1981; Ogawa et al., 1985). It is important to note that the hippocampal distribution of zinc and enkephalin is identical and confined to mossy fiber zone (Stengaard-Pedersen, 1982). Similar coexistence of zinc with enkephalin, dynorphin and substance P has been demonstrated in marginal division of the striatum (Shu et al., 1990). These data suggest that zinc ions are physiologically important modulators of functions of opiate receptors in the hippocampal mossy fiber system. A relationship between zinc and enkephalin has also been suggested for immune function (Murgo et al., 1985). In vitro, zinc decreased the affinity of opiate receptor for binding of naloxone to rat brain membranes (Baraldi et al., 1984). The inhibition is reversed by zinc chelator such as histidine (Hanissian & Tejwani, 1988). In zinc deficiency there is an increase in naloxone binding to brain membrane due to increase in the affinity of the receptors (Essatara et al., 1984). Recently Tejwani and Hanissian (1990) studied the effect of zinc on opiate receptor subclasses and showed that zinc inhibits μ receptors but not δ or κ receptors. The inhibition was reversed by histidine. Zinc also decreased the stimulation of opiate receptors caused by magnesium and manganese. They suggested that the lower susceptibility of δ and κ receptors to zinc may be due either to fewer sulphydryl groups in these receptors or to their inaccessibility to binding by zinc. Zinc also increases binding of benzodiazepine agonist diazepam and decreases the binding of antagonist, β-carboline (Mizuno et al., 1983).

REFERENCES

Acker, G.R., Molineaux, C. & Orlowski, M. (1987): Synaptosomal membrane-bound form of endopeptidase 24.15 generates leu-enkephalin from dynorphin$^{1-8}$, alpha- and beta-neoendorphin, and met-enkephalin from met-enkephalin-Arg^{6}-Gly^{7}-Leu^{8}. J. Neurochem. 48,284-292.

Assaf S.Y. & Chung, S.H. (1984): Release of endogenous Zn^{2+} from brain tissue during activity. Nature 308,734-736.

Baba, A., Kihara, T., Lee, E. & Iwata, N. (1981): Activation of rat brain adenylate cyclase by copper plus dithiothreitol. Biochem. Pharmacol. 30,171-174.

Bandopadhyay, R. & de Belleroche, J. (1991): Regulation of CCK release in cerebral cortex by N-methyl-D-aspartate receptors: sensitivity to APV, MK-801, kynurenate, magnesium and zinc ions. Neuropeptides 18,159-163.

Baraldi, M., Caselgrandi, E. & Santi, M. (1984): Reduction of withdrawal symptoms in morphin-dependent rats by zinc: Behavioral and biochemical studies. Neurosci. Lett. Suppl. 18,S371.

Ben-Ari, Y. & Cherubini, E. (1991): Zinc and GABA in developing brain. Nature 353,220.

Chausmer, A.B., Chausmer, A.L. & Dajani, N. (1991): Effect of mitogenic and hormonal stimulation on zinc transport in mixed lymphocyte cultures. J. Am. Coll. Nutr. 10,205-208.

Cunningham, B.C., Mulkerrin, M.G. & Wells, J.A. (1991): Dimerization of human growth hormone by zinc. Science 253,545-548.

Dreosti, I.E. (1989): Neurobiology of zinc. In Zinc in Human Biology, ed. C.F. Mills, pp. 235-248. London: Springer-Verlag.

Dvergsten C.L., Johnson, L.A. & Sandstead, H.H. (1984): Alterations in the postnatal development of the cerebellar cortex due to zinc deficiency. III. impaired dendritic differentiation of basket and stellate cells. Dev. Brain Res. 16,21-26.

Ebadi, M. & Hama, Y. (1986): Zinc-binding proteins in the brain. Adv. Exp. Med. Biol. 203,557-570.

Ebadi, M., Wilt, S. Ramaley, R., Swanson, S. & Mebus, C. (1984): The role of zinc-binding proteins in regulation of glutamic acid decarboxylase in brain. Prog. Clin. Biol. Res. 144A,255-275.

Ellis, S. & Nuenke, J.M. (1967): Dipeptidyl arylamidase III of the pituitary. Purification and characterization. J. Biol. Chem. 242,4623-4629.

Essatara, M.B., Morley, J.E., Levine, A.S., Elson, M.K., Shafer, R.B. & McClain, C.J. (1984): The role of the endogenous opiates in zinc deficiency anorexia. Physiol. Behaviour 32,475-478.

Forman, B.M. & Samuels, H.H. (1990): Dimerization among nuclear hormone receptors. New Biol. 2,587-594.

Frederickson, C.J., Howell, G.A. & Kasarskis, E.J. (eds) (1984): The neurobiology of zinc, Parts A & B. New York: Alan R. Liss.

Garfinkel, D. (1986): Is aging inevitable? The intracellular zinc deficiency hypothesis of aging. Mol. Hypothesis 19,117-137.

Gromov, L.A. & Serdiuk, E.A. (1990): The analgesic activity of coordination compounds of methionine enkephalin with divalent metals. Farmakol. Toksikol. 53,24-25.

Gulya, K., Kovacs, G.L. & Kasa, P. (1991): Partial depletion of endogenous zinc level by (D-pen2, D-pen5)enkephalin in the rat brain. Life Sci. 48,PL57-62.

Halas, E.S. Wallwork, J.C. & Sandstead, H.H. (1982): Mild zinc deficiency and undernutrition during the prenatal and postnatal periods in rats. Effects on weight, food consumption and brain catecholamine concentrations. J. Nutr. 112,542-551.

Hanissian, S.H. & Tejwani, G.A. (1988): Histidine abolishes the inhibition by zinc of naloxone binding to opioid receptors in rat brain. Neuropharmacology 27,1145-1149.

Henkin, R.I. (1976): Trace metals in endocrinology. Med. Clin. N. Am. 60,779-797.

Howell, G.A., Welch, M.G. & Frederickson, C.J. (1984): Stimulation-induced uptake and release of zinc in hippocampal slices. Nature 308,736-738.

Klasing, K.C. & Johnstone, B.J. (1991): Monokines in growth and development. Poult. Sci. 70,1781-1789.

Kozlowski, H., Masiukiewicz, E. Potargowicz, E. et al. (1990): Ovulation-inducing activity of luliberin (LHRH) complexed by copper(II), nickel (II), and zinc (II) ions. J. Inorg. Biochem. 40,121-125.

Lee, C.M. & Snyder, S.H. (1982). Dipeptidyl-aminopeptidase III of rat brain. Selective affinity for enkephalin and angiotensin. J. Biol. Chem. 257,12043-12050.

Marzullo, G. & Friedhoff, A.J. (1977): An inhibitor of opiate receptor binding from human erythrocytes identified as a glutathione-copper complex. Life Sci. 21,1559-1568.

Marzullo, G. & Hine, B. (1980). Opiate receptor function may be modulated through an oxidation-reduction mechanism. Science 208,1171-1173.

Mizuno, S., Ogawa, N. & Mori, A. (1983): Differential effects of some

transition metal cations on the binding of β-carboline-3-carboxylate and diazepam. Neurochem. Res. 8,873-880.
Murgo, A.J., Plotnikoff, N.P. & Faith, R.E. (1985): Effect of methionine enkephalin plus ZnCl2 on active T cell rosettes. Neuropeptides 5,367-370.
Ogawa, N., Mizuno, S., Fukushima, M. & Mori, A. (1985): Effects of guanine nucleotide, transition metals and temperature on enkephalin receptors of rat brain membranes. Peptides 6 (suppl 1),23-28.
Pekary, A.E., Lukaski, H.C., Mena, I. & Hershman, J.M. (1991): Processing of TRH precursor peptides in rat brain and pituitary is zinc dependent. Peptides 12,1025-1032.
Peters, S., Koh, J. & Choi, D.W. (1987): Zinc selectively blocks the action of N-methyl-D-aspartate on cortical neurons. Science 236,589-593.
Pfeiffer, C.C. & Braverman, E.R. (1982): Zinc, the brain and behavior. Biol. Psychiatry 17,513-532.
Prohaska, J.R. (1987): Functions of trace elements in brain metabolism. Physiol. Rev. 67,858-901.
Rajan, K.S., Colburn, R.W. & Davis, J.M. (1976): Distribution of metal ions in the subcellular fractions of several rat brain areas. Life Sci. 18,423-432.
Rogers, J.M., Keen, C.L. & Hurley, L.S. (1985): Zinc, copper, and manganese deficiencies in prenatal and neonatal development, with special reference to the central nervous system. In Metals Ions in Neurology and Psychiatry, ed. S. Gabay, J. Harris & B.T. Ho, pp. 3-43, Vol. 15, New York: A.R. Liss.
Saito, T., Itoh, T., Satoh, H. & Saito, K. (1988): Copper and zinc distribution in eight regions and subcellular fractions of rat brain. J. Trace Elem. Exp. Med. 1,33-40.
Sever, L.E. & Emanuel, I. (1973): Is there a connection between maternal zinc deficiency and congenital malformations of the central nervous system in man? Teratology 7,117-118.
Shu, S.Y., McGinty, J.F. & Peterson, G.M. (1990): High density of zinc-containing and dynorphin B- and substance P-immunoreactive terminals in the marginal division of the rat striatum. Brain Res. Bull. 24,201-205.
Skidgel, R.A. & Erdos, E.G. (1985): Novel activity of human angiotensin I converting anzyme: Release of the NH_2- and COOH- terminal tripeptides from the luteinizing hormone-releasing hormone. Proc. Natl. Acad. Sci. USA 82,1025-1029.
Stengaard-Pedersen, K. (1982): Inhibition of enkephalin binding to opiate receptors by zinc ions: possible physiological importance in the brain. Acta Pharmacol. Toxicol. Copenh. 50,213-220.
Stengaard-Pedersen, K., Fredens, K. & Larsson, L.I. (1981): Inhibition of opiate receptor binding by zinc ions: possible physiological importance in the hippocampus. Peptides 2 (Suppl 1),27-35.
Tejwani, G.A. & Hanissian, S.H. (1990): Modulation of mu, delta and kappa opioid receptors in rat brain by metal ions and histidine. Neuropharmacolgy 29,445-452.
Turner, A.J. (1986): Strategies for the inhibition of neuropeptide-metabolizing enzymes. Biochem. Soc. Trans. 14,399-401.
Wallwork, J.C. (1987): Zinc and the central nervous system. Prog. Food Nutr. Sci. 11,203-247.
Wallwork, J.C., Botnen, J.H. & Sandstead, H.H. (1982): Influence of dietary zinc on rat brain catecholamines. J. Nutr. 112,514-519.
Westbrook, G.L. & Mayer, M.L. (1987): Micromolar concentrations of Zn2+ antagonize NMDA and GABA receptors of hippocampal neurons. Nature 328,640-643.
Xie, X. & Smart, T.G. (1991): A physiological role for endogenous zinc in rat hippocampal synaptic neurotransmission. Nature 349,521-524.
Yokosawa, H., Endo, S., Ogura, Y. & Ishii, S-I. (1983): A new feature of angiotensin-converting enzyme in the brain: hydrolysis of Substance P. Biochem. Biophys. Res. Commun. 116,735-741.

Metal Ions in Biology and Medicine, vol. 2. Eds. J. Anastassopoulou, Ph. Collery, J.C. Etienne, Th. Theophanides. John Libbey Eurotext, Paris © 1992, pp. 265-268

Active oxygen species, free radicals and pathophysiologic conditions. The pharmacochemical approach

Panos N. Kourounakis, Eleni Rekka, Vassilis J. Demopoulos, Ekaterini Tani, Ioanna Andreadou, Elena Alexandrou

Department of Pharmaceutical Chemistry, School of Pharmacy, University of Thessaloniki, Thessaloniki 54006, Greece

INTRODUCTION

Since the appearance of life, oxygen has been utilized by aerobic organisms. It is the final electron acceptor almost in all metabolic processes. In eucariotic organisms, the coupling of the oxidation of the respiratory chain with the phosphorylation of ADP constitutes the energy source for the preservation of life. Most of the oxygen consumed by the biologic systems is reduced, in a four electron transfer process, to water, by the cytochrome oxidase (Comporti, 1989). Oxygen is also consumed by the P-450 enzyme family. The main role of this group of enzymes is the elimination of the lipophilic, in the physiologic pH, xenobiotics from the body. The microsomal enzymes utilize oxygen for transformations to the oxidized xenobiotic and water, in two successive one electron reductions (Ruckpaul et al., 1989).

GENERATION OF FREE RADICALS AND THE MOLECULAR MECHANISM OF THEIR TOXICITY

The electron transport chains in mitochondria and in the endoplasmic reticulum can also reduce oxygen partially, by the transport of only one electron, resulting in the generation of active oxygen species, like hydrogen peroxide, superoxide anion radicals and hydroxyl radicals:

$$O_2 \xrightarrow{e} O_2^{\cdot -} \xrightarrow[2H^+]{e} H_2O_2 \xrightarrow[HO^-]{e} HO^{\cdot} \xrightarrow[H^+]{e} H_2O$$

Other systems, the prostaglandin cascade, that of xanthine oxidase, produce active oxygen species, like $O_2^{\cdot -}$. In most of such systems, the role of metals (Fe, Mo, Cu) is very important (Walsh, 1979). Fundamental molecular structures, such as cellular membranes, proteins and nucleic acids, contain moieties that are highly susceptible to radical attack. It is accepted that free radicals can act either directly, by covalent binding to membrane lipids and proteins, principally of the endoplasmic reticulum with a possible enzyme inactivation, or indirectly, through an interaction with the unsaturated fatty acids of the biological membranes, resulting in the initiation of lipid peroxidation. The peroxidation of the polyunsaturated fatty acids decreases the fluidity of membranes, an important property for their physiologic function. Furthermore, the formation of hydroperoxides in the hydrophobic region of phospholipids leads to the creation of hydrophilic centres, and thus the protein-ligand interaction is altered. Among the final products of lipid peroxidation, carbonyl compounds, e.g. malondialdehyde, exert cytotoxic action. These compounds can move from the site of their production and act at distant sites. They interact with functional -SH groups, among them with glutathione, thus inactivating a principal defensive system of the body. Alterations of the intracellular Ca homeostasis and activation of PLA_2 are further consequences of lipid peroxidation (Comporti, 1989). Among free radicals and active oxygen species, HO· is very reactive and one of the strongest oxidizing agents. Physiological processes, such as phagocytosis, involve the formation of HO·, and their toxicity is apparently due to the subsequent reactions of this species.

Hydroxyl radicals have been shown to cause DNA strand breaks and to induce K^+ loss from cell membranes (Fridovich, 1988).

DEFENSE OF THE BODY AGAINST OXYGEN TOXICITY AND FREE RADICAL ATTACK

The aerobic cells have developed defensive mechanisms in order to overcome the noxious effects of oxygen. Some of them are the free radical scavenging enzymes, other enzymes like catalases, dismutases, the development of enzymes responsible for the repair of oxidative damage. Antioxidants are important agents in controlling or preventing free radical reactions. In biological systems, physiologically occurring antioxidants (glutathione, tocopherols, ascorbic acid), synthetic agents (BHT, BHA, propyl gallate), various natural products or drugs (flavonoids, catechols, vitamins A and E, phenothiazines) have been proven useful. The exact mechanism of antioxidant action varies with the specific reaction. It may include prevention of allylic hydrogen abstraction from a α-methylene carbon, inhibition of hydroperoxide cleavage, scavenging of free radicals, chelation of transition metals or combination of the above (Scott, 1985). The disturbance of the pro-/anti- oxidant balance of the body in favour of the former is known as "*oxidative stress*". The consequences and prevention of oxidative stress is one of the main objectives of drug research.

PATHOPHYSIOLOGIC CONDITIONS CAUSED BY OR LINKED WITH ACTIVE OXYGEN SPECIES AND FREE RADICAL ATTACK.

Oxygen toxicity and oxygen generated free radicals are gaining remarkable attention recently, and considerable research work is devoted to the effects of free radicals on organisms. Many drugs activate oxygen during their oxidoreductive cycle in the body. In halogenated hydrocarbons, a reductive dehalogenation or homolytic fusion occurs, resulting in free radical generation. These react either with oxygen, in an addition reaction leading to highly reactive peroxy radicals, or they react with polyunsaturated fatty acids, forming new free radicals, which subsequently participate in addition reactions with oxygen. Furthermore, irradiation, supersonification, airborne chemicals, ozone, environmental pollutants (nitrous oxides, heavy metals, condensed polycyclic aromatic hydrocarbons, agrochemicals) may evoke oxidative damage. If the cellular defensive enzyme system against free radicals is disturbed, oxygen activation causes direct cytotoxicity. Actually, this is the molecular mechanism of action of certain drugs. Bipyridyl herbicides (e.g. paraquat) act via an oxygen activation mechanism (Dodge, 1971).

The sarcoplasmic reticulum and the sarcolemma are highly susceptible to free radicals during myocardial injury. Free radical mediated destruction of sarcoplasmic membranes is one of the cellular processes involved in arrhythmias generated during myocardial ischemia and reperfusion (Fridovich, 1988).

Lipid peroxides are implicated in atherosclerosis and vascular disorders. Microangiopathy associated with diabetic complications is accompanied by higher than normal lipid peroxides in plasma (Yoshioka et al., 1989).

Oxygen activation may also be an important factor in aging and in conditions related to age (cancer, parkinsonism, cardiovascular diseases, some mental disorders), as well as in rheumatoid arthritis, other immune complex injuries, and in conditions like certain convulsions and bowel diseases (Marx, 1987).

THE PHARMACOCHEMISTRY OF FREE RADICALS

The main objective of Pharmacochemistry is the discovery of new or better drugs. The best way to achieve this is by rational drug design, handled by several approaches. In this article, examples of research work conducted in our laboratory are shown, in which attempts are made to: **a)** Investigate the possible relationship of free radical activity on inflammation, on vascular or ocular pathophysiologic conditions (:direct or indirect elucidation of the pathobiochemistry of a disease). **b)** Elucidate the mechanism of action of certain toxic agents, e.g. ethanol, and to early detect the nature of the caused damage. **c)** Find relationships between structure - physicochemical properties and action (therapeutic or noxious). **d)** Design structures based on the above with high probability to acquire a protective - therapeutic action, or, at least, to possess the predicted biologic property. In our experiments, lipid peroxidation was induced by the ascorbic acid (0.2 mM) / Fe^{2+} (10 μM) system, and was determined as the 2-thiobarbituric acid reactive material (Rekka et al., 1989). The formaldehyde formed during the oxidation of DMSO by

Fe^{3+}/ascorbic acid was determined by the method of Nash (Nash, 1953) and used to detect hydroxyl radicals (Klein et al., 1981). The determination of the HO· scavenging activity of compounds was expressed as their competition with DMSO for these radicals.
Inflammation is connected to free radical phenomena through: a) The arachidonic acid cascade, leading to prostaglandins and related compounds. b) During phagocytosis, cells like polymorphonuclear leukocytes and macrophages, act by reducing oxygen to active oxygen species. These destroy the pathogens which are phagocytosed. However, they may also cause, extracellularly, damage to other cells. Thus, this process may contribute to tissue damage and malignant abnormalities which accompany inflammation and other autoimmune disorders (Flohé et al., 1985). We thus considered it interesting to examine some novel, basic in character, ethylenediamine derivatives with anti-inflammatory activity. Thus, N-[(1-phenacetyl)propyl]ethylene diamine and N-[(1-cyclohexyl-1-hydroxy)butyl]ethylene diamine presented good anti-inflammatory activity and action against free radicals, as expressed by prevention of lipid peroxidation, or by scavenging hydroxyl radicals. Honey bee venom is known to ameliorate pathologic conditions like rheumatoid arthritis. Therefore, we examined the effect of bee venom on active oxygen species and interleukine production. It was found that it prevented significantly lipid peroxidation and showed very good scavenging activity for HO·. In addition, it prevented directly interleukin-1 production (Rekka et al., 1990).

The presence of lipid peroxides in atherosclerotic aorta has been confirmed, and the accumulation of the complex of lipid peroxides with protein has been claimed to be one of the pathogenic causes of arteriosclerosis. It has been reported that chemically reactive products, like malondialdehyde, released during lipid peroxidation, convert LDL, the major carrier of plasma cholesterol, to an abnormal form, and that receptor-mediated clearance of this altered LDL produces cholesterol ester deposition in cells of atheroma (Haberland et al., 1988). Garlic powder has been found to reduce significantly blood cholesterol and pressure, having an overall beneficial action in atherosclerosis. Thus, we examined the protective effect of standardised garlic powder, alliin and diallyldisulfide on non enzymatic lipid peroxidation of liver microsomal membranes, and their HO· scavenging activity. We demonstrated that under conditions that permit natural alliin found in garlic powder to be converted to allicin, garlic powder presented considerable antioxidant activity, inhibiting lipid peroxidation by about 50% at a concentration equivalent to 0.18 mM allicin (Kourounakis & Rekka, 1991). Diallyldisulfide presented about the same activity at 1mM concentration. Alliin showed poor antioxidant activity, but was an efficient HO· scavenger (Kourounakis & Rekka, 1991). Benzoflavone derivatives (hydroxyethyl rutosides) have been claimed to possess a beneficial action on vascular disorders. We, therefore, examined the effect of a series of such derivatives on lipid peroxidation and as HO· scavengers. We found that many of these compounds acquire both actions (Rekka & Kourounakis, 1991).

The multiple involvement of free radicals in inflammation has already been mentioned. Since some pyrrole-1 and pyrrole-2 acetic acid derivatives are analgesics / anti-inflammatories, we decided to synthesise 2-, 4- or 5-benzoylpyrrole-3-acetic acids, to investigate the antioxidant and HO· scavenging activity, and their aldose reductase inhibitory action, as they present structural similarities with known inhibitors of this reductase. Hyperglycaemia is considered responsible for the complications of diabetes, partly because glucose reacts with proteins resulting to destruction of functionally important proteins. This process is believed to involve oxygen free radical production (Wolff et al., 1991). Our results showed that 5-benzoylpyrrole-3-acetic acid was the most active, the 4-benzoyl derivative the least, while the 2-derivative was somewhat less active than 5-benzoylpyrrole-3-acetic acid as an anti-inflammatory (rat paw carrageenan edema test), a HO· radical scavenger (Demopoulos et al., 1990) and an aldose reductase inhibitor (using a crude preparation of the rat lens enzyme). These three properties go in parallel.

It has been suggested that CNS and immune system are connected via opioid mediators. We examined the effect of 2-*n*-pentyloxy-2-phenyl-4-methyl-morpholine (a ligand of the analgesic receptor, which was synthesised in our laboratory), on immune responses, inflammation and interleukine production, and on lipid peroxidation and HO·. We found that this novel compound possessed a significant action on all tested parameters (Hadjipetrou-Kourounakis, L. et al., 1989; 1992).

As mentioned earlier, the hepatotoxicity of many compounds is mediated via free radical processes. Similar mechanisms may also be responsible for ethanol hepatotoxicity. Because of the wide interest in ethanol toxicity, its participation in numerous interactions with xenobiotics, and in particular its interaction with the microsomal enzyme system, we examined the effect of EtOH on liver microsomal lipid peroxidation and hepatic drug metabolic function. We then examined the effect of the coadministration of vitamins C and E with ethanol on the above parameters. We found that ethanol caused significant peroxidation of the liver lipids, and induced aromatic nitro-reductase. Coadministration of tocopherol prevented hepatic lipid peroxidation caused by ethanol and augmented significantly the nitroreductase. This effect is not shown by ascorbic acid (Tani & Kourounakis, 1991).

We have thus demonstrated that, via the free radical pharmacochemistry, we could elucidate the pathophysiologic mechanisms of certain disorders (inflammation) or toxic action (alcohol hepatotoxicity), confine the interconnection of CNS and immune system by opioid ligands (morpholine derivatives), find new therapeutic properties of compounds (vitamin E), suggest the molecular mechanism of the biologic action of compounds (hydroxyethyl rutosides, active ingredients of Allium sativum), and synthesise new compounds with predicted pharmacochemical properties (benzoyl-pyrrole-acetic acids).

REFERENCES

Comporti, M. (1989): Three models of free radical-induced cell injury. *Chem.-Biol. Interact.* 72, 1-56.

Demopoulos, V.J., Rekka, E. & Retsas, S. (1990): Synthesis of 2-, 4- and 5-benzoylpyrrole-3-acetic acids and study of their in vitro effects on active oxygen species. *Pharmazie* 45, 403-407.

Dodge, A.D. (1971): The mole of action of the bipyridylium herbicides, paraquat and diquat. *Endeavour* 30, 130-135.

Flohé, L., Beckmann, R., Giertz, H. & Loschen, G. (1985): Oxygen-centered free radicals as mediators of inflammation. In *Oxidative Stress*, ed. H. Sies, pp. 403-435. London: Academic Press.

Fridovich, I. (1988): The biology of oxygen radicals: Threats and defenses. In *Oxygen radicals in the pathophysiology of heart disease*, ed. P.K. Singal, pp. 1-11. Boston: Kluwer Academic Publishers.

Haberland, M.E., Fong, D. & Cheng, L. (1988): Malondialdehyde-altered protein occurs in atheroma of watanabe heritable hyperlipidemic rabbits. *Science* 241, *215-218.*

Hadjipetrou-Kourounakis, L., Karagounis, E., Rekka, E. & Kourounakis, P. (1989): Immunosuppression by a novel analgesic- opioid agonist. *Immunol.* 29, 449-458.

Hadjipetrou-Kourounakis, L., Rekka, E. & Kourounakis, A. (1992): Suppression of adjuvant induced disease (AID) by a novel analgesic- opioid agonist which also possess antioxidant activity. *Ann. New York Acad. Sci.*, in press.

Klein, S.M., Cohen, G., & Cederbaum, A.I. (1981): Production of formaldehyde during metabolism of dimethyl sulfoxide by hydroxyl radical generating systems. *Biochemistry* 20, *6006-6012.*

Kourounakis, P.N. & Rekka, E.A. (1991): Effect on active oxygen species of alliin and Allium sativum (garlic) powder. *Res. Comm. Chem. Pathol. Pharmacol.* 74, 249-252.

Marx, J.L. (1987): Oxygen free radicals linked to many diseases. *Science* 235, 529-532.

Nash, T. (1953): The colorimetric estimation of formaldehyde by means of the Hantzsch reaction. *Biochem. J.* 55, *416-421.*

Rekka, E., Kolstee, J., Timmermann, H. & Bast, A. (1989): The effect of some H_2-receptor antagonists on rat hepatic microsomal cytochrome P-450 and lipid peroxidation in vitro. *Eur. J. Med. Chem.* 24, *43-54.*

Rekka, E., Kourounakis, L. & Kourounakis, P.N. (1990): Antioxidant activity of and interleukin production affected by honey bee venom. *Arzneim.-Forsch./Drug Res.* 40, 912-913.

Rekka, E. & Kourounakis, P.N. (1991): Effect of hydroxyethyl rutosides and related compounds on lipid peroxidation and free radical scavenging activity. Some structural aspects. *J. Pharm. Pharmacol.* 43, 486-491.

Ruckpaul, K., Rein, H. & Blanck, J. (1989): Regulation mechanisms of the activity of the hepatic endoplasmic cytochrome P-450. In *Basis and Mechanisms of Regulation of Cytochrome P-450*, eds. K.Ruckpaul and H. Rein, pp. 3-65. London: Taylor & Francis.

Scott, G. (1985): Antioxidants in vitro and in vivo. *Chemistry in Britain* 21, 648-653.

Tani, Ek. & Kourounakis, P.N. (1991): Effect of ethanol and of its interactions with ascorbic acid and tocopherol-Ac on PNBA reduction. *Proc. Pharmacy World Congress*, Washington D.C., CS-148.

Walsh, C. (1979): In Enzymatic reaction mechanisms, ed. C. Walsh, pp. 432-500. New York: Freeman.

Wolff, S.R. Jiang, Z. Y. & Hunt, J. V. (1991): Protein glycation and oxidative stress in diabetes mellitus and ageing. *Free Radical Biology and Medicine* 10, 339-352.

Yoshioka, T., Fujita, T., Kanai, T., Aizawa, Y., Kurumada, T., Hasegawa, K. & Horikoshi, H. J. (1989): Studies on hindered phenols and analogues. 1. Hypolipidemic and hypoglycemic agents with ability to inhibit lipid reroxidation. *J. Med. Chem.* 32, *421-428.*

Metal Ions in Biology and Medicine, vol. 2. Eds. J. Anastassopoulou, Ph. Collery, J.C. Etienne, Th. Theophanides. John Libbey Eurotext, Paris © 1992, pp. 269-274

Immunotoxicologic effects of heavy metals on human skin

K. Nordlind, S. Lidén

Department of Dermatology, Karolinska Hospital, S-104 01 Stockholm, Sweden

The human skin creates an unique milieu to study immunotoxicologic effects of heavy metals due to the simple methods of application and many possibilities to investigate tissue reactions. Heavy metals may cause different inflammatory reaction types in the human skin, the most common being of contact allergic and irritant nature. Lichenoid, granulomatous and vasculitis reactions are also found. In addition, some tissue reaction types may change to other types, like, e.g., eczematous reactions developing into lichenoid reactions.
There are important problems regarding the inflammatory skin effects of heavy metals, like the mechanisms for the start of the inflammatory processes and the handling of these processes by the surrounding tissue, i.e. why is the reaction selflimiting in one individual, while turning into a chronic reaction persisting for several months in another? In this context it should be pointed out that there are similarities in the reaction patterns with other conditions with stress to the skin like after, e.g., virus and bacteria.
In the present study heavy metal salts were tested on the human skin by routine patch testing procedure, biopsies were taken after 3 days from positive patch test reactions and then studied by using immunohistochemistry and antibodies to different inflammatory cells and mediators.

The inflammatory tissue infiltrates after heavy metal salts are composed of different cell types, where major parts are played by mononuclear leucocytes. When studying allergic and irritant patch test reactions and using an indirect peroxidase technique, a majority of the T lymphocytes were $CD4^+$ (helper/inducer) compared to $CD8^+$ (suppressor/cytotoxic), moreover a majority being $UHCL\text{-}1^+$ ('memory') compared to $Leu18^+$ ('naive'), in both types of reactions. It might be expected that the infiltrates in the irritant reactions could have another ratio of lymphocyte subtypes than allergic reactions, and indeed different results have been reported earlier as regards helper/inducer and suppressor/cytotoxic T lymphocytes (Ralfkiaer and Lange Wantzin, 1984; Avnstorp et al., 1987). As regards 'memory' and 'naive' T lymphocytes, Sterry et al. (1990) reported a dominance of 'memory' T lymphocytes in contact allergic tissue reactions and that this dominance was not due to in situ maturation of 'naive' into 'memory' T cells, but rather reflected a selective migration of 'memory' T lymphocytes into the dermis. In the healthy tissue it is predominantly 'memory' T cells which localize to nonlymphoid tissues including the skin, and they are also the predominant cell type within inflammatory lesions (for refs see Mackay, 1991) including dermal cellular infiltrates in other inflammatory skin diseases as well as malignant cutaneous T-cell lymphomas (Bos et al., 1989).

Of considerable interest is the presence of gamma/delta T cells, i.e. T lymphocytes with TcR gamma/delta heterodimers in association with the invariant CD3 complex (Brenner et al., 1986), in the cellular infiltrates after mercuric chloride and gold chloride, often showing epidermotropism, while not being seen in normal skin and in very small number in reactions to nickel sulfate and to silver nitrate. The gamma/delta T cells had gene segments of V delta 2 and gamma V 2 (a) in addition to being $CD4^-8^-$ and thus might have the same phenotype as gamma/delta T cells in the peripheral blood (Hochstenbach and Brenner, 1990).
Gamma/delta T cells have been reported to be able to react with superantigens like, e.g., staphylococcal enterotoxin (Rust et al., 1990), gamma V 2 (a) cells mediated the recognition. A role for gamma/delta T lymphocytes in potential autoimmune reactions has been suggested (Rajagopalan et al., 1990) and in that respect the presence of such cells in lichenoid reactions to gold chloride and mercuric chloride, which was obtained in some of our patients, is of interest. On the contrary, gamma/delta T cell have been shown to exert a negative effect on the immune response, resulting in induction of antigen-specific tolerance (Sullivan et al., 1986). Putative gamma/delta T lymphocytes down-regulated the immune responses to inert protein antigens being presented via intact epithelial surfaces in the respiratory tract (McMenamin et al., 1991). Thus, these cells might have a role for maintenance of homeostasis at skin and mucosal surfaces.

Gamma/delta T cells have been associated with recognition of heat shock proteins (hsp) and especially of the 65kD class (Fisch et al., 1990). Hsp synthesis may be induced after different cellular stress conditions, e.g., heat, microbiological agents and heavy metals (for refs see, e.g. Lindquist, 1986; Kochevar et al., 1991). Of the hsp, the 60 kD family has been suggested as being potential target for autoimmune responses and could provide a link between the stress agent and autoimmunity (Lamb and Young, 1990). The localization of the genes for hsp 70 proteins is adjacent to the region of human chromosome 6 containing genes for the class II histocompatibility antigens which might indicate that these proteins have some association with antigen processing and presentation (Sargent et al., 1989). The hsp 90 gene is linked to a minor histocompatibility locus near H-2 in the mouse (Romano et al., 1989). Antibodies to this family, in addition to the members of the hsp 70 family, are elevated in the sera of patients with systemic lupus erythematosus (Minota et al., 1988).
A marked increase in the expression of heat-inducible forms of hsp 70 and 90 has been found in human monocytes during heat shock (Joslin et al., 1991) and a strong reactivity against hsp 65 was obtained within synovial mononuclear cells in inflamed joints and subcutaneous nodules of rheumatoid patients (Karlsson-Parra et al., 1990).
In the present investigation expression of hsp 65-like immunoreactivity was seen in macrophage-like cells in the dermis in both metal-treated and control skin, in addition to diffusely in the dermis, and sometimes in single dendritic epidermal cells. Hsp 72-like immunoreactivity was found in keratinocytes, while hsp 90-like immunoreactivity was found

in cells in the epidermis and in some macrophage-like cells in the dermis, by double staining being HLA-DR$^+$ and Leu 6$^+$. Thus hsp might be associated both with the presentation of antigens in the human skin as well as the following inflammatory processes.

HLA-DR, the class II major histocompatibility complex molecule, and intercellular adhesion molecule (ICAM)-1 are two complexes which are important for T lymphocyte function. In the present investigation keratinocyte HLA-DR expression was found at 3 days, in both allergic and irritant reactions to gold chloride and in allergic but only exceptionally in irritant reactions to mercuric chloride. This is interesting with regard to the findings that lymphocytes from patients with mercury allergy, in the form of oral mucosal lesions adjacent to amalgam restorations, showed a higher level of interferon gamma in their supernatants compared to control patients, after addition of mercuric chloride (Nordlind and Lidén, in preparation). Interferon gamma is an inducer of keratinocyte HLA-DR expression (Basham et al., 1984, Griffiths et al., 1989). Keratinocyte expression of ICAM-1 was found after application of all tested metal salts, gold chloride, mercuric chloride, nickel sulfate and silver nitrate, however, most extensive and including the whole epidermis after gold chloride.
The implication of expression of HLA-DR and ICAM-1 is not clear. The HLA-DR expression might allow the keratinocytes to participate in immunologic responses such as antigen presentation and cytotoxicity, giving an enhancement of the immune reaction (Gaspari and Katz, 1988; Czernielewski, 1988). However, HLA-DR positive keratinocytes might also be involved in the development of antigen-specific tolerance and downregulation of the inflammatory response (Gaspari et al., 1988). In this way chronic tissue damage might be avoided.
ICAM-1 is the specific ligand for the integrin LFA (lymphocyte function-associated antigen)-1, and its upregulation on keratinocytes is believed to relate to the secretion of cytokines, including interferon gamma by activated T lymphocytes and tumor necrosis factor (TNF) alpha by macrophages (Kupper, 1989). It has been suggested that keratinocyte ICAM-1 induction has a generalized role in cutaneous inflammatory reactions, promoting the infiltration of leucocytes into the epidermis (Willis et al., 1991). ICAM-1 expression is obtained in different inflammatory dermatoses and seems to be dependent on the grade of inflammation (Simon and Hunyadi, 1990; Detmar and Orfanos, 1990).

An increasing number of cytokines are being produced in inflammatory conditions by different cell types (for rev. see, e.g., Arai et al., 1990). In the present investigation the expression of IL (interleukin)-6-like immunoreactivity was studied in the positive patch test reactions to the metal salts. By using fixation in Lanas solution, a monoclonal antibody to IL-6 and an indirect immunofluorescence technique (Hökfelt et al., 1973; Johansson and Nordlind, 1984), nerve fibers with expression of IL-6-like immunoreactivity were seen in close contact with dermal inflammatory cells as well as in some fibers with varicosities in the epidermis, the latter only after treatment with heavy metal salts. Besides immunoreactivity localized to nerves, some cells in the infiltrates as well as in the epidermis also showed immunoreactivity. These findings indicate an immunomodulatory and/or nerve trophic effect for IL-6 in the human skin, in general, in inflammatory conditions. A nerve trophic effect for IL-6 has earlier been suggested (Satoh et al., 1988; Benveniste et al., 1990). Moreover, a pruritogenic effect of IL-6 might exist.

Thus, the problems regarding the mechanisms for the start and limitation of inflammatory skin reactions to heavy metals need to be further studied also by using other techniques such as, e.g., in situ hybridization and cell culture systems.

REFERENCES

Arai, K-i., Lee, F., Miyajima, A., Miyatake, S., Arai, N., and Yokota, T. (1990): Cytokines: coordinators of immune and inflammatory responses. Annu. Rev. Biochem. 59: 783-836.

Avnstorp, C., Balslev, E., and Thomsen, H.K. (1989): The occurrence of different morphological parameters in allergic and irritant patch test reactions. In Current Topics in Contact Dermatitis, ed. P.-J. Frosch, A. Dooms-Goossens, J.-M. Lachapelle, R.J.G. Rycroft, and R.J. Scheper, pp. 38-41. Berlin, Heidelberg: Springer Verlag.

Basham, T.Y., Nickoloff, B.J., Merigan, T.C., and Morhenn, V.B. (1984): Recombinant gamma interferon induces HLA-DR expression on cultured human keratinocytes. J. Invest. Dermatol. 83: 88-90.

Benveniste, E.N., Sparacio, S.M., Norris, J.G., Grenett, H.E., Fuller, G.M. (1990): Induction and regulation of interleukin-6 gene expression in rat astrocytes. J. Neuroimmunol. 30: 201-212.

Bos, J.D., Hagenaars, C., Das, P.K., Krieg, S.R., Voorn, W.J., and Kapsenberg, M.L. (1989): Predominance of "memory" T cells (CD4+, CDw29+) over "naive" T cells (CD4+, CF45R+) in both normal and diseased skin. Arch. Dermatol. Res. 281: 24-30.

Brenner, M.B., McLean J., Dialynas, D.P., Strominger, J.L., Smith, J.A., Owen, F.L., Seidman, J.G., Ip, S., Rosen, F., and Krangel, M.S. (1986): Identification of a putative second T-cell receptor. Nature 322: 145-149.

Czernielewski, J. (1988): Class II MHC antigen expression by keratinocytes results from lymphoepidermal interactions. J. Invest. Dermatol. 90: 886-887.

Detmar, M., and Orfanos, C.E. (1990): Tumor necrosis factor-alpha inhibits cell proliferation and induces class II antigens and cell adhesion molecules in cultured normal human keratinocytes in vitro. Arch. Dermatol. Res. 282: 238-245.

Fisch, P., Malkovsky, M., Kovats, S., Sturm, E., Braakman, E., Klein, B.S., Voss, S.D., Morrissey, L.W., DeMars, R., Welch, W.J., Bolhuis, R.L.H., and Sondel, P.M. (1990): Recognition by human V gamma 9/V delta 2 T cells of a GroEL homolog on Daudi Burkitt's lymphoma cells. Science 250: 1269-1273.

Gaspari, A.A., and Katz. S.I. (1988): Induction and functional characterization of class II MHC (Ia) antigen on murine keratinocytes. J. Immunol. 140: 2956-2963.

Gaspari, A.A., Jenkins, M., and Katz, S.I. (1988): Class II MCH-bearing keratinocytes induce antigen-specific unresponsiveness in haptenspecific TH1 clones. J. Immunol. 141: 2216-2220.

Griffiths, C.E.M., Voorhess, J.J., and Nickoloff, B.J. (1989): Gamma interferon induces different keratinocyte cellular patterns of expression of HLA-DR and DQ and intercellular adhesion molecule-1 (ICAM-1) antigens. Br. J. Dermatol. 120: 1-7.

Hochstenbach, F., and Brenner, M.B. (1990): Newly identified gamma delta and beta delta T-cell receptors. J. Clin. Immunol. 10: 1-18.

Hökfelt, T., Fuxe, K., Goldstein, M. and Joh, T.H. (1973): Immunohistochemical localization of three catecholamine synthesizing enzymes: aspects on methodology. Histochemie 33: 231-254.

Johansson O., and Nordlind K. (1984): Immunohistochemical localization of somatostatin-like immunoreactivity in skin lesions from patients with urticaria pigmentosa. Virchows Arch. (B) 46: 155-164.

Joslin, G., Hafeez, W., and Perlmutter, D.H. (1991): Expression of stress proteins in human mononuclear phagocytes. J. Immunol. 147: 1614-1620.
Karlsson-Parra, A., Söderström, K., Ferm, M. Ivanyi, J., Kiessling, R., and Klareskog, L. (1990): Presence of human 65 kD heat shock protein (hsp) in inflamed joints and subcutaneous nodules of RA patients. Scand. J. Immunol. 31: 283-288.
Kochevar, D.T., Aucoin, M.M., and Cooper, J. (1991): Mammalian heat shock proteins: an overview with a system perspective. Toxicol. Lett. 56: 243-267.
Kupper, T.S. (1989): Mechanisms of cutaneous inflammation. Arch. Dermatol. 125: 1406-1412.
Lamb, J.R., and Young, D.B. (1990): T cell recognition of stress proteins. A link between infectious and autoimmune disease. Mol. Biol. Med. 7: 311-321.
Lindquist, S. (1986): The shock protein response. Annu. Rev. Biochem. 55: 1151-1191.
Mackay, C.R. (1991): T-cell memory: the connection between function, phenotype and migration pathways. Immunology Today 12: 189-192.
McMenamin, C., Oliver, J., Girn, B., Holt, B.J., Kees, U.R., Thomas, W.R., and Holt, P.G. (1991): Regulation of T-cell sensitization at epithelial surfaces in the respiratory tract: suppression of IgE responses to inhaled antigens by $CD3^+$ TcR $alfa^-/beta^-$ lymphocytes (putative gamma/delta T cells). Immunology 74: 234-239.
Minota, S., Koyasu, S., Yahara, I., and Winfield, J.B. (1988): Autoantibodies to the heat-shock protein hsp^{90} in systemic lupus erythematosus. J. Clin. Invest. 81: 106-109.
Rajagopalan, S., Zordan, T., Tsokos, G.C., and Datta, S.K. (1990): Pathogenic anti-DNA autoantibody-inducing T helper cell lines from patients with active lupus nephritis: Isolation of $CD4^-8^-$ T helper cell lines that express the gamma delta T-cell antigen receptor. Proc. Natl. Acad. Sci. (USA) 87: 7020-7024.
Ralfkiaer, E., and Lange Wantzin, G. (1984): In situ immunological characterization of the infiltrating cells in positive patch tests. Br. J. Dermatol. 111: 13-22.
Romano, J.W., Seldin, M.F., and Appella, E. (1989): Linkage of the mouse Hsp84 heat shock protein structural gene to the H-2 complex. Immunogenetics 29: 142-144.
Rust, C.J., Verreck, F., Vietor, H., and Koning, F. (1990): Specific recognition of staphylococcal enterotoxin A by human T cells bearing receptors with the V gamma 9 region. Nature 346: 572-574.
Sargent, C.A., Dunham, I., Trowsdale, J., and Campbell, R.D. (1989): Human major histocompatibility complex contains genes for the major heat shock protein hsp 70. Proc. Natl. Acad. Sci. (USA) 86: 1968-1972.
Satoh, T., Nakamura, S., Taga, T., Matsuda, T., Hirano, T., Kishimoto, T., and Kaziro, Y. (1988): Induction of neuronal differentiation in PC12 cells by a B cell stimulatory factor 2/interleukin 6. Mol. Cell. Biol. 8: 3546-3549.
Simon, M. Jr., and Hunyadi, J. (1990): Etretinate suppresses ICAM-1 expression by lesional keratinocytes in healing cutaneous lichen planus. Arch. Dermatol. Res. 282: 412-414.
Sterry, W., Bruhn, S., Kunne, N., Lichtenberg, B., Weber-Matthiesen, K., Brasch, J., and Mielke V. (1990): Dominance of memory over naive T cells in contact dermatitis is due to differential tissue migration. Br. J. Dermatol. 123: 59-64.

Sullivan, S., Bergstresser, P.R., Tigelaar, R.E., and Streilein, J.W. (1986): Induction and regulation of contact hypersensitivity by resident, bone marrow-derived, dendritic epidermal cells: Langerhans cells and Thy-1+ epidermal cells. J. Immunol. 137: 2460-2467.

Willis, C.M., Stephens, C.J.M., and Wilkinson, J.D. (1991): Selective expression of immune-associated surface antigens by keratinocytes in irritant contact dermatitis. J. Invest. Dermatol. 96: 505-511.

Metal Ions in Biology and Medicine, vol. 2. Eds. J. Anastassopoulou, Ph. Collery, J.C. Etienne, Th. Theophanides. John Libbey Eurotext, Paris © 1992, pp. 275-280

Determination of lead by its inhibition of isocitrate dehydrogenase and diagnosis of lead poisoning

R. W. Henkens*+, T. E. Johnston*, M.L. Nevoret*, J. P. O'Daly*, J. Stonehuerner*, Junguo Zhao+

**Duke University, Department of Chemistry, Durham, NC 27706, +Enzyme Technology Research Group, Inc., 710 West Main Street, Durham, NC 27701, USA*

Our objective is to develop reagents and methods for the direct determination of lead in blood. This paper presents the initial results on measuring sub-micromolar concentrations of lead with an enzyme based system. The enzyme serves as a lead sensitive reagent whose activity is inhibited by low levels of lead.

The requirement for direct enzymatic metal analysis in biological samples is the *selective determination* of *trace levels* of metal in a complex sample that can contain inhibitors, activators, masking agents and other modulators. Effective enzymatic methods require selective, highly sensitive enzyme reagents and reactions. Masking agents and additives that facilitate desired metal exchange reactions may be needed. Side reactions with additives and natural ligands in the sample decrease the conditional equilibrium constant with the enzyme reagent and hence reduce the selectivity and sensitivity of the analysis.

The United States Department of Health has declared in its strategic plan for the elimination of childhood lead poisoning that the development of portable, easy-to-use, cheaper instrumentation for blood lead measurement is extremely important. For wide-spread screening of blood lead levels in children, a simple method is required that can be applied directly to a finger-stick sample of blood. The test must be able to reliably measure lead at the critical decision points such as 10 µg/dL, the level that the U.S. Centers for Disease Control define toxicity for children.

We are studying the inhibition of NADP-linked isocitrate dehydrogenase (ICDH) (EC 1.1.1.42) by lead because this enzyme has been shown to be extremely sensitive to lead (Kratochvil et al., 1967; Sheikh and Townshend, 1974). The oxidation of isocitrate on NADP linked isocitrate dehydrogenase-gold sol (ICDH-Au) modified electrodes has been studied with various electron transfer mediators. The amplification effect due to the enzyme catalyzed turnover of substrate facilitates our investigation of isocitrate dehydrogenase (ICDH) inhibition by lead. Based on this inhibition, electroanalytical methods are being developed for the convenient determination of trace lead in whole blood. The specific goal is to develop a device suitable for wide-spread screening of blood lead levels in children and adults.

EXPERIMENTAL SECTION

ICDH was obtained from Sigma Chemical Co. It was dialyzed against $MnCl_2$ solutions ranging in concentration from 0.1 to 10 mM.

A Pine Instruments RD4 bi-potentiostat interfaced to an IBM-386 computer was used for these experiments. The system was controlled with ASYST programs written at Enzyme Technology Research Group, Inc., and electrochemical data were directly collected and processed in the computer. Cyclic voltammograms were obtained in quiescent solution. In steady-state amperometry experiments the potential was set at 0 volts (Ag/AgCl) in quiescent solution, and the steady state current was measured.

The device for measuring lead employs an ICDH modified electrode system. The principles of the electrode system are illustrated schematically in Fig. 1. The electrode's key operational subsystems are: (1) an electron transfer system, (2) a molecular layer of immobilized metal sensitive enzyme, and (3) a membrane. Metal compounds inhibit the enzyme, preventing the electrocatalytic oxidation of the substrate, thus giving a reduction in electrode response proportional to the amount of metal compounds. Selectivity is further enhanced by the appropriate choice of reaction conditions.

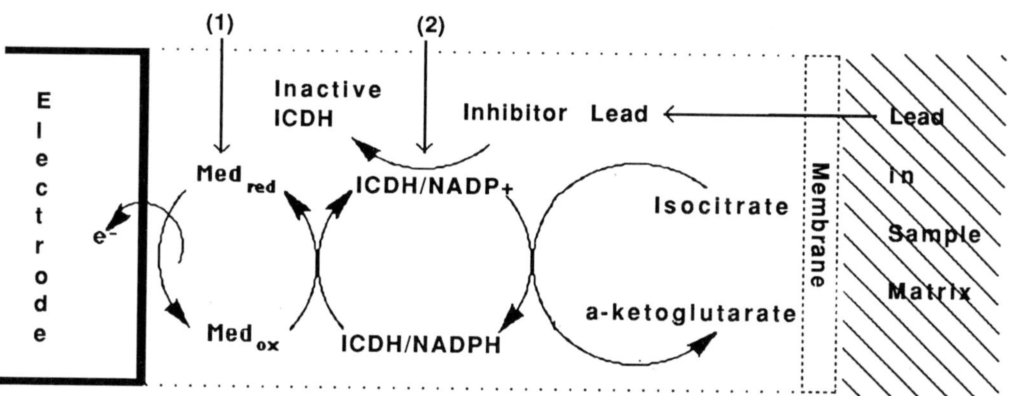

Fig. 1. Schematic diagram of inhibited ICDH electrode for lead compounds.

The electrode cell (Fig. 2) used in this research consists of a carbon rod surrounded by platinum foil and insulated in teflon which contains a silver wire reference electrode. The glassy carbon surface was 3 mm in diameter. The coplanar three-electrode cell was surrounded by a plastic ring that served as a sample holder that normally contains up to 200 µl sample solution. Enzyme reagents are used either free in solution or immobilized using colloidal gold as an enzyme immobilization matrix. In earlier work we have studied the effectiveness of colloidal gold as an immobilization matrix that maintains the activity of redox enzymes for electrochemical applications (Henkens et al., 1987; Crumbliss et al., 1990; Henkens et al., 1991).

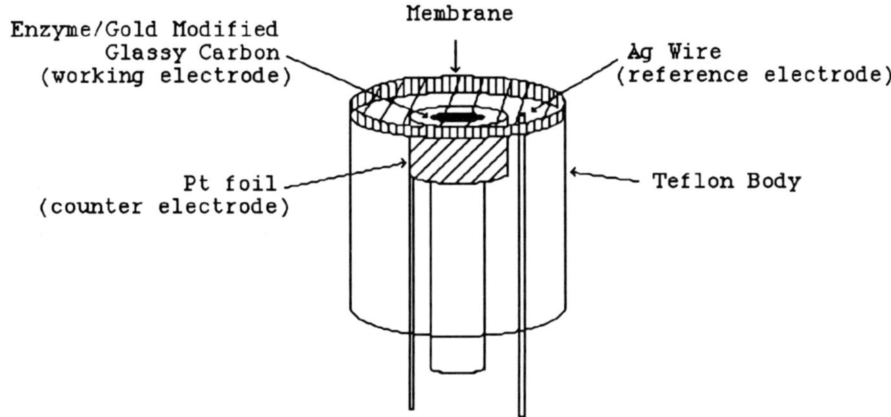

Fig. 2. Diagram of an electrode cell.

Colloidal gold was prepared by the reduction of gold chloride with citrate. The enzyme was then immobilized to yield an ICDH-gold sol by simple adsorption using methods employed previously (Henkens et al., 1991). A small aliquot of the ICDH-gold sol was evaporated onto the working electrode (Fig. 2).

Electrochemical measurements were made by steady-state amperometry at 0 volts (Ag/AgCl) in a buffer solution containing 50 mM Tris at pH 8.5 In some cases N-methylphenazonium methosulfate (NMP-MS) was added to the solution to serve as a mediator. In other cases N-methylphenazonium tetracyanoquinodimethane (NMP-TCNQ) was immobilized on the surface of the working electrode as the mediator.

The percent inhibition of the electrode response by lead was calculated by the signal drop due to the presence of lead divided by the total signal without lead.

Spectroscopic assays were conducted at 340 nm with a Cary 15 spectrophotometer in a manner similar to those reported previously (Kratochvil et al., 1967; Sheikh and Townshend, 1974). Significant deviations include incubation temperature (see Fig. 5) and a typical ΔA/min of 0.05 vs. 0.5.

RESULTS

In the absence of ICDH none of the electrodes tested had a significant response to isocitrate in steady-state amperometry measurements at 0 volts (Ag/AgCl). The colloidal gold-modified glassy carbon electrode showed no catalytic current in cyclic voltammograms recorded with isocitrate.

Experiments were repeated as described above except that ICDH-Au sols were deposited onto the electrode surfaces. The ICDH-Au sol/glassy carbon (HRP-Au/C) electrode showed good current response to varying concentrations of isocitrate in the presence of an electron transfer mediator at 0 volts (Ag/AgCl).

The ICDH exhibited very high sensitivity to lead. In this experiment, the mediator, cofactor and the enzyme were all maintained free in solution. The enzyme was incubated with lead at 25 °C for 10 minutes before addition of NADP and isocitric acid. Response of the ICDH electrode for the determination of 0-50 μg/dL (0-500 ppb) of lead in aqueous solution is shown in Fig. 3. The solid line is calculated on the basis of reversible inhibition by lead using an I_{50} of 2.8 μg/dL.

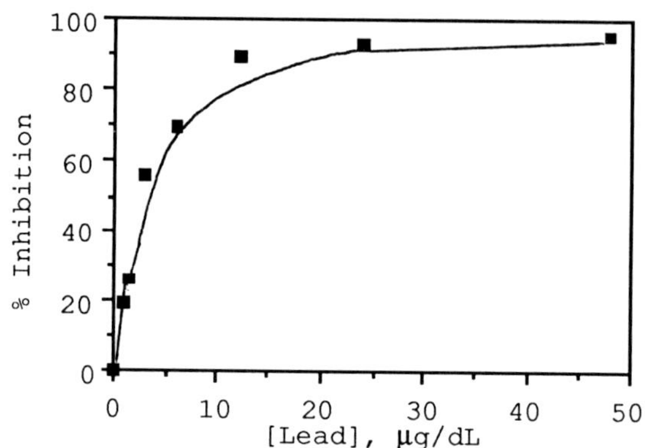

Fig. 3. Response of ICDH to lead by amperometric measurement of percent inhibition vs. lead concentration in unstirred pH 8.5 buffer (50 mM tris, 10 mM KCl) with NMP-MS mediator at 0V/Ag. The electrode material is glassy carbon. The apparent electrode area is 7 mm^2. ICDH was maintained in solution. Percent inhibition was calculated from $(i_0 - i)/i_0$ where i is the measured current in the presence of lead and i_0 is the measured current in the absence of lead.

The excellent response of this electrode to lead is illustrated in Fig. 4 which shows the linear portion of the lead response curve. Lead concentrations of 1 μg/dL or less can be readily determined with this configuration.

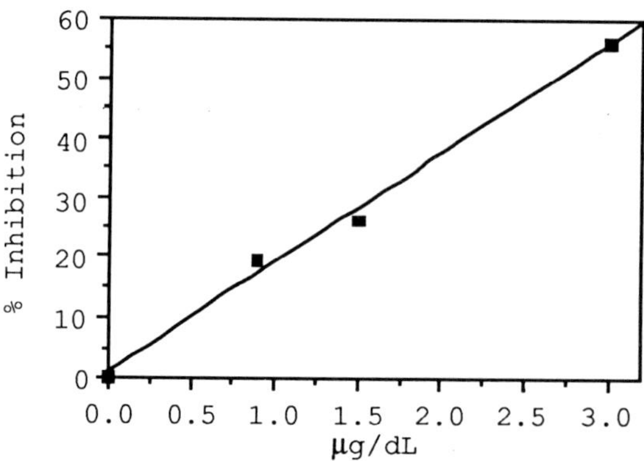

Fig. 4. Same conditions as Fig. 3 but showing linear portion of the lead response curve.

To improve the system in unstirred samples where diffusion rates may limit sensitivity, we have co-immobilized key elements of mediator, NADP and ICDH at the electrode surface. In this way the low usable concentrations of enzyme, cofactor and mediator do not limit the response. The feasibility of co-immobilization of the enzyme, mediator and the cofactor on the electrode surface was shown. In the configuration tested the electrode consists of NMP-TCNQ, NADP, ICDH and polyvinyl chloride added as a binding reagent. This configuration gives a rapid response to isocitrate.

A hemolyzed red blood cell solution without lead does not decrease ICDH activity and when added after lead inhibition does not decrease the extent of inhibition of the enzyme by lead. But the sensitivity for lead is much less in the presence of hemolyzed red blood cells than in water. We are beginning experiments to improve the sensitivity for direct measurement of lead in blood. These experiments will improve the operation of the electrode in blood and characterize metal exchange and masking reagents.

Sheikh and Townshend (1974) showed an incubation time-dependence on the degree to which lead inhibited the activity of ICDH when incubation of the lead and ICDH was conducted at 0 °C in Tris buffer, pH 8.5. They observed that inhibition increased up to an incubation time of 15 minutes after which time the degree of inhibition for 2 µg/dL lead concentration remained constant. We have repeated those spectroscopic studies at an incubation temperature of 25 °C (Fig. 5). Our data, too, show a time dependence of the inhibition, but the controls with no added lead also lose activity with time so that at incubation times in excess of 15 minutes the relative activity of the lead-inhibited sample compared to the control increases (Fig. 5). It must be noted that these are all relative activities, and with incubation times in excess of 15 minutes both the sample and control have lost a large fraction of their initial activities.

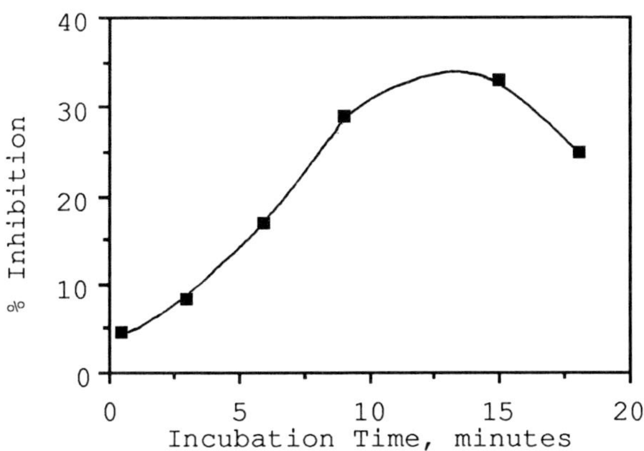

Fig. 5. Time course of ICDH inhibition caused by lead in Tris-chloride buffer, pH 8.5, 8 nM ICDH, 540 nM lead, incubation at 25 °C.

CONCLUSION

We have demonstrated the sensitive measurement of lead in water with an ICDH modified electrode under mild conditions through the amperometric detection of the inhibition of the enzyme catalyzed reaction. This offers an opportunity to build a sensitive electrode test strip for lead in blood. Additional work is needed on improving the sensitivity for lead in blood and on characterizing the effect of blood on electrode response to lead.

REFERENCES

Crumbliss, A.L., Henkens, R.W., Perine, S.C., Tubergen, K.R., Kitchell, B.S., and Stonehuerner, J. (1990): Amperometric Glucose Sensor Fabricated from Glucose Oxidase and a Mediator Co-immobilized on a Colloidal Gold Hydrogel Electrode. *Biosensor Technology: Fundamentals and Applications*, ed. R.P. Buck, W.E. Hatfield, M. Umana, and E.F. Bowden, Chap. 13. New York: Marcel Dekker Publishing Company.

Henkens, R.W., O'Daly, J.P., Perine, S.C., Stonehuerner, J., Tubergen, K.R., Zhao, J., and Crumbliss, A. L. (1991): Electrochemistry of Colloidal Gold Supported Oxidase Enzymes. *J. Inorg. Biochem.* **43**, 120.

Henkens, R.W., Kitchell, B.S., O'Daly, J.P., Perine, S.C., and Crumbliss, A.L. (1987): Bioactive Electrodes Using Metallo-Proteins Attached to Colloidal Gold. *Recl. Trav. Chim. Pays Bas.* **106**, 298.

Kratochvil, B., Boyer, S.L., and Hicks, G.P. (1967): Effect of Metals on the Activation and Inhibition of Isocitrate Dehydrogenase. *Anal. Chem.* **39**, 45-51.

Sheikh, R.A., and Townshend, A. (1974): Application of Enzyme-Catalysed Reactions in Trace Analysis-VII. Determination of Lead and Indium by their Inhibition of Isocitrate Dehydrogenase. *Talanta.* **21**, 401-409.

Metal Ions in Biology and Medicine, vol. 2. Eds. J. Anastassopoulou, Ph. Collery, J.C. Etienne, Th. Theophanides. John Libbey Eurotext, Paris © 1992, pp. 281-286

Lead-toxic and/or essential ?

Rudolf H. Barckhaus, Peter F. Schmidt, Hans J. Höhling

Institute of Medical Physics and Biophysics, University of Münster Hüfferstr. 68, D-4400 Münster, Germany

Lead is a widely distributed heavy metal. Large quantities of lead are added to the atmosphereby engine exhausts and are inhaled in biological systems. The toxicity of this metal has been recognized in recent years, particularly in those countries where it is used in industrial processes.

A morphological characteristic of lead poisoning in men and animals is the formation of intranuclear inclusion bodies in different biological cells.

Lead influences the cytochemical and histochemical metabolism of both the cell and the tissue. Enzymes show a pronounced sensitivity against lead ions (HAMPP et al. 1974). The inhibition of chlorophyll synthesis could be due to toxic effects of lead ions on enzymes involved in chlorophyll synthesis (HAMPP and LENDZIAN, 1974). In urban areas, where exposure to lead is increasing, a far from negligible number of children may be suffering from subclinical lead poisoning with silent brain damage (NEEDLEMAN et al. 1972).

Lead shows different modes of actions (Table 1): Toxicological aspects, influence on the cellular defence mechanism, competition with other elements, but there are also reports on the essentiality of lead.

1. Toxicological aspects (Table 1a, Fig. 1-3)

For the investigation of the toxicological aspects of lead young female wistar rats 1oo-14o g, were divided in two groups. The animal of one group were injected intraperitoneally with lead acetate in sterile water in dodes of 0.20 mg of lead per gram body weight. the rats of the other group were given drinking water containing basic lead acetate in a concentration of 1%. At three an six days after the single dose of lead (group 1), and at 1, 3, and 6 monthsafter the dose of lead in drinking water (group 2), tissue were taken from the cortex of kidney, liver, spleen, duodenum, jejunum, ileum, tibial growth plate, and from the incisors. The samples were (A) shock-frozen for X-ray microprobe analysis, (B) fixed only in glutaraldehyde/formaldehyde, and (C) postfixed with osmium tetroxyde for transmission microscopy. The samples were than embedded in SPURR's medium and in lowicryl K4M.

Thereto tissue blocks of 1-2 mm^3 from the epiphyseal grwoth plate and from kidney were shock-frozen in liquid propane to prevent the growth of ice crystals within the tissue and consequently the dislocation of elements, freeze-dried at -80°C for 8 days, then impregnated in the vacuum with chlorine-free SPURR's medium.

Point measurements of 50 nm gain-diameter respectively microareas ranging from 0.13 x 0.13 µm to 12 x 12 µm were analyzed by microscan and the excited characteristic X-rays were counted and processed with the energy-dispersive system (EDAX).

Table 1. List of the different modes of lead activities.

a) <u>Toxicological aspects</u>	growth plate, kidney (nuclei, mitochondria)	Barckhaus et al. 1991, 1986 Bonucci et al. 1983 Goyer et al. 1970 Goyer and Rhyne 1973 Ricordi et al. 1980
b) Effects on cells	leucocytes macrophages	Baginski 1985 Hilbertz et al. 1986
c) Interaction with other elements	Ca, Fe, Cd, Zn	Mahaffey and Fowler 1977 Mahaffey et al. 1978 Mahaffey and Michaelson 1980 Barton et al. 1978 Willoughby et al. 1972
d) essentiality	lead depletion (anemia, growth depression, disturbances of metabolism, enzyme reductions)	Reichlmayr-Lais and Kirchgeßner 1986 Reichlmayr-Lais et al. 1991

A morphological characteristic of lead poisoning in man and animal is the formation of electron dark inclusion bodies in intracellular compartiments both in nuclei and mitochondria. The lead containing areas composed of proteinand lead and posses-ses dense core from which protein fibrils project outwards (BARCKHAUS et al. 1991; 1986; 1985). It has been suggested that the inclusions are derived either from preexisting intranuclear proteins (RICHTER et al., 1968; GOYER et al., 1973), or from a protein involved in the transport of lead, perhaps a plasma protein (GOYER et al., 1970; GOYER and RHYNE, 1973). One nucleus contains two or more inclusions. After CHOIE and RICHTER (1972) is the development of the intranuclear inclusions an acute manifestation of lead poisoning.
The intoxication of the osteoclasts by lead is after VAN MULLEM and Stadthouders (1974)accompanied by an interference with the normal cellular functions and the osteoclasts undergo an impairment of their function of bone remodelling
RICORDI et al. (1980) examined bone tissue of collie puppies suffering from osseous deformations and spontaneous fractures. Electron microscopical investigations demonstrated lead inclusion bodies frequently in the nuclei and in the cytoplasm of osteoclasts of lead poisoned collie puppies. X-ray microprobe analyses (BONUCCI et al., 1983) showed that the inclusion bodies contained lead. Lead concentration can be reached in the osteoclast when, during bone resorption, they accumulate the lead salts previously incorporatedin the bone matrix. These frequently appear as roundishor oval structures of variable diameter (mean 0.5 µm) consist of protruding filaments and electron-dense granules. These granules contain much higher concentrations of lead than other parts of the inclusion bodies (BONUCCI et al., 1983).

2. <u>Effects of lead on the viability on cells</u> (Table 1b)

There are also reports about the effects of lead and cadmium on viability and phagocytosis of human polymorphnuclear leucocytes (BAGINSKI, 1985). It was demonstrated that the viability of the leucocytes was only slightly decreased after incubation with these metals. However, both metals were found to markedly surpress phagocytic activity of the leucocytes. Thus, indipendent of effects on cell viability the defence mechanisms of human polymorphnuclear leucocytes against infection agents are markedly reduced in presence of lead and cadmium. Investigations of HILBERTZ et al. (1986) with the same metals on the effects on the oxydative metabolism of mouse peritoneal macrophages resulted in a lead concentration dependently suppression of the oxidative metabolism as well as phagocytosis.

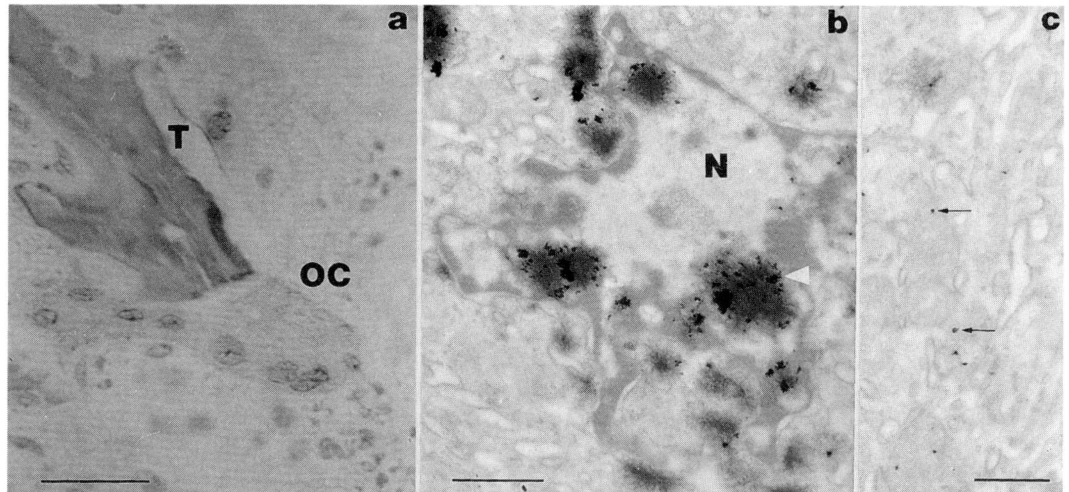

Fig. 1. lightmicroscopical photograph of a large, multinucleated osteoclast (OC) of a growth plate in cloth connection with trabecular bone (T); b) electronmicroscopical micrograph of an osteoclast with intranuclear and intracytoplasmic inclusion bodies with dark lead containing granules (arrow head); c) smaller lead containing granules can be found within mitochondria. bar: a) 2o µm, b-c): 1 µm.

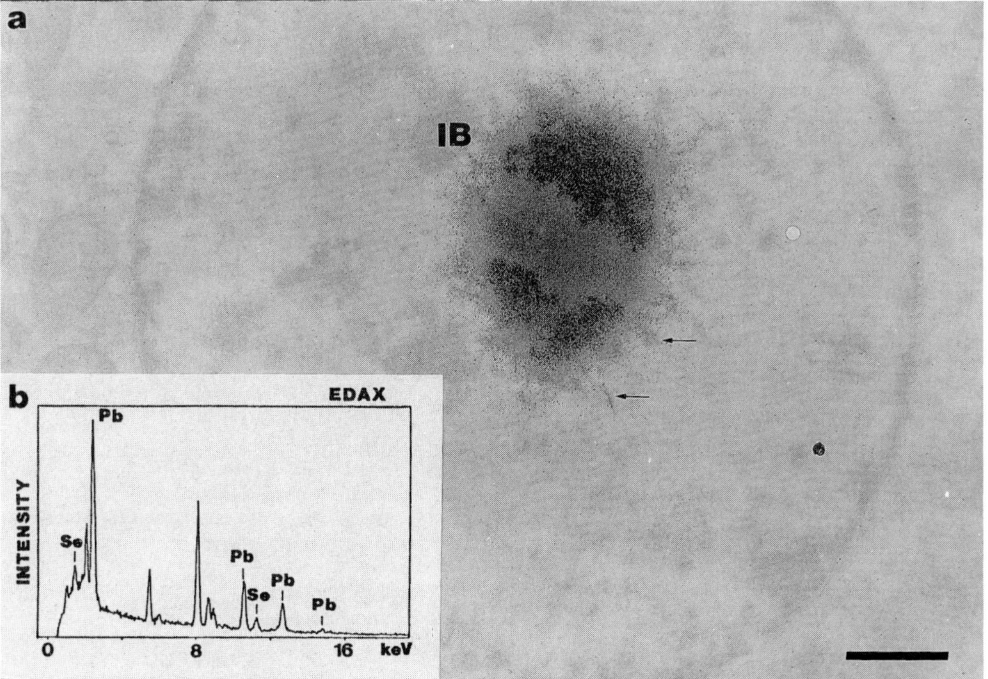

Fig. 2. Intranuclear inclusion body (IB) of a proximal tubular cell of kidney consisting of two dense cores and peripheral microfibrils(arrows); b) electronprobe X-ray microanalysis registered content of lead and selen in above region. Fixed: GA/OsO_4, bar: 1 µm.

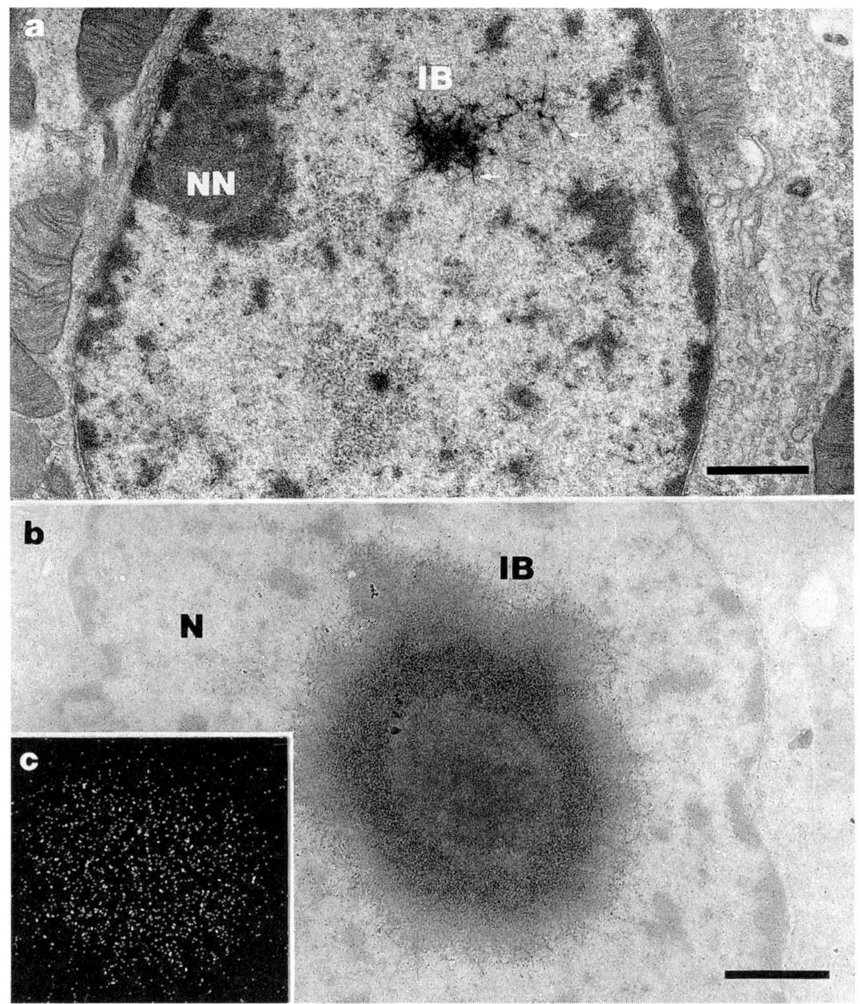

Fig. 3. The appearence of lead containing nuclear structures (IB) can be very different: a) the inclusion body (IB) consists of lead containing osmiophilic fibres (arrows); b) the inclusion body consists of a dark lead containing circular region c) lead distribution pattern (X-ray mapping) of th inner region of the above inclusion body (IB). - Fixed: GA/OsO4; bar: 1 µm.

The data indicate that lead and cadmium may contribute in different ways to the impairment of defence mechanisms in leucocytes and macrophages.

3. Interaction of lead with other elements (Table 1c)

There are also reports of competitions of lead with other elements. Calcium has been shown to compete directly with lead for binding sites on absorptive proteins in the intestinal mucose (BARTON et al., 1978). Iron is similarly antagonistic to lead absorption (MAHAFFEY et al., 1978; Mahaffey and MICHAELSON, 1980).
Other metals that probably reduce lead absorption include cadmium and inorganic arsenic (MAHAFFEY and FOWLER, 1977).
Protective effects of some trace metals may involve a shift in the distribution

of lead in the body rather than an effect on absorption. It was demondtrated , for example, that high levels of dietary zinc protect young horses against the toxic effects of lead on the nervous system. zinc actually increased the concentration of lead in the liver and kidney but lowered the concentration of lead in the brain and bones (WILLOUGHBY et al., 1972)

4. Essentiality of lead (Table 1d)

There are indices that lead could have positive effects on the organism (REICHL-MAYR-LAIS and KIRCHGESSNER, 1986). Lead depletion experiments induced by extreme low-diet could lead to abnormalities (anemia, growth depression and disturbances in iron and lipid metabolism) in the f1-generation of depleted mothers which could be normalized by lead supplementation. These experiments show that lead depletion induces reproducible deficiency symptoms. The symptoms can be prevented and reverted by lead supplementation. Therefore the essential nature of lead seems to be established.
The reason for growth depression of offspring during the nursing period that lead deficiency cause a reduction of the content of different elements in milk (REICHL-MAYR-LAIS et al., 1991). There is a dimunition of effects in the course of lactation.
There are only few informations about the mechanism of element secretion into milk. For Ca it is assumed that its transport is dependent on Ca,Mg-ATPase in gland. Similarly Na,K-ATPase is involved. Both enzymes have reduced activity in red membranes of offspring from lead depleted mother.
Possibly the reduced activity of these enzymes in red cell membrane causes a decrease in cation transport rate through the erythrocyte membrane.

REFERENCES

Baginski B. (1985): Effects of lead and cadmium on viability and phagocytosis of human polymorphnuclear leucocytes. Zbl. Bakt. Hyg. I.Abt. Orig. B 181, 461-468.

Barckhaus R.H., Schmidt P.F. (1991): How can toxic elements (Pb, Ti) be localized in histological sections by electronprobe X-ray microanalysis (EPMA)? In: Histo- and Cytochemistry as a Tool in Environmental Toxicology. Progress in Histochemistry, Vol. 23, No. 1-4. W. Graumann, J. Drukker, (eds.), pp. 332-341.

Barckhaus R.H., Busch Ch., Richter K.-D., Bonucci E., Höhling H.J. (1986): Investigations of intracellular lead concentrations with the X-ray microprobe analysis. Trace elements in medicine 3, 44-45.

Barckhaus R.H., Schmidt P.F., Roessner A., Timm C., Höhling H.J., Grundmann E., (1985): Electronprobe X-ray microanalysis and laser microprobe mass analysis (LAMMA) of titanium in tumor cells of a typical osteoblastic osteosarcoma. Trace elem. medic. 2, 73-76.

Barton J.C., Conrad M.E., Harrison L., Nuby S. (1978): Effects of calcium on the absorption and retention of lead. J. Lab. Clin. Med. 91, 366-376.

Bonucci E., Barckhaus R.H., Silvestrini G., Ballanti P., Di Lorenzo G. (1983): Osteoclast changes induced by lead poisoning (saturnism). Appl. Pathol. I, 241-250.

Choie D.D., Richter G.W. (1972): Lead poisoning: Rapid formation of intranuclear inclusions. Science 177, 1194-1195.

Goyer R.A., May P.M., Krigman M.R. (1970): Lead and protein content of isolated intranuclear inclusion bodies from kidneys of lead-poisoned rats. Lab. Invest. 22, 245-251.

Goyer R.A., Leonard D.L., Moore J.F., Rhyne B., Krigman M.R. (1970): Lead dosage and the role of the intranuclear inclusion body. Ach. envoronm. Hlth. 20, 705-711.

Goyer R.A., Rhyne B.C. (1973): Pathological effects of lead. In Intern. Rev. Exp. Path. 12, 1-77.

Hampp R. Kriebitsch Ch., Ziegler H. (1974): Effects of lead on enzymes of porphy-

rine biosynthesis in chloroplasts and erythrocytes. Naturwiss. 61, 504-505.
Hampp R., Lenzian K. (1974): Effect of lead on chlorophyll synthesis. Naturwissensch. 61, 218-219.
Hilbertz U., Krämer U., De Ruiter N., Baginski B. (1986): Effects of cadmium and lead on oxidative metabolism and phagocytosis by mouse peritoneal macrophages. Toxicology 39, 47-57.
Mahaffey K.R., Fowler B.A. (1977): Effects of concurrent administration of lead, cadmium and arsenic in the rat. Environ. Health. Perspect. 19, 165-171.
Mahaffey K.R., Stone C.L., Banks T.A., Reed G. (1978): Reduction in tissue storage of lead in the rat by feeding diets with elevated iron concentration. In Kirchgessner M. (ed): Proc. Third Int. Symp. Trace. Metal. Metab. in man and animals. Arbeitskreis für Tiernahrung -Storschung, Weihenstephan, pp 584-588.
Mahaffey K.R., Michaelson I.A. (1980): In Needleman HL (ed): The interaction between lead and nutrition in low level lead exposure: The clinical implications of current research. New York: Raven Press, pp 159-200.
Mullem van P.J., Stadhouders A.M. (1974): Bone marking and lead intoxication. Early pathological changes in osteoclasts. Virchows Arch. Abt. B Zellpath. 15, 345-350.
Needleman H.L., Tuncay O.C., Shapiro I.M. (1972); Nature (Lond.) 235, 111.
Reichlmayr-Lais A.M., Kirchgessner M. (1986): Lead - a physiological essential trace element. Trace elem. medic. 3, 34-46.
Reichlmayr-Lais A.M., Eder K., Kirchgessner M. (1991): Lead deficiency: Newer results. In Trace Elements in Man and Animals, Momcilovic B. (ed), 7, 21-22.
Richter G.W., Kress Y., Cornwall C.C. (1968): Another look at lead inclusion bodies. Amer. J. Path. 53, 189-217.
Ricordi M.E., Sivestrini G., Bonucci E. (1980): Inclusion bodies in osteoclasts and lead intoxication. Mineral Metab. Res. 1, 147-150.
Willoughby R.A., MacDonald E., McSherry B.J., Brown G. (1972): Lead poisoning and the interaction between lead and zinc poisoning in the foal. Can. J. Comp. Med. 36, 348-359.

Metal Ions in Biology and Medicine, vol. 2. Eds. J. Anastassopoulou, Ph. Collery, J.C. Etienne, Th. Theophanides. John Libbey Eurotext, Paris © 1992, pp. 287-289

In vitro cytotoxicity of metal ions

M.P. Sauvant*, D. Pépin*, A. Gardes**

**Laboratoire d'Hydrologie et d'Hygiène Faculté de Pharmacie - BP 38, 63001 Clermont-Ferrand Cedex, France. **INSERM U 71, BP 184, 63005 Clermont-Ferrand Cedex 13, France*

INTRODUCTION

Recently there has been an increase in the number and range of in vitro assays, which could evaluate and facilitate rapid screening of environmental pollutants as metal ions. To survey aquatic environmental pollution, some studies advocated the use of toxicological index with microorganisms or chemical and biological methods (BITTON G., 1983) and more recently the use of cultured established cell lines (KFIR R.,PROZESKY O.W., 1981). A great interest must be brought to these methods. Chemical analysis enables to measurement of known toxicants whereas biological assays may be used to detect the presence of known as well as unknown substances. However an evaluation and good knowledges about these techniques and their uses are necessary.

So, the determination of the IC 50 ("Inhibitory Concentration 50") , as an index of the potential toxicity of a substance, is one of the first step in this approach.

The aim of our study is to evaluate the IC 50 of 13 metal ions, frequently found as micropollutants in the environment. For each metal, the IC 50 were determined on an established cell line with 4 assays laying on some different principles : the Neutral Red incorporation assay, the Neutral Red release assay, the M.T.T. assay and the Coomassie Blue assay. Then the results were compared to each other.

MATERIAL AND METHOD

Metal salts tested were : aluminium chloride ($AlCl_3$), barium chloride ($BaCl_2$), cadmium chloride ($CdCl_2$), cobaltous chloride ($CoCl_2$), chromic chloride ($CrCl_3$), copper chloride ($CuCl_2$), ferric chloride ($FeCl_3$), mercuric chloride ($HgCl_2$), manganese chloride ($MnCl_3$), lead nitrate ($Pb(NO_3)_2$), antimony chloride ($SbCl_3$), stannous chloride ($SnCl_4$), and zinc chloride ($ZnCl_2$). They were analytical grade quality and were obtained from MERCK.

An established cell line (fibroblasts - ATCC L-929) was used. Cells were maintained in a 37°C incubator(5% CO_2), in Minimum Eagle's Medium (M.E.M.) supplemented with 5% fetal calf serum, 1% vitamins, 1% non-essential amino-acids, 1% L-glutamine, 1% gentamicin. All products were obtained from GIBCO B.R.L..

Stock cultures were subcultured and seeded in 96-microtiter plate at a density of 2 x $(10)^4$ cells in 0,2 ml complete medium per well.

Twenty-four hours after plating, the cultures were controled and the media were removed from the wells, and replaced with 0,2 ml of fresh complete medium (for control wells) or with 0,2 ml of medium containing test metals at various

concentrations (ranged from (10)-4 to 500 ug/ml). 4 replicate wells were used for each test agent concentration. The dilution of metal were prepared initially with sterile distilled water before each experiment, so that the final concentration of metal solution in the culture medium was always 10% (V/V).
Four in-vitro cytotoxicity assays, which explored various cellular functions, were used : the Neutral Red incorporation assay (lysosomal function), the Neutral Red release assay (membranous function), the M.T.T. assay (mitochondrial function) and the Coomassie Blue assay (amount of cellular proteins). They were conducted respectivily according to BORENFREUND and SHOPSIS' method (1988), to READER et al's method (1989), to DENIZOT and LANG's method (1986) and to SHOPSIS and ENG's method (1985).
All experiments were performed at least three times and the potential toxicities of the metals were compared to control by computing the concentration needed to reduce response by 50%. A linear regression analysis of the data plotted as percent of control versus logarithmic metal concentration and the PROBIT model were used.

RESULTS

In most cases, a relation between the tested doses of metal and the effects on cultured cells were observed. The IC 50 of the metals are given in Table N.1. They are expressed in ug/ml.

METAL	NEUTRAL RED INCORPARATION	NEUTRAL RED RELEASE	M.T.T.	COOMASSIE BLUE
Al	169.0	284.0	218.0	> 500.0
Ba	>500.0	>500.0	>500.0	> 500.0
Cd	1.5	2.2	0.8	1.9
Co	18.0	>100.0	19.0	34.0
Cr	37.0	>500.0	280.0	>500.0
Cu	22.0	>100.0	20.0	22.0
Fe	35.0	45.0	43.0	212.0
Hg	3.9	9.1	3.8	5.5
Mn	28.3	72.9	22.2	34.6
Pb	>500.0	>500.0	98.2	> 500.0
Sb	10.0	>100.0	7.5	30.5
Sn	22.1	20.0	7.9	>100.0
Zn	2.4	>100.0	2.7	29.4

Table N.1 : IC 50 of metals (in ug/ml)

Also, it is possible to define 3 groups of metal according to their relative toxicities
- group 1 : "Low toxicity" (IC50 $\geqslant$ 100 ug/mpl) : Al - Ba - Pb ;
- group 2 : "Moderate toxicity" (10 $\leqslant$ IC50 $<$ 100 ug/ml) : Co - Cu - Fe - Mn ;
- group 3 : "High toxicity" (IC50 $\leqslant$ 10 ug/ml) : Cd - Hg.

Nevertheless, Cr which appears to have a "low toxicity" on 3 tests, has a "moderate toxicity" on the last one. A comparable remark can be done about "moderate" and "low" toxicities for Co, Cr, Nb, Ti and V. Moreover, according to the assays, for one metal, the toxicity can be qualified as "high", "moderate" or "low" ; this situation exists for Sb, Sn and Zn.
The global comparison of the IC 50 obtained for the 13 metal ions on the 4 assays and the calculation of the correlation matrix (which allows the comparison of all the assays) gave always some signifiant relation between the assays took two by two. ($p < 0,01$) (Table N.2).

	NEUTRAL RED INCORPARATION	NEUTRAL RED RELEASE	M.T.T.	COOMASSIE BLUE
COOMASSIE BLUE	0,745 *	0,910 *	0,815*	1
M.T.T.	0,678 *	0,819 *	1	
NEUTRAL RED RELEASE	0,786 *	1		
NEUTRAL RED INCORPARATION	1			

Table N.2 : Correlation matrix for the 4 in vitro cytotoxicity assays (ddl = 12 - * : $p < 0{,}01$)

DISCUSSION

More and more, the in vitro cytotoxicity assays are used as a sensitive technique for the detection of toxicants in the environment and particularly in water. In this study, 4 in vitro assays were tested by exposing an established cell line to known amounts of 13 metals. The basis of 3 of these tests are the incorporation of a supravital dye (Neutral Red or M.T.T.), respectively into the lysosomes and the mitochondrias of viable cells ; then the amount of dye, after specific extraction is quantitated spectrophotometrically and compared to the control. Changes in the accumulation or retention of dye occur when the cell membranes (plasma as well as the very sensitive lysosomal membranes) are injured or damaged. So, the quantification of extracted dye by spectrophotometric analysis is correlated to the number and the viability of the cells.
Cell protein synthesis is a continuous function in actively growing cultures. So, the cellular content of proteins can be considerated as a reflect of the metabolic activity of cells. It must be inhibited by some toxic substances. The Coomassie Blue solution will react with the protein and the developped color is spectrophotometrically evaluated, and correlated to the protein amount.

All of these 4 in vitro assays are rapid, easy, automated and bring a important help to the toxicologist in the screening study of environmental pollutants (BABICH et al, 1986). But, their interlaboratory validation and standardization is necessary. As well as the in vivo LD 50 (lethal dose 50), the exact conditions of determination of an in vitro IC 50 must be specified. This inclued the cell line, the culture conditions as well as the reagents and tested substances. So, that would facilitate the comparison and extrapolation of the results.

REFERENCES

BABICH, H. - SHOPIS, C. et al (1986) : In vitro cytotoxicity testing of aquatic pollutants using established fish cell lines. Ecotoxicol. Environ. Safety 11, 91-99.

BITTON, G.(1983) : Bacterial and biochemical tests for assessing chemical toxicity in the aquatic environment : a review. C.R.C. Critical Reviews in Environmental Control 13 (1), 51-67.

BORENFREUND, E. - SHOPSIS, C. (1985) : Toxicity monitored with a correlated set of cell-culture assays. Xenobiotica, 15, 705-711.

DENIZOT, F. - LANG, R. (1986) : Modifications to the tetrazolium dye procedure giving improved sensitivity and reliability. J. Immunol. Methods 89, 271-277.

KFIR, R. - PROZESKY, O.W. (1981) : Detection of toxic substances in water by means of a mammalian cell culture technique. Wat. Res. 15, 553-559.

READER, S.J. - BLACKWELL, V. et al (1989) : A vital dye release method for assaying the short-term cytotoxic effects of chemicals and formulations. ATLA 17, 28-33.

SHOPSIS, C. - ENG, B. (1985) : Rapid cytotoxicity testing using a semi-automated protein determination on cultured cells - Toxicol. Lett. 26, 1-8.

Metal Ions in Biology and Medicine, vol. 2. Eds. J. Anastassopoulou, Ph. Collery, J.C. Etienne, Th. Theophanides. John Libbey Eurotext, Paris © 1992, pp. 290-294

Enhancing effects of holmium (III) on the monosodium glutamate neurotoxicity*

J. Gao, X.N. Zhao, J. Wu, Z.X. Zhang

Medical School of Nanjing University, Nanjing 210008, P.R. China

INTRODUCTION

It was reported successively by Olney (Olney, 1969) that monosodium glutamate (MSG) was able to induce brain damage and other disturbances in mice. A number of studies have since focused on the pharmacology, physiology and pathophysiology of excitatory amino acids (EAA). Malfunction of EAA neurotransmission has been thought to play a role in neurodegenerative diseases such as Alzheimer′ s disease (Maragos, 1987). Our previous researches showed that the characteristics of analgesic effects by the lanthanide series of elements were similar to those of morphine, and confirmed that morphine had the ability to aggrevate the MSG neurotoxicity (Zhang, 1985; Wang, 1986; Zhao, 1990). At the present study, we employed fluorescent probe Tb^{3+} and transmission electronic microscope to examine the probable enhancing effects of lanthanides such as Ho^{3+} on MSG neurotoxicity, and discuss the possible mechanisms underlying the neurotoxic injury.

EXPERIMENTAL DETAILS

Neonatal mice of both sexes, weighing around 5g, were divided into a variaty of experimental groups at random, and treated with MSG at different doses (0. 25, 1. 0g/kg). The mice in each treatment were injected subcutaneously with saline, MSG, Ho^{3+} (8μmol/L, 5μl/mouse) + MSG or naloxone (5mg/kg) + Ho^{3+} + MSG respectively, and all were killed 6 weeks after the adiministration. The mitochondria and nuclei were obtained according to the density gradient centrifugation procedure from the hypothalamus and hippocampus which were isolated from the mice. The samples for electron-micreoscope observation were prepared simultaneously (Zhao, 1990).

The mitochondrial or the nuclear protein bound Tb^{3+} fluorescent intensity was determined by a Hitachi RF—540 fluorescence spectrophotometer, while thr free K^+ and Ca^{2+} contents in different brain regions were determined by specific ion electrodes (Zhang, 1984).

RESULTS AND DISCUSSION

1. Effects of Ho^{3+} on the changes of protein bound Ca^{2+} levels induced by MSG in hypothalamus and hippocampus

As can be seen in the Table 1 and 2, both the mitochondrial and nuclear protein bound Ca^{2+} were markedly increased following the administration of MSG, and these elevating effects were significantly enhanced by Ho^{3+}, especially in the higher dose of MSG, while the pretreatment of naloxone could block the above changes fully or partially. In the mean time, the same treatments had no effect on the Ca^{2+}-uptake into mitochondria and nuclei in hippocampus

* The Project Supported by National Natural Science Fundation of China

Table 1. Effects of Ho^{3+} on the changes of protein bound Ca^{2+} induced by the lower dose of MSG (0.25g/kg)

Group	Tb^{3+} relative fluorescent intensity			
	Hypothalamus		hippocampus	
	Nul	Mit	Nul	Mit
Control	46.3±2.8	54.8±3.5	51.8±7.2	53.2±7.5
MSG	38.0±4.0[a]	47.5±4.2[a]	53.3±4.4	53.2±6.9
Ho^{3+}+MSG	32.0±3.6[ab]	39.0±3.7[ab]	48.8±5.9	53.2±6.4
Nal+Ho^{3+}+MSG	40.0±3.5[ac]	49.3±5.1[c]	51.2±8.5	50.0±4.1

Values in the Table are means ± S. D. for 5—6 samples.

[a]$P<0.01$ or $P<0.001$, vs the control group

[b]$P<0.05$, vs the MSG group

[c]$P<0.01$, vs the Ho^{3+}+ MSG group

Nul=nucleus Mit=mitochondria Nal=naloxone

Table 2. Effects of Ho^{3+} on the changes of protein bound Ca^{2+} induced by the moderate dose of MSG (1.0g/kg)

Group	Tb^{3+} relative fluorescent intensity			
	Hypothalamus		hippocampus	
	Nul	Mit	Nul	Mit
Control	46.5±1.5	55.3±2.6	48.2±1.7	56.8±3.1
MSG	36.2±2.6[a]	44.0±2.2[a]	49.3±2.5	53.5±4.9
Ho^{3+}+MSG	25.0±3.2[ab]	34.2±2.9[ab]	49.0±2.5	51.5±9.4
Nal+Ho^{3+}+MSG	49.7±5.4[c]	52.5±4.0[c]	48.2±3.9	55.0±5.4

Values in the Table are means ± S. D. for 5—6 samples. Other notes are the same as in Table 1.

[a]$P<0.001$, vs the control group

[b]$P<0.001$, vs the MSG group

[c]$P<0.001$, vs the Ho3+ + MSG group

2. Changes in ultrastructural distribution of Ca^{2+} in hypothalamus and hippocampus

The samples for electron-microscope observation were prepared after the same drug administration as the above. The results in Fig. 1 showed that the increasing electron dense granules occurred in mitochondria and nuclei in hypothalamus (Fig. 1 B, C, F,G)were correlated to the drug influence, i. e. MSG (1. 0g/kg) led to little more precipitate pellets, as compared with the control. while much more precipitate pellets were observed after s. c. Ho^{3+} plus MSG, and both the above alterations could be antagonized by naloxone. Therefore,the drug—induced changes in ultrastructural distribution of Ca^{2+} were exactly consistent with the results described in part 1. Additionally, the ultrastructural distribution of Ca^{2+} in hippocampus region showed no difference compared with the control as well.

3. Changes in K^+ and Ca^{2+} contents in different brain regions of mice after neonatal injection with MSG

Using specific ion electrodes,We assessed the free K^+ and Ca^{2+} contents in cortex,hypothalamus,hippocampus and caudate of mice 6 weeks after the drug administration. The results clearly showed that there was no difference of the free K^+ contents in each discrete brain region,compared with the controls. On the other hand, analogous changes of Ca^{2+} levels appeared only in the hypothalamus (Table 3). These findings provide further evidence that Ca^{2+} play a role of great importance in the neurotoxicity resulting from MSG.

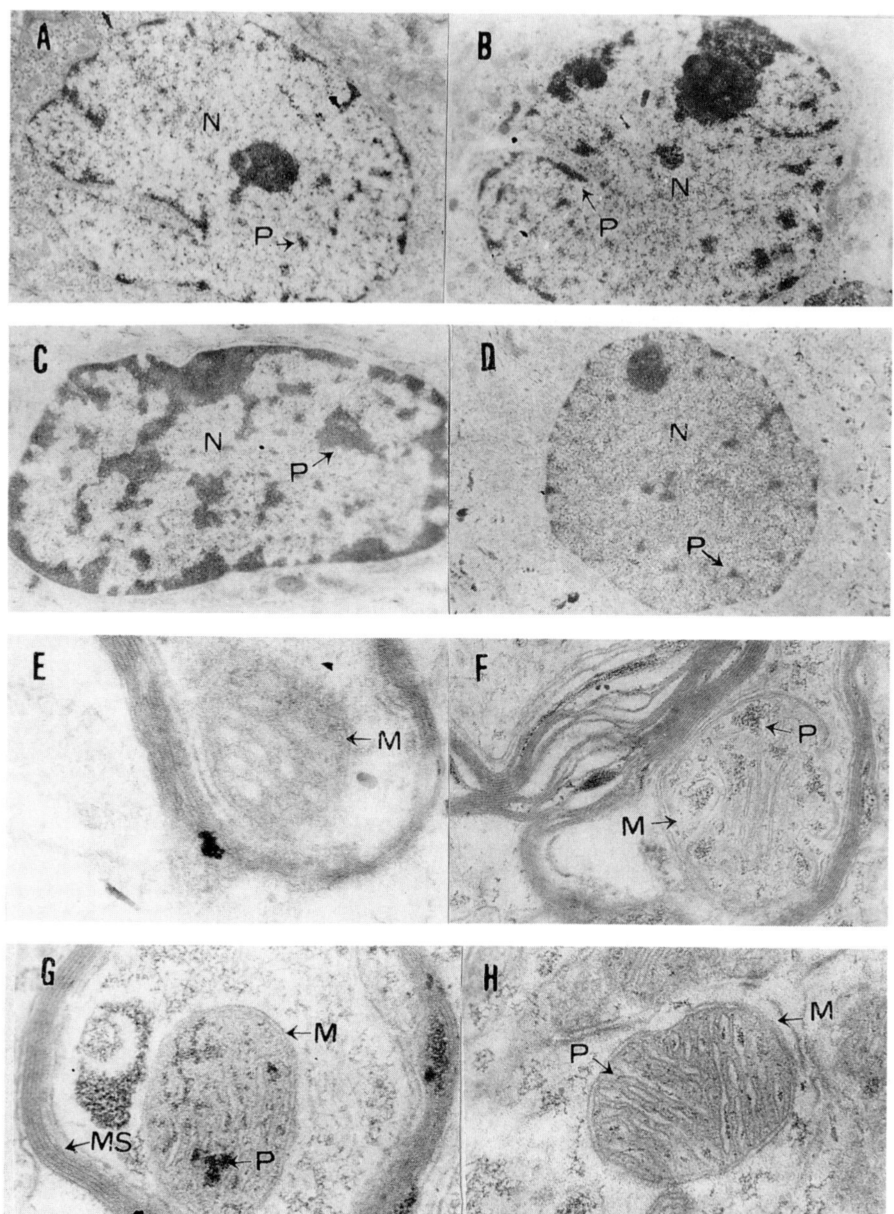

Fig. 1. Ultrastructural distribution of Ca^{2+} in nuclei and mitochondria in arcuate nucleus of mice neonatally treated with MSG. A and E 6 weeks after s. c. saline, showing normal precipitates distribution. B and F showing a number of precipitates in nucleus and mitochondria after s. c. MSG (1. 0g/kg). C and G showing a increase of the precipitates induced by s. c. Ho^{3+} (8μmol/L, 5μl/mouse) before MSG. D and H showing a significant decrease of the precipitates after the treatment with the naloxone (5mg/kg) + Ho^{3+} + MSG. X−ray spectrum element analysis of the precipitate spots confirmed that the main element of the precipitates was calcium. × 40,000 except A (× 8,000), B (× 6,000), C and D (×5,000). P=precipitate pellets N=nucleus M=mitochondria MS=myelin sheath

Table 3. Changes of the free K^+ and Ca^{2+} contents in different brain regions after neonatal injection with MSG (1.0g/kg)

Group	Hypo	Hip	Cortex	Caudate
		K^+ (mg/100g fresh brain)		
Control	224±33	180±69	244±53	187±24
MSG	219±46	188±28	251±61	186±31
Ho^{3+}+MSG	217±28	201±54	263±54	209±55
Nal+Ho^{3+}+MSG	221±44	194±67	261±78	201±37
		Ca^{2+} (mg/100g fresh brain)		
Control	2.1±0.5	1.9±0.2	1.1±0.6	1.6±0.4
MSG	1.8±0.2	2.0±0.4	1.2±0.4	1.6±0.2
Ho^{3+}+MSG	1.2±0.4[ab]	1.8±0.6	0.9±0.2	1.9±0.6
Nal+Ho^{3+}+MSG	1.9±0.7[c]	1.9±0.8	0.8±0.7	1.8±0.4

Other notes are the same as in Table 1.

Hypo=hypothalamus Hip=hippocampus

[a]$P<0.05$, vs the control group

[b]$P<0.05$, vs the MSG group

[c]$P<0.05$, vs the Ho^{3+}+ MSG group

It was known that the characteristics of lanthanide La^{3+} were much similar to those of morphine, and the chemical and physiological properties of lanthanide series of elements were proved to resemble each other (Moeller, 1963; Zhang, 1985). Experiments by Wang et al. (1986) found that although the lower dose of MSG treatment showed no noticeable neuronal damage under microscope, both the ultrastructures and the mitochondrial protein bound Ca^{2+} in hypothalamic arcuate nucleus altered significantly, and the above changes could be obviously enhanced by morphine and lanthanide Tb^{3+}. Therefore, the properties of morphine may be not only similar to those of La^{3+}. The present study proved that another kind of lanthanide Ho^{3+} aggrevated the MSG neurotoxicity as well via the increase in the MSG—induced overloading of protein bound Ca^{2+} not only in mitochondria but in nuclei. These findings indicate that the neuronal injury resulting from MSG may be related to the excessive influx of extracellular Ca^{2+}. At the same time, it was found that the correspondent changes of cations merely belonged to Ca^{2+} and only occurred in hypothalamus. These results also suggest that like morphine, lanthanide series of elements could aggrevate the EAA neurotoxicity as well and both of them probably share the same neuroanatomical site, together with the common ion basis.

REFERENCES

Maragos, W. F., et al., (1987) Glutamate dysfunction in Alzheimer's disease: An hypothesis. Trends in Neurosci. 10:65—67.

Olney, J. W. (1969) Brain lesions, obesity and other disturbances in mice treated with monosodium glutamate. Science 164:719—721.

Wang, G. J. et al., (1986) Enhancing effects of morphine on glutamate neurotoxicity. Chinese J. Pharmacol. Toxicol. 1:57—62.

Zhang, Z. X. et al., (1984) Relationship of brain Ca^{2+} and K^+ contents to electroacupuncture analgesia. Kexue Tongbao 27:1114—1117.

Zhang, Z. X. et al., (1985) Studies on the analgesic effects of lanthanides. J. Less—common Metals. 112:401—409.

Zhao, X. N. et al., (1990) Morphine enhancement of glutamate and kainic neurotoxicity. In: Metal Ions in Biology and Medicine. Eds. Ph. Collery, L. A. Poirier, M. Manfait, J. C. Etienne, John Libbey Eurotext. Paris, pp 156—158.

Zhao, X. N. et al., (1990) ^{45}Ca—uptake, mitochondrial protein bound Ca^{2+} and ultrastructural distribution of Ca^{2+} in some brain regions of mice during drug—induced analgesia. Acta Pharmacol. Sin. 11:112—119.

Metal Ions in Biology and Medicine, vol. 2. Eds. J. Anastassopoulou, Ph. Collery, J.C. Etienne, Th. Theophanides. John Libbey Eurotext, Paris © 1992, pp. 295-298

The relationship between calcium ion and the cytotoxicity of α-quartz

J. Ling*, H.R. Wen*, J.X. Wang*, X.H. Jiao*, Z. Yang*, R.S. Chen*, Z.X. Zhang**, X.N. Zhao**

**Department of Chemistry, Nanjing University, Nanjing 210008, P.R. China. **Medical School of Nanjing University, Nanjing 210008, P.R. China*

ABSTRACT

In this paper, with fluorescence dye Fura–2 / AM and AR–CM cation measurement system to pursue the relationship between Ca^{2+} and the cytotoxicity of α–quartz, we have found that the poisonous function of α–quartz to alveolar macrophage leads to the significant increase of the cytoplasmic free Ca^{2+} concentration ($[Ca^{2+}]_i$) which is due to the innerflow of extracellular Ca^{2+}. Along with this, we have also discussed the reasons of the increase of $[Ca^{2+}]_i$ through the use of Ca^{2+} channel blocker verapamil and the analysis of Ca^{2+}–ATPase activity. The results are mainly as follows:

1. In the Ca^{2+}–medium, the poisonous function of α–quartz to alveolar macrophage leads to the increase of $[Ca^{2+}]_i$. The higher the concentration of the α–quartz dust suspension, or the longer the time of the action, the greater the increase of $[Ca^{2+}]_i$. But in the absence of Ca^{2+}, the phenomenon does not appear. It demonstrates that the increase of $[Ca^{2+}]_i$ is mainly due to the innerflow of extracellular Ca^{2+}.
2. When the action time is 1 h (37℃), verapamil has no significant effect on the increase of $[Ca^{2+}]_i$ caused by α–quartz. However, when the action time is 3 h and 20 h, verapamil can partly inhibit the increase of $[Ca^{2+}]_i$.
3. α–quartz can obviously inhibit the Ca^{2+}–ATPase activity of alveolar macrophage, erythrocytic membrane and mitochondria. The decrease of Ca^{2+}–ATPase activity causes the decrease of active–transport ability of Ca^{2+}. So that the excretion of Ca^{2+} from the cell is inhibited. There is great accumulation of Ca^{2+}in the cell. This leads to the overloading of the cytoplasmic Ca^{2+} and brings about the lesion and even the death of the alveolar macrophage.

INTRODUCTION

The toxicity of α–quartz to alveolar macrophage is the first–step important reaction in the genesis of silicosis[1, 2]. Past researches indicated that Ca^{2+} plays an important role in the toxicity of α–quartz to alveolar macrophage. Our previous studies found that the calcium ion concentration in lung homogenate of rats which had been affected with experimentally silica–induced silicosis increasd significantly[4]. In order to pursue the relationship between Ca^{2+} and the genesis of silicosis, we have detected the concentration of cytoplasmic free Ca^{2+} and the Ca^{2+}–ATPase activities in the poisoning course of α–quartz dust to the rabbit alveolar macrophage. Some interesting results were obtained and preliminary explanations were attempted.

EXPERIMENTS AND RESULTS

1. Macrophages were obtained from lungs of rabbit. They were loaded with 1μmol.dm^{-3}Fura–2 / AM in CO_2 incubator (37℃, CO_2 5%). Macrophages loaded with Fura–2 / AM were exposed to α–quartz in incubator (37℃, $CO_2$5%) for 1 h or 3 h, after 3 h, the 20 h group was incubated at 4℃ for 17 h. $[Ca^{2+}]_i$ was measured in single cell by dule–excitation microfluorimetry with AR–CM–MIC system (SPEX COMP., U. S. A.) and Ca^{2+} fluorescence indicator Fura–2 / AM. $[Ca^{2+}]_i$ was calculated from the ratio (R) of the fluorescence at two different wavelengths according to the previous reported formula[(5)]:

$$[Ca^{2+}]_i = Kd\beta(R - Rmin) / (Rmax - R)$$

where Kd = 137nmol.dm^{-3}(22℃), Rmax, Rmin and β are constants: 7.9 ± 0.42 (n = 10 cells),0.62 ± 0.04 (n = 12 cells), 5.40 ± 0.46 (n = 10 cells).

2. $[Ca^{2+}]_i$ of different action time and diffrent usage of α–quartz dust were measured in the Ca^{2+}–medium (See table 1). The results show that the poiosnous function of α–quartz to macrophage leads to the increase of $[Ca^{2+}]_i$ and $[Ca^{2+}]_i$ increases more greatly when the action time becomes longer or / and the concentration of α–quartz dust suspension becomes higher.

Table 1. The effect of α–quartz on $[Ca^{2+}]_i$ in the Ca^{2+}–medium

group	$[Ca^{2+}]_i$(nmol,dm^{-3})		
	1 h	3 h	20 h
control	119 ± 29(10)	102 ± 16(10)	130 ± 61(8)
α–quartz(100μg / ml)	198 ± 36(8)^{a}	241 ± 60(7)^{a}	265 ± 45(70)^{a}
α–quartz(400μg / ml)	257 ± 86(10)^{a,c}	307 ± 77(12)^{a,c}	496 ± 103(7)^{a,b}
α–quartz(100μg / ml) +veraapamil(5μg / ml)	184 ± 18(9)^{a}	174 ± 28(7)^{a,b}	189 ± 68(10)^{a,b}
α–quartz(400μg / ml) +verapamil(5μg / ml)	207 ± 46(9)^{a}	191 ± 12(9)^{a,d}	232 ± 68(8)^{a,d}

note: 1. each value represents the mean ± S.D.

2. number in parenthesis represents the number of measured cells.

3. a. significantly different from the control, $P < 0.01$.

b. significantly different from α–quartz(100μg / ml), $P < 0.01$.

c. significantly different from α–quartz(100μg / ml), $P < 0.05$.

d. significantly different from α–quartz(400μg / ml), $P < 0.01$.

3. In the Ca^{2+}–medium, when verapamil (its final concentration was 5μg / ml) was added to the cell suspensions, changes of $[Ca^{2+}]_i$ were shown in table 1. It indicates that verapamil can partly inhibit the increase of $[Ca^{2+}]_i$.

4. In the absence of Ca^{2+}, (the other constituents were the same as those of the Ca^{2+}–medium), $[Ca^{2+}]_i$ of different time and different usage of α–quartz dust were measured. Table 2 shows the results. It evinces that $[Ca^{2+}]_i$ of the 400μg / ml α–quartz group decreased significantly when the action time was 20 h.

Table 2. The effect of α–quartz on $[Ca^{2+}]_i$ in the absence of Ca^{2+}

group	$[Ca^{2+}]_i$(nmol.dm^{-3})		
	1 h	3 h	20 h
control	121 ± 26(10)	106 ± 20(10)	114 ± 29(8)
α–quartz(100μg / ml)	130 ± 15(8)	119 ± 19(8)	105 ± 17(10)
α–quartz(400μg / ml)	122 ± 29(11)	123 ± 24(12)	97 ± 24(12)^a

note: 1. a, significantly different from the control , $P<0.05$.

5. Ca^{2+}–ATPase activities were studied of macrophage homogenate, erythrocytic membrane and liver mitochondria exposed to α–quartz dust. The results were shown in table 3 (A indicated the relative activity of Ca^{2+}–ATPase) . It indicates that the cytotoxicity of α–quartz leads to the decrease of Ca^{2+}–ATPase activity. This means the decrease of the active–transport ability of Ca^{2+}.

Table 3. Ca^{2+}–ATPase activity of different samples interacting with α–quartz

group	A of samples(n=4)					
	macrophage		erythrocytic membrane		liver mitochondria	
	2 h	4 h	3 h	6 h	3 h	6 h
control	26.0 ± 0.71	24.0 ± 0.95	20.4 ± 0.79	17.8 ± 1.24	28.2 ± 1.56	27.4 ± 2.00
α–quartz	18.1 ± 2.3^a	16.0 ± 0.93^a	4.5 ± 0.68^b	5.2 ± 0.96^b	18.5 ± 1.37^a	15.5 ± 0.93^b

note: 1. a, significantly different from the control, $P<0.05$.
b, significantly different from the control, $P<0.01$.
2. α–quartz:100μg / ml
3. n represents the number of experiments

DISCUSSION

The experiment results have shown that the cytotoxicity of α–quartz to alveolar macrophage brings about the increase of $[Ca^{2+}]_i$in the Ca^{2+}–medium. And $[Ca^{2+}]_i$ increases more significantly with the prolongation of the action time and the rise of the amount of α–quartz dust, while this effect can only be partly inhibited by calcium channel blocker, verapamil. All these suggest that the innerflow of extracellular Ca^{2+} caused by the excitement of calcium channel is not the only reason of the increase of $[Ca^{2+}]_i$. One of the important ways to deduce $[Ca^{2+}]_i$ is that Ca^{2+}–ATPase of the membrane pumps the redundant Ca^{2+}out of the cells or into some cellular organs (Such as mitochondria). α–quartz causes the obvious inhibition of Ca^{2+}–ATPase activity of cell membrane and mitochondria. Thus the active–transport ability of $Ca^{2+}$of the cell decreases, which leads to the accumulation of cytoplasmic free Ca^{2+}. Past researches have found that cellular organs of macrophage interacted with α–quartz dust undertake structural lesions(6,7). Hence, we think that α–quartz injures the membrane structure and ion modulation mechanism of the cell, which causes the great innerflow of extracellular Ca^{2+}, then the overloading of cytoplasmic Ca^{2+}, thus bringing about the lesion and even the death of alveolar macrophage. So the great innerflow of extracellular Ca^{2+} and the overloading of cytoplasmic $Ca^{2+}$are probably the pathological foundament of silicosis genesis caused by α–quartz dust.

---

* The project is supported by National Natural Science Foundation of China.

REFERENCES

1. Allison A. C. ; et al., (1966): An examination of the cytotoxic effects of silica on macrophages. J. Exp. Med., 124 , 141–161.

2. Heppleston A. G., et al., (1967): Activity of a macrophage factor in collagen formation by silica. Nature, 214, 521–522.

3. Kane A. B. et al., (1980): Dissociation of intracellular lysosomal rupture from the cell death caused by silica. J. Cell Biol., 87, 643–651.

4. Y. Mao, R. S. Chen, et al., (1987): Calcium content of lung and silicosis. Inorganic Chem. (Chinese), 3(4), 12–18.

5. Grynkiewicz G., et al., (1985): A new generation of Ca^{2+} indicators with greatly improved fluorescence properties. J. Biol. Chem., 260, 3440–3450.

6. Merchant R. K., et al., (1990): Silica directly increases permeability of alveolar epithelial cells. J. Appl. Physiol., 68, 1354–1359.

7. Nadler S., et al., (1970): The intracellular release of lysosomal contents in macrophages that have ingested silica. J. Histochem. Cytochem., 18, 368–371.

Metal Ions in Biology and Medicine, vol. 2. Eds. J. Anastassopoulou, Ph. Collery, J.C. Etienne, Th. Theophanides. John Libbey Eurotext, Paris © 1992, pp. 299-303

Mitochondrial calcium and phosphorus accumulation in some brain regions in global cerebral ischemia and reperfusion*

X. Li*, X.N. Zhao*, X.H. Yang*, J. Chen*, M.K. Chen*, Z.X. Zhang*, F.L. Huang**, Q. Shi**, T.H. Zhang**

**Medical School of Nanjing University, Nanjing 210008, P.R. China. **Department of Ultrastructural Pathology, Jinling Hospital, Nanjing 210002, P.R. China*

INTRODUCTION

Intracellular calcium accumulation was extensively studied in relation to cerebral ischemic injury (Kim, 1983), which was observed to be involved in neuroexcitatory mechanism (Rothman, 1986). Investigations of in vitro experiments have revealed that the neurotoxicity involved in cerebral ischemia was associated with delayed calcium accumulation (Marcoux, 1990). In order to clarify whether the neuroexcitation is predominantly responsible for the early ischemic insult, we employed mitochondrial calcium accumulation, which occured in ischemia, as an indicator to study the effect of glutamate on global cerebral ischemia in rat.

MATERIALS AND METHODS

Twenty—four male Sprague—Dowley rats weighing 220—350g were randomly allocated to normal control and ischemic (treated with normal saline or two doses of glutamte) groups. The rats in ischemic group were anesthetized with chloral hydrate (360mg/kg, i. p.). Their vertibral arteries were electrocauterized and the common carotid arteries were isolated (Pulsinelli, 1979). 24 hr later, these awake rats were restrained. After i. cv. normal saline (20μl/rat)or glutamate (20μg/rat, 100μg/rat), their common carotid arteries were occluded for 20 min followed by 2 hr of reperfusion. Then the animals were decapitated; the cortex, hippocampus and hypothalamus were isolated and homogenated in 0. 32 mol/L sucrose to prepare crude mitochondria (Zhao, 1990)for calcium and phosphorus measurement. The mitochondrial calcium and phosphorus contents were determined by Shimadzu VF—320 X—ray fluorescence spectrometer and converted into mg/g protein of mitochondria. Statistical comparisons were made by using analysis of variances with Newman—Keuls test. Differences were considered statistically significant at $P<0.05$.

Rats respectively pretreated with normal saline and glutamate (100μg/rat or 400μg/rat)i. cv. were sacrificed after 20 min of global cerebral ischemia and 6 hr of reperfusion. Their hippocampus and hypothalamus were isolated for ultrastructural study as previously described (Zhao, 1990).

* The Project Supported by National Natural Science Fundation of China and The Analytic Center of Nanjing University

RESULTS

1. Mitochondrial calcium and phosphorus content determinations

Fig. 1. shows that 20 min of global cerebral ischemia and 2 hr of reperfusion resulted in increased mitochondrial calcium concentration in cerebrocortex and hypothalamus, but glutamate in doses of 20μg/rat or 100μg/rat i. cv. failed to intense this alteration.

Hippocampus is one of the regions vulnerable to transient cerebral ischemia, while during 20 min of ischemia and 2 hr of reperfusion, no calcium accumulation was observed. Glutamate administration (20μg/rat, 100μg/rat i. cv.) did not induce the elevation of mitochomdrial calcium level. (Fig. 1.).

Mitochondrial phosphorus contents in these three brain regions presented identical changes with calcium (Fig. 2).

2. Electron—microscope observations

Minute mitochondrial matrix granules were scarcely found in both hippocampus and hypothalamus from normal rats(Fig. 3, A, B). After 20 min of global cerebral ischemia and 6 hr of reperfusion, mitochondrial swelling and granular calcium precipitates occured commonly in these two regions (Fig. 3, C, D). Administration of glutamate oberviously aggrevated mitochondrial abberation in relation to doses (Fig. 3, E, F, G, H).

DISCUSSIONS

Mitochondrial calcium accumulation indicates elevated cytosolic calcium concentration and relates to ischemic injury. The present study shows that mitochondrial calcium contents obviously increased during 20 min of global cerebral ischemia and 2 hr of reperfusion in rat cortex and hypothalamus ,accompanied by the correspondent alteration of mytochondrial phosphorus, while glutamate administration merely induced slight intension in this change ($P>0.05$). However, after 6 hr of reperfusion, deteriorative effect of glutamate on the mitochondrial calcium accumulation and damage was affirmed by electron — microscope observation.

It was reported that extracellular glutamate elevated in rat hippocampus druing 10 min of ischemia followed by 25 min of reperfusion (Benveniste, 1984). Our study shows in rat hippocampus mitochondrial calcium accumulation did not occured till 2 hr after 20 min of ischemia, although extraneous glutamate was administrated. When the reperfusion period was prolonged to 6 hr, mitochondrial swelling and calcification, which were remarkablly intensified by glutamate administration, were observed under electron—microscope.

These results demonstrate that mitochondrial calcium and phosphorus accumulation occurs early in transient ischemic cortex and hypothalamus, but relatively later in hippocampus. Glutamate aggrevates the mitochondrial aberration, but it seems not to predominantly account for the elevation of motochondrial calcium during the early satge of cerebral ischemia.

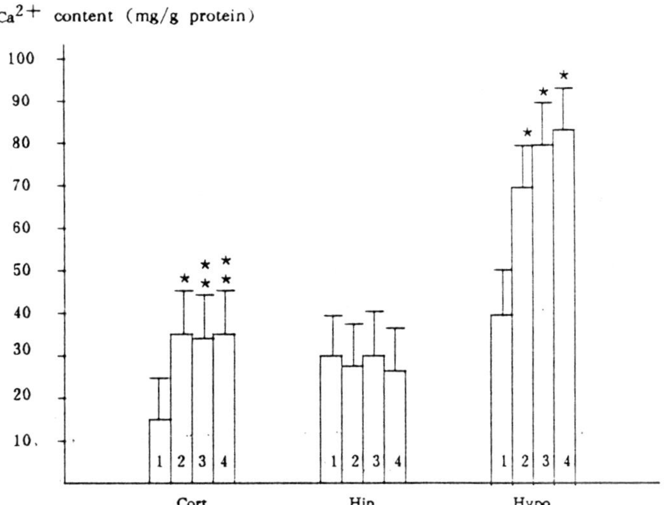

Fig. 1. Mitochondrial Ca^{2+} accumulation resulted from 20 min of global cerebral ischemia and 2 hr of reperfusion

Cort = cortex Hip = Hippocampus Hypo = hypothalamus n = 6

1 = normal control 2 = ischemia group with normal saline

3 = ischemia group with glutamate (20ug/rat)

4 = ischemia group with glutamate (100μg/rat)

• $P<0.05$, vs the control group • • $P<0.01$, vs the Control group

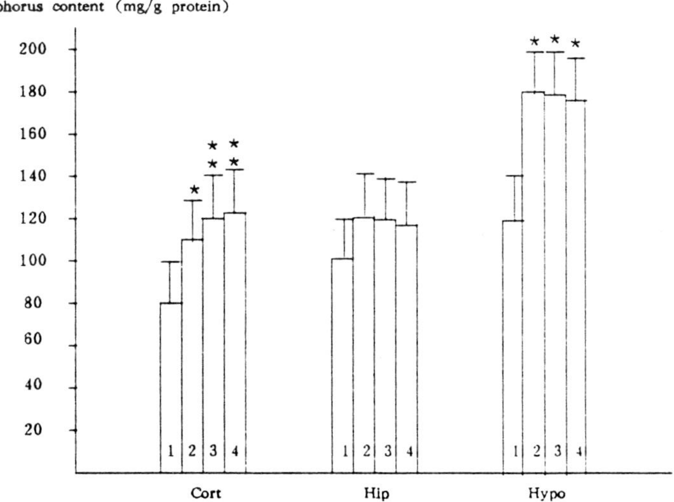

Fig. 2. Increased mitochondrial phosphorus contents induced by 20 min of ischemia and 2 hr of reperfusion

The annotations are the same as those in Fig. 1.

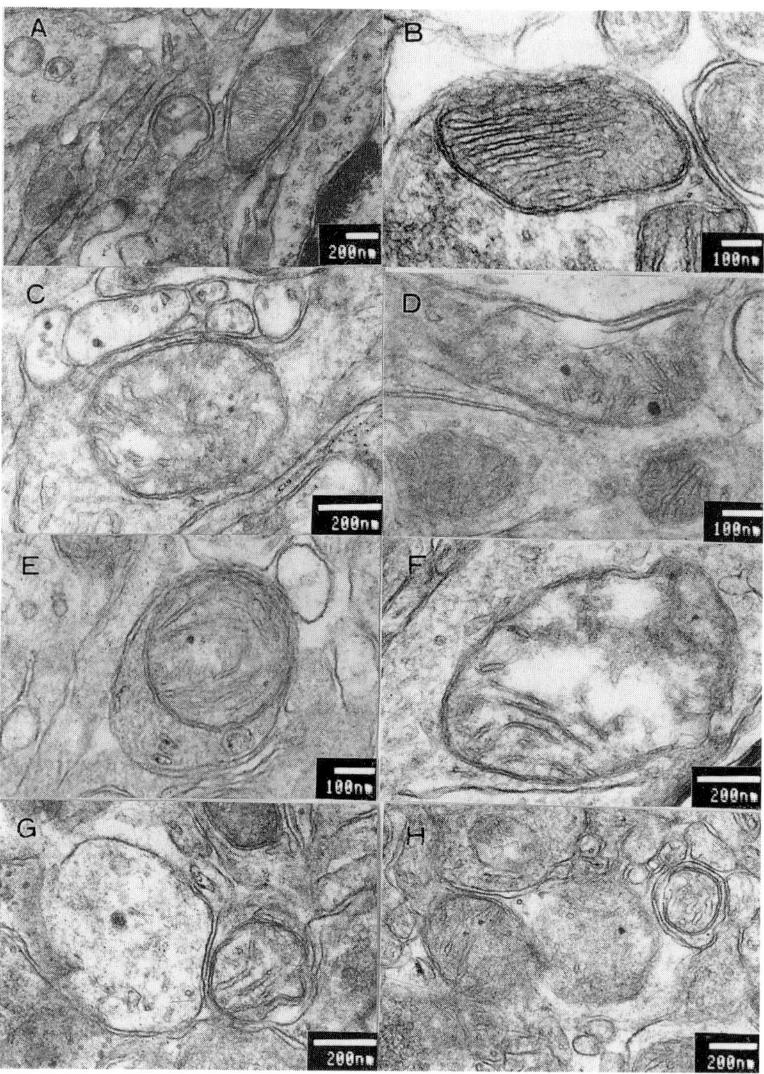

Fig. 3. Electron — microscope observations of rat hipoocampus and hypothalamus neurons A and B show mitochondria from normal rat; C and D show mitochondria in ischemic brain with normal saline; E and F show mitochondria in iachemic brain pretreated with 100μg/rat glutamate i. cv. ; G and H show mitochondria in ischemic brain pretreated with 400μg/rat i. cv.

REFERENCES

Benveniste, H. et al. 1984 Elevation of the extracellular concentrations of glutamate and asparate in rat hippocampus during transient cerebral ischemia monitored by intracerebral microdialysis. J. Neurochem. 43:1369.

Kim, K. M. 1983 In: Pathobiology of Cell Membrane (Ⅲ). Eds. by B. F. Trump and A. U. Arstila, Academic Press, NY, pp127.

Marcoux, F. M. et al. 1990 Hypoxic neuronal injury in tissue culture is associated with delayed calcium accumulation. Stroke 21: Ⅱ—71.

Pulsinelli, W. A. and J. B. Brierley 1979 A new model of bilateral hemispheric ischemia in the unanesthetized rat. Stroke. 10:267.

Rothman, S. M. and J. W. Olney 1986 Glutmate and the pathophysiology of hypoxic—ischemic brain damage. Ann. Neurol. 19:105.

Zhao X. N. et al. 1990 ^{45}Ca—uptake, mitochondrial protein bound calcium and ultrastructural distribution of calcium in some brain regions of mice during drug—induced analgesia. Acta Pharmacol. Sin. 11:112.

Metal Ions in Biology and Medicine, vol. 2. Eds. J. Anastassopoulou, Ph. Collery, J.C. Etienne, Th. Theophanides. John Libbey Eurotext, Paris © 1992, pp. 304-308

Cadmium binding in the soluble contents of the gastrointestinal tract and feces of the rat : HPLC of the extracts after orally aministered ^{109}Cd-labelled phytate, metallothionein and phytochelatin

G.A. Jackl*, G. Reidel**

** GSF-Forschungszentrum f. Umwelt und Gesundheit, Institut für Strahlenbiologie, D-8042 Neuherberg, Germany. ** Nuklearmedizinische Klinik und Poliklinik rechts der Isar der Tu München, D-8000 München 80, Germany*

In foodstuffs the heavy metal cadmium naturally does not occur as an inorganic salt but it is firmly bound to specific binding substances, especially to small polypeptides.
The best known of these compounds are the metallothioneins, small peptides of 7000 dalton which are present in meat (Kägi & Schäffer, 1988), the phytochelatins, peptides of 3500 dalton from green vegetables, roots and tubers (Grill *et al.*, 1987) and phytate, a inosit derivative, which is predominantly found in cereals (Morris *et al.*, 1980) . These compounds can be labelled *in vitro* by partial replacement of stable cadmium using radioactive ^{109}Cd. This label is firmly bound at neutral pH as can be demonstrated by chromatographical methods.
When these substances enter the gastrointestinal tract they may be partially degraded. Thus the Cd-binding may be weakened followed by a new arrangement of the heavy metal ion with digestion products. To identify these Cd-binding compounds, phytate, metallothionein and phytochelatin were labelled with ^{109}Cd and administered to rats which received two different diets based either on soya meal or casein respectively. The soluble extracts of the contents of the stomach, the small intestine and the fecal extracts were analyzed by HPLC. The chromatograms obtained are compared with those from the administered substances and their tryptically digested peptides.

MATERIAL AND METHODS

Cd_3-phytate was synthesized as described by Jackl *et al*, 1985. Rabbit metallothionein (SIGMA-Chemie, Deisenhofen, FRG), a preparation of Cd-phytochelatin (Grill *et al*, 1987), Cd_3-phytate or Cd-chloride respectively were solubilized in 50 mM ammonium acetate buffer, pH 7.4 to a final concentration of 0,2 mg Cd/ml. 10 MBq $^{109}CdCl_2$ (in 0.2 ml 0.1 M HCl) were added to 1 ml of each preparation as a tracer. For tryptic digestion 50 µl of the phytochelatin-, the metallothionein- and the chloride- solutions were incubated for 30 min with an equal part of a trypsin solution (13,000 U/ml).
The biological soya standard diet (Altromin-1324) was derived from soya-, barley-, corn, and wheat- wholemeal and fishmeal. Wheat bran was added for fibre. The semisynthetic casein diet (Altromin C-1000) contained milk proteins and soya oil.

Three weeks after the onset of the semipurified diet the labelled complexes described above (≈5 MBq ^{109}Cd in ≈0,6 ml) were administered to male Wistar rats by stomach tube. Half of the animals were killed after one hour. Stomach and small intestine were prepared and the contents were extracted by brief sonication with 50 mM phosphate buffer pH 7.0. The feces of the other group were collected on the other day and extracted. 50µl samples of the extracts were separated by high performance liquid chromatography (HPLC) on a TSK column (type: G-2000, size 8x300 mm) and analyzed in a well type gamma-counter.

RESULTS AND DISCUSSION

One hour after administration of ^{109}Cd labelled metallothionein, phytochelatin and phytate the contents of the stomach and the intestine were prepared, extracted and the extracts submitted to HPLC. In Fig.1 a and b the chromatograms of the extracts are compared with those of the administered substances and its tryptic digestion products. This is not possible in the case of phytate since it is insoluble at neutral pH.
Below the chromatograms of the original substances at first the chromatograms of the extracts of the soya group are arranged and there below those from the casein group.
^{109}Cd administered as a chloride (vide Fig.1a, left) was present in the stomach independent from the type of diet as free ion. The chromatograms of the intestinal extracts differed dependent on the type of diet: In case of the soya diet the radioactivity accumulated in two peaks of medium molecular weight, in case of the casein diet ^{109}Cd was bound to substances of high molecular weight.
A marked difference between the two diets was found for the feces: in case of the soya diet a high and a low molecular fraction were labelled, in case of the casein diet predominantly fractions of high molecular weight, which partly exceeded those of the soya diet. In case of the phytate (vide Fig.1a, right) in the stomach the major part of labelling was found in small fractions. The rest was free Cd^{2+}. This was independent from the sort of diet.
In case of metallothionein in the stomach of the soya group the binding of the isotope to metallothionein and its peptic digestion products seems to persist. In the casein group the labelling was found in low molecular fractions. In the intestine the labelling was associated exclusively with metallothionein and its degradation products.
After administration of phytochelatin (vide Fig.1b, left) Cd was present in the stomach of both diet groups predominantly as free ion. In the intestinal extracts of the soya group only minor labelling was found in the region of intact phytochelatin. Labelling was distributed over a wide range of fractions. In the casein group however the whole labelling was found in the region of phytochelatin.
The labelling patterns of the feces extracts from all three Cd binding compounds, phytate, metallothionein and phytochelatin resemble to those from the chloride group for the corresponding diets.

CONCLUSIONS

The distribution of cadmium in the soluble contents of the stomach and the small intestine depends on the kind of the administered Cd-binding compound and on the sort of the diet. The applied diet alone is responsible for the distribution of Cd in the feces while the administered compound is of no consequence.

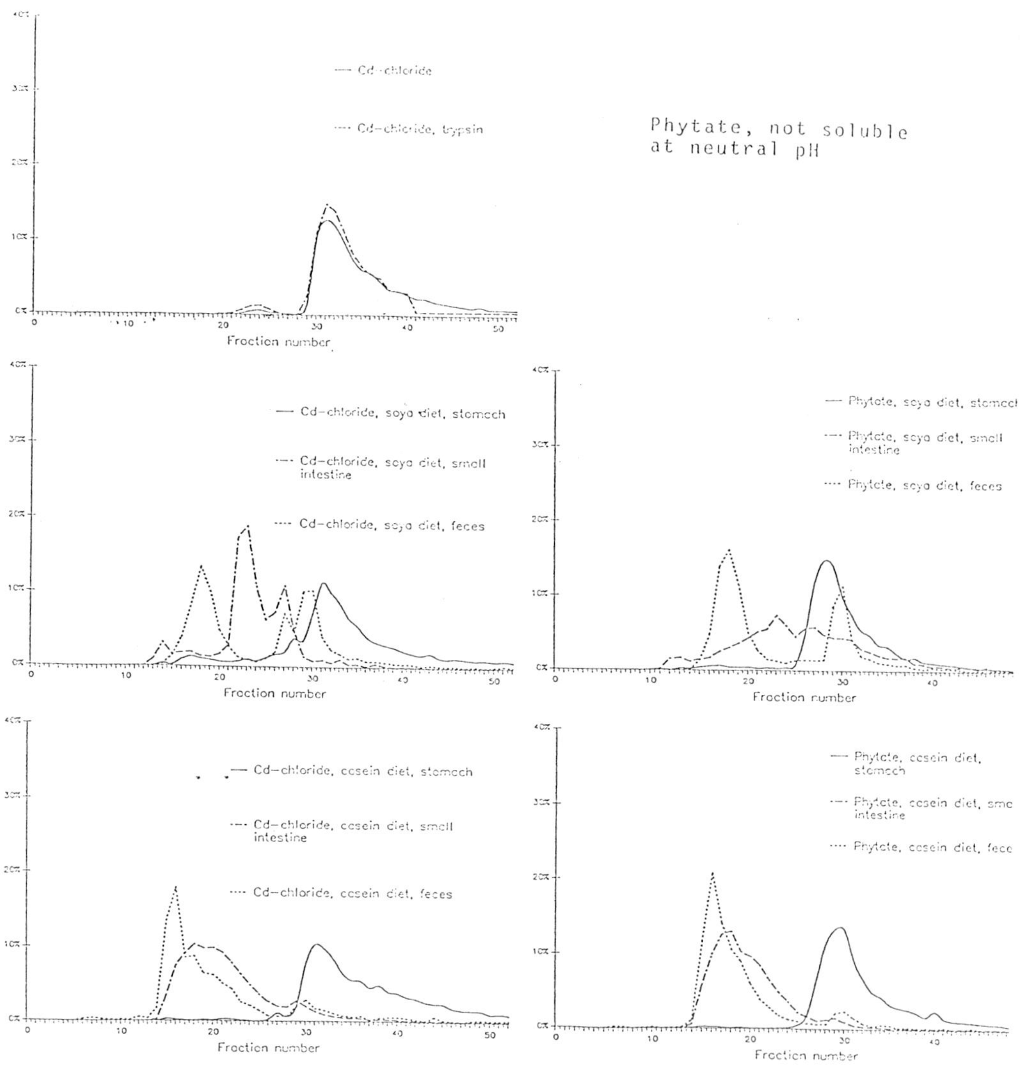

Figure 1 a. Distribution of the ^{109}Cd-radioactivity in the chromatograms

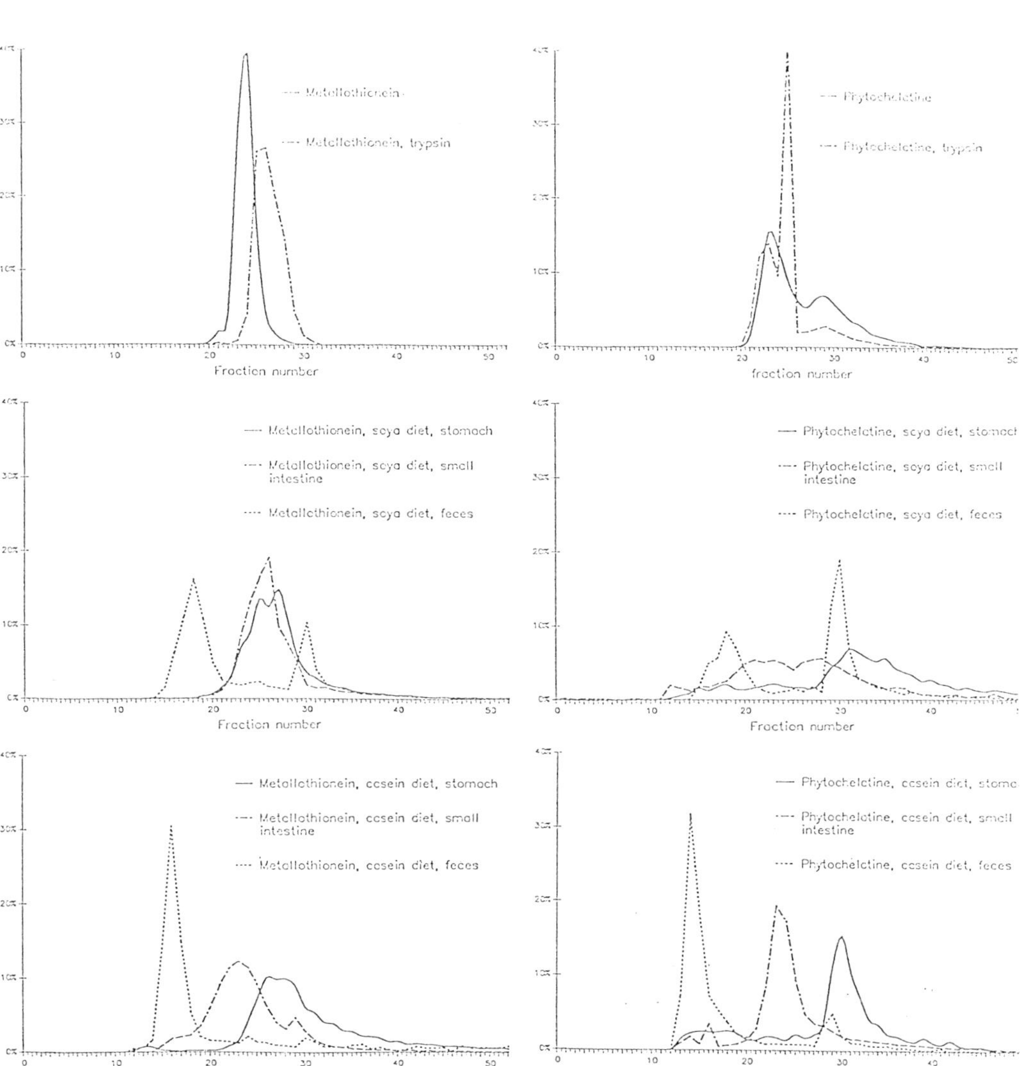

Figure 1 b. Distribution of the ^{109}Cd-radioactivity in the chromatograms

REFERENCES

Grill, E., Winnacker, E.L., & Zenk, M.H.(1987), Phytochelatins, a class of heavy metal binding peptides from plants, are functionally analogous to metallothionein. *Proc. Natl. Acad. Sci. USA, Vol.84,* 439-443

Jackl, G. A., Rambeck W. A. & Kollmer W. E. (1985) Retention of Cd in organs of the rat after a single dose of Cd_3-phytate. *Biol. Tr. Elem. Res.7,* 74-96 5.

Kägi, J.H.R. & Schäffer A.(1988) Biochemistry of metallothionein. *Biochemistry 27,* N° *23,* 8509-8515

Morris, E.R. & Ellis, R. (1980), Effect of dietary phytate/zinc molar ratio on growth and bone zinc response of rsts fed semi-purified diets. *J. Nutr. 110,* 1037-1048

Acknowledgement:
The donation of phytochelatin by Prof. Dr. M.H.Zenk, Ludwig-Maximilians-Universität, München is gratefully acknowledged.

Metal Ions in Biology and Medicine, vol. 2. Eds. J. Anastassopoulou, Ph. Collery, J.C. Etienne, Th. Theophanides. John Libbey Eurotext, Paris © 1992, pp. 309-310

Effect of insulin resistance on cytosolic free sodium in platelets

M. Tepel, S. Bauer, S. Husseini, K. Kisters, K.H. Rahn, W. Zidek

Med. Univ.-Poliklinik, University of Muenster, Albert-Schweitzer-Str. 33, W-4400 Muenster, Germany

Introduction:

Non-insulin-dependent diabetes mellitus (NIDDM) patients show resistance to insulin-stimulated glucose uptake associated with elevated blood pressure (Sowers et al., 1991). Since insulin is known to stimulate sodium transport systems (DeFronzo, 1981) impairment of sodium metabolism may be a possible link between insulin resistance and elevated blood pressure. Therefore in the present study the effect of insulin resistance on cytosolic free sodium concentration ($[Na^+]_i$) was investigated in intact cells using the novel sodium-sensitive fluorescent dye sodium-binding-benzofuran-isophthalate (SBFI).

Methods:

$[Na^+]_i$ was measured in intact platelets from 22 NIDDM patients (15 men, 7 women, aged 43-80 yr) and 26 age-matched healthy control subjects (16 men, 10 women, aged 31-84 yr). The diabetic condition was assessed following accepted clinical criteria of the National Diabetes Data Group (1979). Both systolic and diastolic blood pressure were significantly higher in NIDDM patients compared to healthy control subjects (systolic: 148.0 ± 4.9 mmHg vs 127.3 ± 2.3 mmHg, mean ± SEM, $p<0.001$; diastolic: 86.8 ± 2.6 mmHg vs 79.0 ± 1.0 mmHg, $p<0.01$). Heparinized blood was centrifuged at 240 g for 15 minutes to obtain platelet rich plasma, which was centrifuged at 240 g for 20 minutes, and the platelet pellet resuspended in Hanks balanced salt solution containing 136 mM NaCl, 5.40 mM KCl, 0.44 mM KH_2PO_4, 0.34 mM Na_2HPO_4, 5.60 mM D-glucose, 1 mM $CaCl_2$ and 10 mM N-2-hydroxyethyl-piperazine-N'-2-ethanesulfonic acid, pH 7.4. Measurements of $[Na^+]_i$ using the novel fluorescent dye technique were performed according to recently described methods (Harootunian et al., 1989; Borin and Siffert, 1990). Briefly, the platelet suspension was incubated with 3 μM SBFI-acetoxymethylester (Calbiochem, Frankfurt, Germany) and 0.1% (w/v) non-ionic detergent Pluronic F-127 (Molecular Probes, Eugene, USA) for 60 minutes at 37°C. After centrifugation at 240 g for 10 minutes to remove extraneous dye the platelet pellet was again resuspended in Hanks balanced salt solution. The fluorescence intensity of 1000 μl suspension of SBFI loaded platelets (100,000/μl) in a thermostatized quarz cuvette with constant stirring was measured in a Fluorescence Spectrophotometer Model F-2000 (Hitachi Ltd. Tokyo, Japan) with excitation wavelengths of 340 and 385 nm and an emission wavelength of 500 nm. The fluorescence excitation ratio at 340/385 nm was calculated. The excitation ratio was calibrated in terms of cytosolic free sodium concentration in situ on each platelet preparation by equilibration of intracellular sodium content with known extracellular sodium concentrations in the presence of ionophors. For statistical evaluation of the data Wilcoxon's test was used and two-tailed p values of less than 0.05 were considered to be significant.

Results:

Resting $[Na^+]_i$ was significantly higher in intact platelets from NIDDM patients compared to healthy control subjects (42.6 ± 3.1 mM vs 32.6 ± 2.2 mM, mean ± SEM, $p<0.03$). Inhibition of Na-K-ATPase by 1 mM ouabain for 60 minutes significantly increased $[Na^+]_i$ in platelets from NIDDM patients and from control subjects. Further, there was a significant correlation between $[Na^+]_i$ in resting platelets and ouabain-induced increase of $[Na^+]_i$ ($y=0.77x+38.14$; $r=0.321$, $p<0.05$, Fig. 1).

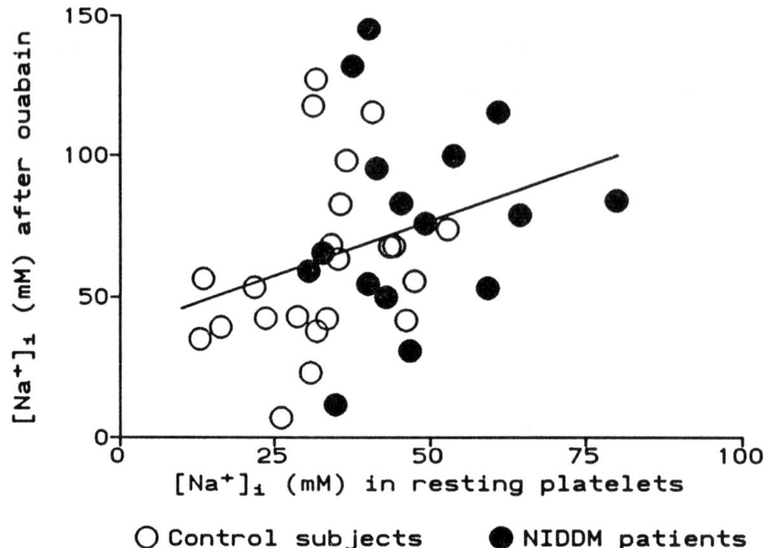

Fig. 1: Correlation of cytosolic free sodium concentration ($[Na^+]_i$) in resting platelets and ouabain-induced increase of $[Na^+]_i$. $[Na^+]_i$ in intact platelets from non-insulin-dependent diabetes mellitus (NIDDM) patients (filled circles) and healthy control subjects (open circles) were measured using the sodium-sensitive fluorescent dye technique. Linear regression line: $y=0.77x+38.14$; $r=0.321$, $p<0.05$.

Discussion:

Using a novel fluorescent dye technique in intact platelets it was shown that $[Na^+]_i$ was increased in NIDDM patients. In addition, inhibition of Na-K-ATPase by ouabain caused a significant rise of $[Na^+]_i$ in platelets. There was a significant correlation between resting $[Na^+]_i$ and $[Na^+]_i$ after inhibition of Na-K-ATPase by ouabain. Since the rise of $[Na^+]_i$ in NIDDM patients may be explained by decreased Na-pumping rates, the correlation between resting $[Na^+]_i$ and ouabain-induced increase of $[Na^+]_i$ point to some compensatory increase in the number of Na-K-ATPase sites. Since Blaustein (1977) hypothesized that increased intracellular sodium may cause accumulation of intracellular calcium, the rise of intracellular sodium may be an early step in the development of hypertension of NIDDM patients.

References:

Blaustein, M.P. (1977): Sodium ions, calcium ions, blood pressure regulation, and hypertension: a reassessment and a hypothesis. Am. J. Physiol. 232, C165-C173.

Borin, M. and Siffert, W. (1990): Stimulation by thrombin increases the cytosolic free Na^+ concentration in human platelets. J. Biol. Chem. 265, 19543-19550.

DeFronzo, R. (1981): The effect of insulin on renal sodium metabolism. A review with clinical implications. Diabetologia 21, 165-171.

Harootunian, A.T., Kao, J.P.Y., Eckert, B.K., and Tsien, R.Y. (1989): Fluorescence ratio imaging of cytosolic free Na in individual fibroblasts and lymphocytes. J. Biol. Chem. 284, 19458-19467.

National Diabetes Data Group (1979): Classification and diagnosis of diabetes mellitus and other categories of glucose intolerance. Diabetes 28, 1039-1057.

Sowers, J.R., Khoury, S., Standley, P., Zemel, P., and Zemel, M. (1991): Mechanisms of hypertension in diabetes. Am. J. Hypertens. 4,177-182.

Metal Ions in Biology and Medicine, vol. 2. Eds. J. Anastassopoulou, Ph. Collery, J.C. Etienne, Th. Theophanides. John Libbey Eurotext, Paris © 1992, pp. 311-312

Serum calcium, magnesium and inorganic phosphorus variations induced by hypoxia and exercise in rats

M. Guerra, J.F. Escanero, L.M. Elósegui, F. Martinez-Sagasti, A. Periset, M. Giménez*

*Departamento de Fisiología. Facultad de Medicina. Universidad de Zaragoza. 50009 Zaragoza. Spain. *Laboratoire de Physiologie de l'Exercice Musculaire, Unité 14 INSERM CO n° 10, 54511 Vandœuvre-Les-Nancy, France*

Introduction.

The exercise-induced effects on serum calcium (Ca), magnesium (Mg) and inorganic phosphorus (Pi) are well known (Hespel et al., 1986; Deuster et al., 1987). However, the variations on serum concentrations of these elements induced by exercise under hypoxia are worse known (Cordova et al., 1988) and the effects a time after exercise under hypoxia remain still unknown. The aim of this paper is to clarify these points.

Material and methods.

A total of 42 male Wistar rats were randomly separated into the following groups: I). Control group, at rest, in air; II). Rats training in air; III). Rats at rest under hypoxia (FIO_2 = 8 %); IV). Rats training under hypoxia; V). Rats in air, training for 15 days and, after, one week at rest; VI). Rats at rest under hypoxia for 15 days and, after, one week at rest in air; VII). Rats training under hypoxia for 15 days and, after, one week at rest in air. To perform the training programme the rats were forced to swim until exhaustion (defined by no swimming during 15 seconds) into a wave-pool (110 x 70 x 70 cm), where the temperature of the water was kept constant (37º C) by a thermostat. The times of entry into the pool and of exhaustion were noted. The day before the blood extractions the animals performed a last session of exercise until exhaustion and, justly, 24 hours after the beginning, were anesthetized (pentobarbital 5 mg/100 g body wt, *ip*) and the blood was obtained from abdominal aorta. Serum Ca and Mg concentrations were determined by atomic absorption spectrophotometry and Pi by colorimetric procedures. The results were treated with a statistic programme (Staw-View) using a MacIntosh.

Results and Discussion.

The results found in this experiment are shown in the following table.

	Calcium	Magnesium	Inorganic Phosphorus
Group I	8.98±0.34	2.38±0.17	8.41±1.03
Group II	8.72±1.2	2.57±0.25	8.59±0.59
Group III	8.22±0.41 a	5.24±0.58 a', b'	8.34±1.32
Group IV	8.44±0.60 a	5.55±1.05 a', b'	7.70±1.52
Group V	8.00±0.58 a, c	4.96±1.84 a, b	9.45±3.24
Group VI	8.19±0.59 a	5.33±1.16 a', b'	9.40±0.99 a, b, d
Group VII	10.06±0.55 a', b', c', d', e'	4.35±0.64 a', b', c'	7.70±1.15 f

Table 1. Results (mean ± standard deviation) of serum Ca, Mg and Pi, expressed as mg/dl.
a ($p<0.05$) and a' ($p<0.01$) in group indicated versus group I (control),
b ($p<0.05$) and b' ($p<0.01$) in group indicated versus group II,
c ($p<0.05$) and c' ($p<0.01$) in group indicated versus group III,
d ($p<0.05$) and d' ($p<0.01$) in group indicated versus group IV,
e ($p<0.05$) and e' ($p<0.01$) in group indicated versus group V and
f ($p<0.05$) and f' ($p<0.01$) in group indicated versus group VI.

The results show that the training in air (group II) do not modify any parameter analyzed; the hypoxia (group III) decreases significantly ($p<0.05$) the serum Ca and increases also significantly ($p<0.01$) the Mg; rats training in hypoxia (group IV) exhibit the same variations that the rats mantained under hypoxia without training.

The rats that performed one training programme and after one week of normal activity (group V) show a significative decrease ($p<0.05$) in serum Ca and an increase also significative ($p<0.05$) in serum Mg, in relation to the control group (group I); the rats that remained at rest for 15 days under hypoxia (group VI) and then a week in air showed the same variations that the rats which stayed only in air (group V) and moreover an significative increase ($p<0.01$) in Pi; and, finally, in the rats training under hypoxia there is an inversion in these changes: serum Ca increases significantly ($p<0.05$) and serum Mg and Pi decrease also significantly ($p<0.05$). These changes may justify the preparation of the elite athletes in heigth before the regular season.

Acknowledgments. This work has been supported by the grant nº 90/0514 from Fondo de Investigaciones Sanitarias de la Seguridad Social (FISss).

References.

Cordova, A., Escanero, J.F. and Gimenéz, M. (1988): Variaciones plasmáticas de calcio, magnesio y fósforo inorgánico en ratas hipoxémicas después del ejercicio. Congreso Nacional de la Sociedad Española de Ciencias Fisiológicas, Tenerife.

Deuster, P.A., Dolev, E., Kyle, S.B, Anderson, R.A. and Schoomaker, E.B. (1987): Magnesium homeostasis during high-intensity anaerobic exercise in men. Am. Appl. Physiol. 62, 545-550.

Hespel, P., Lijnen, P., Fiochi, R., Dennis, B., Lissens, W., M'Buyama-Kabangu, J.R. and Amery, A. (1986): Cationic concentration and trasmembrane fluxes in erythrocytes of humans during exercise. Am. Appl. Physiol. 61, 37-43.

Metal Ions in Biology and Medicine, vol. 2. Eds. J. Anastassopoulou, Ph. Collery, J.C. Etienne, Th. Theophanides. John Libbey Eurotext, Paris © 1992, pp. 313-316

Investigations into the effect of verapamil on the memory consolidation*

W.N. Znang, F.M. Wu, Z.X. Zhnag, X.G. Wang

Department of biology of Nanjing University. Medical School of Nanjing University. Central Laboratory of Nanjing University, Nanjing 210008, P.R. China

INTRODUCTION

Several investigations suggest a particular role of calcium ions (Ca^{2-}) in the induction of long—term potentiation (LTP) (Baimbridge, 1981; Lynch, 1984). Correlated with LTP, the incorporation of radioactive Ca^{2+} into hippocampal slices increased and there was new synthesis of proteins. When an inhibitor of protein synthesis was applied, the development of LTP was blocked either in hippocampal CA1 subfield or in dentate gyrus. It was reported that agents, which block calcium conductance (such as La^{3-}), impaired memory in mice trained in an active avoidance task; while an appropriate dose of Ca^{2+} could counter the amnestic effects of La^{3+} (Mizumori, 1987). The study in our laboratory (in press) showed that bilateral intrahippocampal injection of Ca^{2+} or EGTA markedly attenuated memory retention of mice in a one—trial passive avoidance task and simultaneously reduced the protein synthesis of hippocampal synaptosomes in vitro. In this study, the memorial effects of calcium channel blocker verapamil injection immediately after training in mice were assessed, meanwhile, the effect of verapamil on the protein synthesis of hippocampal synaptosomes in vitro was also observed.

EXPERIMENTAL DETAILS

Male mice weighing 20—22g were used. They were divided at random into verapamil group and saline group.

Behavioral procedures: One—trial passive avoidance (PA) apparatus was similar to that described by Ader et al. (1972), with slight modifications. The step through latency to the dark compartment 24 hr later was recorded as a measure of retention test; high latencies are interpreted as reflecting good retention, and low latencies are taken to indicate poor retention (often amnesia). The results were analyzed according to the Mann—Whitney U—test.

Intrahippocampal injection: The bilateral intrahippocampal injection was carried out approximately according to the method of Mizumori et al. (1987), with the stereotaxic coordinates: A—P—2. 0 and L± 2. 0 mm from bregma, horizontal skull. After training, the mice were immediately given drug injection. The injection needles were lowered 1. 8 mm below the skull. This allowed direct application of the drug to dorsal hippocampus. A volume of 0. 5 μl per side was injected over a period of 88 s. Histological verifica-

* The Project Supported by National Natural Science Fundation of China and The Analytic Center of Nanjing University

tion of injection sites was carried out at the end of the experiment. Frozen sections were stained with cresyl violet, then examined under a light microscope.

Incorporation of ^3H — Leucine into synaptosomal proteins in vitro: Synaptosomes prepared from hippocampi were divided into verapamil group and control group. The incubation with ^3H—Leucine was kept at 37 ℃ for 30 min, and terminated by ice—water bath. Then 12.5% TCA was used for precipitation of the synaptosomal proteins. All the samples were prepared by the conventional method either for the measurement of the total radioactivity incorporated into synaptosomal proteins or for SDS — polyacrylamide gel discelectrophoresis. The total radioactivity incorporated into synaptosomal proteins and ^3H—labeled bands were measured in Beckman LS—9800 liquid scintillation counter.

RESULTS AND DISCUSSION

The passive avoidance results are showed in Table 1. Latencies in the acquisition trial were statistically similar each other in the two groups, the median scores were 6.9 and 9.1 s for verapamil and saline groups, respectively. In the retention trial, the median of latencies in verapamil group were significantly decreased as compared with that in saline group ($p<0.05$), and the median scores were 98.4 and 229.5 s, respectively. The above results indicated that intrahippocampal injection of verapamil impaired memory consolidation, and this corresponded with the report that agents, which block calcium conductance (such as La^{3+}), impaired memory in mice trained in an active avoidance task. (Mizumori, 1987).

Table 1. Effect of verapamil intrahippocampal injection on PA memroy retention

Group	Training latency (s)		Retention latency (s)	
	Median	Interquartile range	Median	Interquartile range
Saline (n=13)	9.1	3.3—29.2	229.5	10.1—300.0
Verapamil (n=9)	6.9	2.3—13.6	98.4 *	15.4—300.0

Verapamil (1.25μg/1μl/mouse) or saline (1μl/mouse) was injected bilateral intrahippocampally immediately after training.

* $p<0.05$, vs the saline group in the retention trial

As can be seen in Fig. 1, verapamil obviously reduced the incorporation of ^3H—Leucine into hippocapmal synaptosomal proteins as compared with saline group ($p<0.01$). By SDS — polyacrylamide gel electrophoresis, a significantly decreased incorporation of ^3H—Leucine in verapamil group was found to occur in synaptosomal proteins with molecular weights in the range of 19—27 KD, 33—34.7 KD and 61—71 KD, when compared with corresponding saline controls (Fig. 2). By comparison of Fig. 1 and Fig. 2, it is obvious that the reduced ^3H—Leu—incorporation into total synaptosomal proteins in verapamil group is resulted from the decreased synthesis of above protein bands with molecular masses of 19—27 KD, 33—34.7 KD and 61—71 KD.

It is generally agreed that long—term memory is dependent on new synthesis of proteins. Our previous study (zhang, 1991) has demonstrated that protein synthesis relied on optimal Ca^{2+} concentration. It is known that there are several types of calcium channels in neuronal membrane, and that the calcium channel blocker can combine with the special site in synaptosomes. Verapamil has been proved to be a member of the phenylalkylamine family of L—type calcium channel blocker. But recently it was demonstrated that verapamil can antagonize the other types of calcium channels. Thus, it is evident that verapamil would affect the synaptosomal functions extensively, and this influence would be certainly expressed in the protein

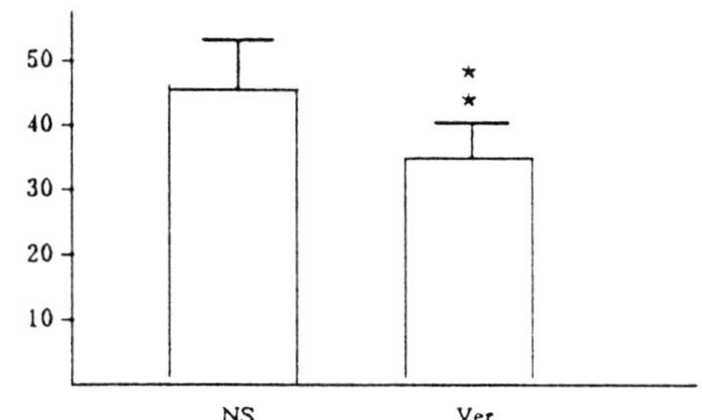

Fig. 1. Effect of verapamil on the incorporation of ^{3}H—leucine into hippocampal synaptosomal proteins. Vertical lines indicate means ± S. D. of 13—15 experiments.

• • $p<0.01$, vs the NS group

NS=normal saline, Ver=verapamil

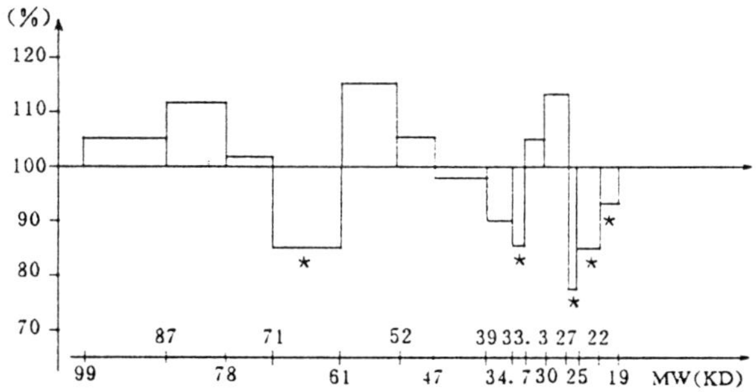

Fig. 2. Changes of ^{3}H—leucine incorporation into SDS—gel fractions of hippocampal synaptosomal proteins after treated with verapamil

Ordinate: % change of specific activity

Abscissa: molecular weight

* $P<0.05$, vs the corresponding controls electrophoretic migration from left to right

metabolism. In the present study, the observation that intrahippocampal injection of verapamil attenuated memory retention in mice trained in a one—trial passive avoidance task, and significantly reduced the incorporation of ^{3}H—Leucine into proteins of hippocampal synaptosomes in vitro suggested that the effect of verapamil on memory consolidation is related with the decreased protein synthesis in hippocampal synaptosomes which probably arised from the alteration of activation of Ca^{2-}-dependent enzymes by blocking the calcium channels in the synaptic membrane.

REFERENCES

Ader, R. , et al. (1972) Retention of a passive avoidance response as a function of the intensity and duration of electric shock. Psychon. Sci. 26, 125—128.

Baimbridge, K. G. et al. (1981) Calcium uptake and retention during long—term potentiation of neuronal activity in the rat hippocampal slice preparation. Brain Res. 221, 299—305.

Lynch, G. et al. (1984) The biochemistry of memory: A new and specific hypothesis. Science 224,

1057—1063.

Mizumori, S. J. Y. et al. (1987) Investigations into the neuropharmacological basis of temporal stages of memory formation in mice trained in an active avoidance task. Behavioral Brain Res. 23, 239—250.

Zhang, W. N. et al. (1991) Relation between the effect of DGAVP on the protein synthesis of hippocampal synaptosomes and the level of calcium ions. Chinese Science Bulletin 36, 243—248.

Metal Ions in Biology and Medicine, vol. 2. Eds. J. Anastassopoulou, Ph. Collery, J.C. Etienne, Th. Theophanides. John Libbey Eurotext, Paris © 1992, pp. 317-318

Convenient enzymatic determination of trace mercury in water

Robert W. Henkens, Junguo Zhao, John P. O'Daly

Enzyme Technology Research Group, Inc., 710 West Main Street, Durham, NC 27701, USA

Certain metals have long been considered as hazardous to health or to pose an environmental threat. Some metals are of particular concern because of toxicity to humans, cadmium, mercury and lead being particular examples. The effects of these metals may not be acute, indeed chronic toxicity is of particular concern because the metals accumulate in the body over a period of long-term exposure. The result, especially in the very young, may be developmental abnormalities both mental and physical.

Our goal is to develop a new technique for the detection and measurement of trace but still dangerous levels of mercury in food and water. In contrast to current methods, the technology will make possible inexpensive, wide-spread testing for mercury contamination.

We report in this paper on the feasibility of detecting nanomolar concentrations of mercury in water with an enzyme based amperometric biosensor. The enzyme serves as an organic reagent whose activity is inhibited by low levels of mercury. Our objective is to develop an enzyme modified electrode for the sensor that has sensitivity to measure nanomolar concentrations for both organic and inorganic forms of mercury with appropriate selectivity and storage characteristics.

An electrode was prepared from colloidal gold adsorbed alcohol dehydrogenase (ADH) using methods employed with other redox enzymes (Henkens et al, 1991). Measurements were made in a microcell 100-200 µl in volume using various concentrations of mercury. Electrochemical measurements were made by steady-state amperometry at 0 volts (Ag/AgCl) in a unstirred buffer solution containing 40 mM phosphate at pH 9.0, using N-methylphenazonium methosulfate as the mediator.

The calibration curve obtained is shown in Fig. 1. The percent response of the electrode caused by mercury inhibition of the ADH was calculated by the signal drop caused by the presence of mercury divided by the total signal without mercury. The excellent response of this electrode to mercury is illustrated in Fig. 2 which shows the linear portion of the dose response curve. The mercury electrode is sensitive to nanomolar concentrations of mercury as can be seen in

Fig. 2 and its selectivity is quite good. The electrode response was irreversible and was specific for mercury in the presence of 20 μM lead ion.

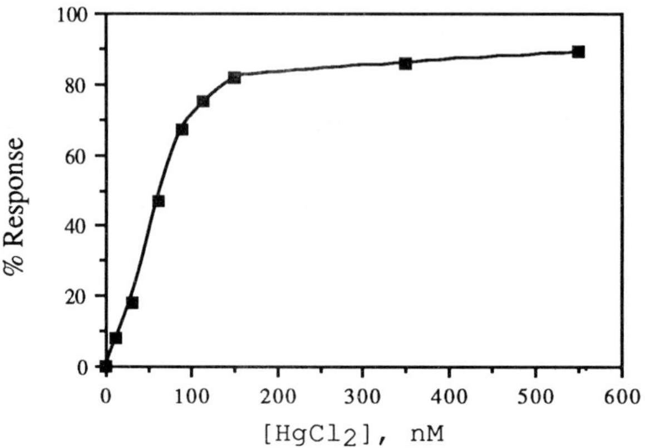

Figure 1. The amperometric response to mercury ion using a colloidal gold/ADH electrode.

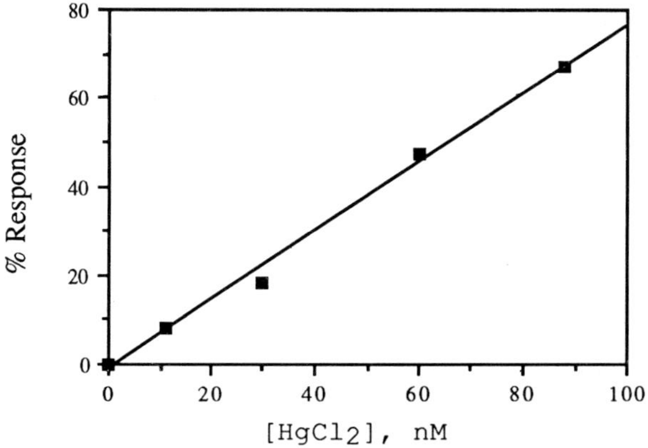

Figure 2. Illustration of the linear response to mercury ion using a colloidal gold/ADH electrode.

REFERENCES

Henkens, R.W., O'Daly, J.P., Perine, S.C., Tubergen, K.R., Kitchell, B.S., and Stonehuerner, J. (1990): Electrochemistry of Colloidal Gold Supported Oxidase Enzymes, *J. Inorg. Biochem.* **43,** 120.

Metal Ions in Biology and Medicine, vol. 2. Eds. J. Anastassopoulou, Ph. Collery, J.C. Etienne, Th. Theophanides. John Libbey Eurotext, Paris © 1992, pp. 319-320

Maternal and developmental toxicity of metavanadate in mice

D.J. Sánchez*, M. Gómez, J.L. Domingo, J.M. Llobet, J. Corbella

*Laboratory of Toxicology and Biochemistry and *Physiology Unit, School of Medicine, University of Barcelona, San Lorenzo 21, 43201 Reus, Spain*

Vanadium is a trace element distributed extensively in nature and used in various heavy industries (steel, oil, etc.), as well as in new fields such as elements in superconductive materials. Thus, although occupational exposure to vanadium is quite common, the general population is also increasingly exposed to this metal mostly in the form of vanadium oxides through the combustion of fossil fuels for energy production. Significant quantities of vanadium are every year released into the atmosphere, into the water and into the soil (Nriagu & Pacyna, 1988).

In spite of the increasing interest of vanadium, the experimental data on its toxicological significance is relatively limited (Parker & Sharma, 1978; Domingo *et al.*, 1985; Cohen *et al.*, 1986). Since information concerning the developmental toxicity of vanadium is particularly scarce (Carlton, 1982; Paternain *et al.*, 1990), in this study we examined the effects of sodium metavanadate in pregnant mice when given ip throughout organogenesis.

MATERIALS AND METHODS

Four groups of 25 plug-positive female Swiss mice (Panlab, Barcelona, Spain) received 0, 2, 4, and 8 mg/kg/day of sodium metavanadate ($NaVO_3$) (Sigma, St. Louis, USA) dissolved in 0.9% saline by ip injection on days 6-15 of gestation. The ip LD_{50} of $NaVO_3$ in mice was previously reported to be 35.9 mg/kg (Llobet & Domingo, 1984). Body weight and food consumption were monitored daily. On gestation day 18, dams were killed by overexposure to ether. Liver and kidney weight, gravid uterine weight, and uterine contents (i.e., number of implantation sites, resorptions, dead and live fetuses) were recorded. Live fetuses were dissected from the uterus, weighed, sexed, and examined for external, internal and skeletal malformations and variations.

RESULTS AND DISCUSSION

Maternal weight gain during treatment (gestation days 6-15), and body weight at termination were only significantly reduced in the 8 mg/kg/day group. However, there was a significant dose-related decreasing trend in weight gain during gestation (days 0-18) as well as in the gravid uterine weight at 2 and 4 mg/kg/day, while no differences among groups were observed in corrected maternal body weight.

Table 1 summarizes the embryotoxic and teratogenic effects of $NaVO_3$ in pregnant Swiss mice. The number of implantation sites per litter, and the sex ratio were similar among groups. In contrast, the number of resorptions and dead fetuses per litter were significantly increased at 4 and 8 mg/kg/day, while the number of live fetuses per litter and the average fetal weight were significantly diminished at these doses. There were no significant increases in the incidence of external or skeletal anomalies, but a significant increase in the incidence of cleft palate was observed at 8 mg/kg/day.

In this study, there was evidence of embryo or fetal toxicity at maternally toxic levels (8 mg/kg/day) and below (4 mg/kg/day). Therefore, the embryofetotoxicity of $NaVO_3$ would be the result of the direct contact of vanadium with the embryonic or fetal tissues. The no-observed-adverse-effect level (NOAEL) for maternal toxicity was 4 mg/kg/day, whereas the NOAEL for developmental toxicity was 2 mg/kg/day.

TABLE 1. Embryotoxic and teratogenic effects in mice treated with sodium metavanadate[a]

	Dose (mg(kg/day)			
	0	2	4	8
No. of litters	20	19	20	22
Implantations/litter	13.14±1.55	14.03±2.17	13.38±1.71	12.59±3.03
Resorptions/litter	0.53±0.66	1.50±1.31	1.84±1.46[b]	8.20±4.57[d]
Dead fetuses/litter	0.15±0.37	0.33±0.49	1.23±0.88[b]	0.93±0.70[b]
Live fetuses/litter	12.46±1.56	12.25±2.22	10.31±3.19[c]	3.40±3.06[d]
Postimplantation loss/ litter (%)	12.12±4.15	12.68±9.71	22.94±17.62[c]	72.99±23.60[d]
Fetal sex ratio (M/F)	1.19±0.45	0.90±0.26	1.05±0.35	1.12±0.58
Fetal body weight (g)	1.15±0.13	1.08±0.13	1.06±0.12[b]	0.94±0.12[d]
No. of fetuses with cleft palate (litters)	0 (0)	2 (1)	5 (4)	16 (10)[d]

[a]Data are presented as means ± SD. [b]Significantly different from control group ($p<0.05$). [c]Significantly different from control group ($p<0.01$). [d]Significantly different from control group ($p<0.001$).

Acknowledgements This study was supported by REPSOL PETROLEO, S.A., Tarragona, Spain.

REFERENCES

Carlton, B.D., Beneke, M.B., and Fisher, G.L. (1982): Assessment of the teratogenicity of ammonium metavanadate using Syrian golden hamsters. *Environ. Res.* 29: 256-262.

Cohen, M.D., Wei, C.I., Tan, H., and Kao, K.J. (1986): Effect of ammonium metavanadate on the murine immune response. *J. Toxicol. Environ. Health* 19: 279-298.

Domingo, J.L., Llobet, J.M., Tomas, J.M., and Corbella, J. (1985): Short-term toxicity studies of vanadium in rats. *J. Appl. Toxicol.* 5: 418-421.

Llobet, J.M., & Domingo, J.L. (1984): Acute toxicity of vanadium compounds in rats and mice. *Toxicol. Lett.* 23: 227-231.

Nriagu, J.O., and Pacyna, J.M. (1988): Quantitative assessment of worldwide contamination of air, water and soils by trace metals. *Nature* 333: 134-139.

Parker, R.D.R., & Sharma, R.P. (1978): Accumulation and depletion in selected tissues of rats treated with vanadyl sulphate and sodium orthovanadate. *J. Environ. Pathol. Toxicol.* 2: 235-245.

Paternain, J.L., Domingo, J.L., Gómez, M., Ortega, A., and Corbella, J. (1990): Developmental toxicity of vanadium in mice after oral administration. *J. Appl. Toxicol.* 10: 181-186.

Metal Ions in Biology and Medicine, vol. 2. Eds. J. Anastassopoulou, Ph. Collery, J.C. Etienne, Th. Theophanides. John Libbey Eurotext, Paris © 1992, pp. 321-322

Evaluation of the effects of DMSA (*meso*-2,3-dimercaptosuccinic acid) on methyl mercury-induced embryolethality in mice

M. Gómez, D.J. Sánchez, V. Piera*, J.M. Llobet, J.L. Domingo, J. Corbella

*Laboratory of Toxicology and Biochemistry and *Anatomy Unit, School of Medicine, University of Barcelona, San Lorenzo 21, 43201 Reus, Spain*

Methyl mercury is the most important form of mercury in terms of toxicity. The major human health effects are neurotoxicity in adults, and toxicity to the fetus of mothers exposed to methyl mercury during pregnancy. Several investigations demonstrated that methyl mercury is embryofetotoxic in various species (Fuyuta *et al.*, 1978; Hoskins & Hupp, 1978; Endo & Watanabe, 1988). Also, exposure to methyl mercury during gestation induced behavioral and neurochemical changes in offspring of rats (Cagiano *et al.*, 1990). In recent years, remarkable advances in the treatment of mercury poisoning have been made. *meso*-2,3-Dimercaptosuccinic acid (DMSA), a water soluble chelating agent structurally similar to BAL, has been reported to be an efficient chelator for the removal of mercury from the mammalian body (Aposhian & Aposhian, 1990). The purpose of the present study was to evaluate whether the embryotoxic effects of methyl mercury can be prevented by DMSA.

MATERIALS AND METHODS

Methyl mercury chloride was obtained from E. Merck (Darmstadt, FRG). DMSA was purchased from Sigma Chemical Co. (St. Louis, MO, USA). Mature Swiss mice (Interfauna, Barcelona, Spain) weighing 30-32 g were mated, and the day on which a vaginal plug was observed was designated day 0 of gestation. All mice were offered Panlab rodent chow (Panlab, Barcelona) and water *ad libitum*.

A series of four DMSA injections was administered subcutaneously to pregnant animals immediately after oral administration (by gavage) of 25 mg/kg of methyl mercury chloride given on day 10 of gestation, and at 24, 48, and 72 hr thereafter. DMSA effectiveness was tested at doses of 0, 80, 160, and 320 mg/kg/injection. The no-observed-adverse-effect level (NOAEL) for DMSA teratogenicity in mice when given subcutaneously was previously found to be 410 mg/kg/day (Domingo *et al.*, 1988). DMSA was dissolved in 5% sodium bicarbonate solutions and given at a pH of approximately 7. Mice in the negative control group were pretreated with 0.9% saline and then post-treated with 5% $NaHCO_3$ solutions.

Dams were killed by overexposure to ether on day 18 of gestation. Uterine horns were opened and the status of uterine implantation sites evaluated, (i.e., number of sites, resorptions, and dead and live fetuses). The body weights of live fetuses were also recorded.

RESULTS AND DISCUSSION

Oral administration of methyl mercury chloride on day 10 of gestation resulted in a high rate of resorptions and dead fetuses. Although not significantly different, fetal body weight was lower in the control positive group than in the negative control group. Recently, Endo & Watanabe (1988) evaluated the protective activity of N-acetylcisteine (NAC) against the embryotoxic and teratogenic effects of methyl mercury with discouraging results. In contrast, in the present study when DMSA was injected at 320 mg/kg, a protective significant effect of the chelator could be observed (Table 1). The number of resorptions and dead fetuses was significantly decreased compared to the control positive group, while the number of live fetuses and fetal body weight did not differ significantly from those in the control negative group.

TABLE 1. Prevention by DMSA of methyl mercury chloride (MMC)-induced embryolethality in mice (mean values ± SD)

	0.9% saline + $NaHCO_3$ (sol)	MMC 25 mg/kg + $NaHCO_3$ (sol)	MMC 25 mg/kg + DMSA 80 mg/kg	MMC 25 mg/kg + DMSA 160 mg/kg	MMC 25 mg/kg + DMSA 320 mg/kg
No. of litters	12	12	15	12	13
Implants per litter	13.33±2.01	13.00±2.21	13.27±2.40	12.92±2.74	13.46±3.86
Live fetuses per litter	11.90±2.70	7.16±5.78[1]	10.40±5.11	9.41±3.44[1]	11.62±3.66[a]
Dead fetuses per litter	0.16±0.29	0.42±0.35[1]	0.13±0.30[a]	0.33±0.45	0.16±0.31[a]
Early resorptions per litter	1.08±1.16	1.25±1.54	1.60±2.77	2.66±2.93	1.38±2.14
Late resorptions per litter	0.25±0.62	4.16±4.78[2]	1.14±3.18	0.50±0.79[a]	0.30±0.48[b]
Mean fetal weight (g)	1.18±0.18	1.12±0.15	1.08±0.20	1.20±0.24	1.24±0.09[a]

[1,2]Significantly different from control negative group; $p < 0.05$, $p < 0.01$, respectively.
[a,b]Significantly different from control positive group; $p < 0.05$, $p < 0.01$, respectively.

The protective activity of DMSA against embryolethality of methyl mercury is very probable due to the chelating action of the groups mercapto of the chelator. Thus, according to the results of this study, DMSA offers encouragement with regard to the therapeutic potential for pregnant women exposed to methyl mercury.

Acknowledgements. This work was supported by the CICYT (Spain) through grant SAL90-0074.

REFERENCES

Aposhian, H.V., and Aposhian, M.M. (1990): Meso-2,3-dimercaptosuccinic acid: Chemical, pharmacological and toxicological properties of an orally effective metal chelating agent. *Annu. Rev. Pharmacol. Toxicol.* 30: 279-306.

Cagiano, R., De Salvia, A., Renna, G., Tortella, E., Braghiroli, D., Parenti, C., Zanoli, P., Baraldi, M., Annau, Z., and Cuomo, V. (1990): Evidence that exposure to methyl mercury during gestation induces behavioral and neurochemical changes in offspring of rats. *Neurotoxicol. Teratol.* 12: 23-28.

Domingo, J.L., Paternain, J.L., Llobet, J.M., and Corbella, J. (1988): Developmental toxicity of subcutaneously administered *meso*-2,3-dimercaptosuccinic acid in mice. *Fundam. Appl. Toxicol.* 11: 715-722.

Endo, A., and Watanabe, T. (1988): Analysis of protective activity of N-acetylcysteine against teratogenicity of heavy metals. *Reprod. Toxicol.* 2: 141-144.

Fuyuta, M., Fujimoto, T., and Hirata, S. (1978): Embryotoxic effects of methylmercuric chloride administered to mice and rats during organogenesis. *Teratology* 18: 353-366.

Hoskins, BB., and Hupp, E.W. (1978): Methylmercury effects in rat, hamster and squirrel monkey. *Environ. Res.* 15: 5-19.

Metal Ions in Biology and Medicine, vol. 2. Eds. J. Anastassopoulou, Ph. Collery, J.C. Etienne, Th. Theophanides. John Libbey Eurotext, Paris © 1992, pp. 323-328

Aluminium exposure and toxicity

José M. Fraga, José R.F. Lorenzo, M. Luz Rey, José R. Cervilla, José A. Cocho

Departamento de Pediatría, Laboratorio de Alteraciones Metabólicas, Hospital General de Galicia, Clínico Universitario, Santiago de Compostela, España

SUMMARY

The aluminium has been implicated as potentially harmful element on the structure and function of severol organ system in humans. The risk of produce disfunctions would be more serious during infancy especially in period of maximum vulnerabity of the brain divelopment. It has been suggested that high aluminaemia decreases erythrocyte activity of the DHPR and that the same effect may occurs on brain DHPR. We report, for the first time, that the elevate ingestion of aluminium with feeds produces a decreasing in the erythrocyte activity of DHPR in newborns.

INTRODUCTION

In recent years there has been considerable research on aluminium as a pollutant that can have toxic effects on the structures and function of various systems within the human organism. Its acute toxicity is now generally recognized, but controversy persists as to the possibility of long-term effects due to its accumulation in the central nervous system and other organs. Association between chronic exposure to aluminium and encephalopathy was first reported thirty years ago (McLaughlin, 1962), and aroused special attention in the 1970s when Alfrey and coworkers related high brain aluminium concentrations to severe neurological disorders in patients on dialysis for chronic renal insufficiency. Aluminium was later also related to the high prevalence of osteomalacia in patients on dialysis, who received aluminium via the dialysis fluid and through oral administration of hypophosphoraemiant gels. Nonrdialysed paediatric patients treated with aluminium gels for renal insufficiency were found to suffer neurological alterations similar to the encephalopathy observed in dialysed patients (Andreoli, 1984), and Sedman (1985) reported that premature newborns fed parenterally had higher concentrations of aluminiun in plasma and urine than orally fed newborns due to contamination of parenteral feed fluids together with poor renal clearance of aluminium.

The scale of the risk of aluminium poisoning became apparent when Freundlich (1985) reported formula milk to be a source of ingestion. Other foodstuffs and drugs were soon added to the list of sources, and the list of pathological effects now includes not only CNS disorders and osteomalacia, but also other osteodystrophies and associated parathyroid lesions, anaemia, lung disorders and skin disease(granulomas and telangiectases).

The mechanism by which aluminium affects cerebral metabolism to produce its neurological effects in unknown. Similarly, it is not clear whether it plays a role in the genesis or evolution of Alzheimer´s disease, though Candy (1986) found deposits of aluminium silicate associated with foci of cerebral degeneration, and Martyn (1989) reported greater incidence of the disease in populations with high aluminium concentrations in their drinking water. More generally, whether aluminium affects cerebral and/or neurological development and cognitive functions is an open question. In favour of this hypothesis is the fact that brain aluminiun levels increase with age, especially in the grey matter, and that accumulation of aluminium in brain cells is very difficult to reverse. If true, the risk to brain function would of course be especially great in cases of high aluminium intake during the first few months of life, when brain growth is more active than at any subsequent time.

Altmann et al (1987) has put forward evidence that aluminium inhibits dihydropteridine reductase (DHPR) in erythrocytes, and has suggested that it may have the same effect on brain DHPR, which would affect the metabolism of neurotransmitters (dopa, norepinephrine, tyrosine and 5-hydroxytryptophan) and so explain aluminium-induced encephalopathy. It has also been reported that, *in vitro* and in laboratory animals, aluminium affects other biochemical agents and functions, including acetylcholinesterase, hexokinase, DNA replication enzymes, calmodulin, L-glutamine transport and gamma-aminobutyric acid transport.

Newborns are exposed to aluminium via four kinds of food or drug: water used for preparing foods and parenteral feeds; commercial foodstuffs with aluminium-bearing additives or contaminants; intravenously administered solutions of amino acids, salts and drugs; and natural products. In this work we evaluated the exposure of newborns to aluminium via food and drugs in our community and examined its relationship to erythrocyte DHPR levels.

METHODS

Aluminium was determined in acidified urine and water, serum, milk and milk powder samples digested with nitric and sulphuric acids. All samples were diluted with a matrix modifier containing nitric acid and Triton X-100; samples were collected in plastic tubes and plastic syringes with stainless steel needles, laboratory ware for reagent preparation was also plastic. Samples were stored at 4ºC pending analysis by atomic absorption spectrometry with electrothermal atomization using a Perkin-Elmer Mod. 1100B spectrometer, an HGA 700 atomicer and pyrocoated graphite tubes with a L´vov platform. Internal quality control was performed using aluminium standards from NIST and IAEA. Our laboratory participates in the Worldwide Interlaboratory Quality Control scheme for aluminium determination run by the Societé Francaise de Biologie Clinique, and has done since the inception of the scheme.

ALUMINIUM IN DRINKING WATER

The aluminium content of water varies widely, and depends on environmental concentrations, the acidity of rainfall and the purification process employer to produce drinking water. The EEC directive of July 15th 1980 on the quality of waters destined for human consumption set a recommended level of 50 μg/l and a maximun admissible concentration of 200μg/l. We found levels of 110-588μgl in tapwater (mean 195μg/l, SD 144μg/l).

ALUMINIUM IN MATERNAL MILK

In fifty samples of maternal milk obtained by expression we found Al levels of 10-42 μg/l (mean 23 μg/l).

ALUMINIUM IN FORMULA MILK

The Al content of formula milk, as ingested by the newborn, depends on both the way it has been obtained and the way it has been prepared for consumption. The following table summarizes our findings.

Table 1.

Milk type (No of samples)	Aluminium content range($\mu g/l$)
Cow´s milk (40)	20-145
Infant formula	
Standard (45)	30-544
Liquid (36)	67-795
For Premature (9)	150-647
Soy-based (11)	372-2530
Hypoallergenic (8)	67-89
Hydrolysed (10)	16-339

PARENTERAL NUTRITION SOLUTIONS

Parenteral formulas containing salts, oligoelements, glucose and amino acids had fairly uniform Al contents: among 23 samples, values ranged from 46 to 90 $\mu g/l$ (mean 65 $\mu g/l$, SD 17 $\mu g/l$).

ADDITIVES FOR PARENTERAL SOLUTIONS

The highest Al concentrations found among parenteral feed additives were those of calcium glucobionate (3238 $\pm$ 243 $\mu g/l$). In glucose additives, values ranged from 495 to 944 $\mu g/l$. The variability among different manufacturers suggests that their products are exposed to different levels of contamination by aluminium.

ALUMINIUM CONCENTRATIONS IN NEONATAL SERUM AND URINE

In 30 newborns with gestational ages of 29-42 weeks, all fed formula milk, Al concentrations in serum ranged from 5 to 38 $\mu g/l$ (mean 15 $\mu g/l$). The highest values were those of the newborns with greatest gestational age. the values found in fourteen newborns who received parenteral nutrition (mean 15.62 $\mu g/l$) did not differ significantly from those of the formula-fed infants (15.11$\mu g/l$) , however, Al concentration tended to increase with the duration of parenteral nutrition.

Al concentrations in urine ranged from 22 to 114 $\mu g/l$, with Al/Cr ratios of 0.2-0.4.

RELATIONSHIP BETWEEN SERUM AL AND ERYTHROCYTE DHPR ACTIVITY

The DHPR activity was assayed according to the method of Narisawa et al (1981). The summary of results is showed in the Table 2.

Table 2. Relationship between serum aluminium levels and erythrocyte DHPR activity in newborns

Group according to Al level (No of cases)	Serum Al (μg/l) mean (SD)	Erythrocyte DHPR (nmol NADH/min/mg Hb) mean (SD)
< 35 (54)	22.5 (8.7)	1.20 (0.23)
> 35 (18)	46.4 (10.7)	1.05 (0.16)
All (72)	28.5 (13.8)	1.16 (0.22)

In a group of 72 newborns, DHPR activity was negatively correlated with serum Al ($r = -0.25$, $p<0.05$). Correlation was closer ($p = 0.003$) in the newborns with serum Al concentrations greater than 35μg/l, suggesting that it may be possible to establish threshold level of aluminaemia above which alteration of DHPR activity becomes more severe.

PRACTICAL IMPLICATIONS: WHAT CAN BE DONE?

Aliminium was long considered to be non - toxic; in 1971 the US Food and Drug Administration still classified it a innocuous. However, subsequent reviews led the FDA´s Endocrine and Metabolic Drug products Advisory Commitee to recommend that the concentrations of aluminium in intravenous additives be limited and specified on product package labels.

The wide variability of aluminium concentrations found in parenteral feeds and other intravenous infusions, and the risk they constitute, suggests that the Al content of these products should be checked periodically, if found to be high, the clinician should seriously consider the reduction or cessation of parenteral nutrition as soon as possible, especially during the neonatal pariod when aluminium overload is most dangerous.

The effects of acute and chronic exposure to aluminium are well established, but long-term effects are still controversial. Pending the availability of conclusive data, it nevertheless seems reasonable, in view of the tendency of aluminium to accumulate in the organism and the high uptake of macromolecules and metals by newborns, to require that food products for infants (especially parenteral feeds and other intravenously administered solutions) have the lowest possible aluminium contents. This requirement should be accompanied by the establishment of Al monitoring programmes in health centres.

This work was supported in part by SM 89-0041 grant from the DGICYT - Ministerio de Educación y Ciencia.

REFERENCES

Alfrey, A.C., Mishell, J.M., Burks, J. (1972): Syndrome of dyspraxia and multifocal seizures associated with chronic hemodialysis. Trans. Am. Soc. Artif. Intern. Organs.18: 257-261.

Alfrey, A.C., LeGendre, G.R., Kaenhny, W.D. (1976): The dialysis encephalopathy syndrome: possible aluminium intoxication. N. Engl. J. Med 294: 184-188.

Altmann, P., Al-Salihi, F., Butter, K., Cutler, P., Blair, J., Leeming, R., Cunningham, J., Marsh, F. (1987): Serum aluminium levels and erythrocyte dihydropteridine reductase activity in patients on hemodialysis. N. Engl. J. Med. 317:80-84.

Andreoli, S.P. Bergstein, J.M., Sherrara , A.J., (1984): Aluminium intoxication from aluminium - containing phosphate binders in children with azotemia not undergoing dialysis. N. Engl. J. Med. 310: 1079 - 1084.

Candy, J.M., Klinowski, J., Perry, R.H., Perry, E.K., Fairbairn, A., Oakley, A.E., Carpenter, T.A., Atack, J.R. Blessed, G., Edwardson, J.A. (1986): Aluminosilicates and senile plaque formation in Alzheimer´s disease. Lancet 327: 354-357.

Freundlich, M., Zillernelo, G., Abitbol, C., Strauss, J., Fangere, M.C., Malluche, H.H. (1985): Infant formula as a cause of aluminium toxicity in neonatal uraemia Lancet 326: 527-529.

Narisawa, K., Arai, N., Hayakawa, H., Tada, K. (1981): Diagnosis of dihydropteridine reductase deficiency by erythrocyte enzyme assay. Pediatrics 68:591-592.

Martyn, C.N. Barker, D.J.P., Osmon, C., Harris, E.C., Edwardson, J.A., Lacey, R.F., (1989): Geographical relation between Alzheimer´s disease and aluminium in drinking water. Lancet 333: 59-62.

Mc. Langhlin, A. L.G., Kazantis, G., King, E., (1962): Pulmanary fibrosis and encephalopathy associated with the inhalation of aluminium dust. Br. J. Ind. Med. 19: 253-263.

Sedman, A.B., Gordon, G.L., Merritt, R.J., Miller, N.L., Weber, K.O., Gill, W.L., Anand, H., Alfrey, A.C. (1985): Evidence of Aluminium loading in infants receiving intravenous Therapy. N. Engl. J. Med. 312: 1337-1343

Metal Ions in Biology and Medicine, vol. 2. Eds. J. Anastassopoulou, Ph. Collery, J.C. Etienne, Th. Theophanides. John Libbey Eurotext, Paris © 1992, pp. 329-330

Efficacy of Tiron on the mobilization of vanadium in diabetic rats after oral aministration of metavanadate

J.M. Llobet, M. Gómez, D.J. Sánchez, J.L. Domingo, J. Corbella, C.L. Keen*

*Laboratory of Toxicology and Biochemistry, School of Medicine, University of Barcelona, 43201 Reus Spain and *Departments of Nutrition and Internal Medicine, University of California, Davis, CA, 95616, USA*

In recent years, it has been demonstrated that the inclusion of vanadate (V^{+5}) and vanadyl (V^{+4}) ions in the drinking water of streptozotocin(STZ)-induced diabetic rats alleviates the diabetic state of the animals (Heyliger *et al.*, 1985; Meyerovitch *et al.*, 1987; Ramanadham *et al.*, 1989). Nevertheless, the improvement of some signs of diabetes (hyperglycemia, hyperphagia, polydipsia) in STZ-treated rats is negated by the severe side effects associated with chronic vanadium administration (Domingo *et al.*, 1991a,b). Moreover, vanadium accumulates in all of the tissues analyzed which would imply an additional risk of vanadium toxicity. Therefore, oral vanadate or vanadyl therapy would be of very limited value (or even inexistent) in the treatment of diabetes.

However, because of the ability of vanadium compounds to diminish the diabetic state of STZ-treated rats, it is worthwhile to consider whether the toxic side effects of this element can be eliminated while maintaining its insulin mimetic properties. Thus, the aim of this investigation was to evaluate the effects of sodium 4,5- dihydroxybenzene-1,3-disulfonate (Tiron), an efficacious chelator in chronic vanadium intoxication (Gómez *et al.*, 1991), on the diabetic status of STZ-treated rats during oral vanadate treatment as well as the effects of vanadium in these animals.

MATERIALS AND METHODS

Diabetes was induced in 40 male Sprague-Dawley rats (200-220 g) by two sc injections (given on days 0 and 3) of STZ (45 mg/kg) in cold 0.1 M citrate buffer (pH = 4.5). Ten rats received citrated buffer alone (control non-diabetic group). Five days later, animals with concentrations of glucose > 250 mg/100 ml were considered diabetic. One group (10 animals) of STZ-induced diabetic rats drank aqueous solutions of NaCl (80 mM), and a second group (30 animals) received for 5 weeks similar solutions to which sodium metavanadate (Sigma, St. Louis, USA) was added until a concentration of 0.20 mg/ml was obtained. After three weeks, ip treatment with Tiron (Sigma, St. Louis, USA) was initiated. Tiron was injected every two days for 2 weeks at 300 and 600 mg/kg/injection. The ip LD_{50} of Tiron has been reported to be 4710 mg/kg (Gómez *et al.*, 1991). During the experimental period, body weight, and food and fluid intake were monitored daily. Blood glucose concentrations were measured on days 4, 14, 27, 31 and 35 of treatment. At the end of the experiment, rats were killed by overexposure to ether and liver, spleen, kidneys, heart, brain, bone (femur), muscle (gastrocnemius) and pancreas were removed for tissue vanadium analyses by AAS (Domingo *et al.*, 1991a,b).

RESULTS AND DISCUSSION

In all of the vanadium-treated groups, food and fluid intake were significantly lower ($p < 0.001$) than in the non-vanadium treated diabetic group. These decreases were independent of the form of vanadate administration: alone or concurrent with Tiron (data not shown). Thus, the improvement in the hyperphagia and polydipsia caused by vanadate was not affected by the treatment with Tiron.

TABLE 1. Blood Glucose Concentrations in the Different Groups of Animals

	Control (non diabetic)	STZ	STZ + $NaVO_3$	STZ + $NaVO_3$ + TIRON (300 mg/kg)	STZ + $NaVO_3$ + TIRON (600 mg/kg)
Day 0	152±34	717±57[1]	677±111[1]	602±134[1]	632±107[1]
Day 4	150±21	699±91[1]	631±160[1]	577±123[1]	597±101[1]
Day 14	149±22	722±129[1]	573±142[1,a]	591±97[1,a]	557±141[1,a]
Day 27	153±15	780±238[1]	533±132[1,b]	503±153[1,b]	494±175[1,a]
Day 31	157±32	739±104[1]	487±151[1,b]	454±195[1,b]	474±80[1,c]
Day 35	166±8	742±65[1]	550±69[1,c]	449±115[1,c]	504±75[1,c]

Results are presented as means (mg/100 ml) ± SD.
[1]Significantly different from control (non-diabetic) group: $p < 0.001$.
[a,b,c]Significantly different from vanadate-untreated diabetic rats: $p < 0.05$, $p < 0.01$, $p < 0.001$.

Table 1 summarizes the effects of orally administered vanadate and ip Tiron on blood glucose levels in the different groups of animals. Treatment with Tiron did not modify the significant improvement of glucose homeostasis caused by vanadate treatment. In contrast, Tiron administration to vanadate-treated diabetic rats resulted in a lower accumulation of vanadium in liver, kidney, heart, bone and muscle (data not shown). Because of the significant efficacy of Tiron in mobilizing vanadium, it suggests that for diabetic rats, the concentrations of metavanadate in drinking water may be substantially increased, which may result in a lowering of glucose levels to those of non-diabetic animals. Although this therapy (oral vanadate + ip Tiron) would not probably be the most adequate for diabetic patients, the encouraging results of this investigation open new possibilities in the search of viable alternative treatment to sc insulin in human diabetes.

Acknowledgements: This study was supported by the CICYT (Spain), through grant SAL91-0023.

REFERENCES

Domingo, J.L., Gómez, M., Llobet, J.M., Corbella, J., and Keen, C.L. (1991a): Oral vanadium administration to streptozotocin-diabetic rats has marked negative side effects which are independent of the form of vanadium used. *Toxicology* 66, 279-287.

Domingo, J.L., Gómez, M., Llobet, J.M., Corbella, J., and Keen, C.L. (1991b) Improvement of glucose homeostasis by oral vanadyl or vanadate teatment in diabetic rats is accompanied by negative side effects. *Pharmacol. Toxicol.* 68, 249-253.

Gómez, M., Domingo, J.L., Llobet, J.M., and Corbella, J. (1991): Effectiveness of some chelating agents on distribution and excretion of vanadium in rats after prolonged oral administration. *J. Appl. Toxicol.* 11, 195-198.

Heyliger, C.E., Tahiliani, A.G., and McNeill, J.H. (1985): Effects of vanadate on elevated blood glucose and depressed cardiac performance of diabetic rats. *Science* 227, 1474-1477.

Meyerovitch, J., Farfel, Z., Sack, J., and Shechter, Y. (1987): Oral administration of vanadate normalizes blood glucose levels in streptozotocin-treated rats. *J. Biol. Chem.* 262, 6658-6662.

Ramanadham, S., Mongold, J.J., Brownsey, R.W., Cros, G.H., and McNeill, J.H. (1989): Oral vanadyl sulfate in treatment of diabetes mellitus in rats. *Am. J. Physiol.* 257, H904-H911.

Metal Ions in Biology and Medicine, vol. 2. Eds. J. Anastassopoulou, Ph. Collery, J.C. Etienne, Th. Theophanides. John Libbey Eurotext, Paris © 1992, pp. 331-332

In vitro cytotoxicity and accumulation of aluminium by cells

M.P. Sauvant*, D. Pepin*, A. Gardes**, M. Bourges***, P. Boumati****

**Laboratoire d'Hydrologie et d'Hygiène - Faculté de Pharmacie, BP 38 63001 Clermont-Ferrand Cedex, France. **INSERM, U 71, BP 184, 63005 Clermond-Ferrand Cedex 13, France. ***Départment de Microscopie Electronique, Faculté de Médecine, BP 38 63001 Clermont-Ferrand Cedex, France. ****Laboratoire de Biophysique, Centre de Microanalyse du CNRS, Faculté de Médecine H. Mondor, 8, rue du Général-Farrail, 94000 Créteil, France*

INTRODUCTION

Aluminium is the third most abundant element in the environment and the potential exposure of human is unavoidable. Substantial accumulation of aluminium over time in humain brain tissue has been established in patients with haemodialysis encephalopathy (ALFREY et al., 1976) or with other neuropathy (PERL et al., 1982). X-ray microprobe analysis allowed to prove the incorporation and the accumulation of Al in the cells (BERRY et al., 1988).
The aim of our study is to investigated in vitro the potential toxicity of Al on an established cell line (fibroblasts, ATCC-L929) by the determination of the growth and the cellular viability, and the incorporation of Al by the cells.

MATERIAL AND METHOD

Cells were cultured at 37°C (5% CO2) in the Minimum Eagle's Medium (M.E.M.) supplemented with 5% fetal calf serum, 1% vitamins, 1% non essential amino-acids, 1% L-glutamine and 1% gentamicin.
Cells were cultured on 96-microtiter plate for the study of the viability evaluated at 24 hours by the Neutral Red incorporation assay (BORENFREUND-SHOPSIS, 1988), the Neutral Red release assay (READER et al, 1989), the M.T.T. assay (DENIZOT-LANG, 1986) and the Coomassie Blue assay (SHOPSIS-ENG, 1985).
For the determination of the cellular growth and Al incorporation, the cultures were realised in Petri dishes. The cells were treated with AlCl3 for 24 and 48 hours, than harvested by trypsination and counted in a haemocytometer. Toxic changes in the appearance and number were first evaluated by direct microscopic examination, then by electronic probe-microanalyser or CASTAING's probe coupled or not to a transmission electronic microscope (respectively the CAMEBAX-probe and the CAMECA MS-46-probe). In the same way, intracellular and cell culture medium of Al-concentration were determined by flameless atomic absorption technics (on PERKIN-ELMER equipment).

RESULTS AND DISCUSSION

The cellular viability decreased when Al-concentration in the culture medium increased. Moreover, after Al treatment, light microscopy revealed a decrease of cellular growth and an increase in the number of granules and vacuoles in the cells. This phenomena was particularly marked in the cells exposed to 100 and 10 ug Al/ml.

Electron microscopy correlated these observations. Many cells contained numerous electron denses particules, especially in cells treated with 100 ug Al/ml. Fine inclusions were in some electrons denses particules, identified as lysosomes. These may be some aluminium-lysosomal precipitates. The number of these granules increased when the Al-dose administred to the cells increased.
The confirmation is brought by the X-ray microanalysis. The analysis of these electron denses particules with the CAMECA MS-46 probe and the CAMEBAX-probe revealed the presence of Al always associated with signals of calcium and phosphorous elements. This X-ray microanalysis enabled to evaluate the chemical composition of mineral inclusions. The in-lysosomal precipitation of Al in the form of phosphorous salts has been evocated and attributed to the action of acid phosphatase (BERRY-HOURDY, 1982).
This in vitro study showed that the cells are abled to tolerate very high quantity of Al. The capture and the lysosomal reaction between Al and P, and secondly the precipitation of these salts, may involved as a detoxification mechanism for Al exposure. This mecanism has already been evocate in vivo for Al and some other metals (GALLE-BERRY, 1980).
And the cytotoxicity of a metal ion did not be limitated to the only determination of a toxicological index, as the IC 50, but must be completed by the determination of the intracellular localization of the metal ion.

REFERENCES

ALFREY, A.C. - LEGENDRE, G.R. et al (1976) : The dialysis encephalopathy syndrome. Possible aluminium intoxication. N. Engl. J. Med. 294, 184-188.

BERRY, J.P. - ESCAIG, F. et al (1988) : Inhaled soluble aerosols insolubilised by lysosomes of alveolar cells. Application to some toxic compounds, electron microprobe and ion microprobe studies. Toxicology 52, 127-139.

BERRY, J.P. - HOURDRY, J. et al (1982) : Aluminium phosphate visualization of acid phosphatase activity. A biochemical and X-ray microanalysis study. J. Histochem. Cytochem. 30, 86-92.

BORENFREUND, E. - SHOPSIS, C. (1985) : Toxicity monitoring with a correlated set of cell-culture assays. Xenobiotica 15, 705-711.

DENIZOT, F. - LANG, R. (1986) : Modifications to the tetrazolium dye procedure giving improved sensivity and reliability. J. Immunol. Methods 89, 271-277.

GALLE, P. - BERRY, J.P. (1980) : The role of acid phosphatases in the concentration of some mineral elements in lysosomes. Electron Microscopy 3, 92-93.

PERL, D.P. - GAJDUSEK, C.M. et al. (1982) : Intraneuronal aluminium accumulation in amyotrophic lateral sclerosis and parkinsonism-dementia of Guam. Science 217, 1053-1055.

READER, S.J. - BLACKWELL, V. et al (1989) : A vital dye release method for assaying the short-term cytotoxic effects of chemicals and formulations. ATLA 17, 28-33.

SHOPSIS, C. - ENG, B. (1985) : Rapid cytotoxicity testing using a semi-automated protein determination on cultured cells. Toxicol. Lett. 26, 1-8.

Metal Ions in Biology and Medicine, vol. 2. Eds. J. Anastassopoulou, Ph. Collery, J.C. Etienne, Th. Theophanides. John Libbey Eurotext, Paris © 1992, pp. 333-337

The silicotic effects of different forms of silica and calcium concentration in lungs of silicotic rats*

Z. Yang, R.S. Chen, Y.X. Yang, X.H. Jiao, A.B. Dai, Z.X. Zhang

Institute of Soil Science, Academia Sinica, Nanjing 210008, P.R. China. Department of Chemistry, Nanjing University, Nanjing 210008, P.R. China. Medical School of Nanjing University, Nanjing 210008, P.R. China

SUMMARY

In this paper, the ζ electric potentials and surface acidic strengths of three different forms of silica — tridymite, α–quartz and amorphous silica, have been measured and compared, and their cytotoxicities to pulmonary alveolar macrophage have been determined. The concentrations of free calcium ion in the rat lungs which had been afflicted with experimentally silica–induced silicosis were measured by ion–selective electrode and Tb^{3+} fluorescent probe. It is found that all above indexes are related more or less closely with the genesis of silicosis.

INTRODUCTION

Silicosis is a debilitating pulmonary disease that afflicts persons who chronically inhale air contain in silica dusts and the pathology has been studied extensively. But, the biological mechanism by which the inhalation of SiO_2 dusts starts a fibrogenic process resulting in silicosis, has not yet been fully understood at the molecular level. Our previous study showed that the concentrtration of Ca^{2+} in lung of silicotic rats increased significantly from the third day after injecttion of α–quartz dust (Y. Mao et al., 1990). On this basis, the characteristics and silicotic effects of different forms of SiO_2 and the relationship between the Ca^{2+} concentrations and genesis of silicosis are to be studied further.

EXPERIMENTS AND RESULTS

1. With micro–electrophoresis method, ζ electric potentials of three forms of silica — tridymite, α–quartz and amorphous silica, were measured. The results were shown in Fig.1.. The higher the pH value, the more negative the ζ electric potential of silica. At pH 7.4, the ζ electric potential of tridymite is the highest and that of amorphous silica is the lowest. According to the pH–ζ curve, the neutral point of tridymite is 1. 3, α–quartz 1. 5, amorphous silica 2,7. Thus, the surface acidic strength of tridymite is the highest, and amorphous silica is the least.

* The project is supported by National Natural Science Foundation of China.

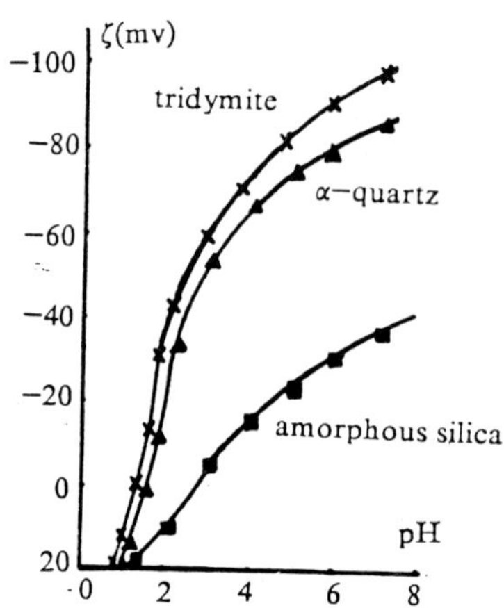

Fig. 1. pH–ζ curve of different forms of silica

2. The cytotoxicities of different silica dust to pulmonary alveolar macrophage (PAM) are different(Table.1). All of them were significantly higher than the control group. But at the beginning, there was no apparent difference. Eight hours later, their cytotoxicities to alveolar macrophage showed significant difference, the order of toxicities being: tridymite > α–quartz > amorphous silica.

Table. 1. Percentage of survival of alveolar macrophage after reacting with different forms of silica

Time(h)	control	tridymite(100μg / ml)	α–quartz(100μg / ml)	amorphous silica(100μg / ml)
2	83.5 ± 2.85	70.4 ± 3.23[a]	72.1 ± 3.65[a]	80.3 ± 4.51
4	75.4 ± 2.58	62.9 ± 4.04[a,d]	67.7 ± 2.18[a]	73.3 ± 3.33
8	73.8 ± 3.03	43.9 ± 4.09[a,c]	50.5 ± 2.37[a]	68.8 ± 4.21[b]
20	64.7 ± 0.81	37.3 ± 2.74[a,c]	44.4 ± 1.40[a]	62.9 ± 3.69
26	63.0 ± 3.90	29.0 ± 3.34[a,c]	39.6 ± 6.51[a]	56.2 ± 2.57[b]
48	59.1 ± 2.78	27.1 ± 3.60[a,c]	36.5 ± 1.87[a]	54.5 ± 1.67[b]

note: each value represents the mean ± S.D., n = 5–8 rabbits / group

a. significantly different from the control, $P < 0.01$

b. significantly different from the control, $P < 0.05$

c. significantly different from α–quartz group, $P < 0.01$

d. significantly different from α–quartz group, $P < 0.05$

3. During the process of genesis of silicosis, the concentration of Ca^{2+} in the lung homogenate of rats after intratracheal injection of various forms of SiO_2 were measured

by ion–selective electrode. The results are shown in Table. 2. The free Ca^{2+} concentration change in lungs is related closely to the genesis of silicosis. It has been well known that the silicosis of rats after injection of tridymite is more serious than that of α–quartz. After injection of silica dust for 3 days, the concentration of free Ca^{2+} in lungs of each group were found to be: tridymite group > α–quartz group > control group. Amorphous silica had no silicotic effect. So, after it was injected into the rat lungs, the Ca^{2+} concentrations in the lungs of this group showed no significant difference from the control. It is shown that, the higher the concentration of free Ca^{2+}in lung, the more serious was the silicosis.

Table.2. Change of free [Ca^{2+}] in lungs of silicotic rats(ppm)

Time(day)	3	10	30	60
control	13.4 ± 2.61	16.1 ± 3.41	12.9 ± 2.70	15.3 ± 3.60
tridymite(50mg / rat)	29.6 ± 6.68^{a,b}	59.3 ± 6.35^{a,b}	54.6 ± 5.13^{a,b}	63.2 ± 5.66^{a,b}
α–quartz(50mg / rat)	21.7 ± 2.47^{a}	40.8 ± 3.39^{a}	26.1 ± 4.10^{a}	45.1 ± 3.52^{a}
amorphous silica(50mg / rat)	12.3 ± 2.10	18.1 ± 2.62	12.3 ± 2.11	16.1 ± 3.50

note: each value represents the mean ± S.D., n = 5–6 rats / group.

a. significantly different from the control, $P < 0.01$.

b. significantly different from α–quartz group, $P < 0.01$.

4. The alveolar macrophage was incubated at 37℃ with α–quartz, the sum content of Ca^{2+} in macrophage was studied by Tb^{3+} fluorescent probe. The results are shown in Table.3. It was seen that the free Tb^{3+}–microphage fluorescence intensity is higher than control. It indicates that the Ca^{2+} in macrophage after α–quartz treatment was lower than that of control. But, after the treatment of α–quartz, the Ca^{2+} concentration in mitochondria that is an important inner Ca^{2+} storage of macrophage did not change significantly.

Table 3. The effect of α–quartz on the fluorescence intensity of Tb^{3}–microphage and Tb^{3+}–mitochondria in macrophage

Sample	fluorescence intensity(I)
Tb^{3+}–Microphage	23.6 ± 0.14
Tb^{3+}–Microphage+α–quartz	31.1 ± 0.58 *
Tb^{3+}–Mitochondria	27.7 ± 0.47
Tb^{3+}–Mitochondria+α–quartz	29.2 ± 1.47

note: each value represents the mean ± S.D., n = 8 rabbits / group

* significantly different from the control, $P < 0.01$.

DISCUSSION

1. The effect of surface acidic strength of silica on the genesis of silicosis

The process of protonation and deprotonation silica surface in aqueous system may be considered as:

$$-\overset{|}{\underset{|}{Si}}-O^- \rightleftharpoons \overset{|}{\underset{|}{Si}}-OH \rightleftharpoons -\overset{|}{\underset{|}{Si}}-OH_2^+$$

The ζ electric potentials on silica surface is dependant on pH of the aqueous system. The higher the pH, the more negative is the ζ electric potential, which means the stronger the surface acidic strengtth. The silanol group on the silica surface reacts with lecithin and other surface matters on PAM. The higher the surface acid stronger the silica reacts with the surface matter on PAM. The ζ electric potential and surface acidic strength of tridymite is the highest, so the reaction tendency of silanol group on its surface is the strongest. Its cytotoxicity to PAM and silicotic effect is the highest.

2. The effect of Ca^{2+} concentration in lungs on the genesis of silicosis

The free Ca^{2+} concentrations in silicotic lungs increase significantly in the initiating period of silicosis. The more serious the silicosis, the higher the free Ca^{2+} concentration in silicotic lung. Thus, the free Ca^{2+} concentration in lung homogenate is an important index in the study on experimental silicosis. The increasing of hydroxyproline content in silicotic lung was used also as an index of determining the genesis of silicosis. Its significant increase only occurs at one month after injection of dust SiO_2. The change of Ca^{2+} concentration is much faster than the change of hydroxyproline content. Therefore, determination of the change of Ca^{2+} concentration in lung is more effective than that of hydroxyproline content.But, why the Ca^{2+} concentration in lung increase when silicosis begins is still not clear. That the macrophage–combined Ca^{2+} concentration decreased significantly show the outflow of Ca^{2+} within the cell of pulmonary after reacting with SiO_2 dust. But the Ca^{2+} concentration out–cell is 10^3 times higher than that of in the cell. thus, only the flow out of in–cell Ca^{2+} can not change the sum Ca^{2+} concentration of lung homogenate. It awaits further studies.

CONCLUSION

It is found that the high negative ζ electric potential and acidic strength on the surface of crystalline silica are important factors that affect the genesis of silicosis. Because of the strong dissociation tendency of the silanol group on the silica surface to give hydrogen ion and negative group, the crystalline silica reacts more readily with the constituents of alveolar matter such as lecithin of cell membrane and amino acid residues of proteins. The acidic strength on tridymite surface is the highest, so its silicotic effect is the strongest.

Sametimes, the change of free Ca^{2+} concentration in lung homogenate is an important index of seriousness of the degree of silicosis.

REFERENCES

Y. Mao et al.(1990), Ca^{2+} and the Starting of Silicosis, Metal Ions in Biology and Medicines, eds. Ph. Callery. et al., John Libbey Eurotaxt, Paris, pp. 148–150.

Metal Ions in Biology and Medicine, vol. 2. Eds. J. Anastassopoulou, Ph. Collery, J.C. Etienne, Th. Theophanides. John Libbey Eurotext, Paris © 1992, pp. 338-339

Cadmium, copper and zinc concentrations in blood plasma and liver tissue in alcohol-toxic liver disease

K. Kisters, C. Spieker, S. Quand Nguyen, M. Tepel, H.P. Bertram*, H. Zumkley, K.H. Rahn, W. Zidek

*Medizinische Polikinik der Universität *Institut für Pharmakologie und Toxikologie W-4400 Münster, Albert-Schweitzer-Str. 33, Germany*

Studies in laboratory animals have shown that cadmium, copper and zinc, which are besides cadmium essential trace elements, have an influence on hepatic drug metabolism. Reduced activity of the metabolizing enzymes in the liver, associated with prolonged drug action, has been demonstrated in zinc-deficient (Becking & Morrison 1970; Becking, 1976) and copper-deficient rats (Moffitt & Murphy, 1973). In man specific syndromes of zinc deficiency have been described (Prasad et al., 1963). In patients with liver disease, serum copper levels are usually elevated and they usually result from impaired biliary excretion of the compound (Hartoma et al., 1977). Cadmium may influence carbohydrate metabolism (Zumkley & Kisters, 1990).

In the present study cadmium, copper and zinc concentrations were determined in blood plasma and in liver tissue of 20 patients with steatosis (A), 12 patients with hepatitis (B) and 8 patients with liver cirrhosis (C). The origin of each liver disease was alcohol-toxic. 11 patients with normal liver function and without alcohol exposition served as controls.
The analysis of trace element content was performed by atomic absorption spectroscopy. An atomic absorption spectroscope of type Perkin Elmer was used.

Results

Cadmium concentrations in blood were measured 0,95±0,48 (A), 0,96±0,60 (B) and 0,86±0,18 µg Cd/l (C) (means±SD, normal range 0,05-1,0 µg Cd/l).
Cadmium concentrations in liver tissue were found 2,57±2,09 (A), 1,77±1,39 (B) and 1,06±0,81 µg Cd/g fresh weight (C) (means±SD, normal range 0,2-4,0 µg Cd/g.f. w.).

Copper concentrations in blood plasma were found 1,25±0,62 (A), 1,04±0,32 (B) and 0,81±0,39 mg Cu/l (C) (means±SD, normal range 0,8-1,3 mg Cu/l). Intrahepatic copper concentration was 9,48±5,78 (A), 15,24±10,13 (B) and 21,92±11,27 µg Cu/g f. w. (C) (means±SD, normal range 2,5-8,0 µg Cu/g f. w.).

Determination of zinc in blood plasma showed 108,7±25,2 (A), 89,4±25,0 (B) and 66,7±31,8 µg% Zn (C) (means±SD, normal range 80-110 µg% Tn). In liver tissue 51,7±36,6 (A), 38,7±35,4 (B) and 54,9±35,8 µg Zn/g f. w. (C) (means±SD, normal range 30-80 µg Zn/g f.w.) were measured.

In controls cadmium, copper and zinc concentrations in blood plasma and in liver tissue were within the normal range.

The findings show elevated intrahepatic copper concentrations in patients with alcohol-toxic liver disease ($p < 0,05$). Furthermore plasma zinc concentration was significantly reduced in patients with alcohol-toxic liver cirrhosis ($p < 0,05$).

References

Becking, G.C., Morrison, A.B. (1970): Hepatic drug metabolism in zinc-deficient rats. In Biochem. Pharmacol. 19: 895-902.

Becking, G.C. (1976): Trace elements and drug metabolism. In Med. Clin. North Amer. 60: 813-830.

Hartoma, T.R., Sotaniemi, E.A., Pelkonen, O., Ahlqvist, J. (1977): Serum zinc and serum copper and indices of drug metabolism in alcoholics. In Europ. J. clin. Pharmacol. 12: 147-151.

Moffitt, A.E., Murphy, S.D. (1973): Effect of excess and deficient copper intake on rat liver microsomal enzyme activity. In Biochem. Pharmacol. 22: 1463-1476.

Prasad, A.S., Miale, A., Farid, Z., Sanstead, H.H., Shulert, A.R. (1963): Zinc metabolism in patients with the syndrome of iron deficiency anemia, hepatosplenomegaly, dwarfism and hypogonadism. In J. Lab. clin. Med. 61: 537-549.

Zumkley, H., Kisters, K. (1990): Spurenelemente, Wissenschaftliche Buchgesellschaft Darmstadt: 30-39.

Metal Ions in Biology and Medicine, vol. 2. Eds. J. Anastassopoulou, Ph. Collery, J.C. Etienne, Th. Theophanides. John Libbey Eurotext, Paris © 1992, pp. 340-342

The role of calcium in the analgesia induced by buprenorphine*

Z.X. Zhang, H. Liao, X.N. Zhao, X.Li, J. Chen, C.X. Wang

Medical School of Nanjing University, Nanjing 210008, P.R. China

INTRODUCTION

The calcium ion is one of the factors indispensible to nociception. Our serial researches showed that the analgesia induced by acupuncture and drugs was associated with the decrease in free calcium level and the increase in calcium binding to mitochondrial protein in some brain regions, and a great deal of calcium precipitate simultaneously occured at the myelin sheath and mitochondria in these regions, while all these effets were antangonized by pretreatment with ruthenium red (Xie, 1988). Since ruthenium red is a nonspecific calcium channel blocker with complex physiological actions, we employed verapamil (Ver), a specific calcium channel blocker, and buprenorphine (Bup), an analogue of morphine, to study the relation between the mitochondrial protein bound calcium in some brain regions and drugs-induced analgesia in order to clarify whether the drug-induced and the acupuncture-induced analgesia share a common ion basis and a similar mechanism of actions.

EXPERIMENTAL DETAILS

Mice of both sexes (25 ± 2g) were randomly divided into various experimental groups. The pain threshold was tested by the radiation tail-flick procedure, and the degree of analgesia was calculated by the equation: $DA(\%) = 100(TL-BL)/(10-BL)$

Where BL is the baseline latency; TL, the test latency. The mice were killed by disjointing cervical vertebrae and the fluorescent spectrum of mitochondrial protein bound Tb^{3+} in discrete brain regions was determined with a Hitachi RF-504 fluorescent spectrophotometer (xie, 1988). The samples were prepared for electron-microscope observation according to the procedures (Shi, 1988). In order to identify the chemical constituents of the electron dense precipitate, unstained sections were mounted on Formvar-coated copper grids and analyzed with Link-860 X-ray energy dispersive spectrography operated at 120 kV, counted 200 s.

RESULTS AND DISCUSSION

Data in table 1 show that verapamil had influence on neither the pain threshold nor the mitochondrial protein bound calcium levels in various brain regions. Bup in the lower dose induced analgesia, but caused no significant changes in the mitochondrial protein bound calcium in the three brain regions.

* The Project Supported by National Natural Science Fundation of China and The Analytic Center of Nanjing University

Table 1 Effect of verapamil on the lower dose of buprenorphine-induced Ca^{2+}-uptake by mitochondria in discrete brain regions in vivo

Treatment	DA(%)	Tb^{3+} relative fluorescent intensity		
		PAG	Hypo	Hip
Control	6.6±5.8	20.4±4.0	18.9±4.6	20.7±4.1
Ver	7.9±2.8	22.5±5.8	22.4±7.0	22.2±4.0
Bup	17.6±8.0[a]	18.7±3.5	24.0±4.9	22.4±5.2
Ver+Bup	7.9±4.4[b]	22.5±4.3	23.7±3.7	19.3±2.2

Verapamil (8μg/mouse) was injected i. cv. 15 min before Bup (0. 2mg/kg i. p.). Values in the table were means ± S. D. for 6-7 mice.

[a] $P<0.05$ as compared with the control group

[b] $P<0.01$ as compared with the Bup group

Bup at 0. 4mg/kg remarkably elevated the pain threshold and decreased the Tb^{3+} fluorescent intensity in PAG and hypothalamus (hypo), which indicated the increase in mitochondrial protein bound calcium in these regions. Preinjection of verapamil decreased the mitochondrial protein bound calcium to the level of the control group. The mitochondrial protein bound calcium in the hippocampus (Hip) was not significantly affected by the above treatments (Tab. 2).

Table 2. Effect of verapamil on the moderate dose of buprenorphine-induced Ca^{3+}-uptake by mitochondria in discrete brain regions in vivo

Treatment	DA(%)	Tb^{3+} relative fluorescent intensity		
		PAG	Hypo	Hip
Control	6.7±5.6	19.8±2.5	18.9±4.0	17.5±2.6
Bup	22.1±8.8[b]	12.7±2.8[a]	12.8±4.0[a]	13.7±3.8
Ver+Bup	8.4±4.5[b]	18.0±4.2[b]	16.8±2.4[b]	18.7±6.4

Buprenorphine (0. 4 mg/kg) was injected i. p. Other treatments and notes are the same as those in table 1.

[a] $P<0.05$ as compared with the control group

[b] $P<0.01$ as compared with the Bup group

Analogous phenomena resulted from the above treatment when Bup was at 0. 8mg/kg (Tab. 3).

Table 3 Effect of verapamil on the higher dose of buprenorphine-induced Ca^{2+}-uptake by mitochondria in discrete brain regions in vivo

Treatment	DA(%)	Tb^{3+} relative fluorescent intensity		
		PAG	Hypo	Hip
Control	6.7±5.8	30.5±2.8	30.5±2.7	29.5±3.8
Bup	41.0±10.9[b]	26.4±4.2[a]	25.1±5.0[a]	28.5±1.6
Ver+Bup	8.2±2.7[c]	31.9±1.8[b]	30.1±4.1[b]	28.5±3.5

Buprenorphine (0. 8 mg/kg) was injected i. p. Other treatments and notes are the same as those in table 1.

[a] $P<0.05$ as compared with the control group

[b] $P<0.05$ as compared with the Bup group

[c] $P<0.01$ as compared with the Bup group

The changes in ultrastructural distribution of calcium ion in these brain regions after administration of Bup in the same doses were also studied. The analogous results were obtained in PAG and Hypo (Fig. 1).

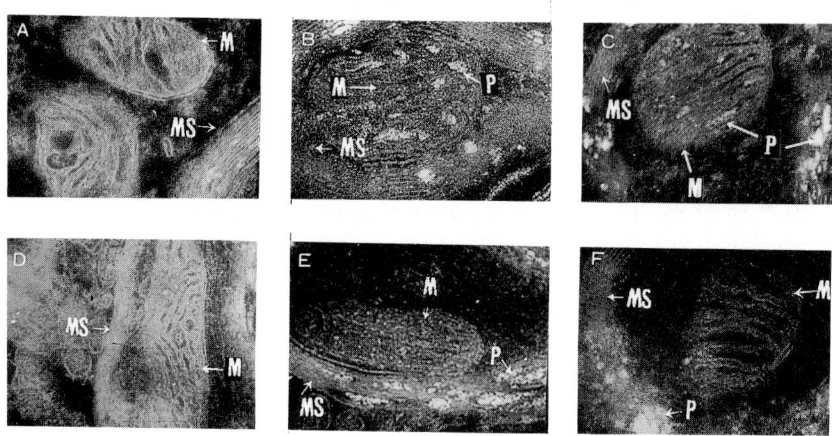

Fig. 1. Ultrastructural distributions of calcium in PAG and Hypo induced by i. p. buprenorphine (Bup, 0. 8mg/kg) in mice. A) and D) were the case of 30 min following i. p. saline, which showed that PAG and Hypo were normal. B) and E) showed a great number of the precipitate pellets at myelin sheath and in mitochondria after i. p. Bup, C) and F) showed significant decrease of the precipitate pellets at these sites induced by i. cv. verapamil (8μg/mouse) before Bup. × 40,000 except C) and F) (×50,000). M =mitochondria; MS=myelin sheath; P=precipitates

Bup is a highly lipophilic derivative of oripavine. It is structurally similar to morphine. Here the findings show that during the Bup-analgesia, the mitochondrial membrane bound calcium and the subcellular calcium distribution relevantly change in PAG and Hypo, and these changes can be reversed by verapamil, while the mitochondrial protein bound calcium in the Hip is not affected by the above treatments. Analogous findings from morphine and acupuncture analgesia were previously reported (Xie, 1988; Shi, 1988). This suggests that the calcium in PAG and Hypo seems relatively specific to drug or acupuncture analgesia which is probably related to the transmembrance transport of calcium.

REFERENCES

Shi, S. L., W. N. Zhang, C. Q. Zhao, Z. X. Zhang, 1988, The effects of electroacupuncture, morphine and Tb^{3+} on the ultrastructural distribution of Ca^{2+} in the discrete brain regions of mice. J. Nanjing University, 24, 505.

Xie, X. Y., X. X. Li, Z. X. Zhang, M. J. Huang, R. S. Chen, 1988, The changes of mitochondrial protein bound Ca^{2+} in some brain regions under the conditions of electroacupuncture or morphine analgesia and the analgesic tolerance. Acta Physiol. Sin., 40 553.

Metal Ions in Biology and Medicine, vol. 2. Eds. J. Anastassopoulou, Ph. Collery, J.C. Etienne, Th. Theophanides. John Libbey Eurotext, Paris © 1992, pp. 343-345

Relationship of lanthanides analgesia and the analgesic tolerance to some brain regions calcium levels*

Z.X. Zhang, N.X. Zhao, X.Li, H. Liao, X.X. Li

Medical School of Nanjing University, Nanjing 210008, P.R. China

INTRODUCTION

A number of reports have indicated that calcium ion may interact with opioids. Calcium decreases the analgesic effect of morphine (Harris, 1975), whereas calcium antagonists enhance the morphine—induced antinociception (Schmidt, 1980). There are also data suggesting that these actions of the opioids might be mediated by altering calcium disposition. It has been reported in recent years that acupuncture, morphine and the lanthanide—induced analgesia not only very similar, but well parallel to the changes in calcium ion of some brain regions (Zhang, 1987). Thus, there is considerable evidance to point out that calcium is closely involved in the action of narcotic drugs, but the nature of this interaction remains unclear. The present study has been undertaken to observe whether naloxone might antagonize the antinociceptive activity of lanthanide samariun (Ⅲ), and to know the role of mitochondrial protein bound calcium in discrete brain regions in the lanthanide—induced analgesia and the analgesic tolerance.

EXPERIMENTAL DETAILS

Mice of both sexes, weighing around 25g, were divided into a variaty of experimental group at random. Pain was tested by the radiation tail—flick procedure and the degree of analgesia was calculated by the equation:

$$DA(\%)=100(TL-BL)/(10-BL)$$

where TL is the test latency, and BL, the baseline latency. The analgesic tolerance was estimated by comparing the daily analgesic effect induced by samarium for 6 consecutive days. The ^{45}Ca radioactivity and the fluorescent spectrum of the mitochondrial protein bound Tb^{3+} in discrete brain regions were determined with a FJ—2101 double channel liquid scintillation spectrometer (Zhang, 1987) and a Hitachi RF—504 fluorescent spectrophotometer (Xie, 1988) respectively.

RESULTS AND DISCUSSION

As can be seen in Fig. 1, after injection i. cv. of Sm^{3+} the analgesic effects were enhanced. Addition of naloxone could effectively antagonize the effects. The pain threshold of the Sm^{3+} plus naloxone group at the 1st or 2nd phases was still higher than that of the control group respectively, but compared with that of the Sm^{3+}—treated group, the pain threshold was significantly reduced. The analgesic effect of the Sm^{3+} plus naloxone group decreased gradually, and concurrently the ^{45}Ca levels in the PAG, hypothalamus (Hypo) and caudate (Caud) regions increased 120 min after administration of naloxone. The Sm^{3+} or naloxone plus Sm^{3+} had no effect on the ^{45}Ca levels in both the cortex (Cort) and the hippocampus (Hip) regions (Tab. 1).

In the other experiment, the animals were made tolerant by the daily injection i. cv. of Sm^{3+} (4μmol/L,

---

* The Project Supported by National Natural Science Fundation of China and The Analytic Center of Nanjing University.

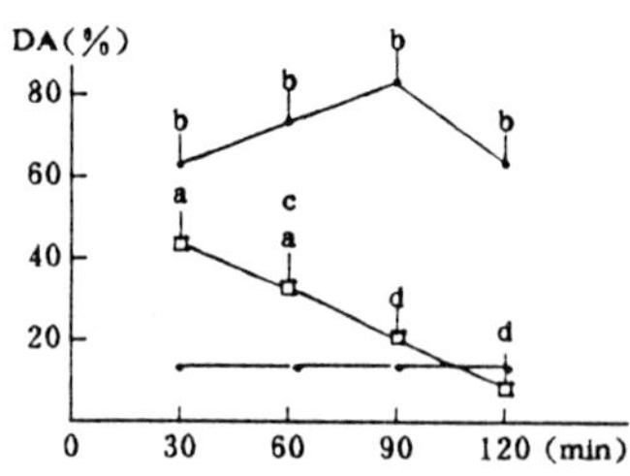

Fig. 1. Naloxone antagonism to the Sm^{3+} — induced analgesia

Saline (— • —, 5μl/mouse or 0. 1ml/mouse) was injected i. cv. or i. p.. Sm^{3+} (— • —, 8μmol/L, 5μl/mouse) was injected i. cv. and naloxone (—□—, 5mg/kg) was injected i. p. 10 min before administration of Sm^{3+}. Analgesia was determined respectively at 30, 60, 90, 120 min after drugs administration. Each value represents the ±S. D. M. for 10 animals.

[a]p<0. 05, vs the control group.

[b]p<0. 01, vs the control group.

[c]p<0. 05, vs the Sm^{3+} group.

[d]p<0. 01, vs the Sm^{3+} group.

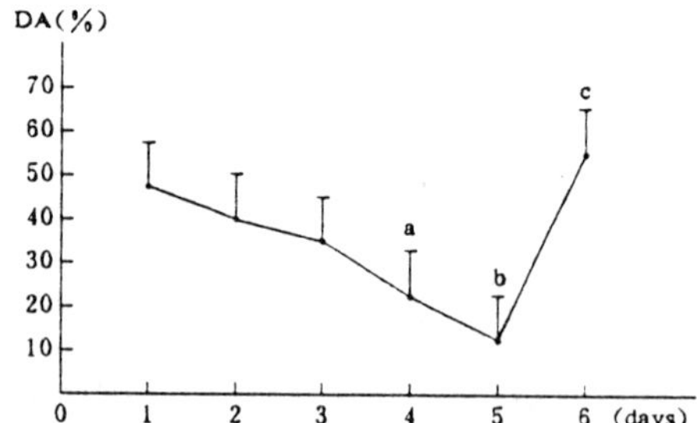

Fig. 2. Effect of EGTA on the SM^{3+} — induced analgesic tolerance

Each value represents the ±S. D. M. for 10 animals.

[a]p<0. 05, vs the 1st day.

[b]p<0. 01, vs the 1st day.

[c]p<0. 05, vs the 5th day.

5μl/mouse) for 6 days. EDTA (4μmol/L, 0. 1ml/mouse) was injected i. p. 10 min before administration of Sm^{3+} on the 6th day. They were killed by decapitation on the 1st, 5th and 6th days respectively, and the mitochondrial protein bound calcium in discrete brain regions was measured. The results, given in Fig. 2 and Tab. 2, show that the pain threshold decreased on the 4th day after the daily administration of Sm^{3+}, and a significant analgesic tolerance to Sm^{3+} was elicited on the 5th day. At the same time, the mitochondrial protein bound calcium in both the PAG and the Hypo regions, compared with that on the 1st day, significantly decreased, i. e. , the Tb^{3+} relative fluorescent intensity increased. After administration of EGTA which has a much higher affinity to Ca^{2+} than to Mg^{2+} on the 6th day, the analgesic tolerance to Sm^{3+} was effectively antagonized, and concurrently the mitochondrial protein bound calcium in the two regions virtually returned to the levels of the 1st day control group. The above treatment had no significant effect on the mitochondrial protein bound calcium in the Hip region. The analogous results were obtained by the same treatment of Ho^{3+} and La^{3+} as well.

Table 1. Changes in ^{45}Ca levels of discrete brain regions during naloxone antagonism to the Sm^{3+}-induced analgesia

Treatment	^{45}Ca (cpm × 10^3/mg protein)				
	Cort	Hip	Hypo	PAG	Caud
Saline	236. 18±34. 17	204. 27±37. 24	297. 28±31. 47	251. 14±16. 12	238. 44±17. 37
Sm^{3+}	224. 81±22. 42	198. 30±30. 52	231. 64±21. 24[a]	172. 83±16. 51[b]	182. 74±13. 87
Nal+Sm^{3+}	218. 64±11. 83	172. 69±28. 43	284. 17±12. 83[c]	234. 17±12. 64[d]	249. 87±16. 14[c]

Saline (0. 1ml/mouse) containing 2960 KBq/kg of ^{45}Ca was injected i. p. Sm^{3+} (8μmol/L. 5μl/mouse) was injected i. cv. and naloxone (Nal. 5mg/kg) containing 2960 KBq/kg of ^{45}Ca was injected i. p. 10 min before administration of Sm^{3+}. After measurement of the final pain threshold at 120 min the animals were killed by decapitation. Each value represents the ±S. D. M. for 10 animals.

[a]p<0. 05, vs the control group. [b]p<0. 01, vs the control group.

[c]$p<0.05$, vs the Sm^{3+} group. [d]$p<0.01$, vs the Sm^{3+} group.

Table 2. Effects of EGTA on the Sm^{3+}-induced analgesic tolerance and the mitochondrial protein bound calcium levels in discrete brain regions

Treatment	DA(%)	Tb^{3+} relative fluorescent intensity		
		Hip	PAG	Hypo
Sm^{3+} (1st day)	48.4±11.2	48.3±6.8	30.4±3.8	29.4±4.1
Sm^{3+} (5th day)	8.4±12.3[a]	45.4±7.9	51.2±6.3[b]	49.7±5.4[b]
EGTA+Sm^{3+} (6th day)	56.7±9.6[c]	50.1±4.4	34.8±5.1[d]	31.2±3.8[d]

Each value represents the ±S. D. M. for 10 animals

[a]$p<0.05$, vs the 1st day, [b]$p<0.01$, vs the 1st day.

[c]$p<0.05$, vs the 5th day, [d]$p<0.01$, vs the 5th day.

The PAG region has been reported to be a sensitive site for the antinociceptive action of morphine (Jacquet, 1974), and our previovs and present studies have indicated that both calcium and naloxone can reduce the analgesic effects not only induced by morphine but by the acupuncture. The findings suggest that the effects of calcium are not peculiar to morphine but likely to extend to various agents and other ways, such as acupuncture which may produce analgesia and the analgesic tolerance. It is also clear that PAG is by no means a unique sensitive site, but other regions, at least the Hypo and Caud areas, are sensitive, too, to the antinociceptive action of morphine, because morphine, lanthanides and acupuncture all could induce the same changes in calcium concentrations in the PAG, Hypo and Caud regions.

REFERENCES

Harris, R. A., Loh, H. H. and Way, E. L., (1975) Effect of divalent cations, cation chelators and an ionophore on morphine analgesia and tolerance, J. Pharmacol. Exp. Ther. 195, 488.

Jacquet, Y. F. and Lajtha, A. (1974) Paradoxical effects after microinjection of morphine in the PAG in the rat, Science, 185, 1055.

Schmidt, W. K. and Way, E. L. (1980) Hyperanalgesic effects of divalent cations and antinociceptive effect of a calcium chelator in naive and morphine-dependent mice, J. Pharmacol. Exp. Ther. 212, 22.

Xie, X. Y., Li, X. X., Zhang, Z. X., Huang, M. J. and Chen, R. S. (1988) The change of mitochondrial protein bound calcium in some brain regions under the conditions of electroacupuncture or morphine analgesia and the analgesic tolerance, Acta Physiol. Sin. 40, 553.

Zhang, Z. X. Zhang Y. Z., Jia, S. P., Lu, X. J., Yu, R. R., Wang, X. G. ang Chen, R. S. (1987) Role of calcium in electroacupuncture analgesia and the development of analgesic tolerance to electroacupuncture and morphine, Sci. Sin. (Series B), 30, 974.

Metal Ions in Biology and Medicine, vol. 2. Eds. J. Anastassopoulou, Ph. Collery, J.C. Etienne, Th. Theophanides. John Libbey Eurotext, Paris © 1992, pp. 346-348

Enhancing effects of the lanthanide Tb^{3+} on glutamate neurotoxicity in mice : morphological observation*

X.D. Han, H. Liao, X.N. Zhao, X. Li, C.X. Wang, Z.X. Zhang

Medical School of Nanjing University, Nanjing 21008, P.R. China

INTRODUCTION

Monosodium glutamate (MSG) damaged the arcuate hypothalamic nucleous (AN), and resulted in many changes of transmitter system in the brain after animals were injected subcutaneously (s. c.) or intraperitoneally with high doses of MSG (Olney, 1969; Kizer, 1977). It has been reported that morphine can enhance glutamate neurotoxicity, and this effect can be reversed by naloxone (Wang, 1986). Because the lanthandies are similar to morphine in the respect of pharmacology (Zhang, 1985), the present study examnied morphologically whether the lanthanide Tb^{3+} have also enhancing effects on glutamate neurotoxicity, and whether naloxone can reverse thses effects.

EXPERIMENTAL AND DETAILS

72 mice of 7—9 days of age, weighing 5. 5 ± 0. 7g, were devided at random into a variety of experimental groups and treated with different doses of MSG (0. 25, 1. 0, 2. 5g/kg). The mice in each treatment were injected s. c. with saline, MSG, Tb^{3+} (0. 8μmol/kg) + MSG or naloxone (5mg/kg) + Tb^{3+} + MSG, respectively. The lanthanide Tb^{3+} was injected s. c. 15 min before MSG, and naloxone was administered s. c. 10 min before Tb^{3}. All neonatal mice were housed with their dams after tretment and were killed 6 hr. post—tratment by transcardial perfusion fixation with formalin solution (10%). The brain was removed and embedded in wax, and serial cornal sections, 10 μm thick, were cut and stained with cresyl violet (Wang, 1986).

RESULTS AND DISCUSSION

1. The effect of the lower dose of MSG (0. 25g/kg) on the AN

As can be seem in Figure, treatment with the saline (A), Tb^{3+} (B) or naloxone (C) alone had no effect on the AN.

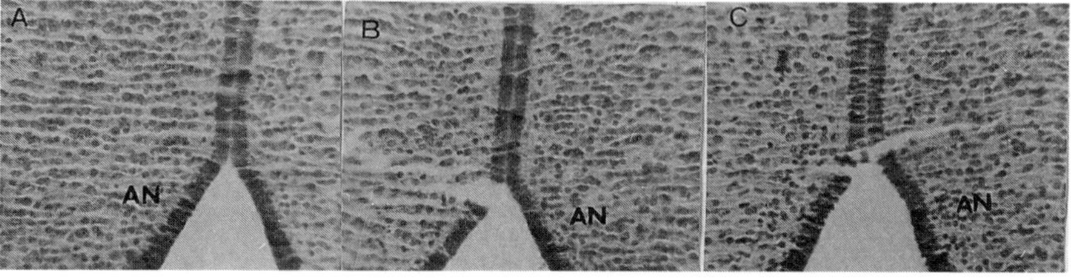

* Project Supported by National Natural Science Fundation of China

Treatments with the lower dose of MSG (Fig. D), the Tb^{3+} + MSG (Fig. E) or the naloxone $+Tb^{3+}$ + MSG (Fig. F) had no effects on the AN as well.

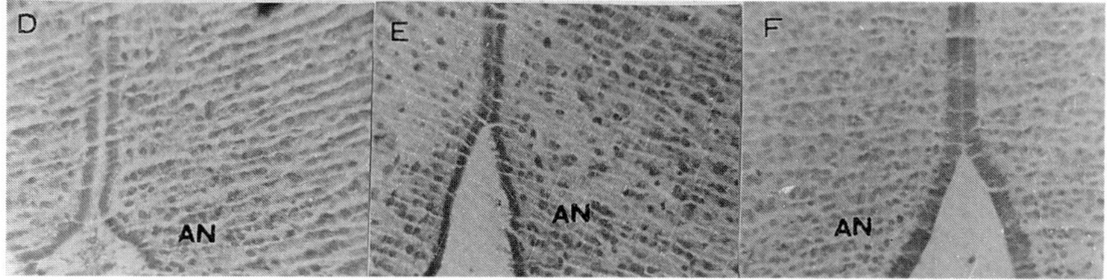

2. The effect of the moderate dose of MSG (1. 0g/kg) on the AN

The moderate dose of MSG induced the nuclear contraction of neurons in the AN (Fig. G), as compared with the saline group , and pretreatment with the same dose of Tb^{3+} obviously damdged great number of neurons in the AN. (Fig. H), as compared with the corresponding controls. The elevating effects was reversed by naloxone (Fig. I)

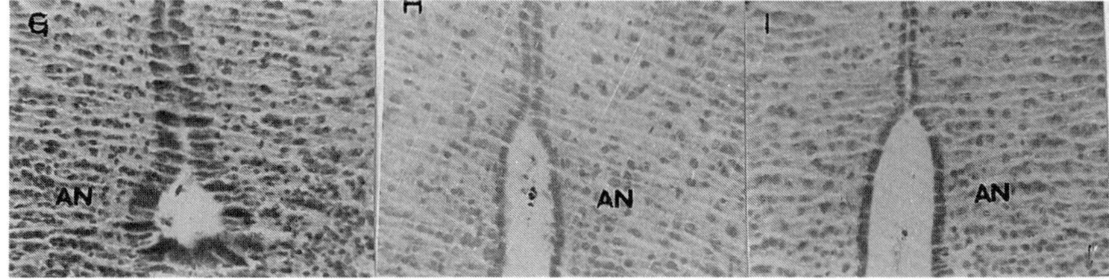

The higher dose of MSG (2. 5g/kg) had much significant effect on the AN (Fig. J), and the effects of the above doses of Tb^{3+} and naloxone on the MSG neurotoxicity were similar to the that induced by the moderate dose of MSG (Fig. K. L.).

It has been reported that The higher dose of MSG can damage the arcuate hypothalamic nucleus of neonatal mice (Olney,1969; Kizer, 1977). It is suggested that MSG made neuron overexciting,and led to the cellular injury even death by combining to the specical receptor of neurons (Olney, 1983; Roberts, 1983). Our previous researches showed that MSG damaged the arcuate hypothalamic nucleus, and the effect could be enhanced by morphine. At the same time, the excessive influx of extracellular Ca^{2+} was found, these effects could be reversed by naloxone (Wang, 1986). It was suggested that the MSG—induced neurotoxicity might be related to cytoplasmic free Ca^{2+} overloading, and induced cellular injury even death due to influx of the excessive extracellular Ca^{2+}(Zhao, 1990). The present study proved that lanthanide Tb^{3+} also elevated the MSG neurotoxicity, and this enhancing effect could be reversed by naloxone as well. Because the characteristics of lanthanides were similar to those of morphine in many respects (Zhang, 1985), and the chemical and physical properties of lanthanide series of elements were resemble to Ca^{2+}. Thus, increase in intracellular Ca^{2+} concentrations in nerve cell which occur follwing

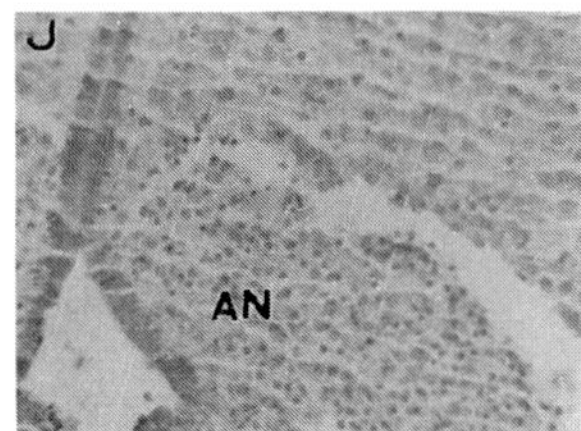

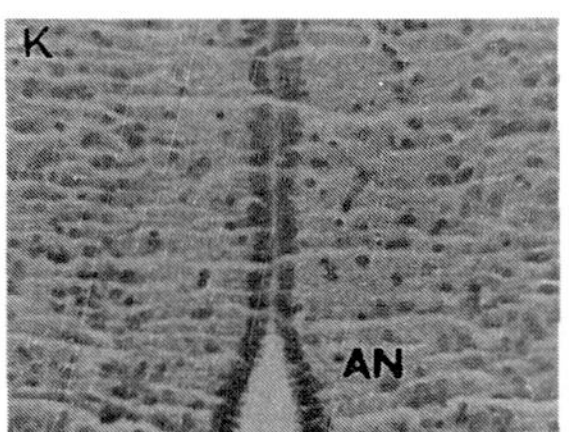

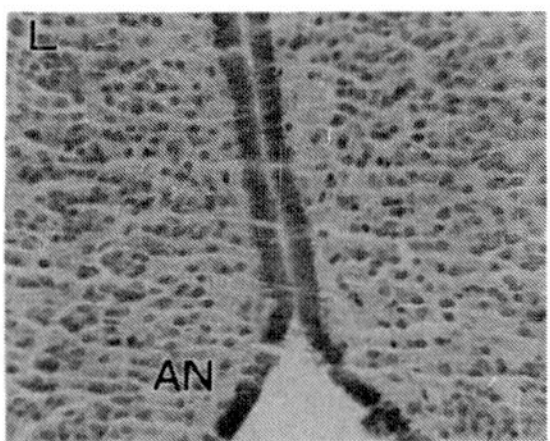

MSG are intimately linked to the neuronal injury.

REFERENCES

Kizer, J. S. et al. (1977) Neurotoxic amino acids and structurally related analogs. Pharmacol. Rew. 19:301.

Olney, J. W. (1969) Brain lesions, obesity and other disturbances in mice treated with monosodium glutamate. Science 164:719.

Olney, J. W. (1983) 《Wenner—Gren. Int Sym Ser》 Vol. 39, P 82, ed. by Fuxe, Macmillan Press, London.

Roberts, P. J. (1983) 《Wenner—Gren. Int Sym Ser》 Vol. 39, P 66, ed. by Fuxe, Macmillan Press, London.

Wang, G. J. et al. (1986) Enhancing effects of mophine on glutamate neurotoxicity in mice. Chinese Journal of Pharmacol. and Toxicol. 1:57.

Zhang, Z. X. et al. (1985) Studies on the analgesic effects of lanthanides. Journal of Less Commom Metals 112:401.

Zhao, X. N. et al. (1990) Morphine enhancement of glutamate and kainic acid neurotoxicity. In: Metal ions in Biology and medicine. Eds. by Ph. Collery et al., John Libbey Eurotext, Paris, p156.

6 NUTRITION

Metal Ions in Biology and Medicine, vol. 2. Eds. J. Anastassopoulou, Ph. Collery, J.C. Etienne, Th. Theophanides. John Libbey Eurotext, Paris © 1992, pp. 351-353

Magnesium and drinking water for health

S. Missailidis*, J. Anastassopoulou*, M. Polissiou**, P. Tarantilis**, Th. Theophanides

**National Technical University of Athens, Laboratory of Radiation Chemistry-Biospectroscopy, Zografou Campus, Zografou 157 73, Athens. **Agricultural University of Athens, Laboratory of General Chemistry, Tera Odos 75, Athens, Greece*

Most of us know that magnesium builds strong muscles and produces energy. But how many people know that magnesium helps bilions of cells in our body, in the heart, lungs, muscles, kidneys, brain, blood or bone? Magnesium delivers the energy by activating the production of a special substance called adenosine triphosphate (ATP), which extracts energy from the foods we eat and delivers it to the bilions of cells. Not many of us know that magnesium is a catalyst or activator to many living chemical processes. If our body is deficient in magnesium this may result in desease or serious discomfort.

Studies in Eastern Finland have shown a higher rate of coronary heart disease than western Finland. The avarege content of magnesium in Finland's soil is low especially in the eastern areas (Marier). Magnesium was also low in the diet and drinking water in the eastern areas. Researchers in Finland and other countries (England, Wales, Sweeden, Canada and USA) found that death rates from heart disease are lower in areas with hard water (hardness of water is the ammount of magnesium and other minerals per liter).

Magnesium and Drinking Water

It is interesting to relate human health and drinking water composition of minerals. However, it is more reliable to give emphasis on the individual chemical constituents of water instead of sole reliance on hardness measurments. This was recomended by the U.S. National Academy of Sciences (1962). The waterborne magnesium is of great importance as is shown from epidemiological studies in United States and Canada. It was found that high-mortality regions had almost no magnesium in the drinking water. The low mortality regions contained more than 10 mg/l. Furthermore, hard waters can contribute as far as 27% of the dietary intake of magnesium.

The magnesium content of drinking water in Greece has been analysed in several localities (Tarantilis) and it was found that magnesium is in most cities above the 10 mg/l threshold. However, recent surveys showed that some localities tended to contain less than 10 mg/l

(Table). It would be interesting to study the mortality rate in these localities and compare them to those localities, where the water tended to contain more than 10 mg/l. Thus magnesium-rich mineral water slould be used as cardioprotective and in therapy.

In the Table is shown the amount of magnesium in mg/l in drinking water for Greek cities. In addition, the calcium content has also been analysed in the drinking water and related to magnesium. The ratio of Mg/Ca is also given. It is shown that in several Greek cities the magnesium content in drinking water is less than 10 mg/l. These areas should then be investigated further for mortality rates.

Table: Magnesium and Calcium contents in drinking water in Greek cities.

City	Magnesium mg/l	Calcium mg/l	Ratio Mg/Ca
ATHENS	7	36	0.19
AGRINIO	5	43	0.12
CHIOS	36	108	0.29
GIANITSA	8	69	0.12
HALKIDA	30	108	0.28
IRAKLIO	27	72	0.38
IOANNINA	6	56	0.11
KARDITSA	7	36	0.19
KALAMATA	26	66	0.39
KORFOU	51	253	0.20
KORINTHOS	72	47	1.53
LAMIA	4	48	0.08
LARISSA	39	119	0.33
LEUKADA	5	53	0.09
MYTILINI	43	47	0.91
PATRA	70	417	0.17
PREVEZA	14	92	0.15
SAMOS	22	86	0.26
SERRES	19	92	0.21
TRIPOLI	8	103	0.08
VOLOS	43	92	0.47
XANTHI	12	21	0.57

Magnesium-ATP Interactions

Recent studies of Mg-ATP interactions (Tajmir-Riahi) have centered the attention on the behavior of ATP in a magnesium environment. How magnesium ions deliver energy by activating this molecule? It is supposed that magnesium ions are hydrated, $Mg(H_2O)_6^{++}$ in a biological milieu and that interaction of these ions with ATP take place through hydrogen-bonding systems with the water hydrogens and the electronegative atoms of ATP, such as the oxygens of the phosphates, and the nitrogens of the base and may be, in some cases, the oxygens of the sugar. These contact interactions may give place to more direct interactions leading to more stable complexes, $Mg(H_2O)_5$-ATP, $Mg(H_2O)_4$-ATP, where one or two water molecules have been substituted by ATP sites, predominently phosphate negatevily charged oxygens. At high Mg:ATP ratios, base sites becomes competitive. In a study conducted in our Laboratory the preparation of magnesium-ATP complexes at various Mg:ATP ratios varying from 1:5 and 5:1 gave two types of complexes of the formulae, Mg.ATP and Mg.2ATP. The structures of these two types of complexes are being investigated by Fourier Transform Infrared Spectroscopy (FT-IR) and Mass Spectrometry. Chemical analysis and other data are indicative of the above formulae. Preliminary FT-IR spectra show that magnesium ions are bound to phosphate groups of the ATP molecule and perturb the α, β and γ phosphate oxygen vibrations. In higher Metal-Ligand ratios there are multinuclear complexes of mixed stocheometry, nMg-ATP.

The metal-nucleotides complexes and their chemistry has been investigated and the role of metal ion complexes in the storage and transport of energy or other molecules by forming ternary complexes. These studies provide new insights into the magnesium-biological molecule interactions.

REFERENCES

Marier J.R.,(1990), Dietary Magnesium and Drinking Water: Effects on Human Health Status, in Metal Ions in Biological Systems, ed. H. Sigel, Marcel Dekker, Inc., Vo 26, p. 85-103, New York.

Tajmir-Riahi A.H., Bertrand M.J. and Theophanides T.,(1986), Synthesis Structure, Proton-Nuclear Magnetic Resonance, and Fourier Transform Infrared Spectroscopy of Several Transitions and Non-tran-sition Metal-adenosine-5'-triphosphate Complexes, Can. J. Chem.64: 960

Tarandilis P., Haroutonian S. and Polissiou M.,(1990), Magnesium Cacium Content of Drinking Water, Fruits, Salt and Saffron of Greece, in Metal Ions in Biology and Medicine, eds., Collery Ph., Poirier L.A., Manfait M., Etienne J-C., p. 177-179, John Libbey Eurotext, Paris.

U.S.National Academy of Sciences, (1979) Geochemistry of Water in Relation to Cardiovascular Disease, Washington, D.C.

Metal Ions in Biology and Medicine, vol. 2. Eds. J. Anastassopoulou, Ph. Collery, J.C. Etienne, Th. Theophanides. John Libbey Eurotext, Paris © 1992, pp. 354-357

Relationship between calcium and dietary habits of patients with stroke

G. Perrakis, G. Panotopoulos, O. Koromila, P.N. Adamopoulos

Department of Internal Medicine, Preventive Medicine Unit, Alexandra Hospital, Greece

Since ancient times, man knows the important influence of nutrition on health.

This influence, quantitively and qualitively, has today an increasing interest in relation to the prevention of many diseases.

One of these diseases is stroke. Stroke represents the third cause of death in developed countries after heart diseases and cancer (6,2). It is also the second cause of invalidity in these countries after automobile accidents. It is obvious that medical, social and economic interest for the prevention of stroke is very large.

The purpose of this study is to investigate the role of serum calcium during the process of stroke and correlate it with dietary habits of patients suffering from stroke.

No similar study was found in the recent literature.

MATERIALS AND METHODS

The material of this study is formed from 351 persons, divided into two groups: A and B.

Group A: is formed by 230 patients suffering from stroke, recovered at Alexandra Hospital, Athens Greece during the period of January 1989-December 1991. Criteria for the selection of patients in this group was the medical history of the patients and the presence of focal semeiology from nervous system characteristic of the disease.

After a clinical examination and laboratory control patients with neurologic symptoms of metabolic, infective or other causes were excluded. Whenever the condition of the patient permitted, computerized brain tomography was used to locate the damage.

Group B: Is the control group and is formed by 121 healthy persons who were selected at random from a representative group of healthy Greek people. Criteria for the selection of patients in this group was age and sex which had to be similar to those of patients in Group A.

In both groups the height (in meters) and body weight (in kilograms) was recorded. When it was impossible to take the measurement of the height and weight of patients in group A the measurement of the height and weight was provided by relatives. From this, Body Mass Index (weight/height^2), one of the most acceptable indexes of obeseity, was calculated.

After 14 hours of fasting, blood was taken to control biochemical variables among which was serum calcium. The blood analysis was made in the laboratory of Preventive Medicine Unit of Alexandra Hospital, which is submitted in the quality control of World Health Organization.

The members of the study had to answer to a questionnaire on dietary habits containing 16 usual foods in Greece. The questionnaire used is similar to that of World Health Organization for cardiovascular diseases. In the case of incapacity of the patient to answer the questionnaire, information was collected from his family (wife, children, etc).

The questionnaire facilitated in reporting the dietary habits with regards to the frequency of consuming meat, fish, starch, pulse, rice, vegetable, fresh salad, fruits, cheese, olive oil, seed oil, vegetable fat, butter, eggs, yogurt and milk.

Corresponding to number 1 was the daily consumption of the above items; to number 2 the consumption of every second day; to number 3 the consumption of twice a week; to number 4 weekly consumption and to number 5 the rare consumption of the above foods.

"T-test" was used for the statistical evaluation of the findings in the study.

RESULTS

From the 351 persons in the study, 230 of these suffered from stroke. They were 121 men (52,6%) and 109 women (47,4%) and formed group A. The rest 121 were healthy people, 66 men (54,5%) and 55 women (45,5%) and formed group B.

The mean age of patients of group A was 71,38 years, Standard Deviation (SD) was 11,25 and Standard Error (SE) was 0,79. In group B the mean age was 69,75 years, SD was 9,24 and SE was 0,83. No statistic differences was found in the age between the two groups ($P < 0,3$).

Body Mass Index (BMI) expressed in weight/height^2 in group A was 26,71, SD 3,94 and SE 0,3 vs the mean BMI 26,75, SD 3,31 and SE 0,3 in group B. There was no statistic difference among the two groups ($P < 0,475$).

The anthropometric characteristics of the two groups are shown in fig. I.

Sex	Group A Mean	± SE	Group B Mean	± SE	P <
male	121		66		
female	109		55		
age (years)	71,3	0,8	69,7	0,8	0,3
Body Mass Index (weight/height²)	26,7	0,3	26,7	0,3	0,475

Fig. I Anthropometric characteristics of groups A and B.

Figure II represents the statistically important differences in the frequency of consumption of items between the two groups.

	Kind of food	P <
more	milk	0,001
	yogurt	0,005
	cheese	0,001
less	olive oil	0,001

Fig. II. Patients with stroke consume statistically

Regarding serum calcium the mean value in patients of group A was 10,18 mg%, SD 0,44 and SE 0,028. In group B the mean value was 10,15 mg%, SD 0,42 and SE 0,038. There was no important statistical difference between the two groups.

DISCUSSION

The findings of the present study regarding the dietary habits of patients with stroke denote that patients with stroke have different habits in comparison to healthy people.

Statistically, patients with stroke consume more frequent products such as milk, yogurt and cheese and less frequent olive oil. That means that patients of group A consume foods rich in animal fat and contemporaneously consume less vegetable fat. These dietary habits should indicate an influence in the lipidemic profile of these patients, a topic not discussed in the present study.

These foods are also rich in calcium. Calcium, especially intracellular, seems to have an important role in the necrosis´ process of the nerve cells, particularly during cerebral ischemia (9).

Calcium plays an important role in the level of nerve synapsis in the process of stimulation-answer, and in the control of important biochemical routes of the cellular metabolic mechanism.

During cerebral ischemia, following a malfunction of the K+ - N+ pump, there appears a massive influx of calcium in the nerve cell(3).

When intracellular calcium increases pathologically, reactions are activated from it, and escape from the normal cellular control and destroy the cellular skeleton and the structures of cell membrane and alterate the function of receptors and ion channels. Furthermore,

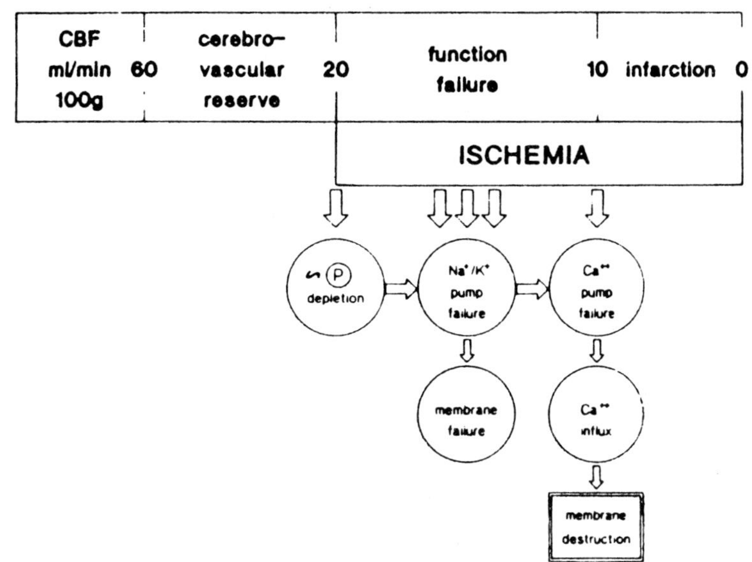

Fig. The Ischemic cascade. Values of cerebral blood flow (CBF) are approximations obtained from experimental data. (see Ref. 3)

calcium perhaps activates endonucleoses that destroy DNA, and provokes damages in the mitochondres, interrupting the production of ATP.
It is also suggested that the administration of calcium channel antagonists like nimodipine, flunarizine and others, in patients with stroke, decreases the necrosis of the nerve cells and reduces further damage of nervous tissue (1,4,5,7,8).

In the present study patients of group A do not present higher serum calcium in comparison to healthy persons. It was impossible to calculate intracellular calcium. Bet we note the coincidence of the recent literature and the findings of the present study on dietary habits of patients with stroke.

REFERENCES

1. Cohan S.L. (1990):Pharmacology of Calcium Antagonists: Clinical relevance in Neurology. Eur. Neurol.30(suppl.2),28-30.
2. Fratiglioni L. et al., (1983):Mortality from cerebrovascular disease. International comparisons and temporal trends. Neuroepidemiology 2,101-116.
3. Gelmers J.H. (1987):Effect of calcium antagonists on the cerebral circulation. Am. J. Cardiol. 59,173B-176B.
4. Gelmers J.H. et al., (1988):A controlled trial of nimodipine in acute ischemia stroke. The New Eng. J. Med.318,203-207.
5. Hulser P.J. et al., (1990):Treatment of acute stroke with calcium anatagonists. Eur. Neurol.30(suppl.2),35-38.
6. Molmgren R. et al., (1987):Geographical and secular trends in stroke incidence. The Lancet.21,1196-1200.
7. Morel N. & Godfraind T. (1990):Cerebrovascular effect of calcium anatagonists. Eur. Neurol.30(suppl.2),10-15.
8. Sandercock R. (1987):Important new treatment for acute ischemia stroke? Br. Med. Jr. 295,1224-1225.
9. Siesjo B.K. (1990):Calcium in the brain under physiological and pathological conditions. Eur. Neurol.30(suppl.2),3-9.

Metal Ions in Biology and Medicine, vol. 2. Eds. J. Anastassopoulou, Ph. Collery, J.C. Etienne, Th. Theophanides. John Libbey Eurotext, Paris © 1992, pp. 358-364

Dietary iron and colorectal cancer risk

Richard L. Nelson*, Faith Davis, Phyllis Bowen, J. Walter Kikendall

**Department of Surgery, room 2204 ; m/c 957 University of Illinois Hospital 1740 West Taylor Street Chicago, Illinois 60612, USA*

INTRODUCTION

Intestinal exposure to ingested iron may be a principal determinant of human colorectal cancer risk. Evidence exists associating iron with both the initiating and promoting phases of carcinogenesis as well as somatic defenses against early cancers through hypoferremia (progression or proliferation). Iron intake and the ingestion of associated foods that greatly effect iron bioavailability and absorption (phytate, tannin, ascorbate and alcohol) vary widely between high risk and low risk countries as well as within the United States. These variances in intake may explain not only the gradients in risk between populations, but the crossover in risk between sexes related to age within the United States. Human and rodent studies support the above hypothesis and are reviewed herein. In addition, new epidemiologic data that demonstrate increased risk of colonic precancerous lesions (adenomas) related to increased body iron stores will be presented (Nelson, 1992c). These new data imply that, in addition to increased iron ingestion, colonic neoplastic risk may be related to genetic syndromes of iron absorption (Nelson, 1992b). They are also amongst the first data that demonstrate concordance of nutritional risk factors between colonic adenomas and cancer, adding support to the adenoma/carcinoma sequence theory (Nelson, 1992a). This review will begin with a general overview of iron nutriture.

BACKGROUND; GENERAL CONTROVERSIES OF IRON NUTRITURE

Iron plays a complex and essential role in human nutrition and metabolism. Besides its role in oxygen transport and utilization, iron is necessary for the function of a number of enzymes, including those involved in immune competence and cellular division (Arthur, 1987). All living cells, prokaryotic and eukaryotic, require iron (Crosby, 1977). There is even evidence that iron sulfides may have been a primary energy source for microbes at the time of the origin of life on earth (Williams, 1990).

A complex system of regulation of absorption, transport and storage of iron has evolved in order to maintain adequate supplies of iron for the above functions in a usable form and yet also avoiding the toxic side effects of iron exposure. Nevertheless iron deficiency, manifested principally as microcytic anemia, is common throughout the world, indeed it is called by many physicians the most common deficiency disorder in the world (Hallberg, 1989). Though not commonly a direct cause of mortality, morbidity is substantial, if often subtle. Weakness, lethargy, impaired physical performance, poor pregnancy outcome, impaired cognitive performance (Dallman, 1989; Lozoff, 1991), unhappiness (Addy, 1986), and poor outcome after surgical operations (Harju, 1988) have been associated with diminished iron stores and anemia. Many of these parameters are reversed with iron therapy, some even before a change in hematocrit is seen, implying that anemia is not the only physiologic explanation of the above symptoms.

The magnitude of this problem (one half billion iron deficient individuals) and the desire to optimize socioeconomic opportunity through optimizing performance, particularly in western societies, has led to broadly based programs of iron supplementation to what is felt to be an iron deficient diet (Finch, 1989), in for instance infant formulas (Comm on Nutr., 1989) and grain flours (Addy, 1986) as well as many other prepared foods. Yet there is inevitably another side to this iron coin. It has been argued that iron deficiency of dietary origin is extremely rare and essentially unknown in adulthood. Iron deficiency in adults arises only from blood loss, hookworm being the most common etiology in the world (an estimated 450,000,000 individuals; Arthur, 1987). Treatment of the primary disorder, whether infestation, ulcer or tumor, should therefore be more efficacious than iron supplementation. The prevalence of iron deficiency anemia in the US has also been questioned by analysis of NHANES II (National Health and Nutrition Examination Survey) data, in which the frequency in adult men was 0.2%, 2.6% in menstruating women and 1.9% in post menopausal women (Cook, 1986).

The extreme consequences of iron overload are more manifestly lethal than deficiency (Harju, 1990). The first and most effective defense against iron overload is the "mucosal break" or intestinal barrier to iron absorption, which is variable and sensitive to the body's iron needs. In a iron sufficient individual only 5 to 10% of dietary iron is absorbed, but up to 40% is absorbed in severe iron deficiency (Crosby, 1977). There is an hereditary disorder of this system of absorption, hereditary hemochromatosis (HH), which with increased iron intakes results in uncontrolled absorption, iron overload, cirrhosis and a 200 fold increase in hepatocellular carcinoma risk. The gene frequency of HH is high, about 10% in Western countries, and the homozygous frequency, being those individuals now identified as diseased, is roughly 1% (Weinberg, 1990). Genetic selectionists may well ponder the potential advantage of this frequency in the pre-vitamin pill era. The frequency of homozygous HH may be greater than iron deficiency anemia in the US in adult males. On this basis the wisdom of population wide iron supplementation has been questioned (Cook, 1986). It is still not known what the health consequences of iron supplementation of HH heterozygotes are (such as tumor incidence), though it is likely that there are differences between these individuals (more than 10% of the US population) and non HH gene carriers.

There are additional reasons to question the wisdom of population wide dietary iron supplementation. All living cells require iron for growth and replication. A principal method of mammalian defense against unwanted microbial invaders is iron withholding, which is defined as follows: Immediately following even a minor inflammatory event, such as minor surgery, serum iron and transferrin saturation drops to subnormal levels. Iron storage and transport proteins are mobilized to further sequester and leach iron from the anatomic region of invasion (such as surgery or abscess or tumor), unless their available iron binding sites are saturated by iron overload. The most important protein in this system seems to be lactoferrin (Weinberg, 1984; Lentendre, 1987). A most graphic example of how the system can be paralyzed by iron supplementation is given by Weinberg:

"On their normal milk diet, these (African) Rift Valley nomads are able to maintain a mean hemoglobin value of 11.7 $\pm$ 0.8 g/dl and a transferrin saturation value of 14 $\pm$ 2.6 %. Their amebiasis infection rate was found to be less than 9%. When investigators fed the Masai 6.2 g of iron (as sulfate) during a 1-yr period, however, the mean hemoglobin value rose to 13.1 $\pm$ 1.2 g/dl and the transferrin iron saturation value rose to 29 $\pm$ 3.1 %. Unfortunately the rate of amebiasis in the iron supplemented test group rose to 83%. Moreover attacks of malaria occurred in 17% of the test group but none of the controls who received no supplemental iron." (Weinberg, 1984)

The anemia of chronic illness may also be a consequence of the iron withholding defense, the correction of which with transfusion may be dangerous for the same reason as iron supplementation. It has even been proposed that the increased incidence of metastases after tumor resection seen when there is perioperative transfusion may be due to iron overload related to transfusion and paralysis of the iron withholding defenses rather then immune suppression related to an as yet unidentified component of autologous blood (Arthur, 1987; Weinberg, 1990).

IRON IN COLORECTAL CANCER RISK; RATIONALE

Superoxide and peroxides are found in all aerobic organisms. Though potent oxidants, there is little evidence for their direct toxicity. However, in the presence of divalent cations, particularly iron, a series of reactions occur, referred to as the Haber-Weiss cycle (or superoxide driven Fenton chemistry):

$$O_2{}^{\cdot -} + Fe^{3+} \longrightarrow O_2 + Fe^{2+}$$

$$Fe^{2+} + H_2O_2 \longrightarrow Fe^{3+} + {}^{\cdot}OH + OH^-$$

Net Reaction:

$$O_2{}^{\cdot -} + H_2O_2 \xrightarrow{\mathbf{Fe}} {}^{\cdot}OH + OH^- + O_2$$

which result in the synthesis of the hydroxyl radical and probably other oxidants (Halliwell, 1984). This cycle has been demonstrated in vitro and in vivo (Imlay, 1988) and has also been found to be sensitive to iron availability in vivo, for iron delivered either parenterally (Dillard, 1984) or enterally (Slivka, 1986). Products of these reactions have been shown to be genotoxic as manifested both through DNA strand breaks and mutagenicity, associating iron with the initiating events of carcinogenesis (Halliwell, 1984; Babbs, 1990). In addition, it is felt that tumor promoters commonly exert their effect through the synthesis of oxygen radicals (Ames, 1983; Farber, 1984; Sun, 1990). Certain chelating agents such as EDTA (ethylenediamine tetraacetic acid) augment $^{\cdot}OH$ synthesis by increasing iron solubility, whereas others, particularly phytate, completely inhibit $^{\cdot}OH$ synthesis by entirely removing the bioavailability of iron (Graf, 1984). Iron therefore can be associated with both the initiating and promoting phases of carcinogenesis as well as the inhibition of the body's iron withholding defenses against early cancers (Weinberg, 1984).

It has been suggested that the protective effect of dietary fiber observed in human colorectal cancer may not be due to alterations in fecal bulk, water content, transit time or pH (Samelson, 1985), but the chelation by the phytic acid within dietary fiber of dietary iron (Graf, 1985). High red meat and high fat western diets are iron rich and also provide copious lipid substrate for peroxidation. In addition roughly half of the population of the United States ingest vitamin supplements which almost uniformly contain iron (Cons. Rep., 1986). Yet adult humans absorb less than 10% of ingested iron (Med. Let., 1978). The remainder of that dietary iron sits within the lumen of the colon with lipids from many sources for a long time (as iron is very constipating) before defecation. Though iron may relate to cancer risk in a number of organs, the colon therefore is a special case because of the luminal milieu. The concentrations of the substrates for the above reactions are much higher than elsewhere in the body (dietary iron and lipids from many sources including diet, bacteria and sluffed mucosal cells), and static due to the relative stasis of the feces. It should be expected therefore that the same reactions described above would occur within the lumen of the colon and that the products of these reactions would also be present in high concentrations in the colon. This has indeed been found to be true (Babbs, 1990).

HUMAN EPIDEMIOLOGIC EVIDENCE RELATING IRON TO COLORECTAL CANCER AND ADENOMATOUS POLYPS

Two studies have data relating iron to colorectal cancer in humans. In the first, body iron stores were analyzed by total iron binding capacity (TIBC) and transferrin saturation (Tf sat.) in the NHANES I cohort, a cohort of 14,407 adults accrued from 1971 to 1975 in the United States, from whom dietary questionnaires, medical examinations and blood samples were obtained. Subjects were followed until 1984 and, among other variables, cancer incidence was analyzed. In 242 men in whom cancer developed, body iron stores were higher (lower TIBC and higher Tf sat.) than in 3113 men who remained free of cancer. Lung, bladder, esophagus and colon were the organs most at risk and perhaps most importantly, there was evidence that dietary iron was also increased in members of the cohort with colon cancer only (Stevens, 1988). In a case control study of rectal cancer, dietary iron intake was positively associated with risk also in men only, though apparently supplemental iron use was not measured in this study, which would make the female data even more difficult to interpret (see below) than the male data (Freudenheim, 1990).

There have been two case/control studies of adenomatous polyps of the colon, the precursors of colon cancer, that included dietary iron data, in Norway and France (Hoff, 1986; Marquart-Moulin, 1987). Both studies showed a decreasing risk of polyps with increasing iron ingestion, significantly so in Norway. Supplemental iron use was not recorded, though this may be the dominant form of iron ingestion. Body iron stores were also not recorded. In our laboratories, we have just investigated the relationship of body iron stores as measured by serum ferritin to adenomatous polyp risk. The population was accrued by colonoscopy from a colorectal screening program for an ongoing case/control study and dietary intervention trial relating to A vitamers. This group included 27 individuals with early cancers, 154 patients with benign adenomas and 169 tumor free controls. Preliminary results of this investigation show a positive correlation of benign adenoma with serum ferritin. When individuals with serum ferritin over 400 were eliminated from the population, being those most likely to have HH, a linear increase in risk was seen with increasing body iron stores.

ODDS RATIO TO FIRST QUARTILE;	1st	2nd	3rd	4th
Adenomatous Polyp	1.0	1.4	2.3	3.4
Cancer	1.0	0.6	1.1	0.2

The pattern was less stabile for cancer, probably due to the small number of cases and the nutritional consequences of the disease. Nevertheless, an increased risk of colonic neoplasia is clearly related to increased iron stores in this population (Nelson, 1992c).

If dietary iron is a major determinant of colorectal cancer risk, an explanation could be provided for an unusual epidemiologic observation. Human colorectal cancer epidemiology is unique among cancers that occur in both sexes, because there is frequently a cross over in risk seen between females and males related to age. Females have a higher risk before age 50 and males a higher risk after age 55 years (Correa, 1977). In all other cancers where there are sex difference in risk, these differences grow (or the risks diverge rather than cross over) with advancing age (Haenszel, p.c.). Female hormonal milieu or use cannot explain this phenomenon, since the greater exposure to estrogens is before menopause, and this should have diminished risk in this age group (Furner, 1989, Chute, 1991). Exposure to supplemental iron does vary significantly between sexes especially before age 50, when women have a far higher pharmacologic iron use than men. This can be seen in data concerning overall vitamin use and the use of specific iron supplements (Moss, 1989). What is striking in these figures is at least the implication that the total pharmacologic iron intake in the US may exceed food sources of iron.

ANIMAL EVIDENCE RELATING IRON TO COLORECTAL CANCER.

Several animal studies have investigated either the role of iron and or phytate in colorectal cancer risk in the form of prospective interventional trials. These studies support the hypothesis that increased exposure to iron, parenteral or dietary, augments colorectal cancer risk and that the phytate component of dietary fiber reverses this effect. In addition, it can be inferred by these results that dietary iron's augmentation of colon tumor induction occurs during the promotional phase of carcinogenesis rather than during initiation (Siegers, 1988, Nelson, 1989, Nielsen, 1987, Shamsuddin, 1988).

CONCLUSIONS & RECOMMENDATIONS

In the future, epidemiologic support for the hypotheses put forth in this review needs to be generated from studies that look at all sources of dietary iron: foods and supplements, as well as foods that effect iron absorption (e.g. calcium, alcohol, ascorbate, phytate and tannins (Hallberg, 1989; Bothwell, 1989)). The relationship of genetic control of iron absorption to cancer risk is certainly suggested by the data and needs to be further investigated. Fecal iron has not been looked at in human population studies and should be. Until more data are available, we may well ask as

Crosby did in 1977, "Who needs iron?" In answering his own question, Crosby stated that "Everything alive needs iron, not too much or it and not too little." Iron supplementation of healthy individuals to improve performance may well have dire health consequences. For now iron supplements are best reserved for medical therapy of a specific illness, symptomatic iron deficiency anemia.

REFERENCES

Addy DP. (1986) Happiness is: iron. Br. Med. J. 292. 969-70.

Ames BN. (1983) Dietary carcinogens and anticarcinogens. Science. 221. 1256-64.

Arthur CK and Isbister JP. (1987) Iron deficiency; misunderstood, misdiagnosed and mistreated. Drugs. 33. 171-82.

Babbs C. (1990) Free radicals and the etiology of colon cancer. Free Rad. Biol Med. 8. 191-200.

Bothwell TH, Baynes RD, MacFarlane BJ and MAcPhail AP. (1989) Nutritional iron requirements and food iron absorption. J. Int. Med. 226. 357-65.

Chute CG, Willett WC, Colditz GA, Stampfer MJ, Rosner B and Speizer FE. (1991) A prospective study of reproductive history and exogenous estrogens on the risk of colorectal cancer in women. Epid. 2. 201-7.

Committee on Nutrition. (1989) Iron-fortified infant formulas. Pediatrics. 84. 1114-5.

Consumer's Rept. The Vitamin Pushers. (1986) 51. 170-5.

Cook JD, Skikne BS, Lynch SR and Ruesser ME. (1986) Estimates of iron sufficiency in the US population. Blood. 68. 726-31.

Cook JD and Skikne BS. (1989) Iron deficiency: definition and diagnosis. J. Int. Med. 226. 349-55.

Correa P and Haenszel W. (1977) The epidemiology of large-bowel cancer. Adv. Cancer Res. 26. 1-140.

Crosby WH. (1977) Who needs iron? NEJM. 297 543-6.

Dallman PR. (1989) Iron deficiency: does it matter? J. Int. Med. 226. 367-72.

Dillard CJ, Downey JE and Tappel AL. (1984) Effect of antioxidants on lipid peroxidation in iron loaded rats. Lipids.19.127-33.

Farber E. (1984) The multistep nature of cancer development. Can. Res. 44. 4217-8.

Finch C. (1989) Introduction: Knights of the oval table. J. Int. Med. 226. 345-8.

Freudenheim JL, Graham S, Marshall JR, Haughey BP and Wilkinson G. (1990) A case-control study of diet and rectal cancer in western New York. Am. J. Epid. 131. 612-24.

Furner SE, Davis FG, Nelson RL and Haenszel W. (1989) A case-control study of large bowel cancer and hormone exposure in women. Cancer Res. 49. 4936-40.

Graf E, Mahoney JR, Bryant RG and Eaton JW. (1984) Iron catalyzed hydroxyl radical formation; stringent requirement for free iron coordination site. J. Biol. Chem. 259. 3620-4.

Graf E and Eaton JW. (1985) Dietary suppression of colonic cancer; fiber or phytate? Cancer. 56. 717-18.

Haenszel W. Pers. comm.

Hallberg L. (1989) Iron in clinical medicine - an update. J. Int Med. 226. 281-3.

Hallberg L, Brune M and Rossander L. (1989) Iron absorption in man: ascorbic acid and dose-dependent inhibition by phytate. Am. J. Clin. Nutr. 49. 140-144.

Halliwell B and Gutteridge JMC. (1984) Oxygen toxicity, oxygen radicals, transition metals and disease. Bioch. J. 219. 1-14.

Harju E. (1988) Empty iron stores as a significant risk factor in abdominal surgery. J. Parent. & Ent. Nutr. 12. 282-5.

Harju E. (1990) Iron in cancer. A review of the present knowledge. in Metal ions in biology and Medicine. Collery P, Poirer LA, Manfait M and Etienne JC, Ed.s pp 45-48. Paris. John Libbey.

Hoff G, Moen IE, Trygg K, Froelich W, Sauar J, Vatn M, Gjone E and Larsen S. (1986) Epidemiology of polyps in the rectum and sigmoid colon. Scand. J. Gastroent. 21. 199-204.

Imlay JA, Chin SM and Linn S. (1988) Toxic damage by hydrogen peroxide through the Fenton reaction in vivo and in vitro. Science. 240. 640-2.

Letendre ED. (1987) Iron metabolism during infection and neoplasia. Cancer & Metas. Rev. 6. 41-53.

Lozoff B, Jimenez E and Wolf AW. (1991) Long-term developmental outcome of infants with iron deficiency. NEJM. 325. 687-94.

Macquart-Moulin G, Riboli E, Cornee J, Kaaks R and Berthe zene P. (1987) Colorectal polyps and diet: a case control study in Marseilles. Int. J. Cancer. 40. 179-88.

Med. Let. (1978) Oral Iron. 20. 45-6.

Moss AJ, Levy AS, Kim I, Park YK. (1989) Use of vitamin and mineral supplements in the United States: current users, types of products and nutrients. Advance Data. Nat. Ctr. for Hlth. Stat. #174.

Neilsen BK, Thompsom LU and Bird RP. (1987) Effect of phytic acid on colonic epithelial proliferation. Cancer Let. 37. 317-25.

Nelson RL, Yoo SJ, Tanure JC, Andrianopoulos G and Misumi A. (1989) The Effect of Iron on Experimental Colorectal Carcinogenesis. Anticancer Res. 9. 1477-82.

Nelson RL. (1992a) Diet and Adenomatous Polyps Risk. Seminars in Colon & Rectal Surgery. 2. 262-268.

Nelson, RL. (1992b) Iron and colorectal cancer risk. Free Radicals in Biol. & Med. 12. 161-8.

Nelson RL, Davis F, Bowen P and Kikendall W. (1992c) Body iron stores and the risk of colonic neoplasia; a case/control study. submitted for publication.

Samelson SL, Nelson RL and Nyhus LM. (1985) Protective role of faecal pH in experimental colon carcinogenesis. J. Roy. Soc. Med. 78. 230-33.

Shamsuddin AM, Elsayed AM and Ullah A. (1988) Suppression of large intestinal cancer in F344 rats by inositol hexaphosphate. Carcinogenesis. 9. 577-80.

Siegers CP, Bumann D, Baretton G and Younes M. (1988) Dietary iron enhances the tumor rate in dimethylhydrazine induced colon carcinogenesis in mice. Can. Let. 41. 251-256.

Slivka A, Kang J and Cohen G. (1986) Hydroxyl radicals and the toxicity of oral iron. Bioch. Pharm. 35. 553-56.

Stevens RG, Jones DY, Micozzi MS and Taylor PR. (1988) Body Iron stores and the risk of cancer. NEJM. 319. 1047-1052.

Sun Y. (1990) Free radicals, antioxidant enzymes and carcinogenesis. Free Rad. Biol. & Med. 8. 583-99.

Weinberg ED. (1984) Iron withholding: a defense against infection and neoplasia. Physiol Rev. 64. 65-102.

Weinberg ED. (1990) Cellular iron metabolism in health and disease. Drug Metab. Rev. 22. 531-80.

Williams RJP. (1990) Iron and the origin of life. Nature. 343. 213-4.

Metal Ions in Biology and Medicine, vol. 2. Eds. J. Anastassopoulou, Ph. Collery, J.C. Etienne, Th. Theophanides. John Libbey Eurotext, Paris © 1992, pp. 365-370

Influence of nutritional intake on zinc, copper, lead and silicium status in chronic alcoholics

P. Pirollet, C. Gillet, F. Paille, M.F. Hutin*, D. Burnel*

*Centre d'Alcoologie, Hôpital Fournier, CO n° 34, 54035 Nancy Cedex. *Service de Chimie Générale, Faculté de Médecine, BP 184, 54500 Vandœuvre, France*

An excessive alcoholic consumption changes serum and tissue concentrations of many trace elements. A previous study demonstrated that serum concentrations of zinc (Zn) and copper (Cu) are lower in alcoholics compared to controls whereas levels of lead (Pb) and silicium are higher (7).

The origin of these disorders is not completely well known. A large intake of alcohol and these results on the basic food are frequently blamed for a primary deficiency.

The present study was designed to extend the previous study (7) :

- by measuring Zn, Cu, Pb and Si intakes in alcoholic patients,
- by comparing the trace elements' status between wine and beer drinkers,
- and by examining its evolution after weaning and an ordinary hospital diet.

METHODS

Subjects

A hundred and forty chronic alcoholics who had just entered a rehabilitation program in our detoxification unit of Nancy hospital participated in the study. All patients were dependent on alcohol according to DSM III R dependence criteria.They included 117 men and 23 women (mean age : 39 ± 9 years, from 21 to 70 years), and exhibited no clinical or biological complications (chronic pancreatitis, encephalopathy, severe hepatic failure). The mean daily alcohol intake was 200 ± 116 g. The withdrawal program began immediately on admission to the hospital unit and was respected for the entirety of their stay. Tranquilizers and oral vitamin supplements (vitamin B1 750 mg per day ; vitamin B6 750 mg per day) were systematically given. Most of them were smokers.

Nutritional evaluation

Alcohol and dietary intakes were determined by a dietican using a 7-day food record and they were calculated by computer (Soft GENI, Micro6®). We defined the wine drinkers (n = 38) and the beer drinkers (n = 22) who drunk 80% or more daily in the form of wine or beer, respectively. The content in trace elements of the alcoholic beverages is variable according to the latters' origins. We examined the concentrations of Zn, Cu, Pb and Si in 12 wines and 4 beers usually drunk in our country.

During the abstinence period, patients were given the ordinary hospital diet (Daily intake : energy = 2300 kcal, protein = 92 g, fat = 96 g, carbohydrate = 266 g, Zn = 12 mg, Cu = 2 mg).

On admission and after 28 days of abstinence, the blood concentrations of the trace elements were examined. They were dosed by emission spectrophotometry on Argon DCP plasma on serum or total blood for Pb. The usual hematologic, electrolytic, renal and hepatic tests were performed. Nutritional status was defined by albumin, retinol binding protein (RbP) and prealbumin dosage.

Statistical analysis

Differences between groups were examined with Student's t test. The results are expressed as the mean and standard deviation.

RESULTS

The body mass index (BMI = weight/height expressed in kg/m2) was 21.9 ± 7.6 for men and 22.6 ± 7.2 for women. The mean serum indicators of nutritional status were above the generally accepted minimun standards (RbP = 0.05 ± 0.01 g/L, Transferrin = 0.25 ± 0,50 g/L, Albumin = 40 ± 4 g/L).

The mean dietary intake averaged over 7-day period was correct. Nonalcoholic energy (2452 kcal ± 1333), protein (109 g ± 60, 17% of total non alcohol calories), fat (95 g ± 60, 33%) and carbohydrate (290 g ± 167, 46%) were normal. The Zn and Cu intakes were respectively 12,67 mg (± 7,40) and 3,32 mg per day (± 1,73). The Pb and Si contents of the food were unknown. The daily food intake of wine and beer drinkers was not significantly different (Table 1).

	W. Drinkers	B. Drinkers	
Energy (kcal/day)	2269 ± 845	2667 ± 1503	$p > 0.05$
Protein (g/day)	100 ± 38	117 ± 79	$p > 0.05$
Fat (g/day)	87 ± 34	94 ± 56	$p > 0.05$
Carbohydrate (g/day)	270 ±120	336 ± 206	$p > 0.05$
Zn (mg/day)	12.00 ± 5.38	13.38 ± 10.04	$p > 0.05$
Cu (mg/day)	3.72 ± 1.71	2.98 ± 1.56	$p > 0.05$

Table 1. Daily food intake in wine and beer drinkers

The mean trace element contents in alcoholic beverages is reported in Table 2. The Zn, Cu and Pb contents of wine was richer than that of beer. The Si content of the beer was higher.

	Wine	Beer	
Zn (mg/l)	0.68 ± 0.25	0.05 ± 0.01	$p < 0.001$
Cu (mg/l)	0.28 ± 0.34	< 0.001	$p < 0.001$
Pb (mg/l)	0.25 ± 0.05	0.16 ± 0.02	$p < 0.01$
Si (mg/l)	17.22 ± 7.16	41.22 ± 10.65	$p < 0.001$

Table 2. Mean trace elements contents in wine and beer.

The capacities of alcoholic beverages was different between wine and beer drinkers (2.2 ± 1.2 L vs 3.7 ± 2.3 L per day). Consequently, the daily Zn and Cu intake was highest in wine drinkers, the daily Si intake was highest in beer drinkers and the Pb intake in alcoholic beverages was identical (Table 3).

	W. Drinkers	B. Drinkers	
Alcool (l/day)	2.2 ± 1.2	3.7 ± 2.3	$p < 0.01$
Alcool (g/day)	196 ± 115	145 ± 95	$p > 0.05$
Alc. (kcal/day)	1374 ± 811	1019 ± 665	$p > 0.05$
Zn (mg/day)	1.41 ± 0.84	0.23 ± 0.18	$p < 0.001$
Cu (mg/day)	0.58 ± 0.35	0.02 ± 0.04	$p < 0.001$
Pb (mg/day)	0.53 ± 0.31	0.60 ± 0.37	
Si (mg/day)	38.90 ± 22.35	150.59 ± 92.21	$p < 0.001$

Table 3. Daily alcohol intake in wine and beer drinkers.

The blood trace element levels in controls and alcoholics are gathered in Table 4 (results of the previous study). In spite of the intake of various trace elements, the type of alcoholic beverage had no influence on their serum levels (Table 5).

	Control	Alcoholic	
Zn (mg/l)	1.06 ± 0.19	0.91 ± 0.18	$p < 0.01$
Cu (mg/l)	1.16 ± 0.44	1.01 ± 0.22	$p < 0.01$
Pb (mg/l)	0.22 ± 0.05	0.27 ± 0.13	$p = 0.03$
Si (mg/l)	0.17 ± 0.01	0.23 ± 0.13	$p < 0.01$

Table 4. Blood trace element levels in controls and alcoholics.

	W. Drinkers	B. Drinkers	
Zn (mg/l)	0.88 ± 0.20	0.95 ± 0.25	$p > 0,05$
Cu (mg/l)	1.00 ± 0.18	0.93 ± 0.13	$p > 0.05$
Pb (mg/l)	0.25 ± 0.11	0.25 ± 0.11	$p > 0.05$
Si (mg/l)	0.19 ± 0.11	0.24 ± 0.14	$p > 0.05$

Table 5. Blood trace element levels in wine and beer drinkers.

After a 28-day period (Table 6.), in spite of weaning and adequate dietary intake, Zn, Cu and Pb levels were unaffected. The Si level was significantly better than that on admission.

	Admission	J28	
Zn (mg/l)	0.91 ± 0.18	0.89 ± 0.17	$p > 0.05$
Cu (mg/l)	1.01 ± 0.22	1.04 ± 0.18	$p > 0.05$
Pb (mg/l)	0.27 ± 0.13	0.27 ± 0.12	$p > 0.05$
Si (mg/l)	0.23 ± 0.13	0.19 ± 0.09	$p = 0,03$

Table 6. Evolution of blood trace element levels.

DISCUSSION

We establish that dependant alcoholics' feeding, exhibited no serious complication, is qualitatively and quantitatively balanced. A large intake of alcohol has no profound effects on basic food intake and the nutrition of the wine or beer drinkers is not different. The fat intake is even better than the mean intake in France.

The Zn level diminution during chronic alcoholism is now widly admitted (7, 8). Spencer and al have shown that Zn intake correlates with protein intake, and that foods high in protein are generally rich in Zn. Indeed, the Zn intake in alcoholics is in tune with the recommended daily dietary intakes for healthy adults (10 to 15 mg per day) (3,4). The Zn intake in alcoholic beverages increases the daily intake to 14.04 ± 7.33 mg per day. There is no dietary deficiency. The serum level of Zn in wine drinkers is not better despite a Zn intake higher. Finally, after a 28 period of weaning and a hospital diet the serum level of Zn do not increase.

The Cu intake is correct, in tune with the recommanded daily dietary intakes for healthy adults (1.5 to 3 mg per day) (3), nevertheless the serum level of Cu is low in chronic alcoholics. In wine drinkers Cu additionnal intake by this beverage does not influence its serum level. The weaning and the hospital diet do not change that.

The alcohol consumption contributes to raise Pb blood level (1), identically in wine and beer drinkers. The wine had been shown up because it is rich in Pb. In fact, the great capacity of beer drunk compensates and the Pb intake by alcoholic beverages is not different between wine and beer drinkers. The pollution of the foods is unknown but the Pb alcoholic intake (0.55 ± 0.35 mg per day) passes beyond the total recommanded week intakes (3 mg per week) (5). Probably, the Pb alcoholic intake contributes to increase blood level and a 28-period of weaning is too short to mobilize the bone stock. The serum level of Si is high in chronic alcoholics. Unfortunately, we cannot determine the Si intake because the Si contents of the foods is not very known. The beer is high Si content and the Si intake in beer drinkers is very high. This intake exceeds the daily intake estimated by Teraoka in Japan, Bowen in England and Varo in Finland (30 to 60 mg per day) (2,6). That can contribute to the high serum level of Si, all the more its level decreases after the weaning period. However the serum levels of Si are not significantly different between beer and wine drinkers and it is likely that others factors arise.

The Zn, Cu, Pb and Si contents are very different in alcoholic beverages but the trace elements' serum levels are identical in wine and beer drinkers. After a 28-day period of abstinence and an ordinary hospital diet, the evolution of serum trace elements levels is variable : Si tends to reach the range of normal values whereas Zn, Cu and Pb are unchanged. The trace element intake seems to play a part of minor importance. There are no Zn and Cu dietary deficiencies and a metabolic origin is more probably. On the other hand, the alcoholic beverages contribute to increase the pollution of the feeding by Pb and Si.

REFERENCES

1 Bortoli A., Fazzin G., Marin V., Trabuio G., Zotti S. (1986) : Relationships between blood Lead concentration and aminolevulinic acid dehydrase in alcoholics and workers industrially exposed to Lead. Arch Environ Health, 41, 251-260.

2 Creac'h P., Adrien J. (1990) : Le silicium dans la chaîne alimentaire et sa localisation dans l'organisme. Med et Nut, 26, 73 - 90.

3 Fidanza R.,Durlach J.,Gueguen J.P. (1989) : Statut nutritionnel en minéraux et oligo-éléments : problèmes et solutions. Med et Nut, 25, 93-107.

4 Harper A. E. (1976) : Basis of recommended dietary allowances for trace elements. In Trace elements in human health and disease. Volume II. Eds A. S. Prasad. Academic Press New York, 371-378.

5 Huel G., Boudene C., Jouan M., Lazar P. (1986) : Assessment of exposure to lead of the general population in French community through biological monitoring. Int Arch Occup Environ Health, 58, 131-139.

6 Pennington J. A. T. (1991) : Silicon in foods and diets. Food additives and contaminants,1, 97-118.

7 Pirollet P., Paille F., Hutin M. F., Corroy A.M., Nabet-Belleville F., Burnel D. (1990) : Effects of chronic alcoholism on trace elements status. Influence of withdrawal program. Trace elements in medicine, 7, 55 (Abs.).

8 Spencer H., Osis D., Kramer L., Norris C.(1976) : Intake, excretion, and retention of Zinc in man. In Trace elements in human health and disease. Eds A. S. Prasad. Academic Press, New York, 345-361.

Metal Ions in Biology and Medicine, vol. 2. Eds. J. Anastassopoulou, Ph. Collery, J.C. Etienne, Th. Theophanides. John Libbey Eurotext, Paris © 1992, pp. 371-376

Influence of ascorbic acid on the gastrointestinal absorption of aluminium

J.L. Domingo, M. Gomez, J.M. Llobet, C. Richart*, J. Corbella

*Laboratoy of Toxicology and Biochemistry and *Department of Medicine, School of Medicine, University of Barcelona, San Lorenzo 21, 43201 Reus, Spain*

It is well documented that small quantities of aluminium are absorbed following the administration of oral aluminium-containing phosphate-binders and antacids (Alfrey, 1985). Although normally, very little aluminium is absorbed from the gastrointestinal tract, when the amount of ingested metal is markedly increased, some of this excess aluminium is absorbed, with a remarkable aluminium retention rate (Lione, 1983; Lote & Saunders, 1991).

Despite large variations in aluminium intake in people with normal renal function, most absorbed aluminium is primarily excreted in the urine. Urinary aluminium excretion increases with increased aluminium loading whether it is from increased gastrointestinal absorption, or intravenous loading in adults or infants (Koo & Kaplan, 1988; Lote & Saunders, 1991). Nevertheless, patients with marked renal insufficiency cannot excrete the absorbed aluminium and are therefore at risk for serious sequelae of aluminium accumulation and toxicity, including encephalopathy, osteomalacia, proximal muscle weakness, and microcytic anemia (Alfrey *et al.*, 1976; Sedman *et al.*, 1984; Bia *et al.*, 1989).

In 1984, Slanina *et al.* reported that the oral administration of aluminium citrate complex resulted in a significant accumulation and retention of the metal in the brain and bone tissues of rats. These results as well as the results of subsequent experiments indicated that the intake of citric acid combined with a prolonged high oral aluminium intake might lead to a tissue accumulation and possible toxic effects of aluminium in the body (Slanina *et al.*, 1984; 1985). Several human studies also showed that citrate is a major factor in the toxicity of orally administered aluminium compounds (Slanina *et al.*, 1986; Molitoris *et al.*, 1989; Mees & Basçi, 1991).

Recently, *in vitro* studies demonstrated that the presence in the gastrointestinal tract of various aluminium-complexing common dietary constituents (citric, ascorbic, malic, oxalic, lactic, gluconic and tartaric acids) in conjuction with gastric acid, solubilizes aluminium cations and may thus result in the equilibrium formation of a soluble complex of aluminium, which by preventing reprecipitation, may result in aluminium absorption and elevated plasma aluminium levels (Partridge *et al.*, 1989).

The aim of the present study was twofold: 1) to assess the effects of ascorbic, citric, malic, oxalic, lactic, gluconic and tartaric acids on aluminium absorption and retention in rats, and 2) to determine in individuals with normal renal function whether ingestion of ascorbic acid together with aluminium hydroxide enhances the gastrointestinal absorption of aluminium compared to ingestion of aluminium hydroxide alone.

METHODS

General

In the first experiment, eight groups of female Sprague-Dawley rats (Panlab, Barcelona, Spain) weighing 200 to 220 g were treated with 281 mg $Al(OH)_3$/kg/day ($\approx$100 mg Al/kg/day) by gastric intubation, five times a week for five weeks. Concurrently, animals in seven groups received ascorbic acid (56.3 mg/kg/day), citric acid (62 mg/kg/day), gluconic acid (62.7 mg/kg/day), lactic acid (28.8 mg/kg/day), malic acid (42.9 mg/kg/day), oxalic acid (28.8 mg/kg/day), or tartaric acid (48 mg/kg/day) in the drinking water. Solutions were prepared daily to adjust the doses to achieve a constant intake by taking into account the differences in body weight and fluid intake. The eighth group served as control, and did not receive any dietary factors in the drinking water. After five weeks, the animals were killed and brain, bone (femur), kidneys, liver, and spleen were removed and kept for aluminium analyses.

In the second experiment, two oral medication regimens were administered to each of thirteen healthy volunteer adults (males, 20-25 years). Ingestion of prescription or non-prescription medications other than the study drugs, was prohibited. Each subject received a three-day course of treatment with each of the following two oral medication regimens dosed three times daily: 1) aluminium hydroxide, 900 mg (Alugelibys, Ibys, Madrid, Spain); 2) aluminium hydroxide 900 mg, plus ascorbic acid, 2g (Roche, Madrid, Spain). A drug free-interval of ten days separated both medication periods. Twenty-four hours urine collection for aluminium determination was obtained during each three-day course.

Analytical methods

Tissue and urine aluminium concentrations were determined by atomic absorption spectrophotometry (Perkin-Elmer Model 4000 and HGA-400 graphite furnace with AS-40 autosampler). For aluminium analysis, 1 ml of urine or about 500 mg of tissue was placed in a 15 ml tube which had been rinsed five times in ultrapure water. Digestion was accomplished by adding ultrapure nitric acid (Suprapur 65%, Merck, Darmstadt, FRG) and heated under pressure at 190° C (Domingo *et al.*, 1987). Samples were then brought to a 10 ml volume with ultrapure water. To eliminate aluminium contamination as much as possible from the environment, all specimen manipulations were performed in a laminar flow hood located in a limited access-room. Procedure blanks (reagents only) were read with each group of samples. Absorbance readings for blanks were substracted from sample readings prior to reference to the standard curve (Slanina *et al.*, 1984; 1985). The coefficients of variation for the different samples were between 4.2 and 7.3%. The percentage recovery under experimental conditions used was found to be 98.2% $\pm$ 8.3%.

Statistics

Data were analyzed using a Kruskal-Wallis one-way analysis of variance with significant F values analyzed further using Mann-Whitney *U* test. A probablity value of $p < 0.05$ was accepted as significant.

RESULTS

Table 1 shows the concentration of aluminium in liver, spleen, kidney, brain, and bone of control and dietary constituents-treated rats. Treatment with ascorbic or citric acids significantly increased the aluminium levels in liver, spleen, brain and bone. Gluconic and lactic acids increased the concentrations of aluminium in spleen, brain, and bone. The levels of aluminium in liver, spleen, and brain were also significantly raised by the intake of malic and oxalic acids, while administration of tartaric acid increased the aluminium concentrations in liver, brain, and bone.

The values for urine aluminium excretion (μg/kg/day) by human volunteers for both treatment periods are summarized in Table 2. The results show that the ingestion of ascorbic acid together with aluminium hydroxide causes threefold increase in urine aluminium excretion compared to ingestion of aluminium hydroxide alone. Similar data are obtained when the results are expressed in μg/g creatinine/day (Table 3). It has been reported that in individuals with normal renal function, most if not all absorbed aluminium is excreted in urine (Koo & Kaplan, 1988; Wilhelm *et al.*, 1989).

TABLE 2
Urinary Aluminium Excretion (μg/kg/day) during Treatment Periods

	Al mean values ± SD		
	Day 1	Day 2	Day 3
$Al(OH)_3$ alone	7.74 ± 2.99	7.85 ± 3.07	7.13 ± 2.23
$Al(OH)_3$ + ascorbic acid	23.46 ± 9.67[a]	21.87 ± 11.62[a]	26.59 ± 14.78[a]

[a]$p < 0.001$ vs. $Al(OH)_3$ alone.

DISCUSSION

In recent years, it has been clearly demonstrated that concurrent ingestion of aluminium compounds and citrate causes a significant increase in the gastrointestinal absorption of aluminium in both healthy subjects and uremic patients (Slanina *et al.*, 1986; Nolan *et al.*, 1990; Walker *et al.*, 1990; Mees & Basçi, 1991). The increased aluminium absorption has been attributed to the chelating properties of citric acid for this metal (Martin, 1986; Domingo *et al.*, 1988; Domingo, 1989). Oral citrate solubilizes Al^{3+}, and an appreciable fraction occurs as a neutral complex that may pass through membranes and provide a vehicle for aluminium absorption into the body (Martin, 1986).Thus, oral consumption of citrate and aluminium compounds to neutralize stomach acid or to bind phosphate results in a higher aluminium absorption and potential accumulation and toxicity.

In the first part of the present study, we found that several aluminium organic chelators that, like citric acid, are frequently present in the diet may also prevent the precipitation of aluminium hydroxide at the pH conditions expected in the intestine (Partridge *et al.*, 1989; Dayde &

TABLE 1

Aluminium Concentrations (μg/g $\pm$ SD) in Tissues of Rats given Aluminium Hydroxide and Various Dietary Constituents

	Liver	Spleen	Kidney	Brain	Bone
Control [$Al(OH)_3$]	0.15 ± 0.19	4.16 ± 2.05	1.55 ± 1.32	ND[d]	2.22 ± 1.19
$Al(OH)_3$ + ascorbic	6.27 ± 4.95[a]	27.32 ± 8.52[c]	6.60 ± 4.76	0.35 ± 0.29[a]	26.31 ± 14.02[c]
$Al(OH)_3$ + citric	6.55 ± 5.19[a]	21.35 ± 7.20[c]	0.78 ± 0.48	0.45 ± 0.37[a]	9.02 ± 2.48[c]
$Al(OH)_3$ + gluconic	1.51 ± 0.36	7.74 ± 2.94[a]	2.01 ± 0.54	0.62 ± 0.33[a]	10.20 ± 5.14[b]
$Al(OH)_3$ + lactic	1.43 ± 0.53	17.36 ± 6.86[b]	4.04 ± 2.21	5.82 ± 5.25[a]	7.77 ± 3.86[a]
$Al(OH)_3$ + malic	3.18 ± 2.77[a]	17.18 ± 9.02[a]	0.80 ± 0.49	0.83 ± 0.55[a]	6.55 ± 4.18
$Al(OH)_3$ + oxalic	3.74 ± 1.58[b]	13.82 ± 5.54[b]	2.12 ± 1.87	0.89 ± 0.42[a]	2.59 ± 1.01
$Al(OH)_3$ + tartaric	3.16 ± 2.19[a]	3.75 ± 2.28	0.43 ± 0.35	2.24 ± 2.53[a]	4.87 ± 1.58[a]

[a]Significance of difference from control [$Al(OH)_3$] group, $p < 0.05$.
[b]Significance of difference from control [$Al(OH)_3$] group, $p < 0.01$.
[c]Significance of difference from control [$Al(OH)_3$] group, $p < 0.001$.
[d]ND= Not detected; detection limit: 0.05 μg/g.

Berthon, 1990). Therefore, these dietary factors enhance the gastrointestinal absorption and retention of aluminium. The administered amounts of citric acid (62 mg/kg/day) correspond approximately with the estimated daily dietary human intakes (Rudman *et al.*, 1980). The quantities in moles of the other compounds are equivalent to the amounts of citric acid. However, citric and ascorbic acids appear to be of most clinical importance as both are available in the diet at relatively high concentrations.

TABLE 3

Comparison of Mean 24-Hour Urinary Aluminium (μg/g creatinine/day) Excretion

	Al mean values ± SD		
	Day 1	Day 2	Day 3
$Al(OH)_3$ alone	18.17 ± 9.29	16.16 ± 6.17	15.13 ± 7.20
$Al(OH)_3$ + ascorbic acid	61.84 ± 24.10[a]	64.42 ± 34.45[a]	73.35 ± 54.02[a]

[a]$p < 0.001$ vs. $Al(OH)_3$ alone.

The results of the second part of this study corroborate that concurrent ingestion of ascorbic acid and aluminium hydroxide is associated with an enhancement in aluminium absorption. Because of the wide consumption of all the above dietary constituents, in order to prevent the risks of aluminium toxicity, it seems quite reasonable that a careful surveillance of the diet of uremic patients who are also taking aluminium-containing medications should be maintained.

Although the effects of citric acid on intestinal aluminium absorption are now well established, especially relevant is also the influence of ascorbic acid on enteral aluminium absorption. Ascorbic acid occurs naturally in plants such as leafy vegetables, citrus fruits and tomatoes. Since ascorbic acid, like citric acid, is considered safe, it (or sodium ascorbate) is also widely used in processed fruits and baked goods to delay or prevent undesirable changes in color, odor, flavor, or texture. Consequently, chronic renal patients should be advised to avoid the concurrent ingestion of ascorbic acid and aluminium compounds.

Acknowledgements. This study was supported by the DGICYT (Spain), through grant PM91-0158. The authors thank the Servei d'Espectroscòpia, University of Barcelona for excellent technical assistance.

REFERENCES

Alfrey, A.C., LeGendre, G.R., and Kaehny, W.D. (1976): The dialysis encephalopathy syndrome. Possible aluminum intoxication. *New Engl. J. Med.* 294, 184-188.

Alfrey, A.C. (1985): Gastrointestinal absorption of aluminium. *Clin. Nephrol.* 24, S84-S87.

Bia, M.J., Cooper, K., Schnall, S., Duffy, T., Hendler, E., Maluche, H., and Solomon, L. (1989): Aluminum induced anemia: pathogenesis and treatment in patients on chronic hemodialysis. *Kidney Int.* 36, 852-858.

Dayde, S. & Berthon, G. (1990): Potential toxicity of presumably insoluble aluminium salts in presence of common dietary acids. *Food Addit. Contam.* 7, S155-S157.

Domingo, J.L., Llobet, J.M., Gómez, M., Tomas, J.M., and Corbella, J. (1987): Nutritional and toxicological effects of short-term ingestion of aluminum by the rat. *Res. Commun. Chem. Pathol. Pharmacol.* 56, 409-419.

Domingo, J.L., Gómez, M., Llobet, J.M., and Corbella, J. (1988): Parenteral citric acid for aluminium intoxication. *Lancet* 2, 1362-1363.

Domingo, J.L. (1989): The use of chelating agents in the treatment of aluminum overload. *Clin. Toxicol.* 27, 355-367.

Koo, W.W.K. & Kaplan, L.A. (1988): Aluminum and bone disorders: with specific reference to aluminum contamination of infant nutrients. *J. Am. Coll. Nutr.* 7, 199-214.

Lione, A. (1983): The prophylactic reduction of aluminium intake. *Food Chem. Toxicol.* 21, 103-109.

Lote, C.J. & Saunders, H. (1991): Aluminium: gastrointestinal absorption and renal excretion. *Clin. Sci.* 81, 289-295.

Martin, R.B. (1986): The chemistry of aluminum as related to biology and medicine. *Clin. Chem.* 32, 1797-1806.

Mees, E.J.D. & Basçi, A. (1991): Citric acid in calcium effervescent tablets may favour aluminium intoxication. *Nephron* 59, 322.

Molitoris, B.A., Froment, D.H., Mackenzie, T.A., Huffer, W.H., and Alfrey, A.C. (1989): Citrate: A major factor in the toxicity of orally administered aluminum compounds. *Kidney Int.* 36, 949-953.

Nolan, C.R., Califano, J.R., and Butzin, C.A. (1990): Influence of calcium acetate or calcium citrate on intestinal aluminium absorption. *Kidney Int.* 38, 937-941.

Partridge, N.A., Regnier, F.E., White, J.L., and Hem, S.L. (1989): Influence of dietary constituents on intestinal absorption of aluminum. *Kidney Int.* 35, 1413-1417.

Rudman, D., Dedonis, J.L., Fountain, M.T., Chandler, J.B., Gerron, G.G., Fleming, G.A., and Kutner, M.H. (1980): Hypocitraturia in patients with gastrointestinal malabsorption. *New Engl. J. Med.*306, 657-661.

Sedman, A.B., Miller, N.L., Warady, B.A., Lum, G.M., and Alfrey, A.C. (1984): Aluminum loading in children with chronic renal failure. *Kidney Int.* 26, 201-204.

Slanina, P., Falkeborn, Y., Frech, W., and Cedergren, A. (1984): Aluminum concentrations in the brain and bone of rats fed citric acid, aluminum citrate or aluminum hydroxide. *Food Chem. Toxicol.* 22, 391-397.

Slanina, P., Frech, W., Bernhardson, A., Cedergren, A., and Mattson, P. (1985): Influence of dietary factors on aluminum absorption and retention in the brain and bone of rats. *Acta Pharmacol. Toxicol.* 56, 331-336.

Slanina, P., Frech, W., Ekstrom, L.G., Slorach, S., and Cedergren, A. (1986): Dietary citric acid enhances absorption of aluminium in antacids. *Clin. Chem.* 32, 539-541.

Walker, J.A., Sherman, R.A., and Cody, R.P. (1990): The effect of oral bases on enteral aluminium absorption. *Arch. Intern. Med.* 150, 2037-2039.

Wilhelm, M., Höhr, D., Abel, J., and Ohnesorge, F.K. (1989): Renal aluminum excretion. *Biol. Trace Elem. Res.* 21, 241-245.

Metal Ions in Biology and Medicine, vol. 2. Eds. J. Anastassopoulou, Ph. Collery, J.C. Etienne, Th. Theophanides. John Libbey Eurotext, Paris © 1992, pp. 377-378

Effects of zinc and copper interactions in rats

Moshe J. Werman, Joseph S. Law, Joseph S. Castro, Sam J. Bhathena

USDA, ARS, BHNRC, Carbohydrate Nutrition Lab. Beltsville, MD 20705, USA

INTRODUCTION

High dietary zinc/copper ratio has been known to have antagonistic effects on copper metabolism (Klevay, 1973) possibly by interfering with intestinal copper absorption (Fischer et al., 1981). In the present study we determine whether the reduction in dietary zinc/copper ratio in copper-deficient rats ameliorates the severity of the symptoms associated with copper deficiency.

METHODS

Forty weanling male Sprague-Dawley rats weighing 45-50 g each were divided into four groups. They were fed ad libitum for five weeks the starch based basal diets (Fields et al., 1983) that were either adequate (6 ppm) or deficient (0.6 ppm) in copper and either low (8 ppm) or adequate (32 ppm) in zinc. Rats were killed by decapitation after an overnight fast. Plasma was separated and liver, heart, pancreas, spleen and testes were excised and stored at -70 C until analyzed. Copper and zinc content in diets and organs were measured by wet and dry ashing (Hill et al., 1986). Plasma glucose, cholesterol, triglycerides (TG), uric acid, alanine aminotransferase (ALAT) and aspartate aminotransferase (ASAT) were measured by enzymatic methods using the automated Centrifichem system. Plasma insulin, adrenocorticotrophic hormone (ACTH), growth hormone (GH), somatomedin-C and corticosterone were determined by radioimmunoassay.

RESULTS

Regardless of dietary zinc levels, rats fed low copper diet exhibited classical symptoms of copper deficiency namely: nondetectable plasma ceruloplasmin activity, reduced hematocrit levels, reduced body weight, pancreatic atrophy, and enlarged liver, heart and testes. In addition, regardless of dietary zinc intake, copper concentrations in liver, heart, spleen, testes and pancreas were significantly lower in rats fed the low copper diets as compared to those fed the copper-adequate diets. However, copper levels tended to be higher in copper-deficient rats fed low zinc than those fed high zinc levels. In contrast, pancreatic copper content in copper-deficient rats was further decreased when the rats were fed the low zinc diet. Among the tissues examined, only the pancreas exhibited reduced zinc content in rats fed the low zinc diets. Regardless of dietary zinc levels, all copper-deficient rats showed increased plasma cholesterol levels and ASAT activity (Table 1). Neither dietary copper levels nor zinc levels altered plasma ALAT activity, glucose, TG, uric acid, insulin, somatomedin-C and corticosterone levels. Regardless of dietary copper levels, rats fed the low zinc diet exhibited lower levels of plasma ACTH and GH as compared to the rats fed the zinc-adequate diets (Table 1).

Table 1- Weight gain, hematocrit and plasma indices of rats fed diets deficient or adequate in copper and low or adequate in zinc.

Dietary Regimen				Plasma parameters				
Copper (mg/kg	Zinc diet)	Wt gain (g)	Hemato (%)	Cerulop (U/L)	Cholest (mg/dL)	ASAT (IU/L)	GH (mg/ml)	ACTH (pg/ml)
6	32	265±15	47±2	107± 7	78±14	131±21	1.5±0.3	124±54
6	8	254±22	45±3	110±11	84±14	115±18	1.3±0.6	98±28
0.6	32	246±19	32±5	nondetected	104±11	156±29	1.7±0.3	103±29
0.6	8	225±32	32±7	nondetected	95±16	137±34	0.9±0.6	82±25
				ANOVA				
Cu		0.0024	0.0001	0.0001	0.0002	0.0082	NS	NS
Zn		0.03	NS	NS	NS	NS	0.02	0.05
Cu*Zn		NS	NS	NS	NS	NS	NS	NS

DISCUSSION

The classical symptoms of copper deficiency observed in this study are in agreement with previous ones (Fields et al., 1983). It is well known that the severity of copper deficiency vary according to the degree and duration of copper deficiency, age, sex, type of dietary carbohydrate source (Fields, 1985) and mineral intake, especially high zinc (Fischer et al., 1981). It has been suggested that zinc antagonizes copper absorption by inducing the synthesis of intestinal thionein that binds newly ingested copper, making it unavailable for metabolism (Oestreicher & Cousins, 1985). Thus, a low zinc intake may increase the absorption of dietary copper. However, lowering the amount of dietary zinc by 4 fold in a copper-deficient diet in order to obtain a low zinc/copper ratio had no beneficial effect on the symptoms of copper deficiency observed in the present study. The data show that the absolute dietary levels of copper and zinc rather than their ratio are important in maintaining normal metabolism.

REFERENCES

Fields, M. (1985): Newer understanding of copper metabolism. Internal Med. 6:91-98.

Fields, M., Ferretti, R.J., Smith, J.C. & Reiser, S. (1983): Effect of copper deficiency on metabolism and mortality in rats fed sucrose or starch diets. J. Nutr. 113:1335-1345.

Fischer, P.W.F., Giroux, A. & L'Abbe, M.R. (1981): The effect of dietary zinc on intestinal copper absorption. Am. J. Clin. Nutr. 34:1670-1675.

Hill, A.D., Patterson, K.Y., Veillon, C. & Morris, E.R. (1986): Digestion of biological material for mineral analysis using a wet and dry ashing. Anal. Chem. 58:2340-2342.

Klevay, L.M. (1973): Hypercholesterolemia in rats produced by an increase in the ratio of zinc to copper ingested. Am. J. Clin. Nutr. 26:1060-1068.

Oestreicher, P. & Cousins, R.J. (1985): Copper and zinc absorption in the rat. Mechanism of mutual antagonism. J. Nutr. 115:159-166.

Metal Ions in Biology and Medicine, vol. 2. Eds. J. Anastassopoulou, Ph. Collery, J.C. Etienne, Th. Theophanides. John Libbey Eurotext, Paris © 1992, pp. 379-380

Copper, chromium and zinc content of foods and diet in a spanish population

M. Schuhmacher, J.L. Domingo, J.M. Llobet, J. Corbella

Laboratory of Toxicology and Biochemistry, School of Medicine, University of Barcelona, San Lorenzo 21, 43201 Reus, Spain

Heavy metals are widely distributed in the environment and it is inevitable that traces of metals can be detected in virtually all plant and animal organisms, and hence in our food. In addition, pollutants discharged into the environment elevate metal concentrations and may ocassionally cause local poisoning accidents. Because of for most people the main route of exposure to heavy metals is through the diet, information about dietary intake is important in assessing risks to human health for heavy metals (Horiguchi *et al.*, 1978).

Copper, chromium, zinc, and their compounds play an important role in many fields of modern industry. Moreover, these elements are also essentials to our health. The aim of the present work was to determine copper, chromium and zinc content in common basic items of the major food groups, as well as to calculate the daily intake of these metals by the population from Tarragona Province, an important industrial and agricultural area of Catalonia (NE, Spain). The north of the Province is basically industrial, whereas the south is essentially agricultural, with an additional important commercial fishing industry in both areas.

MATERIALS AND METHODS

Dietary intake of metals from foods was determined according to two different methods: the total diet study and the duplicate diet study. In the total diet study, a total of 376 food samples from various locations of Tarragona Province were analyzed. The diet was divided into ten groups according to previous studies: meats, fish and seafood, eggs, pulses, cereals, vegetables, roots and tubers, fruits, milk and derivatives, and drinks (Salas *et al.*, 1985; Schuhmacher *et al.*, 1991). For the duplicate diet study, 20 families living in Tarragona Province provided a duplicate of the whole part of their weekly diets. After digestion of food samples, chromium and zinc concentrations were determined by AAS, whereas copper levels were measured by ICP. Chromium, copper, and zinc recoveries were assessed by analyses of Bovine Liver, National Bureau of Standards (SRM 1577) (Bosque *et al.*, 1990; Schuhmacher *et al.*, 1990; 1991).

RESULTS AND DISCUSSION

Pulses was the group with the highest levels of the three metals, while cereals and meat (chromium); cereals, and roots and tubers (copper), and meat (zinc) were also food groups with remarkable contents of these elements. In contrast, vegetables and fruits which are basic foods in the *mediterranean diet*, showed low concentrations of copper, chromium and zinc. The total daily intakes of copper, chromium and zinc by the population of Tarragona Province are shown in Table 1. Total intakes of copper, chromium and zinc were respectively 1156.3 μg/day, 124.6 μg/day, and 7522.9 μg/day, whereas the total intakes obtained through the duplicate diet study were 1119.8 μg/day for copper, 129.0 μg/day for chromium, and 6800.1 μg/day for zinc.

TABLE 1. Food consumption and intake of copper, chromium and zinc by food groups in Tarragona Province, Catalonia, (NE Spain)

Food group	Consumption (kg/day)	Copper intake (μg/day)	Chromium intake (μg/day)	Zinc intake (μg/day)
Meat	0.210	113.0	41.3	4136.9
Fish and seafood	0.063	32.4	9.5	505.1
Eggs	0.041	20.5	5.1	363.8
Pulses	0.017	281.6	5.2	348.2
Cereals	0.170	346.4	34.4	1273.0
Green vegetables	0.155	123.8	10.8	441.9
Roots and tubers	0.990	138.3	5.1	267.1
Fruits	0.170	89.2	4.7	10.9
Milk and derivatives	0.124	1.2	4.2	176.0
Drinks	0.048[a]	9.9	4.3	ND
Total intake	**1.988**	**1156.3**	**124.6**	**7522.9**

[a]l/day. ND: not detected.

The results found through both methods were very similar for copper and chromium, with a relatively small difference for zinc. The daily intakes of copper and zinc by the inhabitants of Tarragona Province were usually lower than those reported for different countries (Horiguchi *et al.*, 1978), and were even lower than the recommended mean values (WHO/FAO). The daily oral intakes for chromium were more similar to the previously reported values, and would be closer to the recommended values (WHO/FAO).

Acknowledgements. This work was supported by the Tarragona County Council, Catalonia, Spain.

REFERENCES

Bosque, M.A., Schuhmacher, M., Domingo, J.L., and Llobet, J.M. (1990): Concentrations of lead and cadmium in edible vegetables from Tarragona Province, Spain. *Sci. Total Environ.* 95: 61-67.

Horiguchi, S., Teramoto, K., Kurono, T., Ninomiya, K. (1978): An attemp at comparative estimate of daily intake of several metals (As, Cu, Pb, Mn, Zn) from foods in thirty countries in the world. *Osaka City Med. J.* 24: 237-242.

Salas, J., Font, I., Canals, J., Guinovart, L., Sospedra, C., and Martí-Hennenberg, C. (1985): Consumption, nutritional habits and nutritional status of the population from Reus. *Med. Clin.* 84: 423-427.

Schuhmacher, M., Bosque, M.A., Domingo, J.L., and Corbella, J. (1990): Lead and cadmium concentrations in marine organisms from the Tarragona coastal waters, Spain. *Bull. Environ. Contam. Toxicol.* 44: 784-789.

Schuhmacher, M., Bosque, M.A., Domingo, J.L., and Corbella, J. (1991): Dietary intake of lead and cadmium from foods in Tarragona Province, Spain. *Bull. Environ. Contam. Toxicol.* 46: 320-328.

7 EPIDEMIOLOGY

Metal Ions in Biology and Medicine, vol. 2. Eds. J. Anastassopoulou, Ph. Collery, J.C. Etienne, Th. Theophanides. John Libbey Eurotext, Paris © 1992, pp. 383-388

Methodological prerequisites and systematical approach to the study of magnesium supplementation in marginal magnesium deficiency

J. Durlach*, V. Durlach**, Y. Rayssiguier***, M. Bara****, A. Guiet-Bara****

**Président SDRM, Hôpital St. Vincent-de-Paul, Paris, 64, rue de Longchamp, F-92200 Neuilly, France. **Clinique Médicale U 52, Reims, France. ***Laboratoire des Maladies Métaboliques, INRA Theix, Ceyrat, France. ****Laboratoire de Biologie de la Reproduction, Université P. et M. Curie, Paris, France.*

INTRODUCTION

Magnesium, the second most abundant intra-cellular cation is a catalytic and structural element of major importance in the human organism. Necessary for the anatomical and functional integrity of various subcellular organelles, it participates in all the major metabolic pathways. It is involved in the regulation of ion metabolisms and in processes of defense i.e. in thermoregulation. Present in all tissues, it participates in the physiology of all systems : neuromuscular, nephrocardiovascular and endocrine particularly (1,2). The main new trends as regards magnesium in health and disease consist in developing protocols of cooperative epidemiological studies of magnesium supplementation in disorders due to magnesium marginal deficiency. These studies appear as the most convincing tool to define the clinical forms of magnesium marginal deficiency in human beings.
But several methodological prerequisites are requested for developing such protocols (3). An approach to the study of the effects of magnesium supplementation in marginal magnesium deficiency should always take into account the established clinical pattern of chronic magnesium deficiency (1,3,4).

1. METHODOLOGICAL PREREQUISITES

Epidemiological trials through oral physiological magnesium supplementation only concern chronic marginal magnesium deficiency. That is why it is necessary to distinguish between the 2 types of magnesium deficits: magnesium deficiency and magnesium depletion between the consequences of chronic marginal magnesium deficiency and of acute magnesium deficiency and also between the diagnostic values of the clinical efficiency of oral and parenteral magnesium load. We will successively analyse these 3 prerequisites.

1.1. Differential diagnosis between magnesium deficiency and magnesium depletion (1,4,5)

In the case of magnesium deficiency, the disorder corresponds to an insufficient magnesium intake: it merely requires oral physiological magnesium supplementation. In the case of magnesium depletion the disorder which induces magnesium deficit is related to a dysregulation of the control mechanisms of magnesium metabolism: either failure of the mechanisms which insure magnesium homeostasis or intervention of endogenous or iatrogenic perturbating factors of magnesium status. Magnesium depletion requires more or less specific correction of its causal dysregulation. Epidemiological trial through oral physiological magnesium supplementation only concerns magnesium deficiency.

1.2. Difference between consequences of chronic marginal and acute magnesium deficiency
Experimental (6) and clinical (1,3,4) forms of chronic magnesium deficiency are better and better identified. But they differ from overt signs of acute deficiency (1,4,5,6,7).
Epidemiological studies of the effects of physiological oral magnesium supplementation should only concern consequences of chronic marginal magnesium deficiency. Large prevalence of the expression of marginal magnesium deficiency in human beings (15 to 20% of the population) seems consistent with the estimation of nutrient deficiency using probability analysis in population where the mean magnesium daily intake is slightly above 4mg/kg/day versus Mg RDA set at 6mg/kg/day (7).

1.3. Significance of magnesium parenteral load and oral magnesium supplementation (1,3-7)
Clinical efficiency of parenteral magnesium administration should not be used as a diagnostic tool attesting to magnesium deficiency. Its pharmacological effects are observed irrespective of magnesium status. Reversely physiological oral doses of magnesium are totally devoid of the pharmacodynamic effects of parenteral magnesium and without clinical effects when magnesium status is normal. Correction of symptoms by this oral magnesium load constitutes the best proof that they were due to magnesium deficiency.

After these 3 prerequisites have been taken into consideration, it is necessary to correctly study the effects of magnesium supplementation in cooperative epidemiological trials to have a good knowledge of the complete record of all the clinical and paraclinical patterns of chronic magnesium deficiency.

2. CLINICAL AND PARACLINICAL PATTERNS OF CHRONIC MAGNESIUM DEFICIENCY

2.1. Open and controlled trials have established the clinical and paraclinical pattern of chronic magnesium deficiency (CMD) (1,3,4,8). Whatever the age nervous consequences can be first studied: clinical and paraclinical symptoms of latent tetany (hyperventilation syndrome, chronic fatigue syndrome, spasmophilia, cryptotetany) with or more often without "idiopathic" mitral valve prolapse (idiopathic Barlow's disease, Da Costa syndrome, soldier's heart, effort syndrome, neurocirculatory asthenia) with or without pseudo-allergy (through peripheral hyperreceptivity) more often than allergy (type I mainly).The non-specific pattern of this symptomatology brings the patient to consult a wide range of specialists as well as general practitioner. It includes non-specific central, peripheral and autonomic manifestations.
The neurotic, or rather, "central" symptoms consist of anxiety, hyperemotionality, fatigue, headaches (and sometimes migraine), insomnia, light-headedness, dizziness, nervous fits, lipothymiae, sensation of a "lump in the throat", of "nuchalgia" and "blocked breathing".

The peripheral signs are acroparaesthesiae, cramps, muscle fasciculations and myalgiae.
The functional disorders include chest pain, sine materia dyspnoea, blocked respiration, precordialgia, palpitations, extrasystolae, dysrhythmias, Raynaud's syndrome, trends to orthostatic hypotension or conversely to borderline hypertension. In fact, the dysautonomic disturbances involve both the sympathetic and the parasympathetic systems.
When the chest pain mimics coronary heart disease, its relief with propranolol and worsening by nitrates may help to distinguish between a benign disorder and a trouble from coronary origin.
The evolution may be studded with various acute paroxymal manifestations which can also sometimes be seen as initial signs of the illness. The major crises of acute tetany or of grand mal -even reduced to a simple loss of consciousness- remain relatively rare. It is more often a question of nervous crises: neurotic, from the "attack of nerves" to the"hysterical crises", or autonomic: lipothymia, reactive hypoglycaemia, pseudo-asthmatic crisis, vagovagal syncope or, on the contrary, paroxysmal tachycardia. Sometimes, centripetal tingling sensations and stiffness of the extremities confer on these nervous crisis a tetanoid character. But, essentially, they all have in common the fact that they occur in a context of fits of anxiety, even sometimes with the impression of imminent death (panic attack), which cause hyperventilation gaseous alkalosis and self perpetuation of the crises.
Physical examination must systematically research the signs of neuromuscular hyperexcitability as well the Chvostek's sign as precordial signs of mitral dyskinesia inducing mitral valve prolapse.
A genuine Chvostek's sign must be systematically sought. With a small (children's) reflex hammer the examiner percusses the soft parts of the cheek at the centre of a line running from ear lobe to the labial commissure, avoiding the lightning contraction of a "false Chvostek's sign" by tapping the bone of the zygomatic apophysis. It is important to consider the quality -and not the intensity- of this clinical criterion of neuromuscular hyperexcitability. It is only its presence or its absence which is significant, respectively quoted 1 or 0.
The examination of the precordial area will be carefully conducted in order to search either for a non-ejection systolic click, or for a mid -to end- systolic or pansystolic murmur, or both, particularly in orthostatism in complete expiration and in the left lateral decubitus position.
Two routine tracings should always be made: a neurophysiological examination (electromyogram (EMG)) and a cardiological examination (echocardiogram (ECC)).
In EMG testing for latent tetany, a Bronck's needle is inserted into the first dorsal interosseous muscle of the left hand. The three classical facilitation tests are used: tourniquet-induced ischaemia lasting 10 min, post-ischaemia lasting 10 min after removal of tourniquet and lastly hyperventilation lasting 5 min. If the EMG shows one (or several) train (s) of autorhythmic activities, "beating" for more than 2 min of one of the three tetanic activities (uniplets, multiplets or complex tonicoclonic tracings) a positive response is defined. As determined for the clinical criterion of tetanic hyperexcitability, this neurophysiological criterion is only considered as a two-class variable. Either its presence or its absence is significant, respectively quoted 1 or 0.
The "excitability index" (EI) is defined as the sum of the two cri-

teria of tetany. It allows different classes among tetanies to be distinguished: one with simultaneous clinical and neurophysiological criteria: EI=2, the others with only one criterion of their tetanic state: EI=1 with two sub-groups, either clinical (through positivity of the Chvostek's sign alone), or electromyographic (through positivity of EMG alone).
The ECC is the best tool for detecting mitral valve prolapse (MVP). With time-motion (TM) mode, three tracings are classical: a "cuplike" tracing of mesotelesystolic MVP (of more than 2 mm), a "hammocking" tracing of holosystolic MVP (of more than 3 mm), an isolated systolic anterior motion (SAM) observed without obstruction nor any septal thickening sign and in the absence of false systolic anterior motion. Two-dimensional echocardiography appears to be more accurate than TM echocardiography. It eliminates a number of artefacts and, particularly, in the section of parasternal longitudinal cut and the apical cut of the four heart chamber. The criterion for mitral prolapse is the billowing of one or both leaflets below the level of the mitral ring. It is very important to assess the leaflet thickness as well as its whole morphology and to appreciate the ventricualr kinetic by calculating:

$$\Delta D = \frac{\text{end diastolic diameter} - \text{end systolic diameter}}{\text{end diastolic diameter}}$$

Pulsed doppler echocardiography allows the detection of associated mitral regurgitation.
Four routine ionic investigations should always be made: plasma Mg (pMg), erythrocyte Mg (eMg), calcaemia and daily calciuria, which can be completed by the research of proteinuria and of urinary infection.
These must first demonstrate normocalcaemia and the absence of hypercalciuria susceptible to induce a secondary magnesium deficit. Next, the evaluation of pMg and eMg with reliable methods, such as atomic absorption spectrophotometry, allows the diagnosis of primary magnesium deficit through hypomagnesaemia in one-third of the cases of latent tetany (LT) due to CMD, with or without MVP. Normal levels do not rule out the diagnosis of CMD. The histograms of LT patients (with or without MVP) and of controls overlap. If the tetanic group reveals gaussian-type magnesaemia curves with significant lower means ($P < 0.001$) both for pMg and eMg, their constitutive elements can be individually hypomagnesaemic (one-third of the cases), normomagnesaemic (almost two-thirds of the cases) and even, although seldom, hypermagnesaemic. Nevertheless one must emphasize the remarkable constancy of magnesaemia which lends importance even to small variations of magnesaemia.
Lymphocyte Mg/cell appears as the most interesting static intra-cellular magnesium item (9).
In particular clinical forms, record should be completed with corresponding clinical and paraclinical explorations. Rhinoscopy in rhinitis, skin tests with not only allergens but also with histamine, acetylcholine and plasma IgE in allergic or pseudo-allergic forms, electroencephalogram and head scan in convulsive forms, psychometric investigations in psychic forms, electronystagmogram and optokinetic test in dizziness, electropolygraphic study of afternoon sleep in dyssomnia, lipid profile in atheromatous dyslipidemias (10).

2.2. Several risk populations require special attention
Pregnant women because of the consequences of deficiency on mother, foetus, neonate and infant (2) and infants born from diabetic mother, (2). Geriatic (11) and sport (12) populations where magnesium deficiency is most often associated with magnesium depletion.
Reversely urinary lithiasis is not a form of marginal magnesium deficiency. Magnesium supplementation has been used in this indication through pharmacological intervention on crystallization factor (1).

2.3. Oral physiological magnesium supplementation
Effect of oral physiological magnesium supplementation is the best tool for establishing the diagnosis of magnesium deficiency.
The magnesium supplementation included in the protocols of cooperative epidemiological studies on the importance of the consequences of marginal magnesium deficiency will not only be studied on extra- and intra-cellular magnesium parameters, but also on all the clinical and paraclinical items. For example stigma of neuromuscular hyperexcitability should be integrated in the protocol of magnesium supplementation concerning allergic, vascular, aging or sport populations.
Magnesium supplementation must not modify energy intake. Soluble magnesium salt in water will be used, with its anion (acid or Na salt) as control (8).
The proper place of magnesium marginal deficiency in the etiopathogeny of diseases will be thus rightly assessed.

CONCLUSION

It is important 1. to identify among the various forms of magnesium deficit those corresponding to a magnesium deficiency,
2. to distinguish between the manifestation of chronic and acute magnesium deficiency,
3. to appreciate the particular diagnostic value of oral physiological magnesium supplementation.

Such are the 3 prerequisites to an adequate systematical approach to epidemiologic intervention trials which only concern chronic marginal magnesium deficiency.
There should be a follow up of the effects of the physiological oral magnesium supplementation not only on magnesium items but also on all the well-know -but non-specific- clinical and paralcinical signs. Its specific efficiency should contribute to highlight the importance of the clinical forms of chronic marginal magnesium deficiency.

REFERENCES

1. Durlach, J. (1988): Magnesium in clinical practice. John Libbey publ. London, pp.360.
2. Durlach, J., Durlach, V., Rayssiguier, Y., Ricquier, D., Goubern, M., Bertin, R., Bara, M., Guiet-Bara, A., Olive, G. and Mettey, R. (1991): Magnesium and thermoregulation. I. Newborn and infant. Is the sudden unexpected infant death syndrome a magnesium-dependent disease of the transition from chemical to physical thermoregulation? Magnesium Res. 4: 137-152.

3. Durlach, J. (1991): Magnesium: clinical forms of primary magnesium deficiency. In: Modern life-styles, lower energy intake and micronutrient status. Ed. Pietrzik K. Springer Verl. London, Berlin, N.-Y., chap. 13: 156-167.
4. Durlach, J., Durlach, V., Rayssiguier, Y., Bara, M.and Guiet-Bara, A. (1991): Recent advances on magnesium in health. Magnesium Res. 4: 204-205.
5. Durlach, J. (1988): Magnesium, a brief historical account. Magnesium Res. 1: 91-96.
6. Kubena, K.S. and Durlach, J. (1990): Historical review of marginal intake of magnesium in chronic experimental magnesium deficiency. Magnesium Res. 3: 219-226.
7. Durlach, J. (1989): Recommended dietary amounts of magnesium: Mg RDA. Magnesium Res. 2: 195-203.
8. Durlach, J. (1992): Chronic fatigue syndrome and chronic primary magnesium deficiency. Magnesium Res. 5: ...-...
9. Durlach, V., Millart, H., Meyer, L., Grulet, H., Gross, A. and Leutenneger, M. (1991): Magnesium status in a group of so-called "spasmophilic" patients. Magnesium Res. 4: 233-234.
10 Durlach, J., Durlach, V., Rayssiguier, Y., Bara, M. and Guiet-Bara, A. (1991): Magnesium and blood pressure. II. Clinical studies (abs.). Magnesium Res. 4: 236.
11 Rayssiguier, Y., Durlach, J., Guiet-Bara A. and Bara, M. (1990): Aging and Magnesium status. In: Metal ions in Biology and Medicine. Eds P. Collery, L.A. Poirier, M. Manfait and J.C. Etienne, John Libbey-Eurotext publ. Paris: 62-66.
12 Rayssiguier, Y., Guezennec, C.Y. and Durlach, J. (1990): New experimental and clinical data on the relationship between magnesium and sport. Magnesium-Res. 3: 93-102.

Metal Ions in Biology and Medicine, vol. 2. Eds. J. Anastassopoulou, Ph. Collery, J.C. Etienne, Th. Theophanides. John Libbey Eurotext, Paris © 1992, pp. 389-394

Public health aspects of trace elements in developing countries

Mohamed Abdulla*, Robert Parr**, Fatima Reis***

Department of Clinical Pharmacology and Therapeutics, Hamdard University, New Delhi 110062, India, International Atomic Energy Agency, A-1400 Vienna**, Austria and LNETI-ICEN-DEEN, Estrada Nacional No. 10, 2685 Sacavem***, Portugal*

INTRODUCTION

During the last few decades, remarkable progress has occurred in the field of trace element research. Recent estimates indicate that most tissues of a living organism contain 40-80 macro and trace elements (Abdulla, Sarkar & Dashti, 1989).Many more trace elements than previously considered essential in human and animal nutrition play crucial role in metabolic processes. At the same time, there is also a growing recognition of the adverse effects of cumulative exposure to small amounts of heavy metals and to large amounts of essential elements. Rapid advances in analytical technology and sophisticated instrumentation introduced during the last few decades have not only helped to recognize the presence of trace elements in living systems and their food chain, but have also added a new dimension to our understanding of their role in health and disease.

The nutritional importance of trace elements has grown rapidly during the last 50 years mainly due to a better understanding of their biological functions.In deficiency states, most trace elements that are known to be essential create health problems. Iron deficiency anemia and goiter are good examples. In terms of people afflicted, the above disorders are close to populations suffering from protein-energy malnutrition. Although starvation and malnutrition are restricted to certain poverty-stricken areas of the world, it has become clearly evident that a sub-clinical deficiency of several minerals and trace elements is fairly common even in affluent countries (Abdulla,1983; Abdulla *et al.*, 1981, 1984; Abdulla, 1986, 1988; Mertz, 1981, 1989; Bruce, 1984).

Except for iodine and iron, trace element nutrition in general has a low priority in developing countries. One reason for this development is the fact that other trace element deficiencies have no characteristic signs and symptoms. From a public health point of view, it is important to assure the general population that the intake of essential trace elements is adequate to meet the requirements. At the same time, the intake of toxic heavy metals must not exceed the permitted levels. It is seldom that these issues are taken up seriously in developing countries by public health authorities. The developing countries that are industrializing in semi-tropical and tropical regions face a long agenda of health problems and as such priorities are given only to issues related to starvation and infectious diseases. Moreover, it is a common belief that the minimum requirements of many essential trace elements are so low that a pure nutritional deficiency rarely occurs in the general population. This paper will discuss some of these important issues with special reference to the population living in developing countries.

RECOMMENDATIONS, METHODOLOGICAL PROBLEMS AND CURRENT INTAKES

Recommendations

One of the basic requirements of nutritional research concerned with trace element nutrition is the knowledge concerning the true intake levels from prepared meals consumed during 24 hours. Barring occupational exposure, the major pathway through which the trace elements enter the human body is via the food chain. Although most of the trace elements in individual food items can be accurately measured today, there is no reliable data for the minimum requirement of several trace elements. One reason for this situation is due to the lack of information concerning the dietary habits. Only limited information is available at present concerning the intake of essential and toxic trace elements from daily diets in developing countries. Without such information, the public health and clinical significance of trace elements cannot be assessed adequately.

Nutritional requirements of trace elements may be influenced by a series of factors related to health, environmental circumstances, and growth and final adult size. The present recommendations that is widely accepted throughout the world is applicable only to healthy populations eating an all-round diet with a relatively high proportion of dairy and meat products. Populations living in the developing world have usually lower body weights and energy intakes. Moreover, diseases in the gastrointestinal tract in tropical and semi-tropical countries may affect the absorption and excretion of a number of trace elements. This in turn may affect the daily requirements. The current recommended dietary allowance (RDA,1980) levels may therefore become unrealistic in developing countries when all these factors are taken into consideration.

According to Beaton (1988) the recommended daily intakes (RDI) should be defined in terms of "basal" and "normative" requirements. <u>Basal requirement</u> is the amount of a trace element needed to prevent a clinically demonstrable impairment of function without any body reserves. <u>Normative storage requirement</u> is the amount of a trace element required to maintain a reserve in the tissues. This reserve can be mobilized to meet essential needs without detectable impairment of function. It has been suggested that the RDIs as previously defined should henceforth be referred to as the safe level of intake. Table I shows the RDIs that exist for a few trace elements.

Methodological Considerations

Information on the dietary intake of trace elements by individuals or groups can be obtained by a number of direct and indirect techniques. Only direct analysis of the actual food consumed during a 24-hour period can provide actual estimate of the dietary intake of trace elements. All other techniques used for the estimation of trace elements have limitations. In order to make valid intake estimates, one should use a combination of techniques (Isacsson, 1980; Varo, 1988). The final choice, however, depends on the available resources. Table II summarizes the various techniques that are commonly used for the estimation of trace element intakes.

Table I. Recommended Daily intake (RDI) of a few trace elements for adults*

Element	Intake Value/day	Remarks
Chromium	50 - 200 μg	estimated safe and adequate intake
Copper	2 - 3 mg	estimated safe and adequate intake
Iron	10 - 18 mg	recommended dietary allowance (RDA)
Iodine	150 μg	RDA
Selenium	50 - 200 μg	estimated safe and adequate intake
Zinc	15 mg	RDA

* For children, adolescents, pregnant and lactating women, the RDI can be different (WHO,1983). The latest recommendations by WHO/FAO/IAEA will be different from these figures. The new recommendations would be available during the end of 1992.

As can be observed from Table II, most techniques have both advantages as well as disadvantages. The data available from developing countries is often based on indirect techniques such as the 24-hour recall. In this technique, the subject participating in the study is asked to recall the types and amounts of food which have been eaten during the past 24 hours. This is a typical retrospective method. It is customary to interpret data from the recall method using standard food tables. Food tables in many developing countries have no data for many trace elements including selenium, chromium and manganese. For toxic elements, there is no information at all. The intakes reported in several developing countries for iron and zinc are often much higher than the true intake from prepared meals (Abdulla, 1986). The health authorities in these often make recommendations based on the scanty information that is available in the country on intake levels. Collection of true data concerning the intake of essential and toxic elements is one of the crucial task of nutrition teams in developing countries.

REPORTED INTAKES OF ESSENTIAL AND TOXIC TRACE ELEMENTS

Based on literature published during the last 20 years, the daily intake of a few selected trace elements for adults are shown in table III. In addition, results from an on-going international atomic energy agency (IAEA) research program on the dietary intake of minor and major trace elements are shown for comparison purposes (Parr *et al.*, 1990, Parr, 1990).

Table II. Methods for the assessment of trace element intakes and sources of errors.

Method	Sources of Errors*	Suitability
Direct methods		
a) Precise weighing b) Market basket c) Duplicate portion	sampling and analytical errors; day to day variation	suited for the estimation of most essential and toxic metals
Indirect methods		
a) Food balance sheets b) Household surveys c) 24-hour and 7-day recall d) dietary dairies; unweighed records e) Weighed intake studies	addition & omission; amount and frequency; food composition table errors	suited for the estimation of macronutrients; unreliable for trace elements; suited for large scale studies
Biological markers		
a) Blood/plasma/serum b) Urine c) Faces d) Hair e) Nail f) specific cell lines g) tissues	invasive: contamination risks; expensive; requires good laboratory facilities	Not suitable for all essential and toxic elements, good for a few elements such as iodine and selenium

* An error likely to occur

Table III. Intake of a few selected trace elements from the global and IAEA study (median values)

Element	daily intake (global data)	IAEA study (11 countries)	unit
Copper	1.5	1,5	mg
Manganese	3.3	5.6	mg
Selenium	51	61	µg
Zinc	9.9	9.8	mg

The results concerning the intake levels of other essential minerals and trace elements are also being computed. The final results of the IAEA study is being completed. When compared with the current recommended levels, the intakes are low for several elements, especially for potassium, magnesium, iron, zinc and selenium. The intake of toxic elements are shown in table IV.

Table IV. Dietary intake of toxic trace elements (median; range)

Element	daily intake (global data)	IAEA study (11 countries)	unit
Aluminum	3.9 (2.3-14)	3.9 - 21	mg
Arsenic	36 (4 - 81)	5.0 - 380	µg
Cadmium	14 (8 -198)	10 - 31	µg
Lead	48 (3 -514)	50 - 340	µg
Mercury	3.8 (0.7-60)	10 - 140	µg

In developing countries, exposure from toxic metals such as lead can be a very serious problem. The levels of pollution of the environment and the adulteration of foodstuffs is almost beyond comprehension.Most capital cities of the developing world are highly polluted. In many cities in India, the air pollution is three times that of the permitted limits. The number of cars, motorcycles and other modes of transport has gone up. In Delhi, for example, about 12 million tons of suspended particles, hydrocarbons, sulphurdioxide, arbonmonoxide and other poisonous gases are spewed into the air. Surveys have been carried out by government agencies, but little has been done concerning the direct effects of pollution on the health of the general population. A recent study in Karachi, Pakistan shows lead levels in the blood of adults almost thrice as that of European populations (40 µg/l) and in children somewhat lower (Manser & Khan, 1989; Buchet *et al.*, 1983). Similar figures are reported from India (Grover, 1989). The use of leaded petrol and uncontrolled emission of exhaust fumes are the major contributing factors for these high levels. The consumption of illicit liquors and food and drinks stored in vessels containing lead are other sources of lead contamination. The high dietary lead intake can interfere with the absorption of other trace elements such as zinc and iron. Clearly much work remains to be done in this area.

REFERENCES

Abdulla, M., Andersson, I., Asp, N-G. *et al.* (1981): Nutrient intake and health status of vegans. Am. J. Clin. Nutr. 34: 11, 2464-2477.

Abdulla, M. (1983): Public health/clinical significance of inorganic chemical elements. In *Nutritional adequacy, nutrient availability and needs*, ed. J. Mauron, pp. 338-355. Basel, Boston, Stuttgart: Birkhauser Verlag.

Abdulla, M., Ally, K-O, Andersson, I. *et al.* (1984): Nutrient intake and health status of lactovegetarians: chemical analyses of diets using the duplicate portion technique. Am. J. Clin. Nutr. 40, 325-338.

Abdulla, M. (1986): Inorganic chemical elements in prepared meals in Sweden. Ph.D. dissertation, University of Lund, Sweden, pp. 6-127.

Abdulla, M. (1988): Nutritional aspects of trace elements. In *Recent progress on trace elements in nutrition*, ed. Y. Itokawa, R. Kawashima, Y. Kotake, T. Matsuno, A. Misaki, Y. Ohta, K. Soda & K. Yamaguchi, pp.71-77. Japan: Trace Nutrient Research Society.

Abdulla, M, Sarkar B. and Dashti, H. (1989); Preface. In *Metabolism of minerals and trace elements in human diseas*, ed. M. Abdulla, H. Dashti, B. Sarkar, H. Al-Sayer & N. Al-Naqeeb, pp. V-V1.London, Tokyo: Smith Gordon, John Libbey, Nishimura.

Beaton, G. (1988): Nutrient Requirements and population data. Proc. Nutr. Soc. 47, 63-78.

Bruce, A. (1984): Selenium in human nutrition and medicine. J. Royal Swed. Acad. Agr. Forestry. 123, 267-271.

Buchet, J.P., Lauwerys, R., Vandervoorde, A. and Pycke, J.M. (1983): Intake of cadmium, lead, manganese, copper, chromium, mercury, calcium, zinc and arsenic in Belgium; a duplicate study. Food Chem. Toxicol. 21:1, 19-24.

Grover, J.K. (1989): Toxicological study of lead in spray paint workers. In *Metabolism of minerals and trace elements*, ed. M. Abdulla, B. Sarkar, H. Dsahti, H. Alsayer & N. Al-Naqeeb. pp. 95-98. London, Tokyo: Smith Gordon; John Libbey; Nishimura.

Isaksson, B. (1980): Urinary nitrogen output as a validity test in dietary surveys. Am. J. Clin. Nutr. 33, 4-12.

Manser, W.T. and Khan A. (1989): Pollution problem in Karachi. In *Metabolism of minerals and trace elements in human disease*, ed. M. Abdulla, H. Dashit, B. Sarkar, H. Al-Sayer, N. Al-Naqeeb, pp. 103-110. London, U.K.: Smith Gordon; Nishimura.

Mertz, W. (1981): The essential trace elements. Science. 213, 1332-1338.

Mertz, W.(1989): Trace element requirements and current recommendations. In *Current trends in trace elements research*, ed. G. Chazot, M. Abdulla & P. Arnad. pp.1-6. London; Tokyo: Smith Gordon; Nishimura.

Parr, R.M. (1990): Recommended dietary intakes of trace elements: Some observations on their definition and interpretation in comparison with actual levels of dietary intake. In *Trace elements in clinical medicine*, ed. H. Tomita, pp. 325-331. Tokyo: Springer-Verlag.

Parr, R.M., Abdulla, M. *et al.* (1990): Dietary intakes of trace elements and related nutrients in elevan countries: Preliminary results from an IAEA-coordinated research program. Paper persented at TEMA-7 meeting in Dubrovnik, Yugoslavia.

Prassad, A.S., Halsted, J.A., and Nadimi, M. (1961): Syndrome of iron deiciency anemia, hypogonadism, dwarfism and geophagia. Am. J. Med. 31, 532-546.

Recommended dietary allowance (RDA, 1980): National Academy of Sciences. 9th edition. Washington, DC.

Varo, P. Althan, G., Ekholm, P., Aro, A. and Koivistoinen, P. (1988): Selenium intake and and serum selenium in Finland: effect of soil fertilization with selenum. Am. J. Clin. Nutr. 48, 324-329.

WHO: (1973): Trace elements in human nutrition. Technical report series No.532, WHO, Geneva.elements and related nutrients in elevan countries: Preliminary results from an IAEA-coordinated research program.

Metal Ions in Biology and Medicine, vol. 2. Eds. J. Anastassopoulou, Ph. Collery, J.C. Etienne, Th. Theophanides. John Libbey Eurotext, Paris © 1992, pp. 395-401

Essential trace metal deficiency and the skeleton

Stanley Wallach, Arthur B. Chausmer

Departments of Internal Medicine and Computer Science, The University of South Florida and the USF College of Medicine, Tampa, FL 33612, USA

INTRODUCTION

Skeletal metabolism encompasses the sum of the processes involved in skeletal development, modeling and remodelling starting during prenatal life and extending to senescence. These processes, which are dependent on bone cell interactions, include endochondral bone formation from a cartilagenous template, intramembranous bone formation, skeletal growth and development (modelling) and finally, remodelling of the adult skeleton. The skeleton accumulates trace metals avidly by virtue of its rich blood supply, large surface area, and unfilled cationic and anionic positions in the crystal lattice of the inorganic hydroxyapatite component. Seven trace elements have been shown to be necessary for normal skeletal metabolism since deficiencies of any of these seven can lead to disruption of osteoblastic and/or osteoclastic function with adverse consequences, as noted in animal and in vitro models. Only two, copper and selenium deficiency, have been clearly implicated in human skeletal diseases, but there are some data suggesting that the other five may play contributing roles in conditions such as osteoporosis. We last reviewed this topic in 1990 (Chausmer 1990) and now wish to update this subject.

BORON

Nielsen and his associates (1990, 1991) have studied the role of boron (B) in mineral and skeletal metabolism extensively, and two recent review articles summarize their findings. Boron deficiency in chicks exacerbates the development of rickets due to a marginal vitamin D intake. Decreased growth, abnormalities of the leg bones, diminished mechanical strength, and an increased serum alkaline phosphatase are observed, and re-feeding B decreases the severity of the rickets and the number of animals affected. In humans, a B deficient diet causes a small but significant decrease in the serum ionized calcium (Ca) and an increase in urinary Ca excretion. The serum 25-hydroxy-vitamin D (calcifediol) level decreases, suggesting that B deficiency in some way reduces vitamin D availability by an unknown mechanism, which might lead to decreased skeletal mineralization, as per the earlier chick experiments. Serum calcitonin and osteocalcin levels increase, possibly as secondary phenomena. These relatively sparse positive data, despite the effort involved in studying B deficiency in animals and humans, suggest a permissive role for B in skeletal metabolism since the effects of B deficiency are only evident in animals who are vitamin D depleted. In the human studies, the actual impact on the skeleton has not been determined.

COPPER

Copper (Cu) plays a key structural and functional role in many enzyme systems, the most important of which relative to the skeleton is lysyloxidase, the enzyme responsible for the pyridinium cross-linkings of the collagen matrix (Chausmer, 1990; Farguharson, 1989; Iguchi, 1990). Lysyloxidase deficiency increases bone collagen solubility and combined other adverse effects of Ca deficiency on osteoblastic function, accounts for the osteopenia, bony fragility, and poor mechanical properties of Cu deficient bone in chick, rabbit, pig, and dog experiments. In the rat, rachitic like changes due to decreased matrix mineralization also occurs, presumably secondary to osteoblast inhibition. Cu deficiency inhibits prostaglandin E_2 induced bone resorption, but has no effect on parathyroid hormone (PTH) stimulated bone resorption.

Two human conditions, infantile Cu deficiency and Menke's syndrome cause osteopenia, bony fragility and fractures. Shaw (1988) has reviewed the skeletal consequences of Cu deficiency in infants due to low birth weight, a Cu deficient diet, and/or the use of total parenteral nutrition devoid of Cu. Schmidt et al (1991) have contributed five recent cases in pre-term infants (25-30 weeks) with Cu deficiency due to a Cu deficient diet. Cu deficient infants manifest osteoporosis, fraying, cupping and spurring of widened epiphyses, subperiosteal hemorrhage with secondary new bone formation, and fractures. Thus, misdiagnoses of accidental injury, child abuse, osteogenesis imperfecta, rickets, and vitamin C deficiency are sometimes made. Careful radiologic examination combined with appropriate biochemical and hematologic studies should permit a diagnosis of Cu deficiency to be made. Cu replenishment usually leads to complete healing of the fractures and partial resolution of the other bony abnormalities. Menke's syndrome is a devastating X-linked genetic disease of boys that poses little problem in diagnosis. Intracellular processing of Cu is defective and is manifested in the skeleton by osteopenia, bone fragility, and occasional fractures. However, the other features of infantile Cu deficiency are not present. Shaw (1988) also mentions a single family with familial Cu deficiency not associated with the extraskeletal features of infantile Cu deficiency or Menke's syndrome but with partial bone changes, and no fractures. These examples are clear-cut examples of the essentiality of Cu to the skeleton. No cases of acquired adult Cu deficiency leading to skeletal abnormalities have been described.

MANGANESE

The data supporting the essentiality of manganese (Mn) to the skeleton has been reviewed by Hidiroglou (1980) and more recently by Strause and Saltman (1987) and Chausmer and Wallach (1990). In both spontaneous and experimental animal models, Mn deficiency results in reduced growth and a variety of cartilagenous and skeletal abnormalities. Perosis in fowl is associated with lax tendons and short, deformed tibiae. In mammals, osteoporosis and deformities of the long bone and joints occur, which in cattle may be manifested by "knuckling" of the joints. The chondrodystrophic joint and tendon abnormalities may be related to deficiencies in Mn-dependent polymerases and glycosyl transferases associated with chondroitin sulfate synthesis and to deficient sulfation of glycosyaminoglycans. The derivation of the skeletal abnormalities is less clear. As a divalent cation, Mn may substitute for calcium (Ca) within the crystal lattice of the bone salt, hydroxyapatite. However, Mn deficient hydroxyapatite is unlikely to be a proximate cause of bone abnormalities. Mn has also been suggest to be an antagonist for Ca as an intracellular messenger. Mn at concentrations above 0.3 mM inhibit in vitro bone resorption whereas concentrations below 0.3 mM stimulate resorption (Stern, 1985). However, it is not likely that Mn deficiency functions in this manner. Strause and Saltman (1987) have provided evidence that Mn deficiency can lead to skeletal abnormalities by interfering with bone cell function. In in vivo models of both bone formation and bone resorption, the presence of severe Mn deficiency is disruptive of bone cell mediated events which could account for the severe developmental defects observed in young Mn deficient animals and in the offspring of Mn deficient mothers.

Several studies have addressed the question as to whether Mn deficiency can be a causal factor in human osteoporosis. Strause et al (1986) fed weanling rats a Mn deficient diet for 12 months and noted hypercalcemia, a rise in serum phosphate levels and a 33% reduction in bone Ca content. Radiologic study of excised bone revealed a punctate pattern of bone loss without disruption of the cortex. Since no histology was done, it is impossible to characterize the osteopenia further. In a human study (Friedman, 1987) healthy young men were fed a Mn deficient diet for 39 days. They too developed hypercalcemia and a rise in the serum phosphate level, but also had an increase in the serum alkaline phosphatase level. The authors speculated that the main effect of Mn deficiency was to promote bone resorption. This conclusion is difficult to reconcile with earlier animal work, but since graded Mn additions to resorbing bone cultures result in biphasic effects on bone resorption (Stern 1985), this theory should be explored further. Strause and Saltman (1987) have presented additional human data in support of a role for Mn deficiency in osteoporosis. In a group of osteoporotic women, they noted a 75% decrease in serum Mn levels compared to controls. The significance of this finding is unclear since their Mn measurements have been criticized as yielding values forty times expected in the control group (Freeland-Graves 1988). Also, the bone Mn content of the osteoporotic patients was not comparably decreased. Most recently, Strause (1991) reported a two year study in non-osteoporotic late post-menopausal women fed a supplement containing Ca, Mn, Zn and Cu. These women gained 1.3% in bone mineral density (BMD), presumably measured by dual photon or X-ray absorptiometry. In contrast, untreated controls lost 2.2% in BMD, a group which was only Ca supplemented lost 0.5% and a group which was only Mn/Zn/Cu supplemented lost 1.6%. These data are tantalizing but do not prove a causal role for Mn deficiency in osteoporosis.

SELENIUM

Selenium (Se) deficiency, a subject of considerable interest in animal and human biology, has not received much attention as to its effects on the skeleton, although a human osteoarthropathy called Kashin-Beck disease has been known in Asia and Eastern Russia for over a century, and is believed by most authorities to be due to Se deficiency (Chausmer, 1990; Whanger, 1989). The disease results in disturbed endochondral bone formation with widespread chondronecrosis, ephiphyseal sclerosis, and disrupted joint development with spurring. Long bone development is also affected with resulting dwarfism. Se supplementation can prevent or reverse many of these features if provided early.

SILICON

The effects of silicon (Si) deficiency in chicks and rats have been recently reviewed by both Chausmer and Wallach (1990) and by Nielsen (1991). Si plays a role in cartilage proteoglycan synthesis as well as in bone matrix (collagen) production and cross-linking, and its mineralization. Si deficiency causes defective endochondral bone formation and growth, with the development of small, poorly formed joints, and skull and long bone abnormalities. These adverse effects are enhanced by superimposed nutritional deficiencies such as Ca deprivation. There has been surprisingly little work done in this area in recent years. Elliot and Edwards (1991) have recently shown that Si supplementation has no effect on growth and skeletal development in chickens. The possible role of Si deficiency in human skeletal diseases is also unclear but recent studies showing that zeolite A, an aluminosilicate mineral, stimulates human osteoblasts suggests possible therapeutic potential in human osteoporosis (Brady, 1991).

VANADIUM

Vanadium (V) has several actions which may be relevant to the skeleton and some evidence exists supporting its essentiality. V exists within the hydroxyapatite crystal lattice as a vanadate (VO_4^{-3}) substituting for phosphate (PO_4^{-3}) (Etcheverry 1984). Both vanadate and vanadyl (VO^{+2}) ions are active in a large number of enzymatic functions within the skeleton (Wallach 1989). Vanadate inhibits both Na, K-ATPases and Ca-ATPases, but not Mg-ATPases (Arnett, 1990;

Bekker, 1990c; Bekker, 1990b). Alkaline and acid phosphatases are also inhibited (Andersson 1984), whereas adenyl cyclase is stimulated. Vanadyl ion inhibits alkaline phosphatases by a different mechanism. Vanadate also serves as a cofactor for several local growth factors critical to the skeleton such as insulin-like growth factor 1 (IGF-1), epidermal growth factor, and transforming growth factor-B (Lau, 1988).

V deposition in the skeleton is greatest in areas of high metabolic activity such as the subperiosteal and endosteal areas, trabecular bone surfaces and the ossification zone of the epiphyseal plate (Wallach, 1989). Vanadate has been shown in vitro to stimulate both osteoblast proliferation (mitogenic effect) and differentiated functions of the osteoblast such as alkaline phosphatase production, matrix collagen synthesis (Lau, 1988), and proteoglycan synthesis (Nielsen, 1991). In contrast to its stimulatory effects on osteoblasts, vanadate inhibits osteoclastic bone resorption induced by PTH, prostaglandin E_2 and calcitriol (Krieger, 1983). This inhibitory effect appears to reside with vanadate inhibition of Ca-ATPase (Bekker, 1990a) so that Ca extrusion from the osteoclast does not occur (Arnett, 1990). Proton pumping into the resorption lacunae is not affected since this depends on Mg-ATPase, which is not inhibited by vanadate at micromolar concentrations. V deficiency probably operates primarily by precluding an osteoblastic response to local growth factors. Chicks maintained on a low V diet have enlarged epiphyseal plates and decreased formation of primary spongiosa (Chausmer, 1990). In goats, Anke et al (1989) has noted swollen, painful joints and skeletal deformities of the forelegs. The histologic appearance of skeletal tissue from V deficient animals has not been reported. No examples of human V deficiency with skeletal abnormalities are known.

ZINC

Zinc is a structural and functional cofactor in over a hundred enzyme systems and is also active in gene expression by serving as the stabilizer of the finger-loop domains in DNA-binding proteins. It would therefore be surprising if Zn deficiency did not influence skeletal metabolism (Chausmer 1989). Both alkaline phosphatase, an osteoblast product, and carbonic anhydrase, the osteoclast enzyme which provides protons for transport into the resorption lacunae require Zn as a cofactor. Widespread disruption of osteoblast function is evident in animal models of Zn deficiency, including decreased collagen production and impaired mineralization. Bone mass and ash content are both diminished, with increased fragility, skeletal malformations and deformities. In two recent studies (Leek, 1988; da Cunha Ferreira, 1989), Zn deficiency in newborn monkeys and rats was induced by feeding the pregnant mothers a Zn deprived diet and continuing it in the newborns. In the monkey model, delayed skeletal maturation and mineralization was noted through three years of age. In the rat studies, 91% of the Zn deficient newborns had multiple skeletal malformations which involved mainly defects in mineralization. A condition known as footrot in ruminants is also due to Zn deficiency.

Yamaguchi and his associates (1988-1991) have published nine studies since 1988 concerning the role of Zn in skeletal metabolism. Using a rat calvarial culture system , inorganic Zn addition enhanced collagen synthesis, glucose consumption and ATP production; and the addition of an organo-Zn compound (B-alanyl-L-histidinato-Zn, AHZ) enhanced DNA, collagen and alkaline phosphatase synthesis as well as mineralization. Zn also potentiated the positive effects of both estrogens and calcitriol on some of these osteoblastic functions. The addition of a Zn chelator decreased collagen and alkaline phosphatase synthesis by 40%. In two in vivo experiments, feeding either AHZ or $ZnSO_4$ to rats also increased differentiated osteoblastic functions and the AHZ also stimulated DNA content, indicating an additional effect on osteoblast proliferation.

Acquired Zn deficiency has been well described in humans but does not appear to influence the skeleton directly. Reversible growth retardation is common but is due to Zn deficiency induced hypogonadism. There is one report of hyperzincuria in human osteoporosis (Herzberg, 1990) but the significance of this finding is unclear since the authors also review previous work in this area and found it to be discrepant. Herzberg et al (1990) speculate that the increased urinary

Zn may represent loss from bone in patients with high turnover osteoporosis and very rapid rates of bone resorption. Two recent animal studies may have relevance to this question. Matzsch et al (1990) have shown that the osteoporotic bone produced in rats by heparin administration is deficient in Zn. Also in rats, Sasahara et al (1990) have reported that the decreased skeletal development and mineralization caused by feeding caffeine is nullified by the co-administration of Zn. The latest human contribution to this subject is by Steidl et al (1990) who noted a large dispersion of values for serum and erythrocyte Zn in osteoporotic patients, with a trend to increased levels compared to nonosteoporotic controls.

REFERENCES:

Andersson, G., Ek-Rylander, B., and Hammarstrom, L. (1984): Purification and characterization of a vanadate-sensitive nucleotide tri- and diphosphatase with acid pH optimum from rat bone. Arch. Biochem Biophys. 228: 431-438.

Anke, M., Groppel, B. Gruhn, K., Langer, M., and Arnhold, W. (1989): The essentiality of vanadium for animals. In Sixth International Trace Element Symposium, Volume 1, Vanadium, eds M. Anke, W. Baumann, H. Braunlich, C. Bruckner, B. Groppel, and M. Grun, pp. 17-27. Jena: Verlagsabteilung der Friedrich-Schiller-Universitat.

Arnett, T.R. and Dempster, D.W. (1990): Protons and osteoclasts. J. Bone Miner. Res. 5: 1099-1103.

Bekker, P.J. and Gay, C.V. (1990a): Characterization of a Ca^{2+}-ATPase in osteoclast plasma membrane. J. Bone Miner. Res. 5: 557-567.

Bekker, P.J. and Gay, C.V. (1990b): Biochemical characterization of an electrogenic vacuolar proton pump in purified chicken osteoclast plasma membrane vesicles. J. Bone Miner. Res 5: 569-579.

Brady, M.C., Dobson, P.R.M., Thavarajah, M., and Kanis, J.A. (1991): Zeolite A stimulates proliferation and protein synthesis in human osteoblast-like cells and the osteosarcoma cell-line MG-63. J. Bone Miner. Res. 6 (Suppl. 1): S139.

Chausmer, A.B. and Wallach, S. (1990): Metabolism of trace metals in animals: Part II: essential trace elements. In Trace Metals and Fluoride in Bones and Teeth, eds. N.D. Priest and F.L. Van de Vyver, pp. 253-270. Boca Raton (FL): CRC Press.

da Cunha Ferreira, R.M., Marguiegui, I.M., and Elizaga, I.V. (1989): Teratogenicity of zinc deficiency in the rat: Study of the fetal skeleton. Teratology. 39: 181-194.

Elliot, M.A., and Edwards, H.M., Jr. (1991): Effect of dietary silicon on growth and skeletal development in chickens. J. Nutr. 121: 201-207.

Etcheverry, S.B., Apella, M.C., and Baran, E.J. (1984): A model study of the incorporation of vanadium in bone. J. Inorg. Bischem. 20: 269-274.

Farquharson, C., Duncan, A., and Robins, S.P. (1989): The effects of copper deficiency on the pyridinium crosslinks of mature collagen in the rat skeleton and cardiovascular system. P.S.E.B.M. 192: 166-171.

Freeland-Graves, J.H. (1988): Manganese: An essential nutrient for humans. Nutr. Today 23: 13-19.

Friedman, B.J., Freeland-Graves, J.H., Bales, C.W., Behmardi, F., Shorey-Kutschke, R.L. Willis, R.A., Crosby, J.B. Trickett, P.C., and Houston, S.D. (1987): Manganese balance and clinical observations in young men fed a manganese deficient diet. J. Nutr. 117: 133-143.

Herzberg, M., Foldes, J., Steinberg, R., and Menczel, J. (1990): Zinc excretion in osteoporotic women. J. Bone Miner. Res. (5. 251-257).

Hidiroglou, M. (1980): Zinc, copper and manganese deficiencies and the ruminant skeleton: a review. Canad. J. Animal Sci. 60: 579-590.

Iguchi, H., Ryuichi, K., Okumura, H. Yamamuro, T., and Kagan, H.M. (1990): Effect of dietary cadmium and/or copper on the bone lysyl oxidase in copper-deficient rats relative to the metabolism of copper in the bone. Bone Miner. 10: 51-59.

Krieger, N.S., and Tashjian, A.H., Jr. (1983): Inhibition of stimulated bone resorption by vanadate. Endocrinology 113: 324-328.

Lau, K.-H.W., Tanimoto, H., and Baylink, D.J., (1988): Vanadate stimulates bone cell proliferation and bone collagen synthesis in vitro. Endocrinology 123: 2858-2867.

Leek, J.C., Keen, C.L., Vogler, J.B., Golubs, M.S., Hurley, L.S., Hendrickx, A.G., and Gershwin, M.E. (1988): Long-term marginal zinc deprivation in monkeys. I.V. Effects on skeletal growth and mineralization. Am. J. Clin. Nutr. 47: 889-895.

Matzsch, T., Bergqvist, D., Hedner, V., Nilsson, B., and Ostergaard, P. (1990): Effects of low molecular weight heparin and unfragmented heparin on induction of osteoporosis in rats. Thrombosis and Haemostasis 63: 505-509.

Nielsen, F.H. (1990): Studies on the relationship between boron and magnesium which possibly affects the formation and maintenance of bones. Magnesium Trace Elem. 9: 61-69.

Nielsen, F.H. (1991): Nutritional requirements for boron, silicon, vanadium, nickel, and arsenic: current knowledge and speculation. FASEB J. 6: 2661-2667.

Sasahara, H., Yamano, H., and Nakamoto, T. (1990): Effects of maternal caffeine with zinc intake during gestation and lactation on bone development in newborn rats. Arch. Oral Biol. 1990: 425-430.

Schmidt, H., Herwig, J., and Greinacher I. (1991): The skeletal changes in premature infants with a copper deficiency. Rofo Fortschr. geb Rontgenstr. Neuen Bildgeb Verfahr. 155: 38-42.

Shaw, J.C.L. (1988): Copper deficiency and non-accidental injury. Arch Dis. Child. 63: 448-455.

Steidl, L., Ditmar, R., and Kubicek, R. (1990): Biochemical findings in osteoporosis. II. Role of zinc. Cas. Lek. Ces. 129: 147-150.

Stern, P.H. (1985): Biphasic effects of manganese on hormone-stimulated bone resorption. Endocrinology 117: 2044-2049.

Strause, L.G., Hegenauer, J., Saltman, P., Cone, R., and Resnick, D. (1986): Effects of long-term dietary manganese and copper deficiency on rat skeleton. V.J. Nutr. 116: 135-141.

Strause, L., and Saltman, P. (1987): Role of manganese in bone metabolism. In Nutritional Bioavailability of Manganese, ed. C. Kies, pp. 46-55. Washington: American Chemical Society Symposium Series 354.

Strause, L. (1991): Trace elements enhance bone-preserving effect of calcium supplement. Geriatrics 46: 67.

Wallach, S. (1989): Biologic essentiality of vanadium with special emphasis on the skeleton. In Sixth International Trace Element Symposium, Volume 1, Molybdenum, Vanadium, eds. M. Anke, W. Baumann, H. Braunlich, C. Bruckner, B. Groppel, and M. Grun, pp. 28-36. Jena: Verlagsabteilung der Friedrich-Schiller-Universistat.

Whanger, P.D. (1989): China, a country with both selenium deficiency and toxicity: some thoughts and impressions. J. Nutr. 119: 1236-1239.

Yamaguchi, M., Oishi, H., and Suketa, Y. (1988): Zinc stimulation of bone protein synthesis in tissue culture. Activation of aminoacyl-tRNA synthetasne. Biochem. Pharmacol. 37: 4075-4080.

Yamaguchi, M., Ozaki, K., and Suketa, Y. (1989a): Alteration in bone metabolism with increasing age: effects of zinc and vitamin D_3 in aged rats. J. Pharmacobio-Dynamics 12: 67-73.

Yamaguchi, M., and Oishi, H. (1989b): Effect of 1,25-dihydroxyvitamin D_3 on bone metabolism in tissue culture. Enhancement of the steroid effect by zinc. Biochem. Pharmacol. 38: 3453-3459.

Yamaguchi, M., and Matsui, R. (1989c): Effect of dipicolinate, a chelator of zinc in bone protein synthesis in tissue culture. The essential role of zinc. Biochem. Pharmacol. 38: 4485-4489.

Yamaguchi, M., Ozaki, K., and Suketa, Y. (1990a): Alteration of glucose consumption and adenosine tri-phosphate content in bone tissue of rats with different ages: the stimulatory effect of zinc. Chem. Pharm. Bull. 38: 1660-1662.

Yamaguchi, M., and Ozaki, K. (1990b): A new zinc compound, beta-alanyl-L-histidinato zinc, stimulates bone growth in weaning rats. Res. Exper. Med. 190: 105-110.

Yamaguchi, M., and Ozaki, K. (1990c): Aging affects cellular zinc and protein synthesis in the femoral diaphysis of rats. Res. Exper. Med. 190: 295-300.

Yamaguchi, M., and Kitajima, T. (1991a): Effect of estrogen on bone metabolism in tissue culture: enhancement of the steroid effect by zinc. Res. Exper. Med. 191: 145-154.

Yamaguchi, M., and Miwa, H. (1991b): Stimulatory effect of beta-alanyl-L-histadinato zinc on bone formation in tissue culture. Pharmacology. 42: 230-240.

Metal Ions in Biology and Medicine, vol. 2. Eds. J. Anastassopoulou, Ph. Collery, J.C. Etienne, Th. Theophanides. John Libbey Eurotext, Paris © 1992, pp. 402-407

Effect of coenzyme Q_{10} supplementation of male rats on cardiac abnormalities associated with a high-fructose, low-copper diet

Charles G. Lewis, Meira Fields*, Willard A. Burns**, Mark D. Lure

*Carbohydrate Nutrition Laboratory, Beltsville Human Nutrition Resarch Center, US Department of Agriculture, Agricultural Resarch Service, Beltsville, MD 20705. *Division of Endocrinology, Georgetown University Medical Center, Washington, DC 20007. **Laboratory service, Veterans Administration Hospital, East Orange, NJ 07019, USA*

INTRODUCTION

Copper deficiency has both direct and indirect effects on the activities of several enzymes of potential importance in maintaining the cardiovascular system. In copper deficient animals a reduction of cytochrome oxidase activity has been considered the cause of respiratory failure of organs (Gallagher 1957; Paynter et al., 1979; Rusinko & Prohaska, 1985). A possible consequence of reduced mitochondrial respiratory enzyme activity might be compensatory mitochondrial enlargement with concomitant heart hypertrophy. The type of carbohydrate in a copper deficient diet is of importance in producing cardiovascular lesions in rats. When sucrose or fructose was the carbohydrate in a copper deficient diet, there was significant heart hypertrophy, mild to severe inflammatory and degenerative changes, severe fibrosis, giant mitochondria with abnormal cristae and destruction of myofibrils (Burns et al., 1990; Redman et al., 1988). These observations were confirmed in rats that received a copper deficient diet containing a mixture of sucrose and starch as carbohydrate (Medeiros et al., 1991). However, if the copper deficient diet contains only starch as the carbohydrate hearts were less hypertropic and had no or mild myocardial lesions (Burns et al., 1990; Redman et al., 1988).

Recently, t-butylhydroquinone (TBHQ) supplementation of a copper deficient diet containing sucrose was reported to ameliorate the cardiac hypertrophy associated with copper deficiency in rats (Johnson & Saari, 1989). The therapeutic effect of TBHQ on the heart was attributed to its antioxidant properties and potential protection against lipid hydroperoxides at the cellular level. Interestingly, coenzyme Q_{10} (another quinone) treatment has beneficial effects on cardiomyopathy (Langsjoen et al., 1988) and cardiac ischemia (Okamoto et al., 1986). Coenzyme Q_{10} is an obligatory member of the electron transport system and is intrinsic to most cells which have mitochondria. In addition to its role as an electron carrier in the electron transport system, coenzyme Q_{10} is thought to play a role in membrane stability, ATP synthesis (coenzyme Q cycle) and inhibition of superoxide radical production during electron transfer activity in mitochondria (Langsjoen et al., 1990). The suggestion has been made that coenzyme Q_{10} may also be involved in non-specific antioxidant reactions which are pharmacological and these reactions can divert coenzyme Q_{10} from its energy production role and be detrimental (Langsjoen et al., 1990). Since copper deficiency may potentiate oxidative cellular damage which may contribute to cardiovascular damage (Johnson & Saari, 1989), the copper deficiency may also lead to coenzyme Q_{10} deficiency by creating a cellular environment that favors superoxide radical production. Therefore, to evaluate the potential that coenzyme Q_{10} deficiency may contribute to the cardiovascular problem of copper deficiency in fructose fed rats, the effect of coenzyme Q_{10} supplementation on some of the classic signs of copper deficiency was evaluated.

MATERIALS AND METHODS

Weanling male Sprague-Dawley rats were housed in quarters maintained at 20°C and 55% relative humidity with 12 hours of light and 12 hours of dark. Rats were randomly assigned to one of two diets containing either 62.7% starch (S) or fructose (F) with 0.6µg Cu/g diet (-Cu). All diets contained the following ingredients (g/kg diet): 627 carbohydrate, 200 egg white solids, 95 corn oil, 30 non-nutritive fiber (cellulose), 35 Cu-free AIN-76 salt mix (formulated in our laboratory to omit cupric carbonate), 10 AIN-76A vitamin mix supplemented with 2mg biotin and 2.7g choline bitartrate. All rats had free access to diet and to distilled deionized drinking water. On Monday-Friday mornings, half of the rats provided with the F-Cu diet were given orally 300mg coenzyme Q_{10}/kg body weight. The S-Cu dietary group was used as the control and they were not provided with coenzyme Q_{10} since we have shown repeatedly that the rats from the S-Cu group do not experince the growth retardation, anemia, cardiovascular problems, morbidity or mortality of the copper deficiency observed in rats fed a fructose containing diet (Burns et al., 1990; Redman et al., 1988).

Fasted rats were decapitated after consuming their respective diets for five weeks. Blood was collected in heparinized tubes and centrifuged to obtain plasma which was removed for the measurement of ceruloplasmin (Schosinsky et al., 1974). Blood collected in capillary tubes was centrifuged for the determination of packed cell volume.

Liver, heart, pancreas and lung were removed quickly, trimmed free of fat and connective tissue and weighed. Tissue and diet minerals were extracted from samples by a method combining dry heat and acid digestion (Hill et al., 1986). Duplicate samples were analyzed by flame atomic absorption spectrophotometry (Perkin-Elmer Model 5000). National Bureau of Standard reference material, bovine liver 1577a, was digested and analyzed along with samples to verify accuracy.

Hearts were washed in ice cold saline, sliced and fixed in Carson's modified Millonig's phosphate-buffered formalin. Following fixation a hemisection of the heart was processed and embedded in paraffin in the usual manner, sectioned at 4µm, and stained with hematoxylin-eosin, periodic acid-Schiff, and Gomori's trichrome. Adjacent areas were embedded in plastic (glycol methacrylate) blocks, cut on a rotary microtome at 0.5-1.0µm and stained with a combined nuclear cytoplasmic stain (Paragon).

Values were analysed by computer using the SAS software system for data analysis (SAS Institute Inc., 1985). Values were considered statistically significant from each other at a p of 0.05 or less by Student's t-test.

RESULTS

Weanling male rats were given their respective diets at 21 days of age when their body weight was 42 ± 3g (mean ± SEM). After 5 weeks, the S-Cu rats were significantly heavier than rats consuming the F-Cu diet and supplementation with coenzyme Q_{10} did not improve body weight (Table 1). When the study was terminated after 5 weeks, 30% of the rats fed the F-Cu diet but not supplemented with coenzyme Q_{10} had died with hemothorax and hemopericardium due to heart rupture at the apex.

Some relative organ sizes are given in Table 1. There were no differences in the relative heart sizes between the two fructose dietary groups but their hearts were significantly larger than the starch dietary group. The relative liver size was largest in the F-Cu rats supplemented with coenzyme Q_{10}, smallest in the S-Cu rats and intermediate in the F-Cu rats. Relative pancreatic sizes of the two groups consuming the F-Cu diet were significantly smaller than the S-Cu rats. Rats fed the F-Cu diet with or without coenzyme Q_{10} had significantly greater relative lung sizes than those fed the S-Cu diet.

Various measures that are typically used to assess copper status are given in Table 2. The hematocrit of rats fed the S-Cu diet was within the normal range for Sprague-Dawley rats but significantly lower for the two dietary groups fed the F-Cu diet. Ceruloplasmin activity was low in the dietary groups fed a copper deficient diet. We typically assay plasma obtained from rats fed a S+Cu diet for 5 weeks as an internal control and we obtained ceruloplasmin activity 10-20 times higher than the values for copper deficient rats in the present study. Liver copper and iron concentrations were similar in the three dietary groups. Interestingly, the lowest lung copper and iron concentrations were observed in the F-Cu dietary group receiving coenzyme Q_{10} supplementation.

Hearts of rats from the three dietary groups were examined for abnormalities by light microscopy (not shown). Heart sections from rats fed the low-copper, high-fructose diet showed myocardial changes which were focal in distribution and variable in severity. The focal nature of the lesions was ascertained in the hemisections of the hearts. The foci were composed of degenerated myocardial fibrils and areas of necrosis with an inflammatory response. These lesions were sometimes located perivascularly. Myocardial vessels did not demonstrate any atherosclerotic changes or vasculitis. No definite lesions could be seen in the rats fed the low-copper, starch diet. Interestingly, lesions were not seen in the hearts from rats fed the low-copper, high-fructose diet and supplemented with coenzyme Q_{10}.

DISCUSSION

Johnson and Saari (1989) have reported that dietary TBHQ supplementation of copper deficient rats ameliorated growth, anemia and cardiac hypertrophy. Although TBHQ and coenzyme Q_{10} are closely related compounds, we did not observe any improvement in these signs of copper deficiency.

The cause of cardiac hypertrophy and lesions with copper deficiency are not known. Cardiac overload due to anemia (Prohaska & Heller 1982), and enlargement of mitochondria and enlargement of myofibrillar mass (Medeiros et al., 1991) have been implicated, but the observations in the present

Table 1. Effect of coenzyme Q_{10} supplementation on body weight and relative organ sizes of copper deficient rats fed dietary fructose.

Diet[1]	S-Cu	F-Cu	F-Cu+Q
Body weight (g)	277 ± 5[3,a]	202 ± 11[b]	185 ± 8[b]
Relative Heart Size[2]	0.46 ± 0.03[b]	0.63 ± 0.05[a]	0.61 ± 0.02[a]
Relative Liver Size	3.0 ± 0.2[c]	4.7 ± 0.2[b]	5.3 ± 0.2[a]
Relative Pancreatic Size	0.51 ± 0.02[a]	0.24 ± 0.02[b]	0.26 ± 0.03[b]
Relative Lung Size	0.53 ± 0.01[c]	0.66 ± 0.02[a]	0.60 ± 0.02[b]

[1]All diets contained 0.6μg copper/g and 627g carbohydrate/kg. S=starch, F=fructose, Q=supplemented with 300 mg coenzyme Q_{10}/kg body weight/day by oral administration. Rats consumed their respective diets for 5 weeks.

[2]Relative organ size = (organ wt x 100)/body weight.

[3]Each value represents the mean ± SEM for 10 rats for S-Cu and F-Cu+Q and 7 rats for F-Cu. Means within a row with different superscript letters are significantly different from each other at a P value of 0.05 or less by Student's t-test.

Table 2. Effect of coenzyme Q_{10} supplementation on copper status measures of copper deficient rats fed dietary fructose.

Diet	S-Cu	F-Cu	F-Cu+Q
Hematocit (%)	44 ± 2[a]	24 ± 3[b]	19 ± 2[b]
Ceruloplasmin (U/l)	3.6 ± 0.7[b]	6.1 ± 0.7[a]	4.6 ± 0.3[a,b]
Liver Cu (μg/g wet wt.)	0.98 ± 0.14	0.75 ± 0.09	0.59 ± 0.05
Liver Fe (μg/g wet wt)	156 ± 16	151 ± 14	157 ± 15
Lung Cu (μg/g wet wt)	1.14 ± 0.13[a]	1.16 ± 0.16[a]	0.78 ± 0.05[b]
Lung Fe (μg/g wet wt)	35 ± 2[a]	30 ± 3[a,b]	27 ± 2[b]

See Table 1 for conditions and descriptions.

study indicate clearly that factors other than copper must be considered since the type of carbohydrate consumed in the diet was of importance. Rats made copper deficient with a diet containing fructose had cardiac hypertrophy while those consuming a diet containing starch did not (Burns et al., 1990; Redman et al., 1988). A copper x carbohydrate interaction was necessary to produce cardiac hypertrophy and while coenzyme Q_{10} supplementation did not prevent the hypertrophy it did prevent the pathology that results from the copper x carbohydrate interaction.

Coenzyme Q_{10} is present in the diet, it is synthesized in cells and it is presumed to be in all cells which have mitochondria and the Golgi complex. The most important function of coenzyme Q_{10} may be as a redox component in electron transfer processes of respiration and coupled phosphorylation. Heart mitochondria from copper deficient rats were enlarged (Burns et al., 1990; Medeiros et al., 1991) and it is tempting to suggest that the therapeutic action of coenzyme Q_{10} observed in the hearts of the F-Cu+Q group was related to the energy-coupling role of coenzyme Q_{10}.

Superoxide radical production and resultant lipid peroxidation has been shown to play a role in producing myocardial damage in a variety of conditions including hypertrophy (Gupta & Singal, 1989). In copper deficiency the activity of superoxide dismutase is greatly diminished (Taylor et al., 1988) and this may lead to increased susceptibility of cells to oxidative damage. Coenzyme Q_{10} is also though to be involved in non-specific antioxidant reactions (Langsjoen et al., 1990). Coenzyme Q_{10} supplementation may provide sufficient coenzyme Q_{10} to "capture" the oxygen radicals generated during cardiac hypertrophy, minimize lipid peroxidation and maintain the integrity of the heart as seen in the F-Cu+Q. group.

Coenzyme Q_{10} has been identified in membranes other than the inner mitochondrial membrane and the functional role of this coenzyme is unknown (Quinn et al., 1980). It has been suggested that coenzyme Q_{10} helps maintain membrane ultrastructure (Quinn et al., 1980). In copper deficiency, heart mitochondria were enlarged and there was disruption of mitochondrial inner and outer membranes (Burnes et al., 1990; Medeiros et al., 1991), and a decline in ATP concentration (Paynter, et al., 1979). It is tempting to speculate that in the present study coenzyme Q_{10} supplementation may have provided sufficient coenzyme Q_{10} to maintain membrane structure and to prevent the cardiac lesions typically seen in rats consuming the low-copper, high-fructose diet.

In summary, although the present study has failed to provide insight into the copper x carbohydrate interaction it has shown that coenzyme Q_{10} supplementation can be of value in maintaining the integrity of the heart under the adverse cellular conditions created by the copper x carbohydrate interaction. It would appear that the protection of the heart provided by coenzyme Q_{10} may be related to it antioxidant capabilities although other possibilities can not be ruled out.

REFERENCES

Burns, W.A., Fields, M., Smith, Jr., J.C. & Reiser, S. (1990): Myocardial lesions in copper deficiency modified by dietary carbohydrates. J. Trace Elem. Exp. Med. 3, 67-77.

Gallagher, C.H. (1957): The pathology and biochemistry of copper deficiency. Aust. Vet. J. 33, 311-317.

Gupta, M. & Singal, P.K. (1989): Higher antioxidant capacity during a chronic stable heart hypertrophy. Circ. Res. 64, 398-406.

Hill, A.D., Patterson, K.Y., Veillon, C. & Morris, E.R. (1986): Digestion of biological materials for mineral analysis using a combination of heat and dry ashing. Anal. Chem. 58, 2340-2342.

Johnson, W.T. & Saari, J.T. (1989): Dietary supplementation with t-butylhydroquinone reduces cardiac hypertrophy and anemia associated with copper deficiency in rats. Nutr. Res. 9, 1355-1362.

Langsjoen, P.H., Folkers, K., Lyson, K., Muratsu, K., Lyson, T. & Langsjoen, P. (1988): Effective and safe therapy with coenzyme Q_{10} for cardiomyopathy. Klin. Wochenschr. 66, 583-590.

Langsjoen, P.H., Folkers, K., Lyson, K., Muratsu, K., Lyson, T., Langsjoen, P. (1990): Pronounced increase of survival of patients with cardiomyopathy when treated with coenzyme Q_{10} and conventional therapy. Int. J. Tiss. Reac. XII, 163-168.

Medeiros, D.M., Bagby, D., Ovecka, G. & McCormick, R. (1991): Myofibrillar, mitochondrial and valvular morphological alterations in cardiac hypertrophy among copper-deficient rats. J. Nutr. 121, 815-824.

Okamoto, F., Allen, B.S., Buckberg, G.D., Leaf, J. & Bugyi, H.J. (1986): Studies of controlled perfusion after ischemia X. Reperfusate composition: Supplemental role of intravenous and intracoronary coenzyme Q_{10} in avoiding reperfusion damage. Thorac. Cardiovasc. Surg. 92, 573-582.

Paynter, D.I., Moir, R.J. & Underwood, E.J. (1979): Changes in activity of the Cu-Zn superoxide dismutase enzyme in tissues of the rat with changes in dietary copper. J. Nutr. 109, 1570-1576.

Prohaska, J.R. & Heller, L.J. (1982): Mechanical properties of the copper-deficient rat heart. J. Nutr. 112, 2142-2150.

Quinn, P.J., Baun, H., Harris, E.J., Franklin, C.S. & Trivedi, P. (1980): The protective role of coenzyme Q_{10} against mercurial and carbontetrachloride toxicity. In Biomedical and Clinical Aspects of Coenzyme Q_{10}, vol. 2. ed. Y. Yamamura, K. Folkers & Y. Ito, pp. 435-446. North-Holland: Elsevier Biomedical Press.

Redman, R.S., Fields, M., Reiser, S. & Smith, Jr., J.C. (1988): Dietary fructose exacerbates the cardiac abnormalities of copper deficiency in rats. Atherosclerosis 74, 203-214.

Rusinko, N. & Prohaska, J.R. (1985): Adenine nucleotide and lactate levels in organs from copper-deficient mice and brindled mice. J. Nutr. 115, 936-943.

SAS Institute Inc. (1985): SAS User's Guide: Statistics, 5th ed., Cary, NC.

Schosinsky, K.H., Lehmann, H.P. & Beeler, M. (1974): Measurement of ceruloplasmin from its oxidase activity in serum by use of o-dianisidine dihydrochloride. Clin. Chem. 20, 1556-1563.

Taylor, C.G., Bettger, W.J. & Bray, T.M. (1988): Effect of dietary zinc or copper deficiency on the primary free radical defense system in rats. J. Nutr. 118, 613-621.

Metal Ions in Biology and Medicine, vol. 2. Eds. J. Anastassopoulou, Ph. Collery, J.C. Etienne, Th. Theophanides. John Libbey Eurotext, Paris © 1992, pp. 408-413

Hepatic iron overload may be responsible for the severity of copper deficiency in rats fed fructose

Meira Fields*, Charles G. Lewis+, W.E. Antholine**, W.A. Burns++, Mark D. Lure+

**Division of Endocrinology, Georgetown University Medical Center, Washington, DC 20007. +Carbohydrate Nutrition Laboratory, USDA, Beltsville, MD. 20705. **National Biomedical ESR Center, Medical College of Wisconsin, Milwaukee, WI. 53226. ++Laboratory Services, Veterans Administration Hospital, East Orange, NJ 07019, USA*

It is well established that nutritional interaction exists between copper and iron (Elvehjem & Sherman, 1932; Sourkes, et al., 1968). Indeed, when dietary copper is unavailable, the copper deficient animals exhibit hepatic iron overload (Elvehjem & Sherman, 1932; Sourkes, et al., 1968; Marston, et al., 1971; Williams, et al., 1985). Iron has long been known to play a major role in the pathogenesis of numerous diseases (Halliwell & Gutteridge, et al., 1984; Braughler, et al., 1986). Iron has been reported to generate free radicals and to accelerate lipid peroxidation under specific conditions (Cantoni, et al., 1989; Braughler, et al., 1986; Rowley & Halliwell 1982).

It has been repeatedly shown that when rats are fed a copper deficient diet that contains fructose, they become sick, emaciated, they develop anemia, heart hypertrophy, heart pathology and they die of the deficiency (Fields, et al., 1984; Redman, et al., 1988). In contrast, copper deficient rats that are fed starch, do not develop these abnormalities and they survive (Fields, et al., 1984; Redman, et al., 1988). Since rats that are fed starch and those that are fed fructose are similarly copper deficient and both exhibit similar levels of hepatic iron overload, but only rats fed fructose are anemic, it seemed likely that it is not copper metabolism, but rather it is the iron that plays a role in the exacerbation of the signs associated with copper deficiency in rats consuming fed fructose. It is suggested that it is not the absolute concentration of hepatic iron, but rather its redox state or the type of the hepatic iron compound that is responsible for the aggravation of copper deficiency when fructose is fed.

This manuscript summarizes data from four separate studies. The results of these studies provide evidence that in copper deficiency, hepatic iron overload plays a role in the severity and the pathology of copper deficiency in rats fed fructose.

1) <u>Electron Spin Resonance (ESR) of the liver</u>

Weanling male and female Sprague-Dawley rats weighing approximately 40-45g each were fed a copper deficienct (0.6μg Cu/g) or copper adequate (6.0μg Cu/g) diets containing 62% fructose or starch for 5 weeks. At the end of the

5th week, the animals were killed and their livers were frozen and stored at -70°C. The 9.1-GHz. 77K liver samples were prepared by pressing the tissue into precision pore pyrex moulds (inner diameter 4mm, length 3 cm), freezing the tissue and then warming the mould until the frozen tissue cylinder could be extracted. These specimens were studied in a finger tip dewar. The ESR Spectra were obtained on a Varian E-9 spectrometer at the National Biomedical ESR Center in Milwaukee, WI. Only copper-deficient male rats that consumed the fructose based diets exhibited reduced body weights, anemia, heart hypertrophy with histopathological changes and some died prematurely due to heart related abnormalities. No anemia, no heart pathology and no mortality occurred in any of the other dietary groups.

In all copper deficient rats, regardless of the type of dietary carbohydrate or the sex of the rat, hepatic iron concentration was nearly two fold the corresponding levels of copper adequate controls (Table 1). Hepatic iron concentrations were further increased in female rats. However, only the spectra of the ESR from livers of male rats fed the fructose diet deficient in copper exhibited a peak at about g=2.03 which was approximately seven fold higher than the corresponding peak from all other copper deficient and adequate animals (Figure 1). This free radical peak was associated with an iron compound. Although copper deficient female rats that consumed fructose exhibited higher concentration of hepatic iron than copper deficient males, their hepatic ESR failed to show the presence of free radicals.

The data of this study clearly show that regardless of differences in absolute concentrations of hepatic iron overload in copper deficient rats, free radicals were present only in the livers of the copper deficient male rats fed fructose.

Table 1. Hepatic copper and iron concentration.

	copper (μg/g wet wt)	iron (μg/g wet wt)
Males		
Fructose-Cu	1.2 ± 0.3	133.4 ± 9.0
Fructose+Cu	4.5 ± 0.05	96.0 ± 4.0
Starch-Cu	1.4 ± 0.3	143.0 ± 23.8
Starch+Cu	4.7 ± 0.2	102.7 ± 5.7
Females		
Fructose-Cu	1.2 ± 0.2	223.5 ± 2.9
Fructose+Cu	5.0 ± 0.09	149.6 ± 15.1

Mean ± SEM

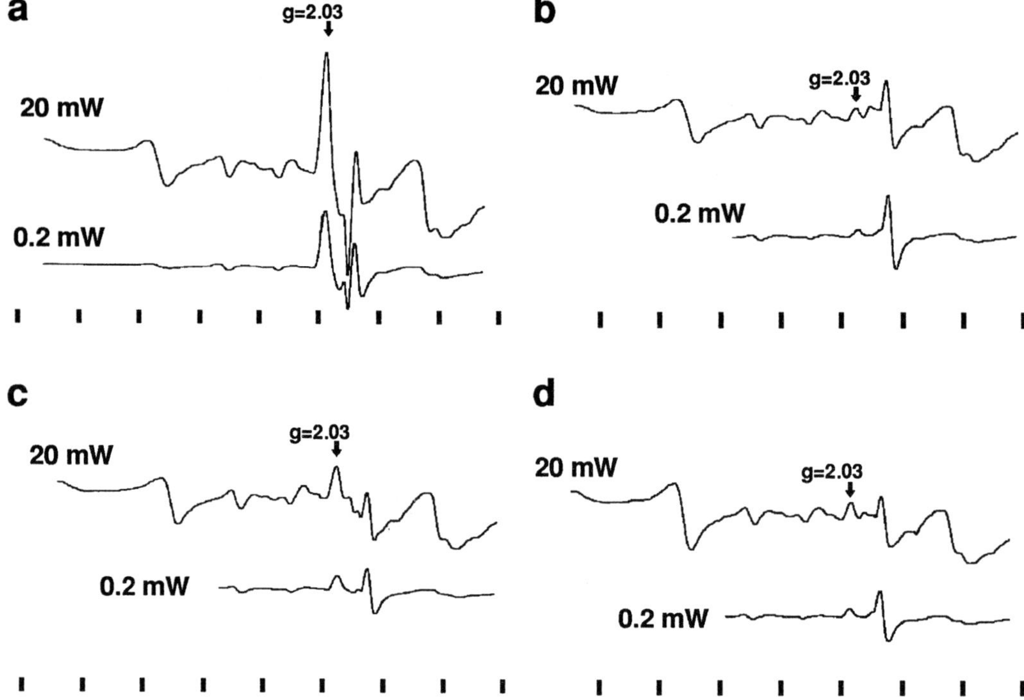

Figure 1. a) Typical ESR Spectrum of liver from a copper deficient male rat fed fructose. b) ESR of liver from a copper deficient female rat fed fructose. c) ESR of liver from a copper adequate male rat fed fructose. d) ESR of liver from a copper deficient male rat fed starch.

2) Deferoxamine (DFX) treatment

Weanling male rats were fed either copper deficient (0.6μg Cu/g) or adequate diets (6.0g Cu/g) containing fructose or starch for 5 weeks. Some of the fructose fed, copper deficient rats were administered daily with a subcutanous injection of 0.1ml saline solution containing DFX mesylate (6.0mg/kg body weight). DFX solution was prepared daily, a few minutes prior to injection.

Copper deficient rats that were fed fructose exhibited heart hypertrophy with histopathological changes, and some died of the deficiency. The administration of DFX to copper deficient rats fed fructose significantly lowered hepatic iron concentration. As a result, no pathological changes were detected in the hearts of rats that had been injected with DFX and none of the rats died.

DFX has been shown to reduce hepatic iron overload both in experimental animals and in humans. In addition, it has been shown to be a powerful inhibitor of lipid peroxidation, OH production and a free radical scavenger (Editorial, 1985; Gutteridge, et al., 1979). The data of this study support the contention that hepatic iron overload in copper deficient rats fed fructose aggravates the signs associated with copper deficiency. Once the concentration of hepatic iron is reduced, the signs associated with the deficiency should be ameliorated.

3) Low dietary iron intake-30μg Fe/g diet

A reduction of hepatic iron concentration can be achieved by lowering the intake of dietary iron. Weanling male Sprague-Dawley rats were fed either a copper deficient (0.6μg Cu/g) or an adequate diet (6.0μg Cu/g) containing fructose or starch for 5 weeks. All diets contained 50μg Fe/g diet. Half of the animals were fed a copper deficient or adequate diets containing fructose or starch that were low in iron (30μg Fe/g). All animals were fed their respective diets for 5 weeks.

The administration of a low iron diet to copper deficient rats fed fructose tended to ameliorate the signs associated with the deficiency. Body weights were higher and the anemia was not as severe as in copper deficient rats fed fructose that was adequate in iron. As expected, hepatic iron concentrations were lower in rats fed the low iron diet than in those fed the adequate iron. However, dietary iron levels of 30μg Fe/g were not low enough to provide full protection against the pathological consequences of copper deficiency. These results prompted us to conduct a second study in which dietary iron was further reduced to 17μg Fe/g diet.

4) Low dietary iron intake-17μg Fe/g

Weanling male Sprague-Dawley rats were fed copper deficient (0.6μg Cu/g) diets containing fructose or starch for 5 weeks. All diets were adequate in iron (50μg Fe/g). Another group of weanling males was fed a copper deficient diet containing 17μg Fe/g diet. The consumption of the fructose diet that was low in both iron and copper prevented hepatic iron overload (Table 2). As a result, these rats did not develop heart hypertrophy, nor did they develop myocardial lesions. In addition, ESR of their livers did not show the presence of free radicals. Furthermore, they survived. In contrast, copper deficient rats that were fed fructose with adequate iron levels developed anemia, heart hypertrophy with histopathological changes and some died of the deficiency. In addition, the ESR of their livers revealed the presence of free radicals.

Table 2. Hepatic copper and iron concentrations following the consumption of an adequate (50μg Fe/g) and a low iron diet (17 μg Fe/g).

	copper (μg/g wet wt)	iron (μg/g wet wt)
50μg Fe/g		
Fructose-Cu	0.75 ± 0.09	150 ± 14
Fructose+Cu	4.72 ± 0.23	80 ± 3
Starch-Cu	0.98 ± 0.13	155 ± 16
Starch+Cu	4.62 ± 0.25	85 ± 4
17μg Fe/g		
Fructose-Cu	0.94 ± 0.1	75 ± 8

Mean ± SEM

Conclusion

The data of these four studies support the contention that iron plays a major role in the exacerbation of copper deficiency in rats fed fructose. Due to fructose metabolism, the combination of hepatic iron overload with copper deficiency creates a toxic environment. Once hepatic iron concentrations were reduced either by DFX or by a low iron diet, the liver did not generate free radicals and the signs associated with the deficiency were ameliorated. Heart pathology was prevented and the animals survived.

REFERENCES

Blake, D.R., Gallagher, P.J. and Potter, A.R. (1984): The effect of synovial iron on the progression of rheumatoid disease. Arthritis Rheum. 27, 495-501.

Braughler, J.M., Duncan, L.A. and Chase, R.L. (1986): The involvement of iron in lipid peroxidation. Importance of ferric to fervous ratios in initiation. J. Biol. Chem. 261, 10282-10289.

Cantoni, O., Furmo, M. and Cattaberi, F. (1989): Role of metal ions in oxidant cell injury. Biol. Trace. Elem. Res. 21, 277-281.

Editorial: Metal chelation therapy, oxygen radicals and human disease. Lancet 1, 143-145.

Elvehjem, C.A. and Sherman, W.C. (1932): The action of copper in iron metabolism. J. Biol. Chem. 98, 309-319.

Fields, M., Ferretti, R.J., Reiser, S. and Smith, J.C. (1984): The severity of copper deficiency in rats is determined by the type of dietary carbohydrates. Proc. Soc. Exp. Biol. 175, 530-537.

Gutteridge, J.M.C., Richmond, R. and Halliwell, B. (1979): Inhibition of the iron-catalysed formation of hydroxyl radicals from superoxide and lipid peroxidation by deferoxamine. Biochem. J. 184, 469-472.

Halliwell, B. and Gutteridge, J.M.C. (1984): Oxygen toxicity, oxygen radicals, transition metals and disease. Biochem. J. 219, 1-14.

Marston, H.R., Allen, S.H. and Swaby, S.L. (1971): Iron metabolism in copper-deficient rats. Br. J. Nutr. 25, 15-30.

Redman, R.S., Fields, M., Reiser, S. and Smith, J.C. (1988): Dietary fructose exacerbates the cardiac abnormalities of copper deficiency in rats. Atherosclerosis. 74, 203-214.

Rowley, D., Halliwell, B. (1982): Superoxide-dependent formation of hydoxyl radicals from NADH and NADPH in the presence of iron salts. FEBS Lett. 142, 39-41.

Sourkes, T.L., Lloyd, K. and Birnbaum, H. (1968): Inverse relationship of hepatic copper and iron concentration in rats fed deficient diets. Can. J. Biochem. 46, 267-271.

Williams, D.M., Kennedy, F.S. and Green, B.S. (1985): Hepatic iron accumulation in copper-deficient rats. Br. J. Nutr. 53, 131-136.

Metal Ions in Biology and Medicine, vol. 2. Eds. J. Anastassopoulou, Ph. Collery, J.C. Etienne, Th. Theophanides. John Libbey Eurotext, Paris © 1992, pp. 414-419

Whole blood concentrations of cadmium in not occupationally exposed citizens (Athens)

Z. Georgiou*, E. Zimalis**, S. Danev***

**Toxicology Laboratory 6 Deligiorgi Str., Athens 10437, Greece. **IKA DKIE, Director of diagnostic center of occupational medecin. 6 Deligiorgi Str., Athens 104 37, Greece. ***Clinical Laboratory G. Sofiiski Str. 1, 1431 Sofia, Bulgaria*

There are two main aspects of the importance of trace elements in biological materials:1. The essential nature of some of the elements for normal growth and health.2.The toxic effects of non essentials.
The earth's crust is the primordial source of all chemical elements of the biosphere.Human civilization and the enormous increase of industrial activity has gradually redistributed many toxic metals from the earth's crust to the environment and increased the possibility of human exposure. Among the various toxic elements Cadmium is specially prevalented in nature due to its high industrial use,increased over the past 30 years.(1,6)

Industries that use cadmium emit it into the atmosphere. Cd contaminates land and natural waters and enters into the food chain of man and animal.(2,7).It is gradually accummulated by ingestion and inhalation so that in a life time an average person living in industrial society accummulates about 30 mg of cadmium in his body.(5) Food is the principal source of cadmium since the intake of cadmium from water and atmospheric air is relatively unimportant(4)
Cigarette smoking significantly increase man's exposure to cadmium. A cigarette generally contains about 2 mg of cadmium from which a remarkable fraction is inhaled and retained in the body.Even previous smokers were found to have a higher blood cadmium levels than non smokers.(8)

The widespread environmental pollution by cadmium is also reflected in the human population and is evidenced by blood cadmium values. Strictly speaking true,normal levels for cadmium in human blood should be zero,assuming that it is non essenntial. However under normal conditions of exposure cadmium concentration is expected to fall below a certain "tolerance limit" i.e a reference level, in relation to which higher values can be appropriately interpreted.(13)

Long term exposure to low air levels of Cd leads to chronic obstructive lung disease and possibly lung cancer.Excessive exposure both via air and food leads to renal tubular disfunction.This is a primarily reabsorption defect in the proximal tubules and it is characteristic effect of cadmium.The first sight of damage is a low molecular weight proteinouria with an increased excretion of β-microglobulins. Aminoacidouria, glucosouria, total proteinouria may occur later.Long term cadmium exposure may also lead to distrurbance of calcium metabolism, osteoporosis and osteomalacia. The syndrome of cadmium induced proteinouria, glucosouria, osteomalacia and or osteoporosis was epidemic in 1950 in a cadmium polluted area of Japan and has been called Itai-Itai disease.(3)

In the human body cadmium concentration ranges broadly from subnanograms per milliliter to a few nanograms per milliliter in biological fluids. Methods used in the past for determination of cadmium blood concentrations as colorimetry or molecular absorption spectrometry were long,complex and inadequate in sensitivity.Nowadays Electrotermal Atomic Absorption Spectroskopy techniques seems to be the methods which offer the greatest possibilities for the determination of cadmium in biological materials.(10)

SUBJECTS AND METHODS

Study population

In the total studied population 506 (272 male and 234 female) healthy Greek adults,not proffecionally exposed to toxic heavy metals were compared. The definite selection of the study population was based on informations gathered by a questionaire recommended by the Scandinavian Commitee of reference values (14) and EPTRV of IFCC (15) mainly related to medical and occupational history.The subjects were devited acording to their smoking habits and sex.

Blood sampling

5 ml venous blood were collected from each participand with venoject vacutainer system in polupropulene metal free tubes with Na EDTA as anticoagulant.The blood samples were kept at 4 C until the analysis which took place within 24 hours after sample collection.The used pippetes tips,tubes and vials in synthetic polymers were washed with 20% Nitric Acid analytical grade,rinsed with ultra pure deionized water and dried in dust free conditions in order to avoid contamination.Only white or blue exchangable tips of automatic pippetes was used since yellow tips contain cadmium.(9)
Blood cadmium concentrations were determined by electrothermal atomic absorption spectrometry.The used method is suggested as standardized method by the subcommittee on Cadmium of the IUPAC Clinical Chemistry Division's Commission of Toxicology. The characteristic concentration of the method is 1.10 /0,0044 A.Precision within a batch is 2%(n=20) and accuracy d=2%. For calibration curves the standard additions method was used and reliability of the method was calculated using Reference

material from Community Bureau of Reference.(11)
Smoking habits were assessed from heath questionnaire. As current smokers were accepted those who smoke more than 10 cigarettes per day.Light smokers (smoking less than 10 cigarettes per day are not included in the present work.

RESULTS AND DISCUSSION

The results obtained are present in next two tables.In table 1 are shown the blood cadmium concentrations in nonsmokers.We didn't found a Gausian distribusion,so we used nonparametric analysis for the determination of reference values.

Table 1. Reference limits of cadmium concentration in whole blood of healthy not proffecionally exposed Athens ser vants.

Parameter	CADMIUM μg/l		
	NONSMOKERS		
	Men	Women	Total
r	136	124	260
Range	0.4-3.0	0.5-2.0	0.4-3.0
Median	0.8	0.9	0.85
0.025 Fractile	0.5	0.5	0.5
90% Confidence interval	0.4-0.5	0.5-0.6	0.5-0.5
0.975 Fractile	1.5	1.6	1.6
90% Confidence interval	1.3-1.6	1.5-2.0	1.4-1.6

In the table 2 are shown the whole blood cadmium concentrations in smokers .We found a Gausian distribusion only in the group of women smokers so for them we used parameter analysis.For the rest groups we used nonparametric analysis as we didn't found gausian distribusion.

Table 2. Reference limits of cadmium concentration in whole blood of healthy not proffecionally exposed Athens servants.

Parameter	CADMIUM μg/l		
	SMOKERS		
	Men	* Women	Total
r	136	111	247
Range	0.5-4.0	0.5-5.0	0.5-5.0
Median	1.6	1.4	1.5
0,025 Fractile	0.542	0.571	0.6
90% Cofidence interval	0.5-0.7	0.645-0.856	0.5-0.7
0,975 Fractile	3.6	2.675	3.58
90% Cofidence interval	3.3-4.0	2.37-3.089	3.2-4.0

* Group with Gausian distribusion.

In smokers the concentrations of cadmium in blood are higher than in non smokers and there is a statistically significant difference ($p>0.001$).
The median whole blood concentration of cadmium in nonsmokers men and women is of the same order or magnitude as in populations not proffecionally exposed to cadmium from India but higher than in other countries as can be seen in Table 3

Table 3. Cadmium concentrations in human blood of some regions of different countries.

COUNTRY	MEDIAN	n	Remarks
Belgium	1.0	89	Nonsmokers
Sweden	0.2	76	Nonsmokers
Yugoslavia	0.5	114	Nonsmokers
Baltimore	0.6	88	Nonsmokers
Japan	1.1	94	Nonsmokers
India	0.9	176	Nonsmokers
This study	0.85	261	Nonsmokers
Belgium	2.0	44	Smokers
Sweden	1.6	84	Smokers
Yugoslavia	3.2	72	Smokers
Baltimore	1.0	60	Smokers
Japan	1.5	79	Smokers
India	1.1	17	Smokers
This study	1.5	247	Smokers

The results presented in table 1 , 2 are gathered from U.S. National Institute of Standard and Technology (13).

Higher blood cadmiun levels in smokers can be explained by the presence of cadmium in tobacco.According Elinder(8) a ciggrette may contain 1-2 μg Cd and a smoker inhale (0.1-0.2 μg) of ca dmium with each smoked cigarette.It is believed that absorption of cadmium from lungs is between 25-50% of total intake which means that for every 20 cigarettes smoked some 0.5-2 μg of ca dmium are absorbed.Moreau(12) found the blood cadmium levels to be elevated in smokers with a doseeffect relationship between the daily consumption of tobacco and the blood cadmium level.In the present study we also found a good correlation between blood cadmium levels and smoking habits as it is shown in Fig 1.

Fig. 1 Correlation between blood cadmium levels and smoking habits.

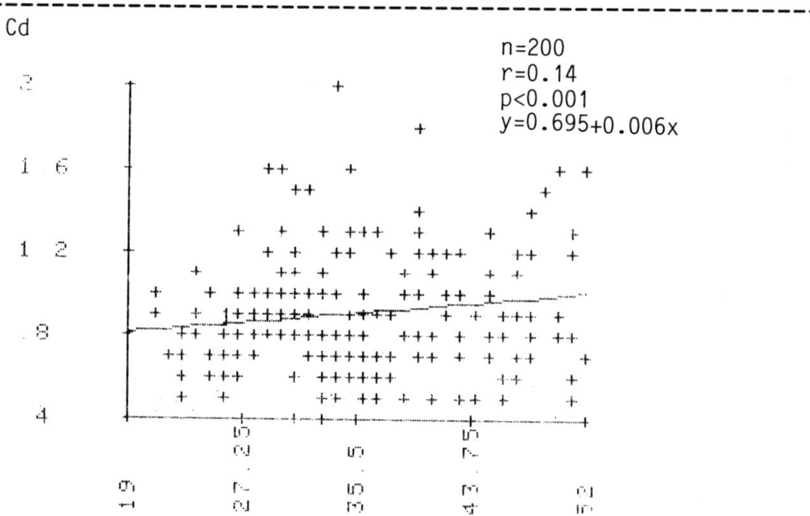

Investigating the cumulative character of toxic metals, we have studied also the influence of age on cadmium whole blood concentration. We have found only a slight correlation in men and women between blood cadmium levels and age (r=0.144, p<0.001) as can be seen in Fig 2.

Fig 2 Correlation between blood cadmium levels and age

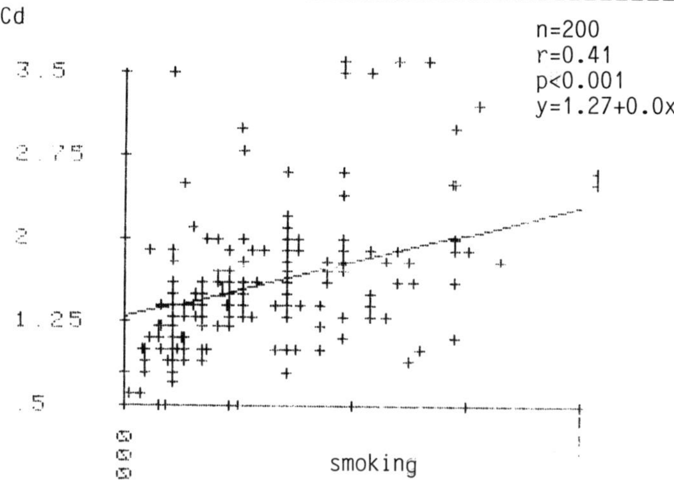

In conclusion we would say that an environmental pollution is evidenced in whole blood concentrations of not proffecionally exposed healthy adults in Athens.This fact may be due to the presence of cadmium emiting factories in the surounds of the city.

References:

1. Chandra Ranjit.(1987):Biological and health implications of toxic heavy metal and essential trace element interactions. Progres in food and nutrition science vol 11.

2. Reilly Conor: Metal contamination of food.

3. Friberg et all.(1986):Handbook of toxicology of metals.2 nd edition Elsevier science publisers.Chater 7 Cadmium.

4. Lauwerys et all (1984):Environmental pollution by cadmium and cadmium body burden.Toxicol.lett.23,287-9.

5. Mc Lellan et all(1978):Measurements of dietary cadmium absorption in humans.J.Toxicol.Environ.Health 4,131-138.

6. Forstner U.(1980):Cadmium,handbook of environmental chemistry.vol3 part A.

7. Hutton M.(1982):Cadmium in the europian community:A prospective assessment of sources of human exposure and environmental impact. MARC Report N=26.Chelsea college London.

8. Elinder et all (1985):Cadmium and health.A toxicological and Epidemiological Appraisal.Ch 3-12.CRC Press Boca Raton Florida.

9. Slavin Walter (1984) Graptite furnance AAS. A source book. Perkin Elmer corporation .

10. Mc Kenzie Smuthe (1988) : Quantitative trace analysis of biological materials.Elsevier

11. Stoeppler et all (1990): Cooperative interlaboratory surveys of the determination of cadmium in whole blood.Fresenius J. Anal.Chem. 338,269-278

12. Moreau et all (1983): Cadmium levels in a general male population with special reference to smoking.Arch. Envir. Healht 38,163-167

13. Iyengar V.et all(1989) : Elemental analysis of biological systems. vol 1 National Bureau of Standarts.Gaithersburg Maryland CRC Press Boca Raton Florida.

14. Solberg H.E.(1983)The theory of reference values.Statistical treatment of collected reference values.Determination of reference limits.J. Clin. Chem.Clin.Biochem.21,749-760

15. Petit Clerc ,C.P.Wilding.(1984):The theory of reference values. Part 2.Selection of individuals for production of reference values.J.Clin.Chem.Clin.Biochem.22,203-208.

Metal Ions in Biology and Medicine, vol. 2. Eds. J. Anastassopoulou, Ph. Collery, J.C. Etienne, Th. Theophanides. John Libbey Eurotext, Paris © 1992, pp. 420-425

Reference limits of selenium concentration in blood serum of a healthy bulgarian sub-population

K. Tzatchev*, Z. Georgiou**, G. Gentchev***

**Mediacal Academy-Department of Clinical Laboratory G. Soffiiski Str. 1, 1431 Sofia, Bulgaria. **IKA DKIE, Toxicology Laboratory 6 Deligiorgi Str., Athens 104 37, Greece. ***Mediacal Academy-Department of Clinical Laboratory G. Sofiiski Str. 1, 1431 Sofia, Bulgaria*

Selenium is now a well recognized essential trace elemen /1/. As a component of the enzyme glytathione peroxidase (EC 1.11.9. glytathion : hydrogen-peroxide oxidoreductase) selenium catalyzes the destruction of peroxides generated during oxidative metabolism in cells/2/. Dietary selenium is necessary to maintain a defence against accumulation of lipid peroxides and free radicals that damag cell membranes.

It is now recognized that some of the diseases common in man are probably related to selenium deficiency/1,3/. Epidemiologiacal studies reveal the importance of selenium in the pathogenesis of cancer/4,5,6,7/ and cardiovascular diseases/8/. It is now know that addition of selenium to the diet effectively prevents juvenile cardiomyopathy, the endemic, condition prevelent in the Chinese provinse of Keshan (Keshan disease). A characteristic feature of that condition is among others, decreased blood and tissue concentration of selenium/9,10/. Previous research made it possible to establish a close relationship between the blood serum levels of selenium and the selenium content of the soil. Low slenium levels are observed among Finns/11/ and New Zeelanders/12/, whereas those of Americans and Canadians are 3 to 4 times higher/13,14/.

The existing geographical differences and the importance of slenium for human health and disease prompt us to investigate in the study reported the selenium levels in blood serum of apparently healthy Bulgarian residents.

MATERIALS AND METHODS

Selenium levels in blood serum were assayed in 294 healthy subjects aged 18-60 years (123 women and 171 men) mainly from Sofia and its surroudings. The examined group included medical personal, students, clerical workers etc whose jobs not involve contact with selenium. A

special questionary designed according the recommendations of Scandinavian Commitee io reference valuew/15/ and EPTRV of IFCC/16/ was used for assessment of the health condition of investigated persons. For the same purpouse the blood of every subject participating in the study was analysed additionaly for same clinical chemistries with Technicon SMA 12/60.
Urine and routine hematologiacal parameters were analysed too.
In the morning between 7-9 o' clock fasting venous blood samples were taken by venopucture into previously checked for contamination polypropilene tubes. After clotting and centrifugation at 1200 x g for 10 min at room temperature the serum was transfered in Eppendorf tubes with caps and stored at -20° C until the analysis.

Serum selenium was determined by electrothermal atomic absorption spectrometry. A modified method of Alfthan er al used/17/.
The measurement was performed on "Perkin-Elmer Zeeman 50000" atomic absorption spectrophotometer. The characteristic concentration of the method is 24.10 g/0,0044 A.s. Precision
within a batch is 5,7%(n=20) and day to day pecision is 7,2% (20 days). The recovery is 97-102%. Additionaly the accurency of the method was checked by determinations of same serum samples with our method and NAA. The results showed very good agrement between the two methods.

All glasware and plastic tubes used for sapling and storage were soaked overnight in 20% nitric acid solution and rinsed with deionized water from "Millipore MIll Q Reagent Water System" and finally checked for contamination with selenium.

The reference limits were estimated with statistical methods recomended by EPTRV of IFCC. For this purpouse was used the original software package "REFVAL"/18/

RESULTS AND DISCUSSION.

The results obtained are presented in Table 1.

Table 1 Reference limits of selenium concentration in blood serum of healthy Bulgarian subjects

Parameter	Selenium (nmol/1)		
	Men	Women	Total
n	171	123	294
Range	341-1329	324-1171	324-1329
Median	722	661	718
0,025 Fractile	444	402	423
90% Confidence interval	422-467	372-431	406-442
0.975 Fractile	1161	1045	1123
90% Confidence interval	1106-1219	986-1108	1080-1168

They show that blood serum selenium conentration of Bulgarian subjects is much lower than those in USA and Canada/13,14/. It is also lower than those found in different European countries (Table 2).

Table 2 Serum selenium levels of the inhabitants of some regions of different European countries (According Thorling et al, 1986/21/)

Region/Country	$\overline{X} \pm S$ nmol/l	n
1. Greece	798 ± 177	21
2. Giessen, FRG	861 ± 127	19
3. Bavaria, FRG	886 ± 127	40
4. Heidelberg, FRG	962 ± 114	23
5. Gothendurg, Sweden	975 ± 139	28
6. Aarhus, Denmark	987 ± 190	58
7. Grenoble, France	1000 ± 190	27
8. Uppsala, Sweded	1025 ± 190	22
9. Unea, Sweded	1038 ± 101	21
10. Paris, France	1038 ± 139	38
11. Barcelona, Spain	1101 ± 177	28
12. Malmo, Sweded	1139 ± 177	52
13. Nederlands	1177 ± 152	36
14. Belgium	1266 ± 114	30
15. Lisbon, Portugal	1291 ± 127	27
16. Ipswish, England	1354 ± 164	20
17. London, England	1379 ± 177	22
This study	721 ± 177	294

The results presented in Table 2 are from collaborative study organized by "The Working Group on Diet and Cancer" under ECP in Leuven, Belgium. All the samples were analysed by fluorimetry in the same laboratory at the Institute of Cancer Research, Aarhus, Denmark.

It is clear that serum selenium level of Bulgarians is the lowest and somewhat near to that for Greece. Recently there are reports for serum selenium levels in Turkey and Yugoslavia which are similae to those found in Bulgaria/19/20/. That is mean that probably all Balkan Peninsula is a selenium deficient region.

Thorling et al/21/found that distribution of the serum selenium values within all the sample areas was close to normal indicating no active regulation of the selenium status in the present range of selenium levels. In our study we have found also Gaussian distribution of serum selenium valves. Thus serum slenium levels correlate direct with soil content of selenium. Since human beings usually do not depend soleley on home grown vegetables and meat from animals raised locally, the effect of a selenium poor soil may not be reflected to quite the same degree in man as in animals. Import of food items produced outside a slelenium-poor region may level out the effect of the local deficiency. Never the less, to some extent the selenium status of people seems to follow the availability of selenium in the soil and quite pronounced differences in serum selenium have been odserved between selenium-rich and selenium-poor countries/12,13/. We havn't data for selenium conent of Bulgarian soils, but as we consider low serum selenium levels and restricted consumption of fish from Bulgarians and restricted import of foods, it is obviously that the content of selenium in the soil especially in Sofia region is low.

We have studied also the influence of gender and age on serum selenium concecntration. Women have lower selenium level and the difference is statisticaly signeficant (p<0,01). We have found only in men a slight correlation between serum selenium level and age (r=0,20 , p<0,20)/Fig. 1/.

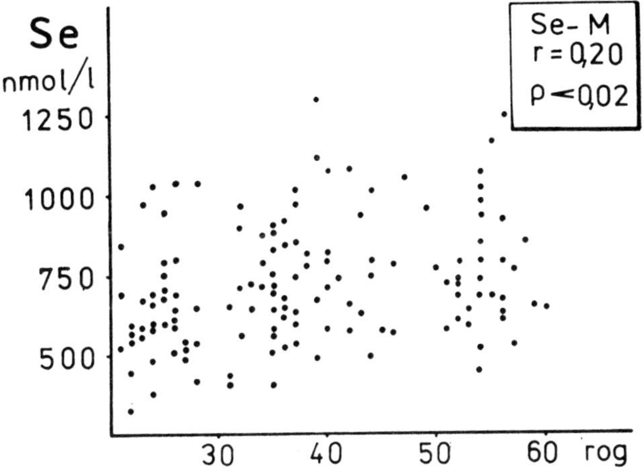

In conclussion we would say that the values from Bulgraria for serum selenium levels are surprisinly low and with the range in individual values within the area it cannot be excluded that boderline deficinecy may be present in part of the population.

References :

1. Lockitch, G., Selenium : Clinical significans and analytical concepts, CRC Crit.Rev.Clin.Lab.Sci., 27, 1989, 6, 483-541.
2. Rotruck, J.T., Discovery of the role of slenium in gluthatione peroxidase, In: J.E.Spallholz, J.L.Martin, H.E. Ganther Eds. Selenium in biology and medicine, Westport, CT. AVI Publishing, 1981, 10-16.
3. Westmark, T.W., Consequences of low selenium intake for man IN: Trace Elements-Analytical Chemistry in Medicine and Biology, Vol. 3, Eds. P. Bratter, P. Schramel, Walter de Grypter, Berlin, New York. 1984, 49-70.
4. Shamberger, K.J., S.A. Tytko, C.E.Willis, Antioxidants and cancer VI. Slenium and age adjusted cancer morality, Arch. Environ. Health, 31, 1976, 231.
5. Sohrauzer, G.N., D.A.White, C.J.Schneider, Cancer morality correlation studies III. Statistical association with dietary selenium intake, Bioinorg.Chem., 7. 1977. 23-35.
6. Cowgill, V.M., The distribution of selenium and cancer morality in the Continental United States, Biol. Trace Elem.Res., 5,1988, 345.
7. Stampfer, M.J., G.A. Colditz, W.C. Willet, The epidemiology of selenium and cancer, Cancer Surv., 6. 1987, 4, 623-633.
8. Salonen, M.J., G.Alfthan, J.Pikkarainen et al., Association between cardiovascular death and myocardial infarction and serum selenium in matched-pair longitudinal study, Lancet, 2, 1982, 175.
9. Keshan Diease Research Group of the Chinese Academy of Science, Observation on the effect of sodium selenite in prevention of Keshan Disease, Chin. Med.J., 92, 1979, 471-476.
10. Chen, X., G.Yang, J.Chen et al., Studies on the relation of selenium and Keshan disease, Biol.Trace Elem. Res., 2, 1980, 91.
11. Westmark, P.Rannu, M.Kirjavinta. I.Lappaleinen, Slenium content of whole blood and serum in adults and children of different ages from different parts of Finland, Acta Pharmacol. Toxicol., 40, 1977, 465.
12. Thomson, C.D, M.F.Robinson, Slenium in human Health and disease with emphasis on those aspects pecullar to New Zeeland, An.J.Clin.Nutr., 33, 1980, 303.
13. Levander, O.A., V.C.Morris, Dietary selenium levels needed to maintain balance in North American adults consuming selfselected diets, An.J.Clin.Nutr. 39, 1984, 809-815.
14. Roekens, E., H.Deelstra, H. Robberecht, Trace elements in human milk, Slenium a case study, Sci.Total.Environ., 42, 1985, 91-108.
15. Alstrom, T., R.Grasbeck, R.Hjem, S.Skandse, Recommendation of reference values in clinical cehemistry and activity report by the commitee on reference values of the Scandinavian Society for Clinical Chemistry and Clinical Physiology, Scand.J.Clin. Lab.Invest., 35, Suppl., 144, 1975.
16. Petit Clerc, C., P.Wilding, The Theory of reference values. Part 2. Selection of individuals for production of refernce values, J.Clin.Chem.Clin.Biochem., 22, 1984, 203-208.

17. Alfthan, G., J.Kumpulainen, Determination of selenium in small

volumes of blood plasma or serum by electrothermal atomic absorption spectrometry, Anal.Chin.Acta., 140, 1982, 221-227.
18. Solberg, H.E., Statistical treatment of collected reference values. Determination of reference limits. J.Clin.Chem.Clin. Biochem., 21, 1983, 11, 749-760. Solbeg, H.E.REFVAL, Techincal report, 1983.
19. Mangubas, K., S.Cin, I.Gokmen et al., Selenium status of normal Turkish children, International Symposium on Selenium, Belgrade, May 12-15, 1991, Abstracts, p.17.
20. Marsimovic, Z., Slenium deficiency in Yugoslavia , International Symposium on Selenium, Belgrade, May 112-15 1991, Abstracts, p.1.
21. Thorling, E.B., K.Overvad, J.Geboers, Selenium status in Europe - Human data a multicenter Study, Ann.Clin.Res., 18, 1986, 3-7.

Metal Ions in Biology and Medicine, vol. 2. Eds. J. Anastassopoulou, Ph. Collery, J.C. Etienne, Th. Theophanides. John Libbey Eurotext, Paris © 1992, pp. 426-427

Influence of sex and age on blood copper and zinc

M. Marrella, R. Gasperini, R. Milanino, U. Moretti, M. Pasqualicchio*, G. Gandini*, E. Trevisani*, R. Vaccari, G.P. Velo

*Instituto di Farmacologia, Università di Verona, Policlinico Borgo Roma, 37134 Verona and *Centro Trasfusionale, ULSS 25, Policlinico Borgo Roma, 37134 Verona, Italy*

Introduction

The research on trace elements in pathology primarily requires a knowledge of the reference values obtained in normal subjects coming from the same geographical area.

When referring to the sexes, it is already well estabilished that in healthy human plasma and whole blood, the copper levels are higher in females than in males (Underwood, 1977). However, as far as we know, less data is available on the levels of plasma and erythrocyte zinc in males and females. Linderman et al. (1971) reports that the plasma zinc values are significantly lower in females than in males and there is no difference in the red cell zinc contents.

Buxaderas and Farré-Rovira (1986) found a slight decrease in plasma and whole blood copper concentrations with aging; in contrast; Bales et al. (1990) found an age related increase of plasma copper. A significant linear decrease in plasma zinc concentrations with increasing age was found (Linderman et al., 1971) while Bales et al. (1990) did not find variation of this parameter with age.

Thus the purpose of this study is to evaluate both plasma and total blood cell (TBC) copper and zinc concentrations on a large number of healthy blood donors divided into groups, based on sex and age.

Material and methods

An age profile of the 593 males and 49 females who participated in this study is shown in table 1. The mean age between males and females was similar in all age groups observed. None of the donors were under pharmacological therapy during the week preceding blood withdrawals. Blood was withdrawn from an antecubital vein and collected into heparinized tubes in the early morning. Haematocrit was assayed automatically by a Sysmec CC 780 instrument. For copper and zinc determinations, all the chemicals used were A.R. grade free from copper and zinc contamination and only copper and zinc free glassware was used. Non-haemolytic plasma was deproteinized by adding an equal amount of a 15% trichloroacetic acid solution. The TBC was acid digested by a procedure which has been previously described (Marrella & Milanino, 1986). Metal determinations were carried out by using flame atomic absorption spectrophotometry (Perkin Elmer 3030 SAA)(Marrella & Milanino, 1986). The values of TBC are referred to as a decilitre of cells because they were corrected for the haematocrit values. Statistic analysis was carried out using the Student's t-test and Pearson's correlation coefficient.

Results

The mean value of haematocrit of each group is shown in table 1; obviously it was higher in males. The concentrations of copper and zinc in the plasma and the TBC of the population examined are shown in tables 2 and 3 respectively.

Concerning the differences between sexes, plasma copper was found to be higher in females than in males in all the age groups of examined. In those under 50 years of age, the plasma zinc was found to be significantly lower in females than males. No variations were found in the TBC copper and zinc levels between males and females.

Aging is accompanied by an increase of plasma copper that was found to be correlated with age in both males and females ($r=0.193$, $P<0.001$ and $r=0.199$, $P<0.01$ respectively). The TBC copper concentration was found to have decreased with aging in both sexes, but only in males was there a significant inverse correlation with age observed ($r=-0.189$, $P<0.01$). The plasma zinc was found to have significantly decreased only in males over 60 years of age. Finally, the TBC zinc concentration was not influenced by age in either of the sexes.

Table 1. Number, mean age and mean haematocrit of 642 blood donors subdivided by age and sex.

Groups (years)	Number M	Number F	Mean Age (years) M	Mean Age (years) F	Mean Haematocrit (%) M	Mean Haematocrit (%) F
20-29	102	10	26.3±2.63	25.8±2.74	45.26±2.65	40.20±3.83 s
30-39	173	9	34.7±2.88	36.9±1.97	45.27±2.33	39.62±1.98 s
40-49	209	19	43.9±2.77	44.5±3.22	45.56±3.19	40.15±1.76 s
50-59	89	11	53.5±2.38	53.4±2.77	44.93±2.78	41.89±1.65 s
60-69	20	0	61.7±1.53	-	45.76±3.30	-

Student t-test: s = $P<0.01$ females versus males.

Table 2. Copper levels in plasma and total blood cells of males (M) and females (F) divided by age.

Groups		Plasma (μg/dl) M	Plasma (μg/dl) F	Total blood cell (μg/dl) M	Total blood cell (μg/dl) F
a)	20-29	87.5±13.08	96.1±13.63	89.9±11.43	86.9±9.30
b)	30-39	93.9±12.26 a^1	103.6±12.43 s^5	86.6±10.51 a^2	86.2±10.9
c)	40-49	96.2±13.79 a^1	110.6±26.65 s^1	86.4± 9.48 a^1	84.8±8.50
d)	50-59	98.4±15.48 a^1,b^2	120.1±13.26 s^1,a^1,b^1	84.4±11.05 a^1	83.3±6.49
e)	60-69	104.3±12.25 a^1,b^1,c^2	-	80.7±10.66 a^1,b^2,c^2	-

Student t-test: $a^1 = P<0.01$, $a^2 = P<0.02$ versus group a; $b^1 = P<0.01$, $b^2 = P<0.02$ versus group b; $c^2 = P<0.02$ versus group c; $s^1 = P<0.01$, $s^5 = P<0.05$ females versus males.

Table 3. Zinc levels in plasma and total blood cells of males (M) and females (F) divided by age.

Groups		Plasma (μg/dl) M	Plasma (μg/dl) F	Total blood cell (μg/dl) M	Total blood cell (μg/dl) F
a)	20-29	101.6±17.88 e^1	88.9±14.05 s^5	1212±165	1180±300
b)	30-39	102.1±14.89 e^1	91.6±15.26 s^5	1240±184	1195±153
c)	40-49	99.8±13.61 e^1	91.4±11.44 s^2	1240±176	1266±180
d)	50-59	98.8±15.15 e^2	96.8± 9.30	1262±184 a^5	1318± 95 b^5
e)	60-69	89.7± 9.92	-	1246±160	-

Student t-test: $a^5 = P<0.05$ versus group a; $b^5 = P<0.05$ versus group b; $e^1 = P<0.01$, $e^2 = P<0.02$ versus group e; $s^2 = P<0.02$, $s^5 = P<0.05$ females versus males.

Discussion

As previously discussed (Underwood 1977)(Buxaderas & Farré-Rovira, 1986) the plasma copper concentration is higher in females when compared with males. The plasma zinc level is lower in females compared to males, but only in those subjects below 50 years of age. The TBC copper and zinc concentrations are the same in both sexes.

The results presented in this paper also show that copper is directly correlated with age. The differences observed among the groups are small, but the trend of increase is constant and the different age groups are often significantly distinguishable. The TBC copper level is inversely correlated with age and the trend observed seems to be rather constant also in this case. The plasma zinc level was found to have decreased only in the group of males over 60 years of age, while zinc concentrations in both plasma and TBC of females were not influenced by age.

In conclusion, the results presented in this paper, showing that both sex and age are capable of influencing the status of copper and zinc in healthy subjects, strongly suggest the use of age and sex matched controls when studying the metabolism of these trace elements in human pathologies.

References

Bales, C.W., Freeland-Graves, J.H., Askey, S., Behmardi, F., Pobocik, R.S., Fickel, J.J. and Greenlee, P., (1990): Zinc, magnesium, copper, and protein concentrations in human saliva: age- and sex-related differences. Am. J. Clin. Nutr. 51: 462-9.

Buxaderas, S.C. and Farré-Rovira, R., (1986): Whole blood and serum copper levels in relation to sex and age. Rev. esp. Fisiol. 42 (2): 213-218.

Lindeman, R.D., Clark, M.L. and Colmore, J.P., (1971): Influence of age and sex on plasma and red-cell zinc concentrations. J. Geront. 26 (3): 358-363.

Marrella, M. and Milanino, R., (1986): Simple and reproducible method for acid extraction of copper and zinc from rat tissue for determination by flame atomic absorption spectroscopy. Atomic Spectroscopy 7 (1): 40-42.

Underwood, E.J., (1977): Copper. In Trace Elements in Human and Animal Nutrition, ed. E.J. Underwood, pp. 56-108. 4th Ed., New York: Academic Press.

Metal Ions in Biology and Medicine, vol. 2. Eds. J. Anastassopoulou, Ph. Collery, J.C. Etienne, Th. Theophanides. John Libbey Eurotext, Paris © 1992, pp. 428-429

Normal values versus real of iron, transferrin and ferritin in Saragonese population (Spain)

M.D. Zapatero Gonzalez, M.L. Calvo Ruata, M. Gonzalez Enguita, B. Gonzalez Ara, A. Garcia de Jalon Comet, E. Ruiz Bajos

Unidad de Nutrición y Metales, Servicio de Bioquimica, Hospital Miguel Servet, INSA-LUD, Zaragoza, España

Iron deficiency is the cause more frecuent of anaemia in the world. According to O.M.S. data 30% of the world population suffer anaemia, especially due to an iron deficiency either inadequate nutritional intake or excessive losses.

In Spain there are few surveys about the prevalence of iron deficiency in normal population.

The porpuse of this work is to study iron status in normal population (0-85 aged) during 1991 in relation to sex and age groups.

MATERIAL AND METHODS

The sample of population that we have studied are healthy inhabitants from Zaragoza distribuied into sex and age groups.

Measurements has been made by the following analytic methods: Iron (Selective Electrode), Transferrin (Kinetic Nephelometry) , Ferritin (E.L.I.S.A.).

RESULTS

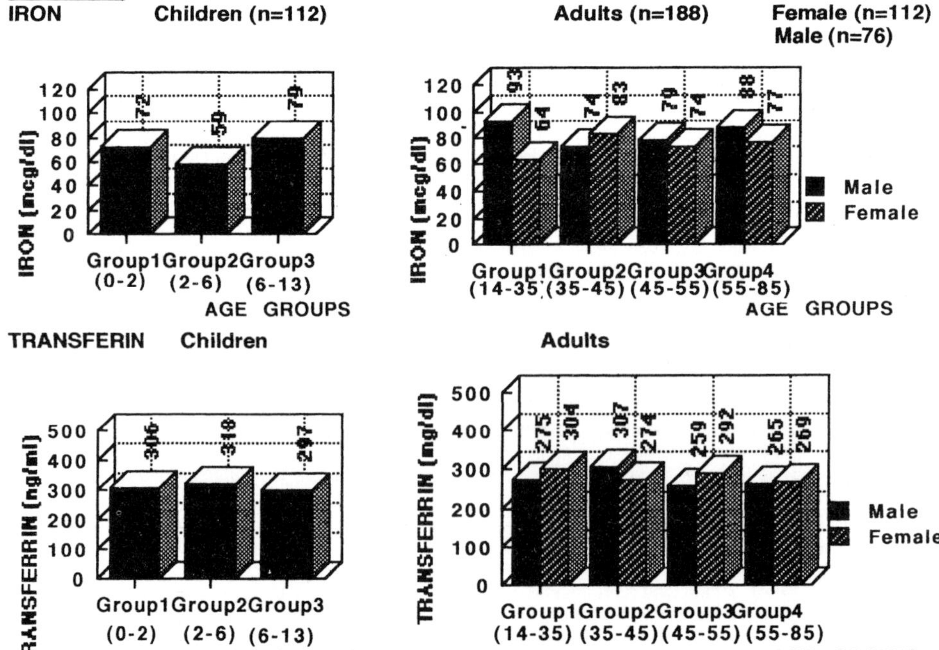

FERRITIN

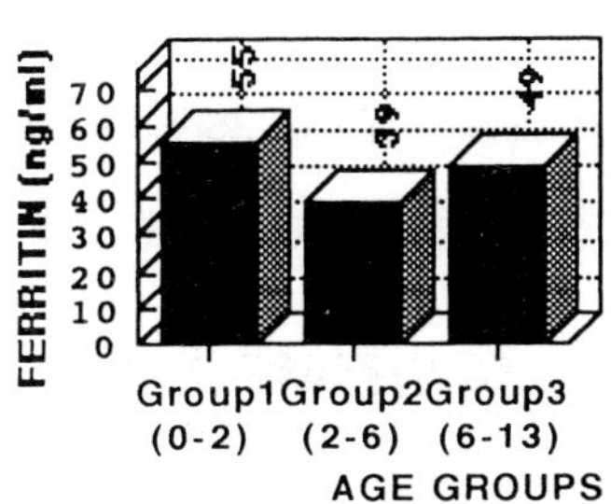

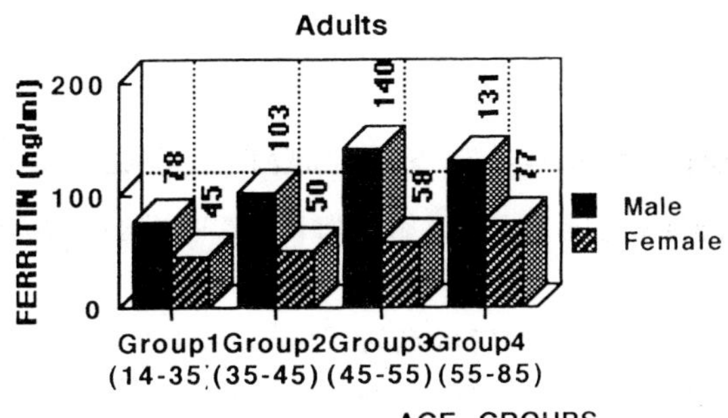

CONCLUSIONS

The transferrin are in a normal range but we can observed a lower serum iron level in our milieu than is described in the bibliography the causes are not well known but the authors think that it could be due to nutritional and socio- cultural changes .

1.- Children:

We have noticed a decrease of the serum iron in the group 2 (2-6 aged), this fact could be due to a change in the nutritional habits and the activity of the children.

Also could influence the routine supplements with oral -Fe during the first year of life to prevent the iron deficiency of the milk.

In the same age group the transferrin is increased to permit a better absortion and the ferritin is decreased in relation to the iron store.

In our milieu the serum iron level in the child population is very variable and it has a repercusssion in the transferrin and ferritin for this reason we have considered the absolute necessity in the practice to make a accurate asses of the iron status and the possible iron deficiency in the 2-6 aged

2.- Adults:

We have observed significatives differences between iron, transferrin and ferritin in relation to sex due to physiological losses of the female.

We have found a positive correlation between ferritin and age, in the same way a negative correlation with the transferrin.

Clasically, in our milieu the female (35-45 aged) are a risk group of iron deficiency, for this reason are supplemented with oral -Fe treatment , this fact could explain the increase of the serum iron level and ferritin in this age group.

In males, the group 2 (35-45 aged) has a decrease of serum iron level with an increase of ferritin and transferrin suggesting not an iron deficiency but a bad distribution of this metal

REFERENCES

De Maeyer, E., and Adiels-Tegman, M. (1985):The prevalence of anaemia in the World.World Health Stat Q 38:302-316.

Hermosa,V.,Mazo,E.,Carril,J.,Cordovilla,JJ.,Luceño.A.,Zubizarreta,A.,(1986):Estudio prospectivo sobre la prevalencia de ferropenia en la población adulta de Cantabria. Med Clin. 87:135-140.

International Nutrition anaemia Consultive Group (1979):Iron deficieny in infancy and Childhood, eds Dallman, PR.,and Simes, MA. (1979): New York : The Nutrition WHO Foundation.

Lopez Gomez, L., Gracia , J.A., and Giralt,M. (1990): Ferropenia hoy y siempre .Sangre.35(4):299-305.

Martin,L.M., Santolaria,F., Gonzalez,G.,et al (1989): Prevalencia de ferropenia y anemia ferropénica en una pobación escolar rural entre 4-15 años. An Esp. Ped.30:159-162.

Metal Ions in Biology and Medicine, vol. 2. Eds. J. Anastassopoulou, Ph. Collery, J.C. Etienne, Th. Theophanides. John Libbey Eurotext, Paris © 1992, pp. 430-431

Levels of some trace elements in autopsy tissues from subjects living in Tarragona province, Spain

M. Schuhmacher, J.L. Domingo, J.M. Llobet, J. Corbella

Laboratory of Toxicology and Biochemistry, School of Medicine, University of Barcelona, San Lorenzo 21, 43201 Reus, Spain

It is well known that various essential metals such as copper, chromium, zinc, cobalt, manganese, iron, etc., play also an important role in a number of fields of modern industry, and consequently these elements are widely dispersed in the environment. Information on the trace metal contents of human tissues is useful for assessing nutrition and for prevention and control of various disease states caused by mineral or trace element imbalance (Saltzman *et al.*, 1990). The main factors influencing the biological effects of trace metals are their actual local concentrations, the eating and drinking habits, the geographical and industrial environment, occupational activity, etc. (Takacs & Tatar, 1987). In the present study, we determined the levels of copper (Cu), chromium (Cr) and zinc (Zn) in kidney, liver, lung, bone and brain autopsy samples taken from subjects living in Tarragona Province (Catalonia, NE Spain). Analysis of the results was made in terms of place of residence, age, sex, and drinking and smoking habits.

MATERIALS AND METHODS

Postmortem analyses of tissue concentrations of Cu, Cr, and Zn were performed on a total of 38 men and 28 women, who at the time of death lived in Tarragona Province. An extensive description of the study areas was recently reported (Bosque *et al.*, 1990). All the subjects were autopsied at the Departments of Pathology of the *Juan XXIII, San Pablo and Santa Tecla* and *Virgen de la Cinta* Hospitals, between May 1990 and June 1991.

Samples of about 1 g (wet weight) of right kidney (cortex separated from the medulla), right lobe of liver and lung, right rib and frontal lobe of brain were predigested with 2 ml of 65% HNO_3 at room temperature overnight. On the following day, the predigested samples were heated at 110° C for 18 hr and 1 ml of $HClO_4$ was added. The mixture was then heated at 150° C for 6 hr and subsequently maintained at 210° C until the ashing procedure was completed. Ashed samples were diluted with 0.1 M HNO_3. Chromium and Zn concentrations were measured by atomic absorption spectrophotometry. Copper levels were determined by inductively coupled plasma atomic absorption spectrometry. The accuracy and precision of the analytical methods were tested with standard reference material (NBS, No. 1577) (Schuhmacher *et al.*, 1991).

RESULTS AND DISCUSSION

The data on Cu, Cr, and Zn concentrations in kidney, liver, lung, bone and brain are shown in Table 1. The highest Cu levels were found in liver and brain, while the highest Cr concentrations were detected in bone and lung. Zinc prevailed in liver and bone. No significant differences in metal tissue concentrations were observed in relation to the place of residence, rural or industrial areas in Tarragona Province. No significant correlation coefficients between Cu, Cr, or Zn, and age or sex were found in the tissues of all these subjects. In contrast, the coefficients were especially remarkable on correlating the levels of Cu and Cr in bone with the drinking and smoking habits of the deceased persons.

TABLE 1. Determination of copper, chromium and zinc concentrations (μg/g wet weight) in human autopsy tissues (Means $\pm$ SD)

Tissue	Copper concentrations	Chromium concentrations	Zinc concentrations
Kidney cortex	1.56 ± 0.51	0.06 ± 0.07	27.08 ± 9.25
Kidney medulla	1.83 ± 0.12	0.04 ± 0.05	35.13 ± 21.64
Liver	4.73 ± 1.66	0.02 ± 0.03	67.32 ± 25.67
Lung	1.02 ± 0.27	0.08 ± 0.05	15.61 ± 8.97
Bone	0.43 ± 0.19	0.12 ± 0.11	49.33 ± 16.01
Brain	4.34 ± 1.24	0.02 ± 0.02	18.00 ± 6.22

In a recent investigation, we showed that the daily intakes of Cu and Zn by the inhabitants of Tarragona Province were even lower than the usually recommended values, while the intake of Cr would be closer to those values (Schuhmacher *et al.*, 1992). Thus, taken together the results of this study with those previously reported (Schuhmacher *et al.*, 1992), it seems clear that the environmental pollution due to Cu, Cr, and Zn would not mean a health hazard for the population of Tarragona Province.

Acknowledgements: This work was supported by the Tarragona County Council, Catalonia, Spain.

REFERENCES

Bosque, M.A., Schuhmacher, M., Domingo, J.L., and Llobet, J.M. (1990): Concentrations of lead and cadmium in edible vegetables from Tarragona Province, Spain. *Sci. Total Environ.* 95: 61-67.

Saltzman, B.E., Gross, S.B., Yeager, D.W., Meiners, B.G., and Gartside, P.S. (1990): Total body burdens and tissue concentrations of lead, cadmium, copper, zinc, and ash in 55 human cadavers. *Environ. Res.* 52: 126-145.

Schuhmacher, M., Bosque, M.A., Domingo, J.L., and Corbella, J. (1991): Dietary intake of lead and cadmium from foods in Tarragona Province, Spain. *Bull. Environ. Contam. Toxicol.* 46: 320-328.

Schuhmacher, M., Domingo, J.L., Llobet, J.M., and Corbella, J. (1992): Copper, chromium, and zinc content of foods and diet in a spanish population. Proceedings of the 2nd International Symposium on Metal Ions in Biology and Medicine. Loutraki, Greece.

Takacs, S., & Tatar, A. (1987): Trace elements in the environment and in human organs. *Environ. Res.* 42: 312-320.

Metal Ions in Biology and Medicine, vol. 2. Eds. J. Anastassopoulou, Ph. Collery, J.C. Etienne, Th. Theophanides. John Libbey Eurotext, Paris © 1992, pp. 432-433

Serum selenium levels in young type I diabetics in a low selenium content area

José R. Cervilla, José A. Cocho, José R.F. Lorenzo, José M. Fraga

Departamento de Pediatría, Laboratorio de Alteracione Metabólicas, Hospital General de Galicia, Facultad de medicina, Universidad de Santiago de Compostela, España

INTRODUCTION

The diabetic angiopathy is a complication that appears earlier and is more frequent in patients with early development of the disease . It´s suppose to be related to lipoperoxidation process (LP) starting at endothelial layer, thromboxan synthesis and platelet aggregation in arteries ,Yagi (1982)
The Selenium (Se)-Glutathion peroxidase system has the postulated role of protecting against cellular peroxidation processes in cooperation with other antioxidant systems .(Cocho et al., 1988). Also, recently has been discovered by Berry et al., (1991) that Selenium is essential in thyroid hormone action, since a Selenium type I iodothyronine deiodinase is responsible for the conversion of thyroxine (T4) to trioidothyronine (T3) to be active in vivo.The geographic situation is the main factor that affect the soil Se content, and therofore in the foodstuffs. Our country Galicia (N.W. Spain) has low Se soil content and so a higher risk of develop "marginal deficiency" of itself (Fraga et al ., 1983; Cervilla et al., 1989)

MATERIAL AND METHODS

We have measured the serum Se (SSe) levels by fluorometry of a group of 12 youngs (7 boys and 5 girls) with symptomatic type I diabetes , ketoacidose, hyperglycemia and glucosuria, aget between 2 1/2 and 14 years, weight (12.5 to 50kg) fed a 1500 to 2500 Kcal/day diet with a total daily dose of 0.3 - 1.3 IU/kg of monocomponent insulin. Their levels were compared with a control group of 89 healthy children with normal development of the same area, aged between 6 and 17 years (47 girls and 42 boys). For statistical analysis the two tail Student test was used.

RESULTS

The SSe levels of diabetic group (Table 1), were significantly higher than control one.There was no statistical differences into the control group by age (6-10 years) versus (more than 10 years)(Table 2).

TABLE 1
Serum Selenium levels (μmol/l) in children

Group	N	mean ±	SD	Range
Diabetics	12	0.91	0.32	0.29 - 1.33
Control	89	0.72	0.20	0.16 -1.20

$p<0.05$

TABLE 2
Serum selenium levels (μmol/l) in children by age

Years	N	mean ±	SD	Range
6-10	46	0.72	0.19	0.32 - 1.11
>10	43	0.71	0.22	0.16 - 1.20
Overall	89	0.72	0.20	0.16 - 1.20

$p > 0.05$

DISCUSSION AND CONCLUSIONS

The higher SSe levels found in children a with diabetes type I may be due to either increasing intestinal absorption or shifting of tissue depot Se to blood current for counteracting a possible excess of LP into the intima of arteries (Gebre-Medhin et al., 1984, 1985). To support this hypotesis should be provide that the intermediate products arising in LP, the lipid peroxides, have been found augmented in adult diabetics with respect to normal ones. Furthermore in diabetic subjects with angiopathy or atherosclerosis like coronary insuficiency or cerebro-vascular accidents, the plasma lipid peroxide levels were higher than in whom the process didn´t developed yet Yagi(1982).Besides that, it´s known that in human atheroma, the lipid peroxides does form or exist and the degree of development itself is correlated with the spreading of LP into the atheroma plaques showed by Yagi (1982).In any case, the increasing of SSe levels is not well understood. The polyuria that occurs in these uncontrolled diabetic children increase at once the Se urinary loss, if one may accept that kidney is the main regulating organ in the Se homeostasis (Kobbah et al., 1988).The increasing of Se intestinal absorption is at least less probable, since the fecal loss is not dependent upon the Se intake (Cocho et al., 1988 ; Gebre- Medhin et al., 1984)

Apparently this situation has no relation to the degree of control of the diabetic disease, because other investigators studying this issue in a low Se area (Northeuropean Country), have found similar higher SSe levels in children with a controlled type I diabetes . Therefore although the increased SSe levels in diabetic children remain unexplained, ours study is the first that confirms the aformentioned selenium status in clildren with type I diabetes.(Gebre - Medhin et al., 1984).

It is interesting to note, that these results show an opposite trend with many other disorders in which Se status has been investigated, since the diseased groups had shown a fairly constant low Se levels or low Se status, Lockitch (1989) and Fraga et al., (1989).

ACKNOVLEDGMENTS

This work has been supported in part by a grant of Social security Investigation Fund (FISS) 90/0540.

REFERENCES

Berry, M.J., Banu, L., and Larsen, P.R. (1991): Type I iodothyronine deiodinase is a selenocysteine-containing enzyme. Nature 349: 438-440

Cervilla, J.R., Fernández-Lorenzo,J.R., Fraga, J.M., Cocho, J.A., and Ramos Martínez, J.I. (1988): Glutathione peroxidase activity in erythrocyter of newborns fed maternal or formula milk. In Proc 2nd intern congr Trace Elem. in Med. and Biol., eds Néve J and Favier A, p. 215. Avoriaz

Cocho, J.A., Cervilla, J.R., y Fraga, J.M. (1988):Selenio. Metabolismo e interés clínico. Rev. soc. Esp. Quím. Clín. 1: 89-93

Fraga, J.M., Cervilla, J.R., Varela Iglesias, J., Peña, J., and Cocho, J.A. (1988): Serum Selenium levels and selenium intakes in newborns. In Proc 2nd Intern. Congr. Trace Elem. in med. and Biol., eds néve J. and Favier A., p.211. Avoriaz: W de Grand Co.

Fraga, J.M., Cocho, J.A., Alvela, M., Alonso Fernández, J.R., Peña, J., and Tojo, R. (1983): Selenium state of children. The selenium content of the serium of normal children and children with inborn errors of metabolism. J. inherit. metab. Dis. 6 . 99-102.

Gebre-Medhin, M., Ewald, U., Olof-Plantin, L., and Tuvemo, T. (1984): Elevated serum selenium in diabetic children. Acta pediatr Scand 73: 109-113.

Gebre-Medhin, M., Kylberg, E., Tuvemo, T. (1985): Dietary intake, trace elements and serum protein status in young diabetics. Acta Paediatr. Sacand 74, suppl. 320: 38-43.

Kobbah, A.M., Hellsing, K., and Tuvemo, T (1988): Early changes of some serum proteins and metals in diabetic children. Acta Paediatr Scand 77: 734-740

Lockitch, G. (1989): Selenium. Clinical significance and analytical concepts. CRC Lab. Sci. 27: 483-541.

Yagi, K. (1982): Assay for serum lipid peroxide level and its clinical significance. In Lipid Peroxides in Biology and Medicine, ed K. Yagi, p. 223 New York: Academic Press.

Metal Ions in Biology and Medicine, vol. 2. Eds. J. Anastassopoulou, Ph. Collery, J.C. Etienne, Th. Theophanides. John Libbey Eurotext, Paris © 1992, pp. 434-435

Environmental level of Tl in blood near zinc smelting works

Jerzy Kwapuliński, Barbara Nowak, Adam Nalewajek, Danuta Wiechula

Silesian University of Medicine, Department of Toxicology Sosnowiec, CP 41200 Jagiellońska 4, Poland

In recent years the attention of researchers has been displayed from acute thallium (Tl) toxicity to the potential health hazards of Tl as a trace pollutant. In Upper Silesia the most important antropogenic sourees of Tl are air emissions and non-ferrous smelting on the industrial humane exposure to Tl predominantly results from ingestion of food and polluted air containing trace amounts of Tl. (Davidson et al.,1974). The program provided for collection of samples of airborne particulate in three different points from smelting plant (500m,1500m,3000m) lokalized at all geographic directions. The average range of the changes Tl content was equal 0.517-2.12 ugTl/g at distance 500 m and 0.031-0.8092 ugTl/g at distance 3000m in east direction from smelting plants. The geometric mean concentrations for thallium were following: site west 500m: 0.5216 ugTl/g.Site East 500m: 1.1583 ugTl/g, site East 1000m: 0.7517 ugTl/g, Site East 3000m: 0.3478 ugTl/g. Table 1.

Table 1. Tl content in deposited dust, ug/g

Distance m	East	South
500	0.0572-0.3055	0.2344-2.6243
1500	0.1327-0.2631	0.0852-1.0
2500	0.0735-0.1119	0.0593-0.3358
	West	North
500	0.1531-2.5337	0.2834-1.6049
1500	0.1042-0.8904	0.0728-0.2866
2500	0.0778-0.2586	0.0534-0.1376

The level of Tl in human blood normally is the range of 0.33-0.59 ug/ml. The highest Tl blood levels were found in subjects living very close to the smelting plants and in workers with longer period of service. The mean content in total population of the investigation workers were following:

0.708 ugTl/ml for 2 years of service
0.323 ugTl/ml for 4 years of service
0.982 ugTl/ml for 7 years of service

2.026 ugTl/ml for 9 years of service
1.025 ugTl/ml for 10-14 years and 1.218 ugTl/ml for 15-34 years of service, 1.253 ugTl/ml for above 35 years of service.
The level of Tl in human blood depends on worker's age period of service and fact of smoking and it grows from 0.127 ugTl/ml to 4.942 ugTl/ml - Table 2,3.

Table 2. The occurence Tl in blood in individual years groups

Groups years	Range of changes ug/cm^3		Mean concentration Tl smokers A	Mean concentration Tl no smokers B
20-25	0.257	0.545	0.449	0.415
26-30	1.175	2.29	0.85	0.454
31-35	0.297	2.808	1.121	1.00
36-40	0.240	2.353	1.201	0.905
41-45	0.316	2.987	1.11	1.093
46-50	0.39	1.705	0.99	1.1
above50	0.442	2.468	1.909	0.985

Table 3. Tl content in blood of smelting workers in relation to the period of service ug/cm^3.

Period of service	Average concentration Tl smokers A	Average concentration Tl no smokers B
1-2	0.558	0.858
3-4	0.355	0.291
5-7	1.362	0.602
8-9	1.729	2.324
10-14	1.1006	0.95
15-34	1.394	1.042
above 34	1.297	1.209

The hypotesis of common source for **Tl** in dust deposited dust suspend and in blood confirmed by high correlation between this metal at the investigation samples. Table 2 sumarizes some data on the environmental blood thallium level in the general population of workers.
The level of thallium in human blood normally is in the range of 0.33-0.59 ug/g.The highest Tl blood levels were found in subjects living very close to the smelting plants and in workers with longer period of service - Table 3.

References

1. Davidson R.D., Natush F.S., Wallace J.R., Evans C.E.: Trace elements in fly ash-dependence of concentration on particle size. Environ.Sci.Techn. 8, 1107-1113,(1974).

Metal Ions in Biology and Medicine, vol. 2. Eds. J. Anastassopoulou, Ph. Collery, J.C. Etienne, Th. Theophanides. John Libbey Eurotext, Paris © 1992, pp. 436-437

Urbanization effects on respiration of experimentally amended soil communities

Photeinos Santas*, Henry C. Merchant

*Department of Biological Sciences, The George Washington University, Washington, DC 20052, USA. * Mailing Address : Division of Biology, Department of Natural Sciences, Southeastern College, 53 Taoiou st., Kifissia, Athens 14561, Greece*

INTRODUCTION

Soil texture, as measured by sand, silt and clay content (Atlas & Bartha, 1981), soil organic matter (Alexander, 1977), soil water content (Burns, 1980) and anthropogenic sources of pollution such as soil lead content (Lagerwerff & Specht, 1970) are among the factors invoked to explain the distribution and abundance of soil biota on a continental, regional and local scales.

The present study attempts to investigate the effects of soil texture, soil organic matter content, added water and lead upon respiration of soil communities near a major highway. Site effects were also assessed by comparing respiration data from two sites (King street and Duke street) on the same highway, selected on the basis of their overall geomorphological similarity but located at different distances from the city (Santas, 1988).

MATERIALS AND METHODS

Each of the above factors (soil clay content, soil organic matter, soil lead content and soil moisture) was studied at two levels (high and low) in a full 2^4 factorial treatment design on each of the two experimental sites. Once a month, 2 g of PbAc and 100 mL deionized water were added to the artificial soil cores designated to the high lead and high water treatment, respectively (Santas, 1988). Soil respiration (expressed in µg C cm^{-2} h^{-1}) was measured in the field three times a month, May through September 1986, by the method of inverted cans and titration of the excess NaOH with HCl. Means were analyzed using Tukey's Honestly Significant Difference. All tests at the 0.01 significance level.

RESULTS AND DISCUSSION

Water and lead acetate did not have any significant effect on soil respiration ($F=0.17$; $df=1$ and 1760; $P>0.01$, and $F=5.93$; $df=1$ and 1760; $P>0.01$, respectively). The lack of significant water effects might be attributed to insufficient water added to the soil cores. Lead concentrations of up to 7500 ppm resulted in no significant reduction of peat soil respiration (Doelman & Haanstra, 1979), probably due to lead adsorption on organic matter; addition of 1000 ppm lead did

1000 ppm lead did not affect respiration of soils artificially amended with kaolinite or montmorillonite (Debosz ***et al.*** 1985). Whether soil biota were adaptated to conditions of increased lead content has not been assessed.

The effects of organic matter on soil respiration depend on soil clay content (F=13.46; df=1 and 1760; P<0.01; Fig. 1). Regardless of clay content, soils rich in organic matter respired significantly more than soils low in organic matter. Addition of clay did not significantly affect respiration of organic soils, whereas respiration of soils low in organic matter was significantly reduced.

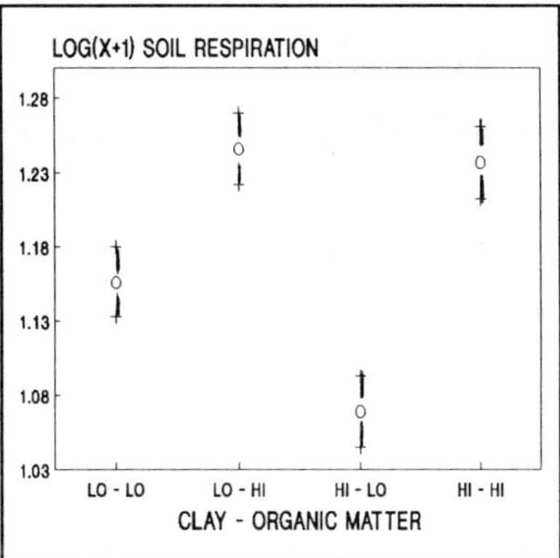

Fig. 1. Means analysis for the effects of the organic matter-by-clay interaction on soil respiration. Means ± 99% JSCI.

The effects of experimental site on soil respiration were not consistent among months (F=8.42; df=4 and 1760; P<0.01; Fig. 2). Despite the apparent similarities between sites, significant between-site differences in lead input are considered responsible for the differences in soil respiration. Traffic volume at King street, the site nearest to the city, was approximately 10,000 vehicles/day more than at Duke street (Virginia Dept. of Highways, *pers. comm.*), the site farthest away from the city. The above results may suggest methods for reclamation of soils severely contaminated by lead.

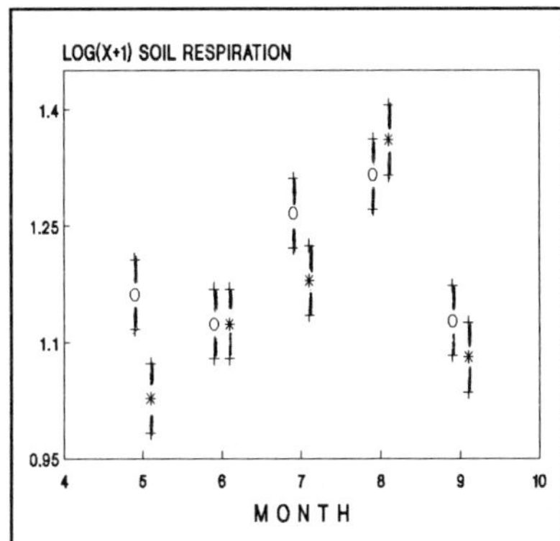

Fig. 2. Means analysis for the effects of the site-by-month interaction on soil respiration. Means ± 99% JSCI. (o: Duke street, *: King street)

REFERENCES

Alexander, M. (1977): Introduction to microbial ecology. New York: John Wiley & Sons.

Atlas, R.M. & Bartha, R. (1981): Microbial ecology. Fundamentals and Applications. Reading, Massachussetts: Addison-Wesley Publishing Co.

Burns, R. G. (1980): Microbial adhesion to soil surfaces: consequences for growth and enzyme activities. In *Microbial communities in soil*, ed. R. C. W. Berkeley, J. M. Lynch, J. Melling, P. R. Rutter & B. Vincent, pp. 249-262. New York: John Wiley & Sons.

Debosz, K. Babich, H. & Stotzky, G. (1985): Toxicity of lead to soil respiration: mediation by clay minerals, humic acids and compost. *Bull. Env. Contam. Toxicol.* 35, 517-524.

Doelman, P. & Haanstra, L. (1979): Effect of lead on soi respiration and dehydrogenase activity. *Soil Biol. Bioch.* 11, 481-485.

Lagerwerff, J. V. & Specht, A. W. (1970): Contamination of roadside soil and vegetation with cadmium, nickel, lead and zinc. *Env. Sci. Tech.* 4, 583-585.

Santas, P. (1988): Effects of clay content, cow manure, lead and water upon roadside soil communities. Washington, D.C.: The George Washington University.

Metal Ions in Biology and Medicine, vol. 2. Eds. J. Anastassopoulou, Ph. Collery, J.C. Etienne, Th. Theophanides. John Libbey Eurotext, Paris © 1992, pp. 438-439

Coexistence of heavy metals in the air and soil in the recreational region in the south of Poland (Wisla)

Barbara Nowak, Jerzy Kwapulinski, Urszula Kosmala, Adam Nalewajek

Silesian University of Medicine, Department of Toxicology Sosnowiec, Jagiellonska 4, Poland

In this work an attempt has been made to determine a quality of the atmospheric air and soil from different emission sources (i. e. motor way, traction of railway, coal fuel combustion in the houses farnace, long term range emission from Tryniec - Czechoslovakia) in Wisła. The program prorided for the collection of 180 samples of airborne and 60 samples of soil particulate in the different points in Wisła.

There are linear emission sources:

1) motor way - average street traffic volume of 324 vehicles / h
2) traction of railway which is in the center of Wisła

The investigation of the heavy metal content in the air and soil were carried out in the quarter of ville (coal fuel comustion) and " clean " area near Wisła (only long term range emission from Czechoslovakia) i. e. peaks Beskidy Mountains. There are surface emission sources. The soil layer area was taken simultanseusly in the points of dust sampling.Table 1.

Table 1. Forecasting the averages values of the metal concentration in the soil [μg/g].

	The quarter of motor way (n=24)	The "clean" area near Wisła (n=96)
Mn	223.3 < 266.4 < 309.5	152.3 < 185.7 < 219.1
Zn	206.2 < 233.3 < 260.4	122.9 < 149.5 < 176.1
Cr	47.7 < 55.2 < 62.7	27.6 < 35.2 < 42.8
Cu	26.6 < 30.5 < 34.4	21.9 < 24.0 < 26.2
Pb	197.3 < 242.4 < 287.2	132.5 < 158.2 < 183.9
Co	17.2 < 18.5 < 19.8	10.9 < 12.5 < 14.1
Cd	2.5 < 2.7 < 2.9	1.0 < 1.6 < 2.2
Ni	38.8 < 43.3 < 47.5	25.3 < 30.7 < 36.1

The all samples were collected during the period 1989 / 90. The dust was mineralized by the means of the mixture of hydrofluoric and nitric acids while the soil was digested in the mixture of the hydrofluoric and perchloric acids. The Atomic Absorption Spectroscopy (AAS) method was used to determine the concentrations of following metals: Pb, Cd, Mn, Cr, Cu, Co, Ni, Zn.

Assuming the value of significance level for normal distribution function equals $\alpha=0.05$ an interval estimation for the average concetrations of metals and dust for different dust emission sources were calculated. Table 2.

Table 2. Forecasting the averages values of the metal concentration in the air [$\mu g / m^3$].

	The linear sources in Wisła (motor way traction of railway) (n=98) Nz=324 vehicles/h	2. The quarter of ville in Wisla (n=36)	3. The "clean" area near Wisła (n=52)
dust	134.8 <151.3 <167.8	23.08 < 47.8 < 71.8	17.6 < 32.9 < 48.1
Mn	0.20 < 0.23 < 0.26	0.14 < 0.15 < 0.16	0.06 < 0.09 < 0.12
Zn	0.45 < 0.49 < 0.53	0.20 < 0.31 < 0.42	0.16 < 0.28 < 0.40
Cr	0.29 < 0.33 < 0.37	0.27 < 0.37 < 0.47	0.15 < 0.18 < 0.21
Cu	0.61 < 0.72 < 0.83	0.26 < 0.29 < 0.32	0.15 < 0.20 < 0.25
Pb	1.67 < 1.83 < 1.99	1.08 < 1.22 < 1.36	0.59 < 0.83 < 1.07
Co	0.15 < 0.17 < 0.19	0.09 < 0.12 < 0.15	0.11 < 0.12 < 0.125
Cd	0.025 < 0.03 < 0.035	0.02 < 0.03 < 0.04	0.01 < 0.02 < 0.03
Ni	0.27 < 0.29 < 0.31	0.16 < 0.25 < 0.34	0.15 < 0.19 < 0.21

n= number of samples
Nz=traffic intensity

Metal Ions in Biology and Medicine, vol. 2. Eds. J. Anastassopoulou, Ph. Collery, J.C. Etienne, Th. Theophanides. John Libbey Eurotext, Paris © 1992, pp. 440-441

Metallothionein and metal levels in urine from a human population in Tarragona, Spain

Jaume Folch, Neus García, José L. Paternain

Unit of Biochemistry, School of Medicine, University of Barcelona, 43201 Reus, Spain

The biological monitoring of toxic metals in a human population allows to prevent harmful effects on public health. Urine, total blood and serum samples are commonly used to carry out the monitorization. Moreover, urine represents the major excretion route for heavy metals, as well as its exposure metabolic indicators.

Metallothioneins (MT) are cytosolic proteins widely spread in the human organism with a high ability to bind divalent metals (Zn, Cu, Cd, Hg, etc...) (Bremner, 1990). Typically, some of the highest concentrations of MT are found in the liver and kidney after metal exposure (Lee et al., 1983). Significative changes in urine MT excretion levels are found closely related with such processes (Sugihira et al., 1986).

Several studies realted with MT excretion have been carried out in human populations living in toxic metal-poluted areas (Tohyama et al., 1982 Sangster et al., 1984; Bem et al., 1988).

The aim of this study was to provide information from MT, Zn and Cu concentrations found in urine from healthy subjects (N=700) living in Tarragona province (NE, Spain). Analysis of the data were made in order to characterize the average values in terms of sex and age groups and, as well, to find correlations between metals and MT levels.

MT concentrations were tested using a radioimmunoassay method. Metal concentrations were determined by computer-controlled sequential inductively coupled plasma spectrometer.

These studies showed average urinary MT concentrations ranged from 20 to 200 μgMT/g creatinine. The highest values were found in female group, with peak values in the age period of 10 to 20 and 45 to 50 years, and only one peak around 40 in male group (Fig. 1). Cu concentrations found ranged from 2 to 28 μg/g creatinine with peak values in the age period of 10 to 20 and 45 to 50 years (only in the female group). Urinary Zn concentrations, ranged from 80 to 450 μg creatinine, showed a similar distribution in the age period of 10 to 20 and 45 to 50 years in the female group. Male Zn and Cu excretion levels showed no significative changes.

Statistically significant differences between MT excretion levels of age and sex groups were found. Furthermore, statistically strong correlations ($p < 0.001$) were found between urine excretion levels of Cu and MT and between Cu and Zn (only within the female group), using a Multiple Correlation Test.

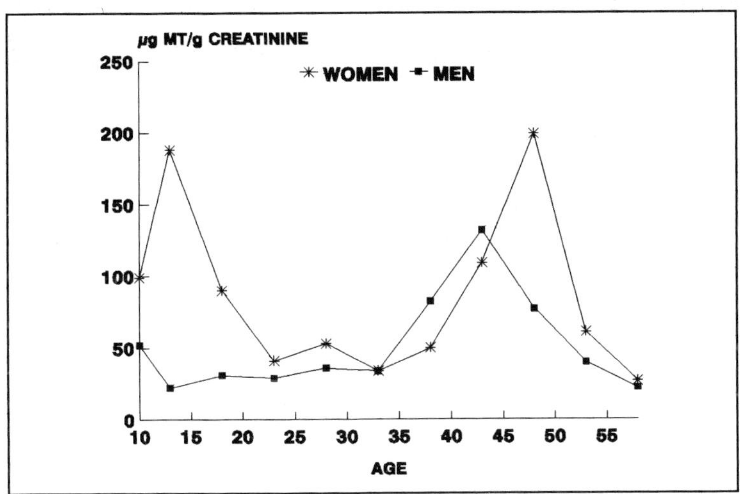

Fig. 1. Urinary excretion of MT in a human population of Tarragona (NE of Spain).

REFERENCES:

Bem E.M., Piotrowski J.K., Sobczak-Kozlowska M., and Dmuchowski C.(1988): Cd, Zn, Cu and metallothionein levels in human liver. *Int Arch Occup Environ Health 60:* 413-417.

Bremner I., and Beattie J.H. (1990): Metallothionein and the trace minerals. *Annu. Rev. Nutr. 10:* 63-83.

Lee Y.H., Shaikh Z.A., and Tohyama C. (1983): Urinary metallothionein and tissue metal levels of rats injected with Cd, Hg, Pb, Cu or Zn. *Toxicology 27:* 337.

Sangster B., de Groot G., Loeber J.G., Derks H.J.G.M., KranjcE. I and Savelkoul T.J.F. (1984): Urinary excretion of Cd, protein, beta-2-microglobulin and glucose in individuals living in a Cd-poluted area. *Human Toxicol. 3:* 7-21.

Sugihira N., Tohyama C., Murakami M. and Saito H. (1986): Significance of increase in urinary metallothionein of rats reatedly exposed to Cd. *Toxicology 41:* 1.

Tohyama C., Shakh Z.A., Nogawa K., Kobayashi E. and Honda R. (1982) Urinary metallothionein as a new renal dysfunction in "itai-itai" disease patients and other Japanese women environmentally exposed to Cd. *Arch Toxicol. 50:* 159-166.

*This work was supported by CICYT, Spain trough project SAL 90-0998.

Metal Ions in Biology and Medicine, vol. 2. Eds. J. Anastassopoulou, Ph. Collery, J.C. Etienne, Th. Theophanides. John Libbey Eurotext, Paris © 1992, pp. 442-443

Urinary N-acetyl-β-D-glucosaminidase activity in occupational Hg and Cr exposition

V. Djurdjic*, L.J. Mandic*, R. Maksimovic**, R. Milivojevic**

**Faculty of Chemistry, University of Belgrade and IOHBIA, Studentski trg 16, POB 550, 11000 Belgrade, Serbia. **Medical Center, Krusevac*

INTRODUCTION

Kidney is an appropriate target organ to toxic injury in chronic exposure to heavy metals. Frequently, precise site of biochemical mechanisms of induced cell injury and early diagnostic parameters of the damage are lacking.

Inorganic Hg and Cr compounds are toxic environmental contaminants and produce marked effects on kidney cell membranes, exibiting nephrotoxicity (Foultres,1983, Stroo & Hook,1977).

In this work the precise site of Hg and Cr renal cell damage were investigated with the aim to find the earliest, specific and sensitive indicator of both metals nephrotoxicity. The activities of N-acetyl-β-D-glucosaminidase (NAG), a lysosomal enzyme, were analysed in urines of workers exposed to inorganic Hg and Cr compounds. The activities of NAG izoenzyme forms were determined, too.

MATERIAL AND METHODS

The study has been performed on two groups of workers manufacturing with inorganic Hg (n=22) and Cr compounds (n=20). Both metal concentrations were determined in urine by AAS-method (Perkin Elmer 1100B) with previous digestion with mixture of acids. The same method was used for Hg blood content determinations. NAG activities were analysed spectrophotometrically by the use of ω-nitrostyril substrate (Yuen et al.1982). The NAG izoenzymes were determined by chromatography on DEAE cellulose.

RESULTS AND DISCUSSION

The contents of blood and urinary Hg and Cr were presented on Fig.1. On the same figure the total NAG activities was presented, too.

On the basis of the data presented it can be seen that besides significant increases of urinary excretion of both metals the significant increases of total NAG activities were found only in exposed to Hg. In workers exposed to Hg significant correlation between blood and urinary metal content was found. Blood Cr levels was not determined because it isn´t good indicator of body Cr status.

More than Cr, readily absorbed Hg exibits a tissue high afinities presenting a cumulative poison (Bomhard et al.,1985). Selective concentration of Hg in kidney cell lysosomes and their damage enhance the urinary total NAG and specific izoenzyme NAG activities. Thus,

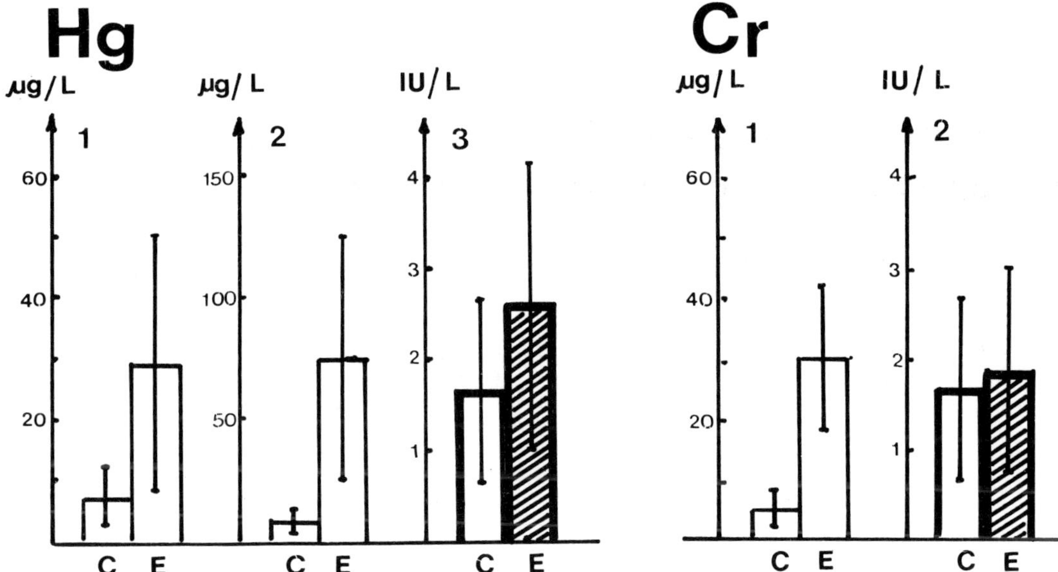

Fig.1. Metal concentrations and NAG activities in nonexposed (C) and exposed (E) subjects. Hg: 1. blood Hg content, 2. urinary Hg content, 3. urinary NAG activities in exposed to Hg. Cr: 1. urinary Cr content, 2. urinary NAG activities in exposed to Cr

activities of membrane bound izoenzyme B-form in exposed to Hg was found to be increased.

During the excretion Cr affects transport processes of renal tubular cell membranes (Berndt,1975). Urinary NAG activities of workers exposed to Cr were not significantly incresed. Being less absorbed and accumulated than Hg, in similar conditions it had not the same nephrotoxic effects.

Hg and Cr have many uses and therefore numerous oppotunities for contamination exist. Although both metals are found to affects tubular kidney cells they exibit different nephrotoxic effects. The total NAG and izoenzyme determinations may serve as early and more sensitive parameters of nethrotoxicity than commonly used.

REFERENCES

Berndt,O.W.(1975):The effect of potassium dichromate on renal tubular transport processes. Toxicol.Appl.Pharmacol.132,40-52

Bomhard,E.,Maruhn,D.,Vogel,O.(1985):Comparative investigations on the effects acute introperitoned Cd, Cr and Hg exposure on the kidney. Uremia Invest,9,131-136

Foultres,E.C.(1983): Tubular sites of action of heavy metals and the nature of their inhibition of amino acids reabsorption. Fed.Proc.42, 2965-2968

Stroo,W.E.,Hook,J.B.(1977): Enzymes of renal origin as indicators of renal nephrotoxicity.Toxicol.Appl.Pharmacol.39,423-434

Yuen,C.T.,Price,R.G.,Chattagoon L.,Richardson A.C.(1982): Colorimetric assays of NAG and β-galactosidase in human urine using newly developed ω-nitrostyril substrates.CCA 125,195-204

Metal Ions in Biology and Medicine, vol. 2. Eds. J. Anastassopoulou, Ph. Collery, J.C. Etienne, Th. Theophanides. John Libbey Eurotext, Paris © 1992, pp. 444-447

Selenium concentration in tumor tissues of neoplasms of the central nervous system

K. Tzatchev, Ch. Tzekov, L. Angelov

Medical Academy-Department of Clinical Laboraty G. Sofiiski Str. 1, 1431 Sofia, Bulgaria

Selenium is an essential trace element in man and in animals. A voluminous literature based on many animal studies shows that under certain condition relatively high dietary levels of selenium can have a protective action against a variety of chemically included and transplantable tumors in rats and mice/1,2/.
A number of geografical observational studies have shown that cancer mortality rates were inversaly related to the geographic distribution of selenium/3,4,5/.

Some case-control have demonstrated lower blood selenium levels among the cancer patients but this finding is not entirely consistent/5/. In our previus study we found diminished serum selenium level in patients with malignant tumors of central nerveous system(CNS)/6/. The mechanisms by which the serum selenium level decreases in various cancerous conditions are still unknown. It has not yet been established whether the reduced selenium level in the serum is a causative factor of the malignant state or a sequela.

In this study the results of the investigation of selenium concentration in tumor tissue of some benign and malignant tumors of CNS are reported.

MATERIALS AND METHODS

The total number of investigated patients with cerebral and extracerebral tumors is 37/(17 men and 20 women aged 4 to 72 years) and their distribution according histology of tumors is presented on Table 1.

Table 1 Distribution of investigated patients according histology of the tumors

Group	n
<u>Bening tumors</u> :	
Meningiomas	16
Neuriomas	3
Craniopharyngiomas	3
Plexuspapilloma	1
<u>Malignant tumors</u> :	
Glioblastomas	13
Meduloblastomas	1

Tumor tissues of the patients with CNS tumors were obtainded at surgical excision and immediately were frozen for later analysis of selenium levels.

Selenium analysis was performed after wet digestion with nitric acid. Fresh tumor tissue was at 65°C for 24 hours. Then the tissue was homogenized and the fat was removed with diethylether for 2 hours. After that 1,0 ml HNO3 was added to 0,1-2,2 g tumor tissues and heated at 80°c in sandbath unitl complete destruction of organic matter. Finally the sample was neutrulized with 1-2 drops of NH3 and diluted to 2-5 ml with deionized water. In resulted solution selenium was determined directly with electrothermal atomic absorption spectrometry with graphite furance using atomic absorption spectrophotometer "Perkin-Elmer Zeeman 5000".

All glasware and plastic tubes used for sampling, storage and sample pretreatment with deionized water from "Millipore Milli Q Reagent Water System".
Statistical analysis was carried out using Student's t-test.

RESULTS AND DISCUSSION

Table 2 presents the results of the tumor tissue selenium levels measurements. The mean selenium concentration of 14 malignant tissue samples (25,11 ± 16,25 nmol/g fresh weight) was significantly higher than that of 23 bening tumor tissue samples (13,98 ± 6,34 nmol/g fresh weight) p<0,02/.

Table 2 Concentration of selenium in the tumor tissue of patients with tumors of CNS

Diagnosis	Se nmol/g f.w. /$\bar{X}$ ± S /
Bening tumors :	
Meningiomas	13,84 ± 5,49
Neuriomas	11,11 ± 10,36
Craniopharyngiomas	15,95 ± 8,84
Plexuspapilloma	18,87
Malignant tumors :	
Glioblastomas	23,55 ± 15,79
Meduloblastomas	45,35

In our previous study we found that serum selenium concentration in patients with malignant of CNS is lower than those with bening tumors or healthy controls/6/. Similar findings are reported in patients with malignant tumor with different localization/7,8/.

Although these studies demonstrate selenium levels after diagnosis of cancer, the lower selenium levels may result from metabolic consequences of the tumor or from poor dietary intake.
Studies to date have shown that most selenium is absorbed from gastrointestinal tract and up to 50% is excreted in urine.
Kogate et al/9/ found that the amount of daily urinary output of selenium was approximately the same between the cancer patients and surgical patients with bening diseases. Thay also found significantly higher selenium concentration in malignant tissue of gastrointestinal tumors than in non-malignant tissue. Tumors are known to concentrate Se and this is the clinical bases for utilization of radioactive selenium for tumor detection. This preferential sequestration of the element may partially reflect the low selenium levels in cancer patients. Our finding support such hypothesis because the malignant tumors of CNS unlike gastrointestnal tumors are enclosed in cranium cavity and in spite of this are the existence of nerveous humoral barrier function they concentrate selenium and influence serum selenium level in the same manner.

The results of the latest case-control studies could't confirm the prediagnostic role of selenium in cancer/10,11,12/. Probably the low serum selenium levels in cances patients is rather consequence than cause of the disease. One of the possible mechanisms by wich the serum selenium decreases in cancer patients is th redistribution of serum selenium and it's concentration in tumor tissue, wich is in a good agreement with our results.

References :

1. Ip, C. Selenium inhibition of chemical carcinogenesis, Fed.Prco. , 44, 1985, 2573-2578.
2. Combs, G.F., Slenium , In: Moon, T.E. M.S.Micozzi, Eds., Nutrition and cancer prevention, New York, Marcel Dekker Inc., 1989, 389-420.
3. Stamfer, M.J., G.A.Colditz, W.C.Willet, The epidemiology of selenium and cancer, Cancer Surv., 6. 1987. 623-633.
4. Levender, O.A. , A Global View of Human Selenium Nutrition, Ann.Rev.Nutr. , 7, 1987, 227-250.
5. Lockithch. G., Selenium: clinical, significance and analytical concepts, CRC Crit.Rev.Clin.Lab.Sci., 27, 1989, 6, 483-542.
6. Philipov, Ph., K.Tzatchev, Selenium concentration in serum of patients with cerebral and extracereberal tumors, Zent.Bl. Neurochirur., 49, 1988, 344-347.
7. K.Tzatchev, M.Tzvetkov, Ch.Kumanov, D.Mladenov, Se level in the serum of patients with prostatic cancer, 7 th Congress of the Wuropian Association of Urology, Budapest, Hungary, June 26-28, Abstracts 1037.
8. Mc Connel, K.V. , R.N. Jager, K.I. Bland , A.J. Blotsky, The relationship of dietary selenium and breast cancer, J.Surg.Onco., 15, 1980, 67-70.
9. Kogata, M., M..Kobayashi, M.Yamamura et al., Slenium levels in malignant and normal tissues of gastrointestinal cancer patients, J. Clin.Biochem.Nutr., 5, 1988, 95-101.
10. Rigstad, J., B.K.Jacobsen, S.Tretil et al., Serum selenium concentration associated with risk of cancer, J. Clin.Pathol., 41, 1988, 454-457.
11. Hunter, D.J., J.S.Moris, M.J.Stamfer et al., A prospective study of selenium status and breast cancer risk , JAMA, 264, 1990, 9, 1128-1131.
12. Overvad, K., D.Y.Wang, J.Olsen et al., Selenium in human mammary cancerogenesis: a Case Control Study, Eur.J.Cancer, 27, 1991, 7, 900-902.

Metal Ions in Biology and Medicine, vol. 2. Eds. J. Anastassopoulou, Ph. Collery, J.C. Etienne, Th. Theophanides. John Libbey Eurotext, Paris © 1992, pp. 448-450

Prevalence of lead poisoning in children consulting at well-child clinics in Paris

C. Alfaro*, P.Lombrail*, C. Vincelet*, M. Delour**, F. Squinazi***, A. Fontaine*, S. Gottot*, M. Brodin*

**Public health service. Hôpital R. Debré, 48, bd Serurier, 75019 Paris, France. **Direction de la Protection Maternelle et Infantile de Paris. ***Laboratoire d'Hygiène de la Ville de Paris*

A lead poisoning epidemic was discovered in Paris in 1985 because of the appearance of cases of encephalopathies (Carlus-Moncomble C. et al, 1987; Cohen R., 1987) . Inquiries in the housing of affected children showed the role of old paintings (Garnier R. & Chataigner R., 1989). This risk is already known in the USA, Belgium (Steenhout A., 1988) and England (Barltrop D., 1972). Young children are particularly concerned when eating or absorbing flakes or dust containing lead. The professional use of lead-containing paintings is prohibited in France since 1948 (Décret, 1948), but the paintings of housing built before may contain high quantities of lead.
Signs of minor poisoning are behavioral troubles, growing disturbances, digestive problems. The intoxication may be totally symptom-free with central nervous disturbances developing silently (McMichael A.J. et al, 1988; Needleman H.L. et al., 1990). Acute encephalopathies may develop with a blood lead level of 800μg/l (Graef T.W. & Lovejoy F.H., 1988). Four percent of US children aged 6 months to 5 years have a blood lead level >= 300μg/l. To be socially disadvantaged is associated with a 5 times higher prevalence (Mahaffey K.R. et al, 1982).

A screening strategy was implemented in Paris in 1987 by the direction of the PMI (well child clinics). The target was the north-east of Paris because of the concentration of poor housing in this area and because the first cases lived there: this is the area I. The first step of the screening consisted in a systematic search of a standard set of clinical signs (Delour M. & Squinazi F, 1989). A measure of the blood lead level and free erythrocyte porphyrins (FEP) had to be done if a child presented one or more signs (Hygiene laboratory of Paris city). In the rest of Paris no systematic screening was done: area II. 1500 children were found to have a toxic lead level (>=150μg/l) in a four years period (between 1987 and 1990); 300 of them had to be oriented to the hospital because of a lead level above 500μg/l or the presence of clinical signs of severity.

The **aim** of our study is to evaluate the prevalence of the lead poisoning in children aged 1 to 4 years consulting at PMI centers, in Paris as a whole and in both areas in the first trimester of 1991.

Population and method: we did a cross-sectional study. The population under study consisted in all the children aged 1 to 4 years (12 to 47 months) registered in PMI centers in Paris. We assembled a sample consisting in 32 clusters with a probability of sampling proportional to the number of the children registered in the 64 PMI centers. The nurses established the list of all the children of the required age registered and still followed in each center. We chose randomly 16 children in each cluster. The size of the sample was calculated to allow a 4% precision for an anticipated prevalence of 10% (multiplied by 2 to take into account the cluster effect). We analyzed the results by area by performing a post hoc stratification. We adopted the strategy of the CDCs for establishing our biological reference. First, we did a capillary testing to find children with FEP >= 350 μg/l. Children with FEP >= 350 μg/l had to undergo a lead level determination on venous blood except if they had had a measure less than 6 months before or had a known poisoning. Cases were defined considering two levels for intervention: blood lead level >= 250 μg/l (CDCs 1985) and >= 150 μg/l (CDCs 1991). Prevalence rates are shown with a 95% confidence interval.

Results: 14 children among the 512 had had a blood lead level determination in the preceding 6 months or >= 150 μg/l. 498 children had to have a FEP level determination. 176 were lost for follow-up, 269 had FEP < 350 μg/l and 53 had FEP >= 350 μg/l. Among those 53, a blood lead level determination was done for 37. The evaluation of the prevalence rate must take into account the high proportion of children lost for follow-up. A minimal hypothesis would consider only the cases discovered during the study. In this case, the prevalence rate is 1.4% (+- 1.4%) for a 250 μg/l level and 5.7% (+- 2.8%) for a 150 μg/l level. An alternative hypothesis would be to consider the children lost for follow-up as they were not different of the children for which we have biological information. With this mean hypothesis, the prevalence rates are 1.9% (+- 1.7%) and 9.6% (+- 3.5%) for the levels of 250 and 150 μg/l respectively. This hypothesis is plausible: the children lost for follow-up have sex and age characteristics not different from the others and the lost for follow-up rates do not differ in areas I and II. The prevalence rates for the 150 μg/l level by area are (minimal and mean hypothesis): 6.6% (+- 3.9%) and 11.5% (+-4.9%) in area I; 4.3% (+- 3.8%) and 6.7% (+- 4.9%) in area II. Finally, we remember that the sensitivity of a FEP level >= 350 μg/l for diagnosing a lead poisoning with a level >= 150 μg/l is 66%. With this additional information, the prevalence rate of the lead poisoning in this population may be as high as 14.3% (+- 3%) in Paris as a whole, 16.3% (+- 4%) in the area I and 10.5% (+- 4%) in the area II.

Conclusions: at least one child in ten in the Paris PMI population is intoxicated at a level of 150 µg/l. The prevalence rate of area II justify the extension of the screening for lead poisoning in children registred in PMI centers, in Paris as a whole.

REFERENCES

Barltrop D. (1972) : Children and environmental lead. In *Lead in the Environment* (Heple P ed.) London, UK : Institute of petroleum :52-60.

Carlus-Moncomble C., Orzechowski C. et al (1987) : Le saturnisme de l'enfant. In *Journées Parisiennes de Pédiatrie,* pp.205-212, eds Flammarion Médecine-Sciences.

Cohen R. (1987) : L'intoxication par le plomb des jeunes enfants -Un problème toujours actuel. *Rev Péd,* 2:83-89.

Décret du 11 décembre 1948 N° 48-1901

Delour M. & Squinazi F, (1989) : Intoxication saturnine chronique du jeune enfant. *Rev Ped* ;25:38-47

Garnier R. & Chataigner R. (1989) : Intoxication saturnine de l'enfant. *J toxicol Clin Exp* ; 9 : 345-349.

Graef T.W. & Lovejoy F.H. (1988) ; Intoxications par les métaux lourds. In : *Harrison TR "Principes de Médecine Interne",* eds Flammarion Médecine-Sciences, pp. 850-855.

Mahaffey K.R. et al, (1982) : National estimates of blood lead levels : United States 1976-1980: Association with selected demographics and socioeconomic factors. *N Engl J Med* ;307:573-579.

McMichael A.J. et al (1988) : Port Pirie Cohort Study: Environmental exposure to lead and children's abilities at the age of four years. *N Engl J Med* ; 319:468-475.

Needleman H.L. et al. (1990) : The long-terme effects of exposure to low doses of lead in childhood. *N Engl J Med* ; 322:83-88.

Steenhout A. (1988) : Exposition urbaine au plomb. *JTCE* ;8:176-189.

Author index

Achevé d'imprimer par Corlet, Imprimeur, S.A.
14110 Condé-sur-Noireau (France) - N° d'Imprimeur : 4590 - Dépôt légal : mai 1992
Imprimé en C.E.E.